AF738078

LOST IN TRANSLATION

Barriers to Incentives for Translational Research in Medical Sciences

LOST IN TRANSLATION

Barriers to Incentives for Translational Research in Medical Sciences

Editors

Rakesh Srivastava
University of Kansas, USA

Wojciech Maksymowicz
University of Warmia and Mazury in Olsztyn, Poland

Wlodek Lopaczynski
National Cancer Institute, USA

World Scientific

NEW JERSEY • LONDON • SINGAPORE • BEIJING • SHANGHAI • HONG KONG • TAIPEI • CHENNAI

Published by

World Scientific Publishing Co. Pte. Ltd.
5 Toh Tuck Link, Singapore 596224
USA office: 27 Warren Street, Suite 401-402, Hackensack, NJ 07601
UK office: 57 Shelton Street, Covent Garden, London WC2H 9HE

Library of Congress Cataloging-in-Publication Data
Lost in translation : barriers to incentives for translational research in medical sciences / editors, Rakesh Srivastava, Wojciech Maksymowicz, Wlodek Lopaczynski.
p. ; cm.
Includes bibliographical references and index.
ISBN-13: 978-9814489065 (hardcover : alk. paper)
ISBN-10: 9814489069 (hardcover : alk. paper)
I. Srivastava, Rakesh K., editor of compilation. II. Maksymowicz, Wojciech, editor of compilation. III. Lopaczynski, Wlodek, editor of compilation.
[DNLM: 1. Translational Medical Research. W 20.55.T7]
R853.Q34
610.72'4--dc23

2013046112

British Library Cataloguing-in-Publication Data
A catalogue record for this book is available from the British Library.

Copyright © 2014 by World Scientific Publishing Co. Pte. Ltd.

All rights reserved. This book, or parts thereof, may not be reproduced in any form or by any means, electronic or mechanical, including photocopying, recording or any information storage and retrieval system now known or to be invented, without written permission from the publisher.

For photocopying of material in this volume, please pay a copying fee through the Copyright Clearance Center, Inc., 222 Rosewood Drive, Danvers, MA 01923, USA. In this case permission to photocopy is not required from the publisher.

Typeset by Stallion Press
Email: enquiries@stallionpress.com

Printed in Singapore by B & Jo Enterprise Pte Ltd

Foreword

It is a great privilege to write a Foreword for this important book evaluating the state of the art in translational research. With 28 chapters and over 600 pages, *Lost in Translation — Barriers to Incentives for Translational Research in Medical Sciences* presents for the first time all the contributions from scientists and clinicians active in various areas of translational research in one volume.

The chapters cover the aspects of translational research in cancer, infectious diseases, nutrition (endocrinology), neuroscience, stem cells and its role in public health and behavioral sciences, clinical practice, its organization and funding in the U.S. and in the world, resources as well as outcomes. Other topics include translational epidemiology, biostatistics and informatics, health services and economics, ethics and legal regulations in the U.S. and internationally. The barriers to incentives for translational research are expertly discussed by the editors, Dr. R. Srivastava, Professor of Pharmacology, University of Kansas; Prof. W. Maksymowicz, Dean of the Faculty of Medical Sciences, University of Olsztyn, Poland; and Dr. W. Lopaczynski, Health Sciences Administrator, NCI, NIH, who are also co-authors of other chapters. The book is enriched by numerous color figures.

This volume brings together many of the world's top experts who have made major contributions to their particular fields. The contributors represent some of the most sophisticated investigators working in basic as well as clinical areas, each contributor having been involved in research in his or her particular area of expertise. Additionally, every chapter is well documented with suitable references.

With their wide circle of acquaintances and international reputations, the editors have been able to bring together a highly distinguished group of individuals. Indeed, we are indebted to them for this book, its excellent planning, systematic organization, and the coverage of so many areas. The book identifies the current state of translational research, and some chapters, such as that by Dr. Terry Moody on cancer, include the currently available therapies and future treatment.

In conclusion, the book provides a comprehensive overview of translational work. It will be most useful as an advanced textbook not only for graduate students, but also for scientists and even clinicians, to continually update their scientific and medical education or simply to get an overview of translational work. A famous Spanish endocrinologist, Gregorio Marañón, once said, "Many books are written, and they come and go and are forgotten if they are not significant." This book, however, will be the gold standard of our time. A seminal contribution to science and medicine, it is destined to become a classic. I hope readers enjoy it as much as I did.

Andrew V. Schally
Nobel Prize in Physiology or Medicine for 1977

From the Editors

This book aims to define translational research and find ways to prioritize and accelerate translational research in the biomedical sciences in order to rapidly turn new knowledge into first-in-human studies. Although translational research means different things to different people, the book represents an effort to bring together international scientists, active in various areas of science driven by translation, to share their opinions and, hopefully, generate new ideas and potential collaborations.

Medical research agencies worldwide have had similar experiences: while there has never been a shortage of basic science discoveries, the perception of divergent ecosystems of basic and clinical research has created a significant gap between basic research achievements and the appearance of new drugs or therapies. However, the obstacles and difficulties in making bench-to-bed translation have not been adequately described.

This book has a simple goal: to provide a comprehensive overview of translational work that includes significant discoveries and pioneering contributions in areas such as immunology, gene therapy, stem cells, and population sciences. It may be used as an advanced textbook by graduate students, and even ambitious undergraduates, in the biomedical sciences. It is also suitable for non-experts, such as medical doctors who wish to have an overview of some of fundamental models in translational research.

Managing the translational enterprise remains a work in progress. The world is changing rapidly, and the scientific field needs to seek new ways to ensure that discoveries get translated for patients efficiently and as quickly as possible. In addition, the expectation is that investment in biomedical research should pay dividends through effective therapeutic solutions. This unique project provides a broad collaborative approach by the international scientific community to present its views and opinions on how to cross barriers to incentives for translational research in the medical sciences.

The studies have been done and the data are in — yet we struggle to understand why it takes so long to translate genome-era discoveries into practice. To this end, the contributors to this book, representing a diverse group of international experts, have attempted to provide a historical perspective on how biomedical science has been driven by translation while progress on the clinical front in disease management has been slower than desired.

The book covers a large variety of topics, from general approaches to integrating emerging science into clinical practice; through organization, prioritization, and review of translational research; to translational science in cancer, infectious diseases, and neuroscience, including stem cells and endocrinology; and to translational epidemiology, biostatistics and informatics, economics, and behavioral sciences.

We would like to thank all of the people who have contributed to this book.Their efforts reflect their commitment to the field of translational research in biomedical sciences.

Wlodek Lopaczynski, MD, PhD
Wojciech Maksymowicz, MD, PhD
Rakesh K. Srivastava, PhD

Contents

List of Contributors

Edyta Adamska
Department of Endocrinology, Diabetology and Internal Medicine, Centre for Clinical Research, Medical University of Bialystok, Bialystok, Poland

Neeraj Agarwal
Department of Internal Medicine, Division of Medical Oncology, University of Utah Huntsman Cancer Institute, Salt Lake City, Utah, USA

Atique U. Ahmed
The Brain Tumor Center, The University of Chicago, Chicago, Illinois, USA

Christopher I. Amos
The Geisel School of Medicine at Dartmouth, Dartmouth College, Lebanon, New Hampshire, USA

Brenda Auffinger
The Brain Tumor Center, The University of Chicago, Chicago, Illinois, USA

Vito A. Baldassarro
Interdepartmental Center for Industrial Research (HST-ICIR), University of Bologna, Bologna, Italy

John R. Barbour
Georgetown University School of Medicine, Washington, DC, USA

L. Kay Bartholomew
University of Texas Health Science Center at Houston, School of Public Health, Division of Health Promotion and Behavioral Sciences, Houston, Texas, USA

Julia Batten
Department of Internal Medicine, Division of Medical Oncology, University of Utah Huntsman Cancer Institute, Salt Lake City, Utah, USA

Mitchel S. Berger
Department of Neurological Surgery, The Brain Tumor Research Center, and the Neuro-Oncology Program of the Helen Diller Family Comprehensive Cancer Center, University of California-San Francisco, San Francisco, CA 94158

Kenneth W. Bueltmann
Advocate Illinois Masonic Medical Center, Chicago, Illinois, USA and University of Illinois at Chicago, USA

Lisa H. Butterfield
University of Pittsburgh Cancer Institute, Pittsburgh, Pennsylvania, USA

Laura Calzà
Interdepartmental Center for Industrial Research (HST-ICIR), University of Bologna, Bologna, Italy

Mitchell S. Cairo
Departments of Pediatrics, Medicine, Pathology, Microbiology and Immunology and Cell Biology and Anatomy, New York Medical College, Valhalla, New York, USA

Mieczysław Chorąży
Center for Translational Research and Molecular Biology of Cancer, Maria Sklodowska-Curie Memorial Cancer Center and Institute of Oncology, Gliwice Branch, Wybrzeze Armii Krajowej 15, 44-101 Gliwice, Poland

Michal Ciborowski
Department of Endocrinology, Diabetology and Internal Medicine, Centre for Clinical Research, Medical University of Bialystok, Bialystok, Poland

Edward P. Cohen
University of Illinois, College of Medicine, Chicago, Illinois, USA

Marek Czosnyka
Neurosurgical Unit, Department of Clinical Neurosciences, University of Cambridge, UK

Zofia H. Czosnyka
Neurosurgical Unit, Department of Clinical Neurosciences, University of Cambridge, UK

Marie Davidian
Department of Statistics, North Carolina State University, Raleigh, North Carolina, USA and Department of Biostatistics and Bioinformatics, Duke University Medical Center, Durham, North Carolina, USA

Mercedez Fernández
Interdepartmental Center for Industrial Research (HST-ICIR), University of Bologna, Bologna, Italy

Maria E. Fernandez
University of Texas Health Science Center at Houston, School of Public Health, Division of Health Promotion and Behavioral Sciences, Houston, Texas, USA

Paul Galardy
Department of Pediatric Hematology/Oncology, Mayo Clinic, Rochester, Minnesota, USA

Ruth Gausche
Hospital for Children and Adolescents, Department for Women and Child Health, Centre for Pediatric Research, University of Leipzig, Leipzig, Germany

Stephen L. George
Cancer Center Biostatistics, Duke University Medical Center, Durham, North Carolina, USA and Department of Biostatistics and Bioinformatics, Duke University Medical Center, Durham, North Carolina, USA

L. Giardino
Interdepartmental Center for Industrial Research (HST-ICIR), University of Bologna, Bologna, Italy, Department of Veterinary Medical Sciences and Health Science and Technologies, University of Bologna, Bologna, Italy and IRET Foundation, Ozzano dell'Emilia, Bologna, Italy

A. Giuliani
Department of Veterinary Medical Sciences and Health Science and Technologies, University of Bologna, Bologna, Italy

Lisa G. Giulino-Roth
Department of Pediatric Hematology/Oncology, Weill Cornell Medical College, New York, USA

Richard M. Goldberg
Comprehensive Cancer Center, The Ohio State University Medical Center, Columbus, Ohio, USA

Stanton Goldman
Division of Pediatric Hematology/Oncology, Medical City Children's Hospital, Dallas, Texas, USA

Maria Górska
Department of Endocrinology, Diabetology and Internal Medicine, Centre for Clinical Research, Medical University of Bialystok, Bialystok, Poland

Ronald Hancock
Laval University Cancer Research Centre, 9 rue McMahon, Québec, QC, Canada G1R 2J6, and Biosystems Group, Institute of Automatic Control, Silesian University of Technology, Gliwice, Poland

Toby T. Hecht
Translational Research Program, Division of Cancer Treatment and Diagnosis, National Cancer Institute, 9609 Medical Center Drive, Room 3W110 MSC 9726, Rockville, MD 20850-9702, USA

Sabine Herget
Hospital for Children and Adolescents, Department for Women and Child Health, Centre for Pediatric Research, University of Leipzig, Leipzig, Germany

Andreas Hiemisch
Hospital for Children and Adolescents, Department for Women and Child Health, Centre for Pediatric Research, University of Leipzig, Leipzig, Germany

Andrew M. Hruszkewycz
Translational Research Program, Division of Cancer Treatment and Diagnosis, National Cancer Institute, 9609 Medical Center Drive, Room 3W110 MSC 9726, Rockville, MD 20850-9702, USA

Jiuping Ji
National Clinical Target Validation Laboratory, Frederick National Laboratory for Cancer Research, Frederick, Maryland, USA

Wieland Kiess
Hospital for Children and Adolescents, Department for Women and Child Health, Centre for Pediatric Research, University of Leipzig, Leipzig, Germany
E-mail: wieland.kiess@medizin.uni-leipzig.de

Sri Lakshmi S. Kollepara
Department of Internal Medicine, DMC-Sinai Grace Hospital, Detroit, Michigan, USA

Antje Körner
Hospital for Children and Adolescents, Department for Women and Child Health, Centre for Pediatric Research, University of Leipzig, Leipzig, Germany

Michael R. Kosorok
Department of Biostatistics, University of North Carolina at Chapel Hill, Chapel Hill, North Carolina, USA and Department of Statistics and Operations Research, University of North Carolina at Chapel Hill, Chapel Hill, North Carolina, USA

Sarah Krasny
University of Texas Health Science Center at Houston, School of Public Health, Division of Health Promotion and Behavioral Sciences, Houston, Texas, USA

Adam Kretowski
Department of Endocrinology, Diabetology and Internal Medicine, Centre for Clinical Research, Medical University of Bialystok, Bialystok, Poland

Dhruv Kumar
Department of Pharmacology, Toxicology and Therapeutics, and Medicine, The University of Kansas Medical Center, Kansas City, USA

Yvonne Lau
NIH Extramural Research Integrity Officer OD/OER/OEP, Bethesda, Maryland, USA

Colleen Ryan Leonard
Independent Consultant, Research Solutions International, LLC, Rockville, Maryland, USA

Maciej S. Lesniak
The Brain Tumor Center, The University of Chicago, Chicago, Illinois, USA

Wlodek Lopaczynski
Bethesda, Maryland , USA

L. Lorenzini
Interdepartmental Center for Industrial Research (HST-ICIR), University of Bologna, Bologna, Italy

Wojciech Maksymowicz
Department of Neurosurgery and Stem Cell Research Laboratory, University of Warmia and Mazury, Olsztyn, Poland

Mark Manak
Department of Diagnostics and Monitoring, US Military HIV Research Program (MHRP), HJF, Walter Reed Army Institute of Research, Silver Spring, Maryland, USA

C. Mangano
Department of Veterinary Medical Sciences and Health Science and Technologies, University of Bologna, Bologna, Italy

Jana Markert
Hospital for Children and Adolescents, Department for Women and Child Health, Centre for Pediatric Research, University of Leipzig, Leipzig, Germany

Maurie Markman
Cancer Treatment Centers of America, Philadelphia, Pennsylvania, USA and Drexel University College of Medicine, Philadelphia, Pennsylvania, USA

Rodney Miles
Department of Pathology, University of Utah, Salt Lake City, Utah, USA

Terry W. Moody
National Cancer Institute, Center for Cancer Research, Office of the Director, Bethesda, Maryland, USA

Jason H. Moore
The Geisel School of Medicine at Dartmouth, Section of Biostatistics and Epidemiology, Dartmouth College, One medical Drive, 7927 Rubin Building, NH 03756, USA

Stefanie Naumann
Hospital for Children and Adolescents, Department for Women and Child Health, Centre for Pediatric Research, University of Leipzig, Leipzig, Germany

Madlen Neef
Hospital for Children and Adolescents, Department for Women and Child Health, Centre for Pediatric Research, University of Leipzig, Leipzig, Germany

Marian L. Neuhouser
Cancer Prevention Program, Division of Public Health Sciences, Fred Hutchinson Cancer Research Center, Seattle, Washington, USA

Erica N. Peters
Friends Research Institute, Baltimore, Maryland, USA and Yale University School of Medicine, New Haven, Connecticut, USA

Roland Pfaeffle
Hospital for Children and Adolescents, Department for Women and Child Health, Centre for Pediatric Research, University of Leipzig, Leipzig, Germany

Russell O. Pieper
Department of Neurological Surgery, The Brain Tumor Research Center, University of California San Francisco, San Francisco, California, USA and Neurologic Oncology Program, Helen Diller Family Comprehensive Cancer Center, University of California-San Francisco, San Francisco, CA94158

Michael D. Prados
Department of Neurological Surgery, The Brain Tumor Research Center, and the Neuro-Oncology Program of the Helen Diller Family Comprehensive Cancer Center, University of California-San Francisco, San Francisco, CA 94158

Belinda Reininger
University of Texas Health Science Center at Houston, School of Public Health, Division of Health Promotion and Behavioral Sciences, Houston, Texas, USA

Zheng Ren
Department of Biostatistics, University of North Carolina at Chapel Hill, Chapel Hill, North Carolina, USA

Esther Rincon
The Brain Tumor Center, The University of Chicago, Chicago, Illinois, USA

Marek Rudnicki
Advocate Illinois Masonic Medical Center, Chicago, Illinois, USA and University of Illinois at Chicago, USA

Sharmila Shankar
Department of Pathology and Laboratory Medicine, The University of Kansas Medical Center, 3901 Rainbow Boulevard, Kansas City, Kansas, USA

Narinder K. Sharma
Department of Pharmacology, Toxicology and Therapeutics, and Medicine, The University of Kansas Medical Center, Kansas City, Kansas, USA

S. Sivilia
Department of Veterinary Medical Sciences and Health Science and Technologies, University of Bologna, Bologna, Italy

Jill P. Smith
National Institute of Diabetes and Digestive and Kidney Diseases, Division of Digestive Diseases and Nutrition, Bethesda, Maryland, USA

Rakesh K. Srivastava
Department of Pharmacology, Toxicology and Therapeutics, and Medicine, The University of Kansas Medical Center, Kansas City, Kansas, USA

Gary Stein
Department of Biochemistry, The University of Vermont Cancer Center, Burlington, Vermont, USA

Eva Szabo
Lung and Upper Aerodigestive Cancer Research Group, Division of Cancer Prevention, National Cancer Institute, National Institutes of Health, Bethesda, Maryland, USA

Srinivas K. Tantravahi
Department of Internal Medicine, Division of Medical Oncology, University of Utah Huntsman Cancer Institute, Salt Lake City, Utah, USA

Tor D. Tosteson
The Geisel School of Medicine at Dartmouth, Section of Biostatistics & Epidemiology, Dartmouth College, One Medical Center Drive, 7927 Rubin Building, Lebanon, NH 03756, USA

Anastasios A. Tsiatis
Department of Statistics, North Carolina State University, Raleigh, North Carolina, USA and Department of Biostatistics and Bioinformatics, Duke University Medical Center, Durham, North Carolina, USA

Peter Ujhazy
National Cancer Institute, Rockville, Maryland, USA

Claire Verschraegen
Department of Hematology/Oncology, The University of Vermont Cancer Center, Burlington, Vermont, USA

Jennifer Irvin Vidrine
University of Texas, MD Anderson Cancer Center, Department of Health Disparities Research, Houston, Texas, USA

Mandy Vogel
Hospital for Children and Adolescents, Department for Women and Child Health, Centre for Pediatric Research, University of Leipzig, Leipzig, Germany

Graham W. Warren
Department of Radiation Oncology, Hollings Cancer Center, Medical University of South Carolina, Charleston, South Carolina, USA and Department of Cell and Molecular Pharmacology and Experimental Therapeutics,

Hollings Cancer Center, Medical University of South Carolina, Charleston, South Carolina, USA

David W. Wetter
University of Texas, MD Anderson Cancer Center, Department of Health Disparities Research, Houston, Texas, USA

Theresa L. Whiteside
University of Pittsburgh Cancer Institute, Pittsburgh, Pennsylvania, USA

Louise Wideroff
National Institute on Drug Abuse, Bethesda, Maryland, USA

Brian Wojcik
Bethesda, Maryland, USA

Fred A. Wright
Department of Biostatistics, University of North Carolina at Chapel Hill, Chapel Hill, North Carolina, USA

Izabella Zandberg
Independent Consultant, Research Solutions International, LLC, Rockville, Maryland, USA

I. Barriers to Incentives for Translational Research

CHAPTER 1

Translational Research: Lost in Complexity

Mieczysław Chorąży and Ronald Hancock†*

INTRODUCTION

The great discoveries in biology and medicine in the last century aroused an unprecedented euphoria and the hope that major questions as to the nature of life and the mechanisms of diseases would be solved in the near future. After the elucidation of the structure of DNA, the subsequent concept that information can flow only unidirectionally from DNA to proteins[1] led the general public as well as biomedical scientists to consider genes as the sole entities responsible for the activities of human organisms in both normal and pathological conditions. An enormous amount of data on normal and mutated genes has been published and collected in data banks during the second half of the past century and the first decade of this century.

Genes are often regarded as autonomous entities independent from other molecules in the cell and from the external environment, and therefore are believed sometimes to determine even the most complex phenotypic traits (genetic determinism).[2] This genocentric manner of thinking postulates that the pathway between a gene (the genotype) and the outcome (the phenotype) has a linear character, so that damage, e.g., by mutation,

*Center for Translational Research and Molecular Biology of Cancer, Maria Sklodowska-Curie Memorial Cancer Center and Institute of Oncology, Gliwice Branch, Wybrzeże Armii Krajowej 15, 44-101 Gliwice, Poland, Tel: +48-32-278-9842; E-mail: *chorazy@io.gliwice.pl*

†Laval University Cancer Research Centre, 9 rue McMahon, Québec, QC, Canada G1R 2J6, and Biosystems Group, Institute of Automatic Control, Silesian University of Technology, Gliwice, Poland; Tel: +1-418-525-4444; E-mail: *ronald.hancock@crhdq.ulaval.ca*

to a gene whose product is essential for the normal phenotype results in a disease phenotype due to modification or absence of the gene's product. In reality, this is an oversimplification because it has been well documented that a single gene can be associated with multiple disorders[3] while an apparently single disorder can be caused by mutations in any one of several genes.[4] We have also learned that only a subset of individuals carrying a mutation are affected by a particular disease and that not all individuals with a given mutation are affected equally (see review in Ref. 5).

This "linear thinking" about the nature of life and disease was propagated by the popular media[6] and inspired the hunt for genes responsible for complex behavioral traits such as IQ, linguistic ability, depth of religious faith, political or sexual preference, or even alcoholism[7] in addition to genes which code for the thousands of enzymatically active and structural proteins, receptors, transcription factors, and others, in cells. Similarly, genetic origins have been proposed for the evolution of personality and of new abilities during development (cultural inheritance) (see reviews in Refs. 8 and 9). This "linear thinking" was at the origin of the belief that knowing the DNA sequence of a patient's genes would allow the development of new therapeutic approaches to combat diseases,[10–12] for example by using new pharmaceuticals that block the activity of a "disease gene," substituting a damaged gene by a new, normal gene (gene therapy), or inactivating or eliminating a "disease protein," which seemed to be easy tasks. Frequently, to convince readers and funding agencies of a correlation between a mutation and a particular, even complex, trait (a disease or the metastatic potential of cancer cells, for example), their relationship is often described as "statistically significant." In the biomedical literature, one can find many example of conclusions of this type that were shown later to be unreliable due to inadequate sample sizes,[13,14] recalling the character in the work of the Scottish poet Andrew Lang, who "uses statistics as a drunken man uses lamp posts ... for support rather than illumination." The story at the molecular level has become infinitely more complex, and it is clear that there exists more than one direction of information flow.[15] For example, the replication and transcription of genes are under the influence of interacting proteins and RNAs that themselves are products of genes. Obviously, a different kind of information flow that goes back and forth between genes and proteins evolved by interactions of macromolecules and emerged to manage and regulate processes in living organisms.

In this chapter, we discuss how, in a biological context, the concept of "translational research" is not adequate to study and understand the vast and subtle complexities of the phenomena of life and disease.

WHAT IS BIOLOGICAL COMPLEXITY?

What differentiates living from inanimate things? Schrödinger's question, "What is Life?"[16] has not lost its significance despite the unprecedented amount of information on the structure and function of cells and the macromolecules of which they are composed that has been collected during the last 60 years. For Emmeche,[17] "something is complex in the ontological sense when it is organized as a system of many non-identical components which themselves have system-like properties (such as being further decomposable), and whose mutual interactions bring forth a kind of collective behavior which is different from the behavior of the parts." Complexity is an inherent property of living organisms that arose at the very beginning of evolution when spontaneous interactions of simple chemical molecules in favorable environmental conditions formed more complex macromolecules, membranes and vesicles, and subsequently "primitive" protocells and later multicellular organisms.[18] Complexity has developed along with evolution and increased with the growth of the number and variety of their components, shaped by the continuous influence of the environment.[19]

The complexity of an organism is not related to the number of genes it contains, a phenomenon termed the G-value paradox,[20] because the transcription of information encoded in a gene into an RNA and then its translation into a protein do not proceed in a simple 1:1:1 manner, as was thought soon after the birth of molecular biology. Mechanisms have evolved to "manipulate" the primary information encoded in genes into abundant "secondary information" by alternative splicing, editing or nonsense-mediated decay (NMD) of messenger RNAs (mRNAs), as illustrated in Fig. 1. The number of protein-coding genes in human cells is about 20,000,[21] but the number of protein species exceeds this number

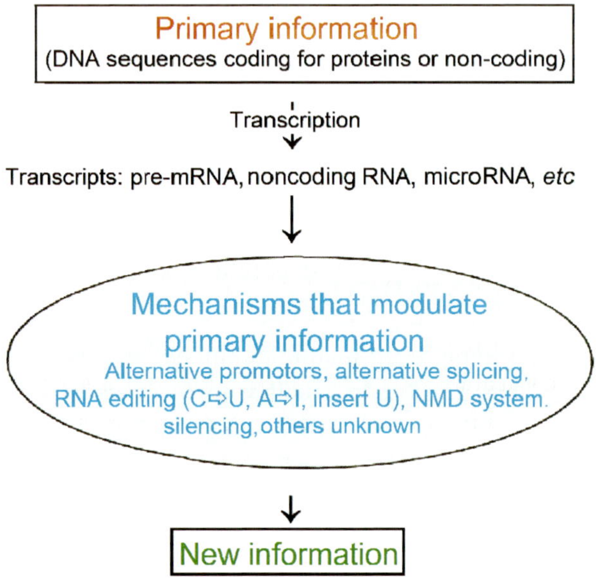

Fig. 1. Steps in the transformation of the primary information encoded in genes (DNA) into new, more enriched information.

by at least 10 times.[22] "We have barely scratched the surface of the myriad ways in which genomic sequences are massaged and manipulated to produce the complex set of physiological events involved in disease and health."[23]

Further, the tertiary structures and functions of proteins do not depend only on their amino acid sequence encoded by a gene, but can be modulated by more than 300 different types of post-translational modification that enlarge their pleiotropic potential, including phosphorylation, acetylation, methylation, sumoylation and glycosylation.[22] The structure of genes and their activity can be modified by epigenetic factors and the environment to a much greater extent than was thought earlier.[24,25] Thus, although genes are an essential source of information, they are not the sole source[26,27]; "the particular presumption is that a 'plan of procedure' for development is itself written in the sequence of nucleotide bases. Is this presumption correct? I want to argue that, at best, it must be said to be misleading, and at worst, simply false."[27]

Analytical Approaches

If living systems were based only on interactions of matter and energy, reductional analysis, the decomposition of the whole into its components and their characterization, should provide an understanding of the essence of life. This was the philosophy underlying the Human Genome Project (HGP), the Encyclopedia of DNA elements (ENCODE) project, the National Cancer Institute Cancer Genome Anatomy Project, and others, which have provided remarkably comprehensive and detailed knowledge of the genes of living organisms.

But reductionist analyses of the parts of a system, although a useful tool, cannot provide us with an understanding of how it works at higher levels, because the entire system is not the simple summation of its parts.[28,29] A simple reductionist analysis of organs, cells and chemical molecules, and further of atoms and electron spins, is not sufficient to explain the properties of such complex systems as the phenomena of life, and in particular the complexity of a human with his entire potential and cultural heritage.[30] One should therefore not expect that we would be able to predict phenotypic effects at the highest level of complexity even if we have the complete physicochemical characteristics of the molecules in cells and of the rules that govern their interactions. "Neither simple nor complex quantitative measure of complexity will in themselves bring us an understanding of complex living systems ... Perhaps what we should be seeking is another idea of what 'understanding' a complex system could be like, other than the reductive top-down decomposition and the corresponding bottom-up re-synthesizing."[17]

A more appropriate and successful concept to understand living systems is that termed "emergence," which is the antithesis of the reductionist approach.[31–33] A reductionist analysis of water would not inform us about its characteristic property of wetness, because this is an emergent property only shown when many millions of water molecules interact under the proper environmental conditions; we would only learn that it is a molecule composed of one atom of oxygen and two of hydrogen. Similarly, semipermeability is not a property of any of the individual components of a semipermeable membrane. Life is a *sui generis* example of emergence that has evolved from inorganic matter over milliards of years to its recent forms[18] with the emergence of new properties as changes occurred in the structures of dynamic networks of interacting molecules under the influence of the environment and with time.

Hierarchical Levels

One universal component of complexity is the hierarchical organization seen in all living systems around us, from the structure of cells and organisms to communities of ants and humans to ecosystems. The human organism, like all living creatures, is built from atoms that form the basal hierarchical level and are further decomposable into subatomic particles and forces. Atoms interact and organize into molecules that represent the next, higher level and interact to form the structural and functional units of life, cells and the further hierarchical levels of tissues, organs and organisms. But the properties of higher hierarchical levels are not completely reducible to those of lower levels. Structural and functional complexity increase from lower to higher hierarchical levels (Fig. 2) and lower levels

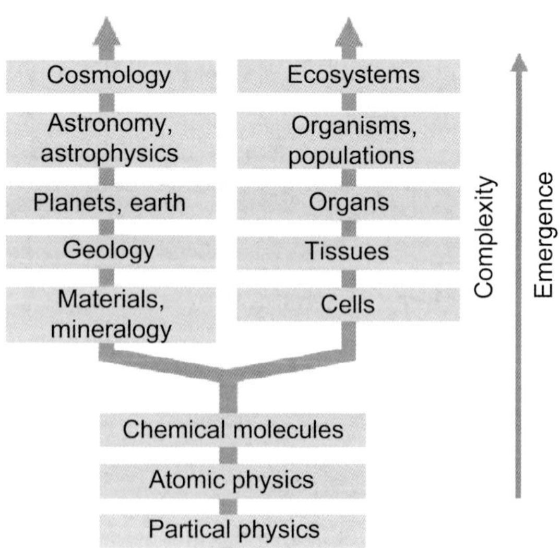

Fig. 2. Hierarchical organization of nonliving and living systems (adapted from Ref. 36). The three lower levels are common to inanimate and living systems, and bifurcation at the level of chemical molecules leads to the evolution of more complex living systems with corresponding emergent properties.

are subordinated to, and restricted by, higher levels so that they are constrained and may lose some autonomy. A holistic look at humans reveals that at their lower hierarchical levels they are similar or identical to the corresponding level in animals, but the highest levels, particularly the central nervous system, show an extreme and unique level of complexity.[34,35]

Self-organization

A further fundamental and universal feature of complexity in living organisms is "self-organization," the spontaneous assembly of molecules into ordered structures and systems. Self-organization of structural and functional complexes such as membranes and vesicles by spontaneous self-recognition, and selection of the combinations most suitable thermodynamically and functionally, must have played a central role in the formation of the first life forms.[37,38] Self-assembly is involved in the formation of numerous crucial structural components of cells, including the cytoskeleton,[39,40] membranes,[41] centromeres,[42] the nuclear lamina,[43] and structures in the nucleus.[44] Our understanding of a further aspect of complexity, the development of asymmetry (symmetry breaking) is also very limited[45]; this generates the patterns necessary for initiating morphogenetic processes that form and differentiate tissues and organs,[46] "a first step of complexity generation."[47] For example, in epithelial cells, apical-basal polarity is created by the development of two surfaces that differ in structure and functions.

THE COMPLEXITY OF NETWORKS IN CELLS AND ORGANISMS

Systems Biology

Biological functions do not arise only from properties of individual molecules but predominantly from the interactions between them,[48] and interaction and integration of molecular processes are the bases of the functioning of living cells.[49] "Every object that biology studies is a system of systems."[50] Living cells and organisms are complex systems that have the "capacity to exist as metabolically self-sustaining wholes"[51] and can replicate and form lineages. At the molecular level, complexity is reflected in the thousands of macromolecules that cells contain, mainly proteins, DNA, RNA, lipids, and so on.

Most proteins interact with other macromolecules in networks that are responsible for metabolism, signaling, regulation, transcription, translation, etc. Description of these interactions in quantitative terms allows mathematical modeling of networks, and "systems biology" is providing essential tools to understand living organisms and to reveal a holistic view of how they work as a whole in normal[52–56] and pathological[57,58] conditions. The structure and functioning of the metabolic, transcriptional regulation, signaling, and other networks in the cell, and the interplay between them, are described in detail in Refs. 59 and 60. The realization that the final outcome of a functioning network is the result of interactions of many molecules and cannot be attributed to the features of any single component is having a major impact in biology, and especially in medicine, since a pathological phenotype can no longer be interpreted as the structural or functional failure of the product of a single gene.

Disease Networks

Relatively few diseases, for example, cystic fibrosis and hemophilia, can be ascribed to perturbations of a single gene. Instead, "a disease is rarely a consequence of an abnormality in a single gene, but reflects the perturbation of the complex intracellular and intercellular networks that link tissue and organ system"; and further "... the impact of specific genetic abnormality is not restricted to the activity of the gene product that carriers it, but can spread along the links of the network and alter the activity of gene products that otherwise carry no defects"[48] (see also Refs. 60 and 62). "Network medicine" is a seminal new concept based on systems biology.

Models of networks and the topology of their components can reveal whether a certain gene could be involved in the etiology of a particular multicausal disease.[63,64] Disease networks can reveal the tendency of genes (or their products) to form local clusters or "disease modules" whose connections (links) indicate molecular relationships between disease-associated cellular components.[65] These modules may overlap with one another, reflecting phenotypes where individuals with a particular disease have further signs typically found in other diseases, and their interconnections reveal common factors involved in pathogenic mechanisms, for example, shared genes or their products (Fig. 3). A map termed the human "diseasome" has been elaborated on the basis of such network patterns.[65,66]

Equilibrium States and Attractors

A central concept derived from systems modeling approaches is that the stability of the structures and properties of living cells reflects stable equilibrium states that are the result of specific programs of expression of many mutually regulating genes.[67] In contrast, mutations in individual genes have only a minor influence on the overall properties of large networks.[68] A network of genes can potentially create numerous distinct stable programs of gene expression or equilibrium states (Fig. 4) which are likely to correspond to the specific stable programs of gene expression that characterize different types of differentiated cells and are termed "attractors."[58,67] It is noteworthy that among these repertoires of potential stable gene expression programs are phenotypes that are characteristic of cancer cells but normally are not expressed.[58]

Complex Responses in Cells and Organisms

The emergent phenomena that are characteristic of higher levels of life cannot be predicted simply from the properties of lower levels, because the interrelations between the parts and the levels are not linear but rather follow algorithmic rules and routes whose outcomes can be predicted only in terms of probabilities.[69–74] The model where the phenotypes of cancer cells are determined by modulation of networks of genes rather than mutations of single genes[58,65] is a significant advance in understanding carcinogenesis. This concept clarifies why only a subset of individuals carrying a mutation may be affected, why patients'responses to therapy may differ,[3,4] and why a single gene may be associated with multiple phenotypes. The more than 10 distinct disease phenotypes caused by different mutations in the gene coding for the nuclear envelope protein lamin A, which specifically affect striated muscle, adipose tissue or peripheral nerves, or produce syndromes of premature aging, provide striking examples of the latter phenomenon.[75]

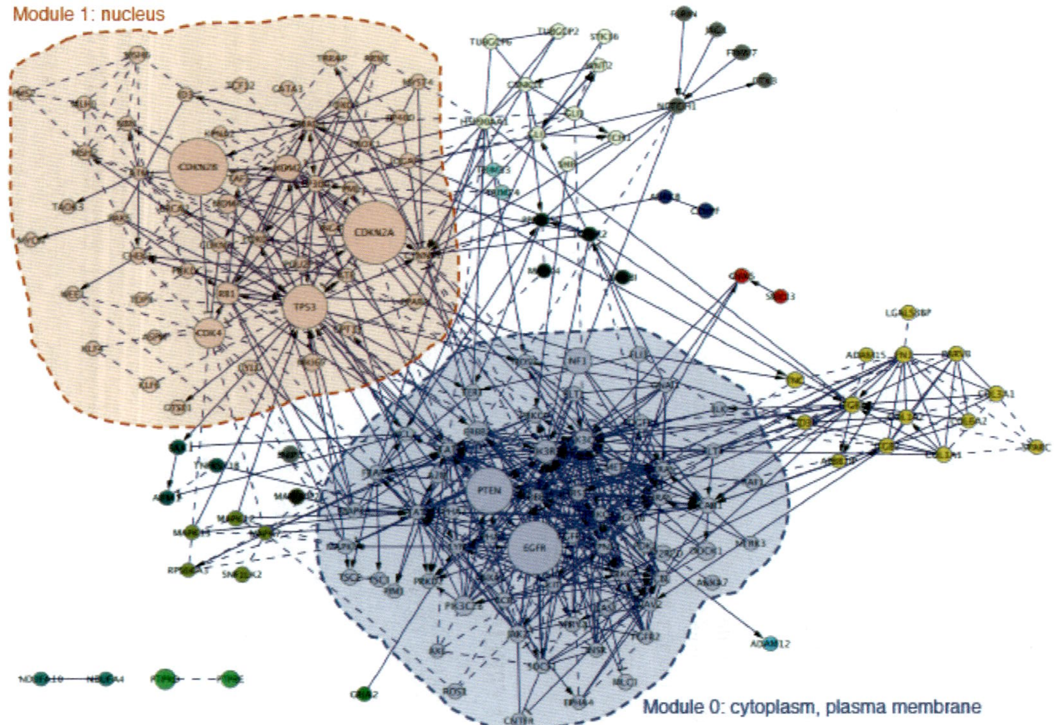

Fig. 3. A network of genes whose sequence is altered in human glioblastomas. Most genes with recurrent mutations form clusters (nodes) whose size is shown proportional to the number of samples in which the sequence of the corresponding gene was altered. The links between clusters show functional relationships of the proteins produced by these genes. Reproduced from Ref. 61 under the BioMed Central Open Access license agreement and with the kind permission of Dr. G. Wu.

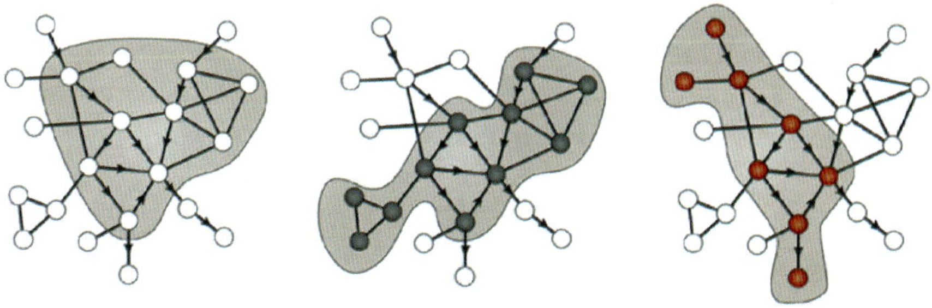

Fig. 4. The concept of disease as a consequence of rearranged connectivity in a functional subnetwork module. (A) A topological module (brown), a locally dense neighborhood of the interactome where the nodes (white) show a higher tendency to interact with one another than with nodes outside the module. (B) A functional module, a network neighborhood in which there is a statistically significant segregation of nodes with related functions (gray) in the same network neighborhood. (C) A disease module with alternative connections between nodes (red) as a result of mutations, deletions, copy number variations, or expression changes of genes which can be linked to a particular disease phenotype. Modified from Ref. 65, reproduced with the kind permission of the publisher and of Dr. A.-L. Barabási.

SERENDIPITY, A CRUCIAL FACTOR IN BIOMEDICAL RESEARCH

One of the central ideas underlying the concept of translational research is that once the genetic structure of a patient is known, it should be possible to eliminate their disease by replacing their aberrant gene by a new, normal gene (gene therapy), by developing new pharmaceuticals that block its activity, or by inactivating its aberrant product. There are only very limited data to support the proposition that this strategy will be successful. Instead, abundant evidence shows that key discoveries that pave the way for new therapies are predominantly the result of serendipitous observations.[76–80]

As observed by Kornberg, "investigations that seemed totally irrelevant to any practical objective have yielded most of the major discoveries of medicine ... and the pursuit of curiosity about the basic facts of nature has proved throughout the history of medical science to be the most practical, the most cost-effective route to successful drugs and devices. No matter how counterintuitive it may seem, basic research is the lifeline of practical advances in medicine."[78] Seminal discoveries that form the foundations of present biomedical sciences, for example, the discovery of X-rays, penicillin, the tumor suppressor protein p53, cisplatin, DNA sequencing methods, and more recently the development of proteasome inhibitors for successful therapy of multiple myeloma,[79] were consequences of curiosity[80] and would not have been made in a translational research context.

THE LIMITS OF TRANSLATIONAL RESEARCH

It has become clear that the priority for further understanding of the order and disorders of living systems is to explore the complexities of the networks that determine their activities, an enterprise for which genocentric thinking is no longer adequate. Our knowledge of the basic levels of molecular structures, interactions and dynamic processes is so scarce that higher hierarchical levels with their emergent properties cannot yet be reconstructed. Singer[35] observes that "for fundamental reasons ... it is difficult to foresee how any intervention or control will affect the behavior of a complex system. ... If it is a straightforward system with primarily linear dynamics, then hierarchical structures might be appropriate. If, however, the system is highly complex with strong nonlinear behavior, then we should rely on its self-organizational power and creativity, and not succumb prematurely to the illusion that we can selectively intervene." This difficulty in predicting the behavior of higher hierarchical levels of living systems has a deep practical significance in medicine: the physician may be unable to evaluate and predict the behavior of a patient because he sees a Cartesian machine composed of individual parts rather than an integrated system with complex interactions of cells, tissues and organs.

The power of thinking in terms of gene networks rather than single mutations is illustrated by new insights into the complex responses seen in some human disorders when a single gene can be associated with multiple phenotypes, only a subset of individuals carrying a mutation are affected, or patients' responses to therapy differ.[3,4] A convincing model derived from experimental and computational studies is that these different responses reflect different types of perturbation of the interactions of a mutated protein with its partners in networks.[5] A mutation that results in truncation or loss of stability of a protein effectively eliminate it from a network, but amino acid substitutions that only alter its intermolecular interactions may give rise to partially functional products whose interactions in networks are altered and thus lead to quite different phenotypic consequences. The unexpected results of many experiments using gene knockouts are consistent with this idea.[81] This model based on network properties provides a molecular explanation for complex genotype–phenotype relationships as well as for different responses and unexpected secondary effects of therapies.

Translational research strategies are inherently inappropriate to explore potentially seminal directions such as the preceding examples, because available technologies and reductionist thinking are essentially their only ingredients.[82] Van Regenmortel[83] has offered a succinct comment from the field of research on HIV therapies: "a common problem with many of these innovations is that their potential risks and unwanted side effects tended to be overlooked initially, as was the case for gene therapy. There is probably a more fundamental reason for these failures: namely, that most of these approaches have been guided by unmitigated reductionism." Translational research strategies may be appropriate for certain challenges in certain circumstances,[84] but we should be aware that their introduction may mask agendas that reflect the views of administrators or individuals whose understanding of creative science is limited. At a time when clinical medicine is placing more and more importance on "evidence-based" approaches, it is paradoxical that research funding should be oriented towards a strategy whose "evidence base" shows very little proof of its efficacy compared with the demonstrated productivity of creativity driven by curiosity, which must continue to be the foundation of biomedical research.

(*The viewpoints expressed in this article are those of the authors and may not reflect those of the institutions in which they work.*)

REFERENCES

1. Crick F. (1970) Central dogma of molecular biology. *Nature* **227**: 561–563.
2. Roubertoux PL, Carlier M. (2011) Good use and misuse of "genetic determinism". *J Physiol Paris* **105**: 190–194.
3. Coppieters F, Lefever S, Leroy BP, De Baere E. (2010) CEP290, a gene with many faces: Mutation overview and presentation of CEP290base. *Hum Mutat* **31**: 1097–1108.

4. Shy ME, Garbern JY, Kamholz J. (2002) Hereditary motor and sensory neuropathies: A biological perspective. *Lancet Neurol* **1**: 110–118.
5. Zhong Q, Simonis N, Li Q-R, *et al.* (2009) Edgetic perturbation models of human inherited disorders. *Mol Syst Biol* **5**: 321.
6. Petersen A. (2001) Biofantasies: Genetics and medicine in the print news media. *Soc Sci Med* **52**: 1255–1268.
7. Conrad P, Weinerg D. (1996) Has the gene for alcoholism been discovered three times since 1980? A news media analysis. *Social Probl* **8**: 3–25.
8. Bickle J. (2003) *Philosophy and Neuroscience: A Ruthlessly Reductive Account.* Kluwer Academic, The Netherlands.
9. Munafo MR, Flint J. (2011) Dissecting the genetic architecture of human personality. *Trends Cogn Sci* **15**: 395–400.
10. Cramer F. (2001) Gene technology in humans: Can the responsibilities be borne by scientists, physicians, and patients? *Interdiscipl Sci Rev* **3**: 162–166.
11. Jaroff L. (1992) Seeking a God-like power. *Time* **58** (special Fall issue).
12. Hayden EC. (2012) Sequencing set to alter clinical landscape. *Nature* **482**: 288.
13. Wacholder S, Chanock S, Garcia-Closas M, *et al.* (2004) Assessing the probability that a positive report is false: An approach for molecular epidemiology studies. *J Natl Cancer Inst* **96**: 434–442.
14. Ioannidis JPA. (2005) Why most published research findings are false. *PLoS Med* **2**: e124.
15. Ellis GFR. (2008) On the nature of causation in complex systems. *Trans R Soc S Afr* **63**: 1–16.
16. Schrödinger E. (1944) *What Is Life? The Physical Aspect of the Living Cell.* Cambridge University Press, Cambridge.
17. Emmeche C. (1997) Aspects of complexity in life and science. *Philosophica* **59**: 41–68.
18. Morowitz HJ. (2002) *The Emergence of Everything.* Oxford University Press, Oxford.
19. Vinicius L. (2010) *Modular Evolution: How Natural Selection Produces Biological Complexity.* Cambridge University Press, Cambridge.
20. Hahn MW, Wray GA. (2002) The g-value paradox. *Evol Dev* **4**: 73–75.
21. Clamp M, Fry B, Kamal M, *et al.* (2007) Distinguishing protein-coding and noncoding genes in the human genome. *Proc Natl Acad Sci USA* **104**: 19428–19433.
22. Jensen ON. (2004) Modification-specific proteomics: Characterization of post-translational modifications by mass spectrometry. *Current Opin Chem Biol* **8**: 33–41.

23. Jogalekar A. (2012) The perils of translational research. *Sci Am* (http://blogs.scientificamerican.com/the-curious-wavefunction/2012/11/26/the-perils-of-translational-research).
24. Powers DA, Schulte PM. (1998) Evolutionary adaptations of gene structure and expression in natural populations in relation to a changing environment: A multidisciplinary approach to address the million-year saga of a small fish. *J Exp Zool* **282**: 71–94.
25. Turner BM. (2009) Epigenetic responses to environmental change and their evolutionary implications. *Philos Trans R Soc Lond B Biol Sci* **364**: 3403–3418.
26. Lewontin R. (2001) *It Ain't Necessarily So: The Dream of the Human Genome and Other Illusions.* New York Review Books, New York.
27. Keller EF. (1999) Elusive locus of control in biological development: Genetic versus developmental programs. *J Exp Zool* **285**: 283–290.
28. Polanyi M. (1968) Life's irreducible structure. *Science* **160**: 1308–1312.
29. Johnson S. (2002) *Emergence. The Connected Lives of Ants, Brains, Cities and Software.* Penguin Press, London.
30. Cohen IR. (2000) *Tending Adam's Garden.* Academic Press, San Francisco.
31. Van Regenmortel MH. (2004) Reductionism and complexity in molecular biology. *EMBO Rep* **5**: 1016–1020.
32. Korn RW. (2005) The emergence principle in biological hierarchies. *Biol Phil* **20**: 137–151.
33. Macklem PT. (2008) Emergent phenomena and the secrets of life. *J Appl Physiol* **104**: 1844–1846.
34. Mainzer K. (2007) *Thinking in Complexity. The Computational Dynamics of Matter, Mind, and Mankind.* Springer, London.
35. Singer W. (2007) Understanding the brain. *EMBO Rep* **8**: S16–S19.
36. Ellis GFR. (2006) On the nature of emergent reality. In: P Clayton, PCW Davies (eds), *The Re-emergence of Emergence*, Oxford University Press, Oxford, pp. 79–107.
37. Lehn J-M. (2004) Supramolecular chemistry: From molecular information towards self-organization and complex matter. *Rep Progr Phys* **67**: 249–265.
38. Bensaude-Vincent B. (2009) Self-assembly, self-organization: Nanotechnology and vitalism. *Nano Ethics* **3**: 31–42.
39. Huber F, Käs J. (2011) Self-regulative organization of the cytoskeleton. *Cytoskeleton* **68**: 259–265.
40. Kirschner M, Gerhart J, Mitchison T. (2000) Molecular "vitalism". *Cell* **100**: 79–88.
41. Simons K, Sampaio JL. (2011) Membrane organization and lipid rafts. *Cold Spring Harb Perspect Biol* **3**: a004697.

42. Mogliner A, Craig E. (2010) Towards a quantitative understanding of mitotic spindle assembly and mechanics. *J Cell Sci* **123**: 3435–3445.
43. Gerace L, Huber MD. (2012) Nuclear lamina at the crossroads of the cytoplasm and nucleus. *J Struct Biol* **177**: 24–31.
44. Hancock R. (2013) New models of the nucleus. *Int Rev Cell Mol Biol* (in preparation, to be published in summer 2013).
45. Iden S, Collard JG. (2008) Crosstalk between small GTPases and polarity proteins in cell polarization. *Nat Rev Mol Cell Biol* **9**: 846–859.
46. Li R, Bowerman B. (2010) Symmetry breaking in biology. *Cold Spring Harbor Perspect Biol* **2**: a003475.
47. Kirschner M, Mitchison T. (1986) Beyond self-assembly: From microtubules to morphogenesis. *Cell* **45**: 329–342.
48. Barabási AL, Oltvai ZN. (2004) Network biology: Understanding the cell's functional organization. *Nat Rev Genet* **5**: 101–113.
49. Westerhoff HV, Palsson BO. (2004) The evolution of molecular biology into systems biology. *Nat Biotechnol* **22**: 1249–1252.
50. Jacob F. (1974) *The Logic of Living Systems.* Allen Lane, London.
51. Dupré J, O'Malley MA. (2009) Varieties of living things: Life at the intersection of lineage and metabolism. *Philos Theor Biol* **1**: e003.
52. von Bertalanffy L. (1969) *General Systems Theory: Foundations, Development, Applications.* G. Braziller, New York.
53. O'Malley MA. (2012) Evolutionary systems biology: Historical and philosophical perspectives on an emerging synthesis. *Adv Exp Med Biol* **751**: 1–28.
54. Bellomo N. (2008) *Modeling Complex Living Systems. A Kinetic Theory and Stochastic Game Approach.* Birkhäuser, Basel.
55. Trewavas A. (2006) A brief history of systems biology. *Plant Cell* **18**: 2420–2430.
56. Bray D. (2003) Molecular networks: The top-down view. *Science* **301**: 1864–1865.
57. Faratian D, Clyde RG, Crawford JW, Harrison DJ. (2009) Systems pathology — Taking molecular pathology into a new dimension. *Nat Rev Clin Oncol* **6**: 455–464.
58. Huang S, Ernberg I, Kauffman S. (2009) Cancer attractors: A systems view of tumors from a gene network dynamics and developmental perspective. *Sem Cell Dev Biol* **20**: 869–876.
59. Buchanan M, Caldarelli G, De Los Rios P, *et al.* eds. (2010) *Networks in Cell Biology.* Cambridge University Press, Cambridge.
60. Wang E. ed. (2010) *Cancer Systems Biology.* Chapman and Hall/CRC.

61. Wu G, Feng X, Stein L. (2010) A human functional protein interaction network and its application to cancer data analysis. *Genome Biol* **11**: R53.
62. Soto AM, Sonnenschein C. (2004) The somatic mutation theory of cancer: Growing problems with the paradigm? *BioEssays* **26**: 1097–1107.
63. Shin CJ, Wong S, Davis MJ, Ragan MA. (2009) Protein–protein interaction as a predictor of subcellular location. *BMC Syst Biol* **3**: 28.
64. Gohlke JM, Thomas R, Zhang Y, *et al.* (2009) Genetic and environmental pathways to complex diseases. *BMC Syst Biol* **3**: 46.
65. Barabási AL, Gulbahce N, Loscalzo J. (2011) Network medicine: A network-based approach to human disease. *Nat Rev Genet* **12**: 56–68.
66. Goh KI, Cusick ME, Valle D, *et al.* (2007) The human disease network. *Proc Natl Acad Sci USA* **104**: 8685–8690.
67. Kauffman S. (1969) Homeostasis and differentiation in random genetic control networks. *Nature* **224**: 177–178.
68. Aldana M, Balleza E, Kauffman S, Resendiz O. (2007) Robustness and evolvability in genetic regulatory networks. *J Theor Biol* **245**: 433–448.
69. Audet J. (2010) Adventures in time and space: Nonlinearity and complexity of cytokine effects on stem cell fate decisions. *Biotechnol Bioeng* **106**: 173–182.
70. Ricard J. (2010) Systems biology and the origins of life? Part II. Are biochemical networks possible ancestors of living systems? Networks of catalysed chemical reactions: Non-equilibrium, self-organization and evolution. *Comptes Rendus Biologies* **333**: 769–778.
71. Jura A, Wegrzyn P, Jura J, Koj A. (2006) Regulatory mechanisms of gene expression: Complexity with elements of deterministic chaos. *Acta Biochim Pol* **53**: 1–10.
72. Toole J, Page SE. (2011) Predicting cellular automata. *Complex Systems* **19**: 343–362.
73. Hanel R, Pöchacker M, Thurner S. (2010) Living on the edge of chaos: Minimally nonlinear models of genetic regulatory dynamics. *Philos Transact A Math Phys Eng Sci* **368**: 5583–5596.
74. Anbar M. (2001) What is life? *IEEE Eng Med Biol Mag* **20**: 15–19.
75. Bertrand AT, Chikhaoui K, Yaou RB, Bonne G (2011) Clinical and genetic heterogeneity in laminopathies. *Biochem Soc Trans* **39**: 1687–1692.
76. Kingdon M. (2012) *The Science of Serendipity: How to Unlock the Promise of Innovation in Large Organizations.* Wiley, London.
77. Walter P. (2010) Walking along the serendipitous path of discovery. *Mol Biol Cell* **21**: 15–17.

78. Kornberg A. (1995) Of Serendipity and Science. *Stanford Medicine* (summer) (http://www.rockefeller.edu/pubinfo/Pasteur/Kornberg_essay.html)
79. Goldberg AL. (2012) Development of proteasome inhibitors as research tools and cancer drugs. *J Cell Biol* **199**: 583–588.
80. Neufeld EF. (2011) From serendipity to therapy. *Annu Rev Biochem* **80**: 1–15.
81. Mazzocchi F. (2008) Complexity in biology. Exceeding the limits of reductionism and determinism using complexity theory. *EMBO Rep* **9**: 10–14.
82. Hait WN. (2003) Barriers to translational research: The perils of Pauline. *Abstracts, 94th Annual Meeting of the American Association for Cancer Research*, Washington, DC, USA (July 11–14, 2003) (http://forums.lymphoma.com/archive/index.php/t-9534.html).
83. Van Regenmortel MH. (2012) Basic research in HIV vaccinology is hampered by reductionist thinking. *Front Immunol* **3**: 194.
84. Curran T. (2005) Lost in translation: The future of cancer research? *Clin Cancer Res* **11**: 4644–4645.

CHAPTER 2

Methylation, Methionine and Metaphors

Claire Verschraegen[*,‡] *and Gary Stein*[†]

2.1. INTRODUCTION — WHAT IS TRANSLATION?

Word origin: trānslātiōn (s. of trānslātiō) a transferring, equivalent to trānslāt(us) + -iōn.[1]

Trans•late /trans 'lāt/ –Verb

(i) Express the sense of (words or text) in another language.
(ii) Be expressed or be capable of being expressed in another language: "shiatsu" literally translates as "finger pressure."

Synonyms: interpret – render – construe
Translational – Adjective
Translationally – Adverb
Translation – Noun

A step in protein biosynthesis wherein the genetic code carried by mRNA is decoded to produce the specific sequence of amino acids in a polypeptide chain. The process follows transcription in which the DNA sequence is copied (or transcribed) into an mRNA. Eukaryotic mRNA

*Department of Hematology/Oncology, The University of Vermont Cancer Center, Burlington, Vermont, USA
†Department of Biochemistry, The University of Vermont Cancer Center, Burlington, Vermont, USA
‡Corresponding author. Claire Verschraegen, Department of Hematology/Oncology, The University of Vermont Cancer Center, 89 Beaumont Ave, Given Building E-214, Burlington, VT 05405, USA; Tel: +1-802-656-5487; Fax: +1-802-656-5414; E-mail: *claire.verschraegen@vtmednet.org*
[1] Merriam-Webster dictionary. *www.merriam-webster.com/dictionary*

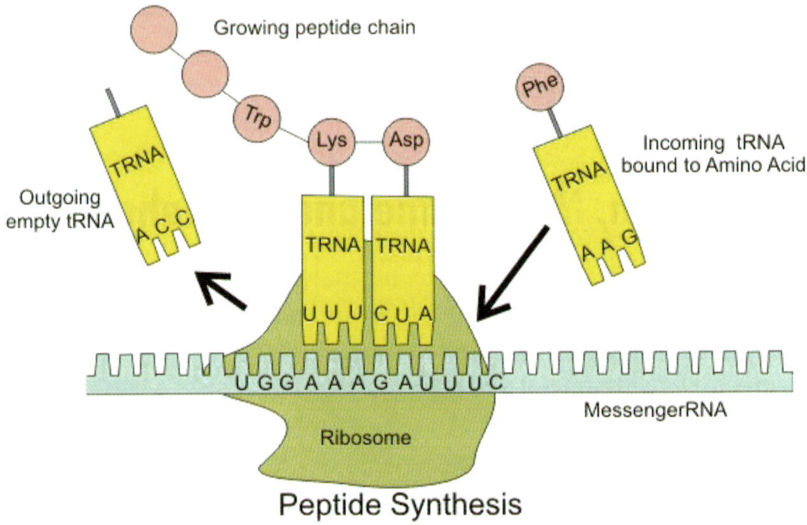

Fig. 1. Schema of the four steps in protein translation.

precursors must be processed in the nucleus (e.g., capping, polyadenylation, splicing) before they are exported to the cytoplasm for translation where the ribosomes are located.

Protein translation consists of four steps (Fig. 1):

(1) *Activation or amino acid charging of tRNA*: The correct amino acid is covalently bonded to the correct tRNA: Specific enzyme aminoacyl tRNA synthetases bind tRNA by the anticodon and the amino acid. The enzyme then forms a covalent bond between the carboxyl group of the amino acid and the hydroxyl groups of the pentose sugar of the tRNA. The aminoacyl tRNA synthetase recognizes the specific tRNA not because of the anticodon but because there are specific recognition sites on the tRNA.

(2) *Initiation*: The small subunit of the ribosome binds to the 5′ end of mRNA with the help of initiation factors and leads to the assembly of active ribosome and the reading of the first mRNA codon: This occurs once per polypeptide chain. The mRNA start codon in eukaryotes is usually AUG, coding for a N-terminal methionine, which is then cleaved off. Eukaryotic mRNA has a special cap at the 5′ end of the mRNA which is recognized by a cap-binding protein. Eukaryotes also

have 10 initiation factors, called eIF1, eIF2, to eIF10. These initiation factors modulate the plasticity of the ribosome units to induce optimal translation.

(3) *Elongation*: The next aminoacyl-tRNA in line binds to the ribosome along with GTP and an elongation factor. Three steps are involved. First, the proper aminoacyl-tRNA from cytoplasm transfers to the A-site of the ribosome. Second is the peptidyl transfer, where the new amino acid links covalently to the growing polypeptide chain. And last, the translocation, where the tRNA moves from the A-site to the P-site with a simultaneous movement of mRNA by three nucleotides. Thus, elongation, which depends on eukaryotic elongation factors, is a three-step microcycle. The initiator tRNA occupies the P-site in the ribosome, and the A-site is ready to receive the new aminoacyl-tRNA, adding a new amino acid to the nascent polypeptide chain.

(4) *Termination*: The A-site of the ribosome faces a stop codon (UAA, UAG or UGA). The reaction ends.

2.2. BUT IS THIS THE WHOLE STORY?

Beyond protein translation lies the "supercomplex" of molecular interactions that direct the cellular mechanism into the physiological mechanisms necessary for life. When these processes are going awry, cancer cells may emerge with a poisonous gift for immortality. Because there is no life without death — You must be willing to die in order to live (Yoruba proverb, West Africa) — immortality is incompatible with healthy living. The work of the scientist is to understand these processes at the molecular and cellular level, and the role of the clinician is to modify the environment at the human level, to deliver therapeutics to cancer patients in order to regain some (= cancer remission) or full (= cancer cure) homeostasis of the "supercomplex." Many questions remain incompletely answered:

- What is the "catalytic" event(s) leading a cell on the cancer path?
- What are the intrinsic versus extrinsic factors leading to this event?
- What host factors must be considered?
- What strategies can be employed to target cancer cells?
- What are the hurdles to implementing this targeting clinically?

2.3. THE BENCH SCIENTIST VIEW

Parameters of biological control that are compromised with the onset and progression of tumorigenesis provide a blueprint to enhance capabilities for cancer prevention, early detection, therapy and survivorship. There is longstanding recognition that genetic perturbations contribute to cancer biology and pathology. Point mutation, deletions, gene amplification and intra- as well as inter chromosomal rearrangements and translations are classical molecular lesions that are linked with cancer in an obligatory manner. These genetic changes provide definitive molecular diagnostics for tumors, are informative for therapeutic options, and can be indications of remission, cure or relapse. Evidence is accruing that compromised epigenetic control is linked to the initiation and progression of solid and liquid tumors.[1,2] Genetic and epigenetic involvements in cancer are not mutually exclusive and are becoming increasingly understood. Rather, there is a synergy between inheritable changes in gene expression that are DNA-encoded and those that are transmitted from parental to progeny cells during mitotic division through non-DNA-encoded mechanisms. Parameters of epigenetic control include posttranslational modifications of histones, DNA methylation and noncoding RNAs. More recently, mitotic bookmarking has emerged as a novel dimension to epigenetic regulation.[3,4]

2.3.1. Histone Modifications

For the past half century, there has been an appreciation for the epigenetic regulatory contribution of histone modifications to the control of gene expression.[5,6] Acetylation, methylation and phosphorylation of these basic (arginine- and lysine-rich) chromosomal proteins that package DNA as chromatin have been extensively studied. Compelling evidence has documented the role of histone modifications in mediating chromatin organization that determines gene activation or suppression and the extent that genes are transcribed. Mechanistically, modified histones influence accessibility of gene regulatory domains to factors that control transcription. The dynamic and physiologically responsive addition and removal of acetate (HATs and HDACs) and phosphate (kinases and phosphatases) and methyl (methylases and demethylases) moieties from histone proteins reinforce the biological and clinical implications of epigenetic mechanisms.

2.3.2. DNA Methylation

Methylation of DNA sequences selectively modifies genomic architecture and frequently represses gene expression by rendering regulatory domains of gene promoters inaccessible to transcription factors.[7,8] There are abundant examples of methylation that mediate gene silencing and are instrumental for development, differentiation, tissue remodeling and reprogramming pluripotency. For example, methylation in a CpG island of the retinoblastoma (Rb) gene, a tumor suppressor gene common in human cancers, was first discovered in 1989.[9] In 1994, the idea that CpG island promoter hypermethylation could be a mechanism of gene inactivation was proposed to explain the modulation of the Von Hippel-Lindau (VHL) gene which undergoes methylation-associated inactivation.[10] Somatic inactivation of the VHL tumor suppressor gene is associated with a familial type of clear cell renal cell cancer. CpG island hypermethylation as a common mechanism of inactivation of the tumor suppressor gene was confirmed when studying $p16^{INK4a}$ in human cancers.[11] Many other methylation sites also play a role in various oncogeneses.[12] With new, powerful and user-friendly techniques, such as sodium bisulphite modification[13] and methylation-specific PCR,[14] the list of candidate genes with putative aberrant methylation of CpG islands has grown exponentially.[15]

2.3.3. Noncoding RNAs

RNA-mediated gene silencing is strikingly illustrated by chromosome X inactivation, which involves Xist (X-inactive specific transcript) RNA.[16] More recently, noncoding RNAs that have been shown to control gene expression include microRNAs and long noncoding RNAs. MicroRNA involvement in control of gene expression is broad-based.[17,18] Beyond the well-studied involvement in development there are also compelling examples of microRNA-related mechanisms that support transformation and tumor progression.[19]

2.3.4. Mitotic Bookmarking

Recent findings indicate that tissue-specific transcription factors remain associated with target gene loci on mitotic chromosomes.[20] Mitotic bookmarking provides a mechanism to sustain tissue-specific gene expression by transferring gene regulatory complexes from parental to progeny cells during mitotic division. Tissue-specific transcriptional machinery that supports the myeloid, muscle, adipocyte and osteoblast phenotypes is mitotically transmitted. This novel dimension to control of gene expression extends beyond biological regulation. Mitotic bookmarking contributes to establishing and sustaining the AML leukemia phenotype. The AML leukemia 8:21 translocation fusion protein is retained with target genes on mitotic chromosomes.[21] Co-regulation of tissue-specific and ribosomal genes by the 8:21 translocation fusion protein functionally modifies control of proliferation and phenotype that leads to alterations in growth control and regulation of protein synthesis.

2.3.5. Dreams of Clinical Applications

The clinical relevance of epigenetic control as observed in the laboratory is being translated into applications for both cancer diagnosis and therapy.[22] Epigenetic signatures that are based on cohorts of modified histones and DNA methylation with involvement of functionally related genes will provide novel dimensions to cancer diagnosis and prediction of responsiveness to therapy.[23–26] The specificity for such epigenetic signatures, at least in part, reflects the combinatorial organization of the regulatory machinery. Additional refinements might lead to increased specificity and minimal "off-target" consequences. The discovery of histone and DNA modifying factors are now applied to the treatment of solid tumors and leukemias. HDAC inhibitors (romidepsin and vorinostat) are used for treating patients with cutaneous T-cell lymphoma.[27] These compounds also block proliferation and induce differentiation of erythroleukemia cells. DNA methylation inhibitors (azacytidine and decitabine) have been tested clinically and approved for myelodysplastic syndromes.[28] In phase III studies of patients with myelodysplastic syndrome treated with azacytidine, observed response rates ranged from 30 per cent to 60 per cent, most interestingly with documented improved survival compared with either supportive care or cytotoxic chemotherapy when treatment is continued over long periods of time, again a departure from the principles of standard chemotherapy dosing.[29,30] Early phase III studies of decitabine yielded similar responses to chemotherapy treatments. These trials used a limited number of treatment cycles, and no effect of survival was noted.[31,32] However, when unlimited number of cycles of decitabine are administered,[33] patients experienced high response rates (40 per cent complete response, over 70 per cent total response) and prolonged survival.

However, cancer therapy based on epigenetic parameters of control remains an emerging strategy. Refinement of these concepts and their clinical applications has a long way to go. Thus exploiting regulatory parameters of epigenetic control to restore quiescence and phenotype to tumor cells is an approach that requires further development. It is realistic to anticipate the emergence of links between epigenetically modified components of control in tumors with alterations in proliferation, growth and phenotype that translate to strategies for restoration of biological function in tumor cells.[34,35]

2.4. THE CLINICIAN INVESTIGATOR VIEW

2.4.1. The Necessity of Methionine

The chemistry of methionine as the initiator amino acid of protein formation has been exploited in patients to prevent cancer growth. This is facilitated by the fact that methionine, being an essential amino acid, must be present in food in sufficient amounts for survival. Thus, feeding cancer patients a diet low in methionine was tested in a clinical trial. Eight patients with a variety of metastatic solid tumors enrolled in a phase I clinical trial of a commercially available methionine-free medical food served as the primary dietary protein source for all patients. The prescribed diet contained 0.6–0.8 g of protein, 25–35 kcal, and 2 mg of methionine per kilo gram per day. Participants consumed the experimental diet for an average of 17.3 weeks (range 8–39 weeks), which lowered the plasma methionine levels by 58 per cent (from 21.6 ± 7.3 to 9 ± 4 μM within 2 weeks), with no changes in serum albumin and prealbumin levels or calorie counts. There was a weight loss of approximately 0.5 per cent of body mass index (0.5 kg) per week. Enteral dietary methionine restriction was found to be safe and tolerable in adults with metastatic solid tumors and resulted in a significant reduction in plasma methionine levels. Additionally, two patients benefited with a decrease of tumor burden.[36] One practical problem is the price of such a diet, about US$1,000 per month.

Another way to reduce methionine content is to decrease access to this amino acid enzymatically.[37] Methioninase is an enzyme that specifically degrades methionine and homocysteine, thereby inhibiting the growth of a variety of cancer cells *in vitro* and *in vivo*.[38,39] Recombinant methioninase was tested in a phase I clinical trial. Patients in the trial experienced no significant toxicity, and plasma methionine levels fell dramatically, as expected.[40] The antitumor activity of methioninase was not assessed in the trial. A polyethylene glycol conjugation of methioninase has been developed to reduce the potential antigenicity and lengthen the half-life of the recombinant enzyme.[41–43]

2.4.2. The Hope for Gene Reactivation

Our group has tested two combinations involving modulation of methylation in patients with advanced cancers. The first study involved the combination of azacytidine with erlotinib. The epidermal growth factor receptor (EGFR) is a validated target in malignancy with available specific drugs. The hypothesis was that an epigenetic therapy might reactivate the EGFR membrane receptor expression and thus enhance the anti-proliferative effect of erlotinib. The main objective of this phase I study was to evaluate the combination of erlotinib and 5-azacytidine, a demethylating agent at low dose, for safety and maximal tolerated dose (MTD). Thirty patients with advanced solid tumors were treated in a standard 3 + 3 cohort design. Erlotinib was dosed at 150 mg daily, and 5-azacytidine was escalated by increasing the number of daily doses of 75 mg/m^2 per cycle. Patients were followed for dose-limiting toxicity and efficacy was assessed by RECIST criteria. Common non-hematologic toxicities included rash, diarrhea, nausea and fatigue; the majority of adverse events were grade 2 or less. The recommended dose for phase II study is erlotinib 150 mg daily by oral administration and 5-azacytidine 75 mg/m^2 subcutaneously daily on days 1–4 and 15–18 of a 28-day cycle. Partial responses were seen in one patient each with lung and ovarian cancers, and stable disease was observed in 11 patients. Two patients with lung and larynx cancer had prolonged stable disease. While the combination of erlotinib and 5-azacytidine was well tolerated and had some interesting clinical activity in lung, head and neck, and ovarian cancers, the mechanism of action could not be assessed for practical reasons.[44]

Hydralazine and procainamide, both weak hypomethylating agents, have demonstrated the ability to reverse aberrant promoter methylation at concentrations that could be achieved clinically. Valproic acid causes hyperacetylation of histones H3 and H4. In a phase I trial of women with cervical cancer, a partial reversion of a panel of aberrantly silenced genes was demonstrated at all dose levels tested, with gene re-expression in three-quarters of the informative cases.[45] *In vitro*, hydralazine is not cytotoxic, although valproic acid is, and this effect is potentiated by the addition of hydralazine.[46,47] The combination of hydralazine and valproic acid also increases the cytotoxicity of several standard agents, such as gemcitabine, cisplatin, topotecan and doxorubicin.[48] In our study of the combination of valproic acid with hydralazine, we observed a patient with advanced melanoma whose disease stabilized for over 14 months at low doses of hydralazine. In this study, valproic acid dosing was titrated to therapeutic levels prior to initiating hydralazine in escalating doses per cohort. Valproic acid was administered orally at 250 mg every 8 hours for 7 days, then at 500 mg for 7 days. The dose was then titrated to obtain a serum level between 0.4 mM and 0.7 mM. On day 14, hydralazine was started orally at a dose of 25 mg daily continuously. Patients were assessed after 28 days. If no dose-limiting toxicities were observed in three patients, then the next cohort was initiated. The dose of hydralazine was doubled by cohorts of 3 + 3 patients until a dose of 200 mg per day was reached. Afterwards, the dose per cohort was increased by 100 mg up to a maximum dose of 400 mg/day. While the response rate seen in this study did not justify further investigation, the fact that a prolonged effect was seen in a patient with melanoma remains intriguing (Jones D, personal communication).

2.4.3. Dreams of Cancer Cure

With the advent of a newly discovered biological aspect of gene control, a fury of clinical trials has taken place in the last 10 years. Table 1 lists many such trials. As we are entering the molecular age of cancer understanding, the biological classification of tumors based on the epigenetic "snapshot" is far from applicability in a busy clinical setting. Unfortunately, with the lack of targeted biomarkers that would lead to selecting the right drug for the right cancer among the right patient population, these efforts have yielded results that are not yet satisfying. Response rates are usually similar to the ones seen with chemotherapy. Although epigenetic modulation might be an additional treatment option for assiduous patients, adverse events are still in the unacceptable range, alas accepted because, psychologically, the disease is still worse than any available therapy's anticipated side effects. Despite such difficult obstacles in this course against death, efforts must continue to understand our patients and their cancer better, and we must keep trying new strategies, continue to collect tumor and data, and promote new ideas into actions that seem, at times, as formidable as the rock of Sisyphus. Staying the course will eventually shed more hopeful light on the mystery of cancer. "Each grain of that stone, each mineral flake of that night-filled mountain, in itself forms a world. The struggle itself toward the heights is enough to fill a man's heart. One must imagine Sisyphus happy."[49]

2.5. WHAT IS LOST IN TRANSLATION?

Dietary restriction for the treatment of cancer is not a new concept,[61–62] but selective diet manipulations, in this case amino acid restriction, have not been extensively studied. *In vitro* and *in vivo* studies of essential amino acid manipulation found alterations of tumor growth in surroundings lacking methionine, isoleucine or valine.[64] A methionine-free diet is life saving for people with vitamin B6 non-responsive homocystinuria or with hypermethioninemia and is available commercially. A wide variety of cancer cell lines are methionine dependent even in the presence of homocysteine, but normal cells survive in the growth medium where methionine is replaced by homocysteine.[65] Animals fed diets with homocysteine instead of methionine suffer no ill effects and grow normally.[66,67]

Table 1 Selected Recent Clinical Results with DNA Methylation Inhibitors

Treatment	Dosage	Indication	Results	Comments	References
Azacytidine	75 mg/m^2 SQ, daily × 7, q4 weeks	MDS	CR 7%, PR 16%	Improved progression-free survival compared to supportive care.	Ref. 30
Azacytidine	75 mg/m^2 SQ, daily × 7, q4 weeks	MDS	CR 17%, PR 12%	Improved survival compared to conventional therapy.	Ref. 29
Azacytidine for maintenance	subcutaneous 60 mg/m^2 daily × 5, q4 weeks until relapse	High-risk MDS, chronic MMC leukemia and acute myeloid leukemia syndromes in CR after induction chemotherapy	Median overall survival, 20 months	CR duration was not associated with CDKN2B methylation status or karyotype. Hypermethylation of CDH1 was significantly associated with low CR rate, early relapse, and short overall survival.	Ref. 50
Azacytidine + phenylbutyrate	Aza 25–75 mg/m^2 SQ, daily for 5–14 days, q4 weeks + Phenylbutyrate 375 mg/kg/d IV, CI × 7 days beginning on the final day of Aza	MDS and AML	CR 14%, PR 3%	Tumor suppressor gene hypomethylation more pronounced in responders.	Ref. 51
Azacytidine + valproic acid + ATRA	Aza 75 mg/m^2 SC, daily × 7, q4 weeks + valproic acid 50–75 mg/kg PO days 1–7 + ATRA 45 mg/m^2 PO days 3–7	Poor prognosis or relapsed or refractory leukemias	CR 22%	Higher response rate in previously untreated patients. Correlation between valproic acid levels and response.	Ref. 52

(*Continued*)

Table 1 (Continued)

Treatment	Dosage	Indication	Results	Comments	References
Azacytidine + valproic acid	Aza 100 mg/m^2, daily × 5 + valproic acid titrated to serum level 80–110 mg/ml)	Poor prognosis or relapsed leukemias and MDS	CR 29%, PR 8%	Higher response rate in previously untreated patients.	Ref. 53
Azacytidine + valproic acid	Aza 20–95 mg/m^2 SQ, daily × 10, q4 weeks + valproic acid titrated to plasma levels of 75 to 100 μg/mL	Relapsed refractory solid tumors	SD 25%		Ref. 54
Azacytidine + erlotinib	Aza 75 mg/m^2 SQ daily days 1–4 and 15–18 q4 weeks + erlotinib 150 mg/day	Relapsed refractory solid tumors	SD 40%		Ref. 44
Decitabine	15 mg/m^2 IV over 3 hours q8h for 9 doses, q6 weeks	MDS	CR 24%, PR 10%		Ref. 32
Decitabine	15 mg/m^2 IV over 3 hours q8h for 9 doses, q6 weeks	MDS	CR 9%, PR 8%	Improved progression-free survival compared to supportive care.	Ref. 31
Decitabine	5–20 mg/m^2 IV over 1 hour daily × 10	Poor prognosis or relapsed or refractory leukemias	CR 18%, PR 6%, HI 8%	Greater response rate at lower doses. Flat hypomethylation dose-response past 150 mg/m^2 total dose.	Ref. 55
Decitabine	3 dose schedules, most patients treated at 20 mg/m^2 IV over 1 hour daily × 5, q4 weeks	MDS	CR 34%, PR 1%	Improved survival compared to chemotherapy in a case-control study. Association between *P15* reactivation and response.	Ref. 33

(*Continued*)

Table 1 (Continued)

Treatment	Dosage	Indication	Results	Comments	References
Decitabine	15–20 mg/m^2 IV over 1 hour daily × 10 (some patients also received valproic acid)	AML	CR 16%, PR 12%	Correlation between ER reactivation and response. Addition of valproic acid did not impact responses.	Ref. 56
Decitabine	2.5–20 mg/m^2 IV over 1 hour daily × 5–10 days	Relapsed or refractory solid tumors	PR 4%, Minor response 11%, SD 46% (at 4 weeks)	No correlation between tumor and peripheral blood mononuclear cell hypomethylation after therapy.	Ref. 57
Decitabine + valproic acid	Decitabine 15 mg/m^2 IV over 1 hour daily × 10 + valproic acid 25–50 mg/kg PO days 1–10	Poor prognosis or relapsed or refractory leukemias	CR 19%	Higher response rate in previously untreated patients. Correlation between valproic acid levels and response.	Ref. 58
Decitabine + interleukin 2	Decitabine 0.1–0.3 mg/kg SQ d days/week for 2 weeks + interleukin 2 600,000 IU/kg IV q8h × 14 doses on weeks 3 and 6	Metastatic melanoma and renal tumors	CR 6%, PR 12%, SD 18%		Ref. 59
Decitabine + carboplatin	Decitabine 45–135 mg/m^2 IV × 1, q4 weeks + carboplatin AUC 5–6 IV d8	Relapsed or refractory solid tumors	PR 3%, SD 9%	Hypomethylationof MAGE-A1 documented in tumors.	Ref. 60

SQ, subcutaneously; IV, intravenous; CI, continuous infusion; ATRA, all-trans retinoic acid; MDS, myelodysplastic syndrome; MMC, myelomonocytic; AML, acute myelogenous leukemia; CR, complete response; PR, partial response; SD, stable disease; MAGE-A1, melanoma antigen family A1; ER, estrogen receptor; CDKN2B, cyclin-dependent kinase inhibitor 2B; CDH1, cadherin-1.

Examples of dietary methionine effects were clinically studied in healthy, cancer-free people. In one study, the methylation of DNA on the initiation or progression of colon cancer in relationship to dietary folate and methionine was assessed in a cohort of 47,931 US male health professionals. The hypothesis was that deficient intakes of folate or methionine and high consumption of alcohol, an antagonist of methyl-group metabolism, would increase the risk of colon neoplasia. The dietary intake of these healthy men was recorded during 1 year on a validated, semi-quantitative food-frequency questionnaire. During the next 6 years, 205 new cases of colon cancer were documented. Current alcohol intake was directly related to risk of colon cancer, and folate and methionine intakes were weakly inversely associated with risk of colon cancer. Combinations of high alcohol and low methionine and folate intakes yielded striking associations for total colon cancer (RR = 3.30, 95% CI = 1.58–6.88) comparing low-methyl diets with high-methyl diets among nonusers of aspirin. Among men with high intakes of folate or methionine, alcohol levels of more than two drinks daily were not associated with risk of colon cancer, suggesting a protective effect. While such studies have clear limitations, inadequate intakes of folate and methionine might increase the risk of colon cancer.[68] Unfortunately, such epidemiologic studies are not mechanistically linked to laboratory observations, which weaken the conclusions that one could draw for a healthy lifestyle focused on cancer avoidance.

In another study of the associations between dietary intakes of methionine and B vitamins (i.e., riboflavin, niacin, vitamin B6, folate and vitamin B12) with lung cancer risk (The Shanghai Women's Health Study), 74,941 healthy women that had never smoked were followed for a median of 11.2 years. Lung cancer was diagnosed in 428 women. Again, baseline dietary intakes were derived from a validated, interviewer-administered food frequency questionnaire. Concurrent with the US study of colon cancer in healthy men, dietary riboflavin intake (HR = 0.62; 95% CI = 0.43–0.89; p trend = 0.03 for the highest quartile compared with the lowest) and a higher than median intake of methionine (HR = 0.78; 95% CI = 0.60–0.99) were inversely associated with lung cancer risk in these healthy women.[69]

While a restriction of methionine in the diet might be helpful to prevent cancer growth, in healthy people a lack of methionine might lead to the development of cancers. How cancer growth is affected is not as simple as preventing protein generation. Determining the molecular mechanisms for the tumor specific growth inhibitory effects of methionine restriction requires an in-depth understanding of the specialized functions of methionine. One such function of methionine is as a donation pool of major methyl groups for methylation of DNA, RNA, proteins, and other molecules. Epigenetic modifications lead to specific phenotypical expressions. The role of methylation is to stabilize DNA by compacting the chromatin structure, thus rendering cells less susceptible to DNA-damaging agents. Cytosine methylation within CpG islands is one of the classical mechanisms by which gene expression is regulated.[70] The loss of methylated cytosines reduces the chromatin stability and decreases binding sites for methyl-specific DNA-binding proteins.[71] This reduction in methyl-directed protein binding increases the access of oxidant on DNA sequences and induces more enzyme-induced DNA strand breakage.[72] In animal models, severe and prolonged methyl deficiency through dietary restriction of methionine, choline, homocysteine and folate induces global demethylation of normal liver DNA and causes increased susceptibility to DNA strand breaks.[73] Interestingly, hypermethylation is much more common in tumors than in normal tissues.[74] In cancer cells, focal DNA hypermethylation silences several growth inhibitory and pro-apoptotic genes at the transcription level.[73]

Methylation might be a double-edged sword. In cancer cells, inhibition of DNA methylation by methionine restriction may increase susceptibility to lethal DNA damage or "liberate" tumor suppressor mechanisms. But in normal cells, the opposite might be true, where demethylation renders cells more susceptible to carcinogenetic elements in the environment. The understanding of the methylation equilibrium of genes and associated proteins might lead to a better definition of appropriate treatments against cancer cells, while sparing the normal cellular methylation balance.

In current practice, clinicians have access to the hypomethylating nucleoside analogs, azacytidine and decitabine. These nucleoside analogs are incorporated into cells by specialized and efficient transporters. Azacytidine was tested in early clinical trials in the 1970s and 1980s but deemed too toxic when used in the classical cytotoxic model of chemotherapy administration revolving around the Skipper–Schabel–Wilcox log-kill model.[75]

Epigenetic modifiers work at low doses, as evidenced by differentiation seen after chronic low dose azacytidine *in vivo*. Hypomethylation induced by these agents is now correctly identified as a low dose treatment effect. The advantages of metronomic treatment in older patients with leukemia brought these drugs back to life clinically, and DNA methylation became the new therapeutic target once the mechanisms of action were better understood. The DNA hypomethylating property is limited to cytosine analogs with 5′ modifications of the ring.[76] Upon enzymatic phosphorylation of azacytidine to 5-aza-CTP and 5-aza-dCTP, incorporation into RNA and DNA occurs. This leads to the formation of irreversible covalent bonds with DNA methyltransferases, which result in bulky DNA/protein adducts and inhibition of DNA synthesis. At high doses, this metabolic process causes cell death, but at low doses, repair occurs through excision and proteasome degradation, resulting in DNA repair. This removal of DNA methyltransferases results in hypomethylation of newly synthesized DNA by passive demethylation. Decitabine functions similarly to azacytidine in inhibiting and degrading DNA methyltransferases. The absence of new methylation might lead to recovery of gene function, and this hypothesis has been tested in many clinical trials. Unfortunately, the initial response to these demethylation agents is often short-lived.[77]

Various non-nucleoside analog drugs might also inhibit DNA methylation, including procainamide, hydralazine, and other compounds. How these drugs affect hypomethylation and their role in interfering with the biology of DNA methyltransferases is not clear. Hydralazine inhibits DNA methyltransferase activity but has little or no activity in the down regulation of DNA methyltransferases. A docking protocol used to predict the binding mode of compounds 2′-deoxycytidine, 5-azacytidine and 5-aza-2′-deoxycytidine was applied to study the inhibitory DNA methyltransferase activity of hydralazine. Similar molecular interactions within the binding pocket of cytosine analogs were observed. These interactions involve a complex network of hydrogen bonds with arginine and glutamic acid residues that mechanistically modulate DNA methylation. Despite the different scaffolds of other non-nucleoside DNA methyltransferase inhibitors such as procaine and procainamide, this modeling study reveals similar interactions within the DNA methyltransferase 1 binding site.[78] Inhibitors of DNA methyltransferases are being designed. MG98, an antisense compound directed at DNA methyltransferase 1 that was effective *in vitro*, did not show efficacy in human clinical trials.[79] The dynamics of such a precisely targeted therapeutic approach might shed light on the contradictory results observed by clinicians because of cytotoxic effects competing for demethylating effects resulting in a U-shaped dose-response for hypomethylation induction.[80] Finally, hypomethylation can activate some oncogenes known to be silenced in cancer such as *COX2* or *EGFR*.[81] This lack of specificity makes predictions of clinical outcomes extremely complex.

2.6. CONCLUSIONS

While we understand molecular mechanisms better, we also realize how the complexity of molecular networking, or the "supercomplex," leads to a fine cellular balance that defines the phenotypic role of each cell within an organism. Once this equilibrium is disturbed, the organism tips off balance. Cancer is such an off-balance disease. The recovery of homeostasis involves adjustment of multiple controls, one of them being epigenetics. Perhaps the time has come to think of biology and biological interactions in a relativistic way, akin to quantum theory (Lajos Pusztai, MD, PhD, Juckett lecturer, Vermont, 2013), that helps understand transformation, and its clinical applicability, as a completely new metaphor.

REFERENCES

1. Zaidi SK, Young DW, Javed A, *et al.* (2007) Nuclear microenvironments in biological control and cancer. *Nat Rev Cancer* 7: 454–463.
2. Zaidi SK, Young DW, Montecino MA, *et al.* (2010) Mitotic bookmarking of genes: A novel dimension to epigenetic control. *Nat Rev Genet* **11**: 583–589.
3. Zaidi SK, Young DW, Pockwinse SM, *et al.* (2003) Mitotic partitioning and selective reorganization of tissue-specific transcription factors in progeny cells. *Proc Natl Acad Sci USA* **100**: 14852–14857.
4. Rada-Iglesias A. (2013) Pioneering barren land: Mitotic bookmarking by transcription factors. *Dev Cell* **24**: 342–344.

5. Elsasser SJ, Allis CD, Lewis PW. (2011) Cancer. New epigenetic drivers of cancers. *Science* **331**: 1145–1146.
6. Sadeh R, Allis CD. (2011) Genome-wide "re"-modeling of nucleosome positions. *Cell* **147**: 263–266.
7. You JS, Jones PA. (2012) Cancer genetics and epigenetics: Two sides of the same coin? *Cancer Cell* **22**: 9–20.
8. Bergman Y, Cedar H. (2013) DNA methylation dynamics in health and disease. *Nat Struct Mol Biol* **20**: 274–281.
9. Greger V, Passarge E, Hopping W, *et al.* (1989) Epigenetic changes may contribute to the formation and spontaneous regression of retinoblastoma. *Hum Genet* **83**: 155–158.
10. Herman JG, Latif F, Weng Y, *et al.* (1994) Silencing of the VHL tumor-suppressor gene by DNA methylation in renal carcinoma. *Proc Natl Acad Sci USA* **91**: 9700–9704.
11. Mao L, Merlo A, Bedi G, *et al.* (1995) A novel p16INK4A transcript. *Cancer Res* **55**: 2995–2997.
12. McRonald FE, Morris MR, Gentle D, *et al.* (2009) CpG methylation profiling in VHL related and VHL unrelated renal cell carcinoma. *Mol Cancer* **8**: 31.
13. Clark SJ, Harrison J, Paul CL, Frommer M. (1994) High sensitivity mapping of methylated cytosines. *Nucleic Acids Res* **22**: 2990–2997.
14. Herman JG, Graff JR, Myohanen S, *et al.* (1996) Methylation-specific PCR: A novel PCR assay for methylation status of CpG islands. *Proc Natl Acad Sci USA* **93**: 9821–9826.
15. Esteller M, Corn PG, Baylin SB, Herman JG. (2001) A gene hypermethylation profile of human cancer. *Cancer Res* **61**: 3225–3229.
16. Splinter E, de Wit E, Nora EP, *et al.* (2011) The inactive X chromosome adopts a unique three-dimensional conformation that is dependent on X is tRNA. *Genes Dev* **25**: 1371–1383.
17. Lian JB, Stein GS, van Wijnen AJ, *et al.* (2012) MicroRNA control of bone formation and homeostasis. *Nat Rev Endocrinol* **8**: 212–227.
18. Di Leva G, Croce CM. (2013) miRNA profiling of cancer. *Curr Opin Genet Dev.*
19. Rastinejad F, Conboy MJ, Rando TA, Blau HM. (1993) Tumor suppression by RNA from the 3′ untranslated region of alpha-tropomyosin. *Cell* **75**: 1107–1117.
20. Young DW, Hassan MQ, Yang XQ, *et al.* (2007) Mitotic retention of gene expression patterns by the cell fate-determining transcription factor Runx2. *Proc Natl Acad Sci USA* **104**: 3189–3194.

21. Bakshi R, Zaidi SK, Pande S, *et al.* (2008) The leukemogenic t(8;21) fusion protein AML1-ETO controls rRNA genes and associates with nucleolar-organizing regions at mitotic chromosomes. *J Cell Sci* **121**: 3981–3990.
22. Black JC, Whetstine JR. (2013) Tipping the lysine methylation balance in disease. *Biopolymers* **99**: 127–135.
23. Lima SC, Hernandez-Vargas H, Simao T, *et al.* (2011) Identification of a DNA methylome signature of esophageal squamous cell carcinoma and potential epigenetic biomarkers. *Epigenetics* **6**: 1217–1227.
24. Bianco-Miotto T, Chiam K, Buchanan G, *et al.* (2010) Global levels of specific histone modifications and an epigenetic gene signature predict prostate cancer progression and development. *Cancer Epidemiol Biomarkers Prev* **19**: 2611–2622.
25. Teschendorff AE, Menon U, Gentry-Maharaj A, *et al.* (2009) An epigenetic signature in peripheral blood predicts active ovarian cancer. *PLoS One* **4**:e8274.
26. Widschwendter M, Fiegl H, Egle D, *et al.* (2007) Epigenetic stem cell signature in cancer. *Nat Genet* **39**: 157–158.
27. Rangwala S, Zhang C, Duvic M. (2012) HDAC inhibitors for the treatment of cutaneous T-cell lymphomas. *Future Med Chem* **4**: 471–486.
28. Schecter J, Galili N, Raza A. (2012) MDS: Refining existing therapy through improved biologic insights. *Blood Rev* **26**: 73–80.
29. Fenaux P, Mufti GJ, Hellstrom-Lindberg E, *et al.* (2009) Efficacy of azacitidine compared with that of conventional care regimens in the treatment of higher-risk myelodysplastic syndromes: A randomised, open-label, phase III study. *Lancet Oncol* **10**: 223–232.
30. Silverman LR, Demakos EP, Peterson BL, *et al.* (2002) Randomized controlled trial of azacitidine in patients with the myelodysplastic syndrome: A study of the cancer and leukemia group B. *J Clin Oncol* **20**: 2429–2440.
31. Kantarjian H, Issa JP, Rosenfeld CS, *et al.* (2006) Decitabine improves patient outcomes in myelodysplastic syndromes: Results of a phase III randomized study. *Cancer* **106**: 1794–1803.
32. Wijermans PW, Lubbert M, Verhoef G, *et al.* (2005) An epigenetic approach to the treatment of advanced MDS: The experience with the DNA demethylating agent 5-aza-2′-deoxycytidine (decitabine) in 177 patients. *Ann Hematol* **84**(Suppl 1): 9–17.
33. Kantarjian H, Oki Y, Garcia-Manero G, *et al.* (2007) Results of a randomized study of 3 schedules of low-dose decitabine in higher-risk myelodysplastic syndrome and chronic myelomonocytic leukemia. *Blood* **109**: 52–57.
34. Pasque V, Jullien J, Miyamoto K, *et al.* (2011) Epigenetic factors influencing resistance to nuclear reprogramming. *Trends Genet* **27**: 516–525.

35. Simonsson S, Gurdon J. (2004) DNA demethylation is necessary for the epigenetic reprogramming of somatic cell nuclei. *Nat Cell Biol* **6**: 984–990.
36. Epner DE, Morrow S, Wilcox M, Houghton JL. (2002) Nutrient intake and nutritional indexes in adults with metastatic cancer on a phase I clinical trial of dietary methionine restriction. *Nutr Cancer* **42**: 158–166.
37. Tan Y, Zavala J, Sr., Han Q, *et al.* (1997) Recombinant methioninase infusion reduces the biochemical endpoint of serum methionine with minimal toxicity in high-stage cancer patients. *Anticancer Res* **17**: 3857–3860.
38. El-Sayed AS, Shouman SA, Nassrat HM. (2012) Pharmacokinetics, immunogenicity and anticancer efficiency of Aspergillus flavipes L-methioninase. *Enzyme Microb Technol* **51**: 200–210.
39. Machover D, Zittoun J, Saffroy R, *et al.* (2002) Treatment of cancer cells with methioninase produces DNA hypomethylation and increases DNA synthesis. *Cancer Res* **62**: 4685–4689.
40. Tan Y, Zavala J, Sr., Xu M, *et al.* (1996) Serum methionine depletion without side effects by methioninase in metastatic breast cancer patients. *Anticancer Res* **16**: 3937–3942.
41. Tan Y, Sun X, Xu M, *et al.* (1998) Polyethylene glycol conjugation of recombinant methioninase for cancer therapy. *Protein Expr Purif* **12**: 45–52.
42. Yang Z, Wang J, Yoshioka T, *et al.* (2004) Pharmacokinetics, methionine depletion, and antigenicity of recombinant methioninase in primates. *Clin Cancer Res* **10**: 2131–2138.
43. Tan Y, Xu M, Hoffman RM. (2010) Broad selective efficacy of recombinant methioninase and polyethylene glycol-modified recombinant methioninase on cancer cells *in vitro*. *Anticancer Res* **30**: 1041–1046.
44. Bauman J, Verschraegen C, Belinsky S, *et al.* (2012) A phase I study of 5-azacytidine and erlotinib in advanced solid tumor malignancies. *Cancer Chemother Pharmacol* **69**: 547–554.
45. Chavez-Blanco A, Segura-Pacheco B, Perez-Cardenas E, *et al.* (2005) Histone acetylation and histone deacetylase activity of magnesium valproate in tumor and peripheral blood of patients with cervical cancer. A phase I study. *Mol Cancer* **4**: 22.
46. Chavez-Blanco A, Perez-Plasencia C, Perez-Cardenas E, *et al.* (2006) Antineoplastic effects of the DNA methylation inhibitor hydralazine and the histone deacetylase inhibitor valproic acid in cancer cell lines. *Cancer Cell Int*, **6**: 2.
47. De la Cruz-Hernandez E, Perez-Plasencia C, Perez-Cardenas E, *et al.* (2011) Transcriptional changes induced by epigenetic therapy with hydralazine and magnesium valproate in cervical carcinoma. *Oncol Rep* **25**: 399–407.

48. Coronel J, Cetina L, Pacheco I, *et al.* (2011) A double-blind, placebo-controlled, randomized phase III trial of chemotherapy plus epigenetic therapy with hydralazine valproate for advanced cervical cancer. Preliminary results. *Med Oncol* **28**(Suppl 1): S540–S546.
49. Camus A. *Le Mythe de Sisyphe*, Gallimard 1942.
50. Grovdal M, Karimi M, Khan R, *et al.* (2010) Maintenance treatment with azacytidine for patients with high-risk myelodysplastic syndromes (MDS) or acute myeloid leukaemia following MDS in complete remission after induction chemotherapy. *Br J Haematol* **150**: 293–302.
51. Lin J, Gilbert J, Rudek MA, *et al.* (2009) A phase I dose-finding study of 5-azacytidine in combination with sodium phenylbutyrate in patients with refractory solid tumors. *Clin Cancer Res* **15**: 6241–6249.
52. Soriano AO, Yang H, Faderl S, *et al.* (2007) Safety and clinical activity of the combination of 5-azacytidine, valproic acid, and all trans retinoic acid in acute myeloid leukemia and myelodysplastic syndrome. *Blood* **110**: 2302–2308.
53. Kuendgen A, Bug G, Ottmann OG, *et al.* (2011) Treatment of poor-risk myelodysplastic syndromes and acute myeloid leukemia with a combination of 5-azacytidine and valproic acid. *Clin Epigenetics* **2**: 389–399.
54. Braiteh F, Soriano AO, Garcia-Manero G, *et al.* (2008) Phase I study of epigenetic modulation with 5-azacytidine and valproic acid in patients with advanced cancers. *Clin Cancer Res* **14**: 6296–6301.
55. Yang AS, Doshi KD, Choi SW, *et al.* (2006) DNA methylation changes after 5-aza-2′-deoxycytidine therapy in patients with leukemia. *Cancer Res* **66**: 5495–5503.
56. Blum W, Klisovic RB, Hackanson B, *et al.* (2007) Phase I study of decitabine alone or in combination with valproic acid in acute myeloid leukemia. *J Clin Oncol* **25**: 3884–3891.
57. Stewart DJ, Issa JP, Kurzrock R, *et al.* (2009) Decitabine effect on tumor global DNA methylation and other parameters in a phase I trial in refractory solid tumors and lymphomas. *Clin Cancer Res* **15**: 3881–3888.
58. Garcia-Manero G, Kantarjian HM, Sanchez-Gonzalez B, *et al.* (2006) Phase 1/2 study of the combination of 5-aza-2′-deoxycytidine with valproic acid in patients with leukemia. *Blood* **108**: 3271–3279.
59. Gollob JA, Sciambi CJ, Peterson BL, *et al.* (2006) Phase I trial of sequential low-dose 5-aza-2′-deoxycytidine plus high-dose intravenous bolus interleukin 2 in patients with melanoma or renal cell carcinoma. *Clin Cancer Res* **12**: 4619–4627.
60. Appleton K, Mackay HJ, Judson I, *et al.* (2007) Phase I and pharmacodynamic trial of the DNA methyltransferase inhibitor decitabine and carboplatin in solid tumors. *J Clin Oncol* **25**: 4603–4609.

61. Bos AM, Howard BV, Beresford SA, *et al.* (2011) Cost-effectiveness analysis of a low-fat diet in the prevention of breast and ovarian cancer. *J Am Diet Assoc* **111**: 56–66.
62. Irwin ML, McTiernan A, Manson JE, *et al.* (2011) Physical activity and survival in postmenopausal women with breast cancer: Results from the women's health initiative. *Cancer Prev Res (Phila)* **4**: 522–529.
63. Chlebowski RT, Blackburn GL, Thomson CA, *et al.* (2006) Dietary fat reduction and breast cancer outcome: Interim efficacy results from the Women's Intervention Nutrition Study. *J Natl Cancer Inst* **98**: 1767–1776.
64. Sugimura T, Birnbaum S, Winitz M, Greenstein J. (1959) Quantitative nutritional studies with water-soluble, chemically defined diets. VIII. The forced feeding of diets each lacking in one essential amino acid. *Arch Biochem Biophys* **81**: 448–455.
65. Stern PH, Hoffman RM. (1986) Enhanced *in vitro* selective toxicity of chemotherapeutic agents for human cancer cells based on a metabolic defect. *J Natl Cancer Inst* **76**: 629–639.
66. Kreis W. (1979) Tumor therapy by deprivation of L-methionine: Rationale and results. *Cancer Treat Rep* **63**: 1069–1072.
67. Breillout F, Hadida F, Echinard-Garin P, *et al.* (1987) Decreased rat rhabdomyosarcoma pulmonary metastases in response to a low methionine diet. *Anticancer Res* **7**: 861–867.
68. Giovannucci E, Rimm EB, Ascherio A, *et al.* (1995) Alcohol, low-methionine–low-folate diets, and risk of colon cancer in men. *J Natl Cancer Inst* **87**: 265–273.
69. Takata Y, Cai Q, Beeghly-Fadiel A, *et al.* (2012) Dietary B vitamin and methionine intakes and lung cancer risk among female never smokers in China. *Cancer Causes Control* **23**: 1965–1975.
70. Baylin SB, Herman JG, Graff JR, *et al.* (1998) Alterations in DNA methylation: A fundamental aspect of neoplasia. *Adv Cancer Res* **72**: 141–196.
71. Nan X, Campoy FJ, Bird A. (1997) MeCP2 is a transcriptional repressor with abundant binding sites in genomic chromatin. *Cell* **88**: 471–481.
72. Razin A. (1998) CpG methylation, chromatin structure and gene silencing — A three-way connection. *EMBO J* **17**: 4905–4908.
73. Pogribny IP, Basnakian AG, Miller BJ, *et al.* (1995) Breaks in genomic DNA and within the p53 gene are associated with hypomethylation in livers of folate/methyl-deficient rats. *Cancer Res* **55**: 1894–1901.
74. Stern PH, Hoffman RM. (1984) Elevated overall rates of transmethylation in cell lines from diverse human tumors. *In Vitro* **20**: 663–670.
75. Skipper HE. (1986) Laboratory models: Some historical perspective. *Cancer Treat Rep* **70**: 3–7.

76. Yoo CB, Jones PA. (2006) Epigenetic therapy of cancer: Past, present and future. *Nat Rev Drug Discov* 5: 37–50.
77. Issa JP, Kantarjian HM. (2009) Targeting DNA methylation. *Clin Cancer Res* 15: 3938–3946.
78. Singh N, Duenas-Gonzalez A, Lyko F, Medina-Franco JL. (2009) Molecular modeling and molecular dynamics studies of hydralazine with human DNA methyltransferase 1. *Chem Med Chem* 4: 792–799.
79. Klisovic RB, Blum W, Wei X, *et al.* (2008) Phase I study of GTI-2040, an antisense to ribonucleotide reductase, in combination with high-dose cytarabine in patients with acute myeloid leukemia. *Clin Cancer Res* 14: 3889–3895.
80. Qin T, Jelinek J, Si J, *et al.* (2009) Mechanisms of resistance to 5-aza-2′-deoxycytidine in human cancer cell lines. *Blood* 113: 659–667.
81. Montero AJ, Diaz-Montero CM, Mao L, *et al.* (2006) Epigenetic inactivation of EGFR by CpG island hypermethylation in cancer. *Cancer Biol Ther* 5: 1494–1501.

II. Integrating Emerging Science into Clinical Practice

CHAPTER 3

Integrating Emerging Science into Clinical Medicine

Marek Rudnicki[*,†] *and Kenneth W. Bueltmann*[*]

3.1. INTRODUCTION

Over the last several decades, extensive resources have been dedicated to medical investigations. This has resulted in significant progress in evidence-based knowledge pertinent to preventive, acute and chronic health care. Based on this research, multiple health care innovations have been developed utilizing this basic science knowledge. The new findings enabled better understanding of the pathophysiology underlying multiple medical diseases, drug interactions, application of many procedures, treatments, utility of technology, behavioral interventions and other clinical programs. Implementation of discoveries into medical practice, however, as well as prevention strategies and their resulting outcomes, have not kept pace with research progress and its development. Despite the development of modern investigational technologies, original research encounters a very arduous and challenging road before application into clinical practice. Without effective transformation, the fundamental aspects of quality health care — effective, efficient, current and timely care that could save many lives — cannot be achieved.[1,2]

[*]Advocate Illinois Masonic Medical Center, Chicago, Illinois, USA and University of Illinois at Chicago, USA

[†]Corresponding author: Marek Rudnicki, MD, PhD, Advocate Illinois Medical Center, Department of Surgery, 836 W. Wellington, Chicago, IL 60657, USA; Tel. +1-773-296-5347; Fax +1-774-396-5570; E-mail: *marek.rudnicki@advocahealth.com*

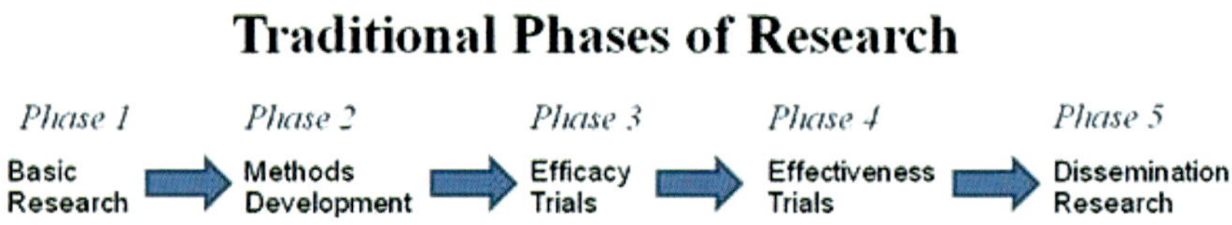

Fig. 1. Traditional phases of research (Based on Refs. 1 and 2).

Time has progressed and multiple models have been developed to describe successful application of research findings into the science of clinical medicine. Several authors have agreed that a five-phase model of integrating research findings into clinical practice might be most informative.[3] These phases include: (a) basic research, (b) methods development, (c) efficacy trials, (d) effectiveness trials, and (e) dissemination trials (Fig. 1).

Many have argued, however, that rigid adherence to the five-phase model may not be necessary. In particular, they have asserted that the five-phase linear perspective has led to a disconnection between efficacy and effectiveness research.[4] The resulting problem is that insufficient attention has been paid to how a program (or product or service) might be applied in the "real world" from the very inception of the program. A program needs to be designed from the onset to be adaptable to multiple populations in multiple settings, which can be delivered by practitioners with minimal specialty training and at the lowest financial cost and in the shortest time possible. In addition, one might counter-argue that not only does programming need to be adapted to systems but systems also need to be adapted to programming.[5]

It is this familiarity and communication between disciplines that has facilitated progress in the last 20 years. Attempts to improve algorithms have resulted in more detailed designs. Assembly of the parts, with sensitivity to current trends in the industry, and more relaxed detail, produces flowcharts that are much easier to understand and follow. From this interaction alone, it can be evinced that even at the present moment, our understanding of translational science is clouded by ambiguity and redundancy. The perception of translational science may therefore be overshadowed by unnecessary technical specification and pose a philosophical barrier to progress in the field. What the models all share is a reciprocality between nodes, and freedom to move information flow forward or backwards depending on the nature of the knowledge at hand.

Other sources of expertise have expanded upon this relationship into more complex models that include additional steps or phases. These methods are not always unique and tend to resemble one another on several levels. In common, these modalities stress a continuity of communication and flow upwards to the patient, as well as a percolation of investigation back to the bench side. Feedback loops cannot be underemphasized. The notion of feedback loops has been proposed in various community research studies that acknowledge the importance of the reach of programming (a phase V function) prior to establishing the efficacy and/or effectiveness of a program and subsequent dissemination.[6]

Work by Glasgow and Khoury has placed an emphasis upon knowledge synthesis within a T4 model (Fig. 2). Five phases are specified, confronting population-based observation and the "discovery" of ideas and technology that can be propelled into basic and clinical investigation (T0). A more versatile designation of T0 may include an interdigitation of observation and reporting, solely to emphasize that the observation can derive from a

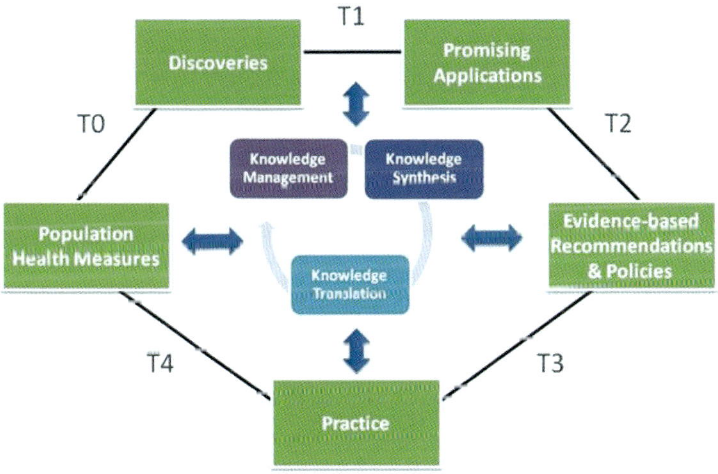

Fig. 2. Incorporation of knowledge integration into the translation continuum.

variety of origins. The first phase (T1) involves research allowing for the development of tests and other clinical interventions. Analysis of outcomes of new interventions is depicted as T2. This phase is concluded by evidence-based guidelines and recommendations by professional organizations and expert panels. It is within this T1–T2 "vortex" that the existence of significant technical, organizational, political and ethical barriers may presently delay or disrupt the translational continuum. Investigation designed to increase uptake and implementation of evidence-based recommendations into practice is considered T3. T4 research involves evaluation of the effectiveness (including cost-effectiveness) of these interventions in practice, in diverse populations and different environments.[7] These authors also stress a dissemination of data with emphasis upon implementing this previously integrated knowledge. It is further conceded that the knowledge must be utilized in order to consider it a valid translation. In this scheme, it is difficult to overlook the centrally placed caption and the pivotal impact that information systems will have upon the progress of translational medicine.

3.2. EFFORTS TO DEFINE TRANSLATIONAL RESEARCH, SCIENCE AND MEDICINE

Translational medicine has been a buzzword that has gained momentum and popularity since its advent in the early 1990s. Since this time, it has evolved to become a significant focus for medical care providers and the practice of evidence-based medicine. Currently, translation is also considered an integral part of all aspects of research and as a relatively new movement in terms of federal funding (e.g., as currently promoted by National Cancer Institute; National Institute on Drug Abuse; National Institute of Environmental Health Sciences; and National Heart, Lung, and Blood Institute). The National Institutes of Health (NIH) offer the following definition:

> "*Translational research includes two areas of translation. One is the process of applying discoveries generated during research in the laboratory, and in preclinical studies, to the development of trials and studies in humans. The second area of translation concerns research aimed at clinical trials*

and other prospective studies, retrospective studies, observational studies, and dissemination and implementation to enhance the adoption of best practices in the community. Cost-effectiveness of prevention and treatment strategies also is an important part of translational science. Bidirectional communication and work processes are integral to each of these two areas of translational research. The comparative effectiveness research of prevention and treatment strategies is also an important part of translational science."[8,9]

In the health professions, translation describes an extended process of how research knowledge that is directly or indirectly relevant to health behavior eventually serves the public. Translational research has been defined as the "process of translating discoveries in the laboratory into clinical interventions for the diagnosis, treatment, prognosis, or prevention of disease with direct benefit of human health."[10] This "new kid on the block" signifies the impressive growth of research and knowledge under the umbrella of "translational medicine."

Within 20 years, the number of publications listed in PubMed has increased from 32 hits in 1992 to 2,362 hits in 2012 (Fig. 3). Additionally, the first month of 2013 boasts 304 manuscripts already accepted for publication. Several new journals have been established to complement the rapidly expanding field of translational medicine [e.g., *Journal of Translational Medicine* (2003), *Journal of Translational Oncology* (2008), *Journal*

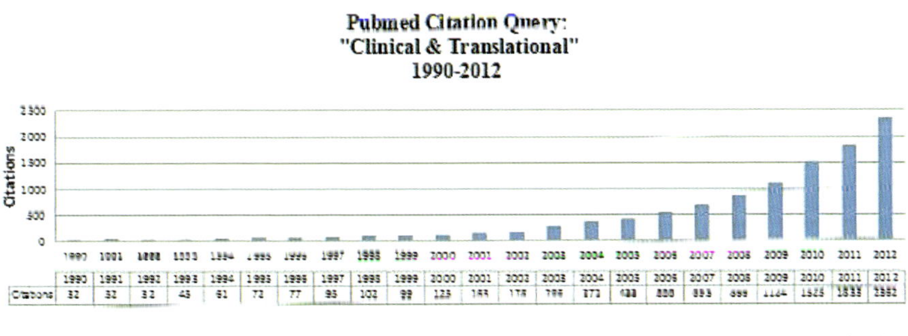

Fig. 3. Publication covering translational medicine increased tremendously over the last twenty years (Data from *www.pubmed.com*, Accessed Feb 5, 2013).

of Translational Research (2009), *Journal of Translational Stroke Research* (2010), *Journal of Translational Psychiatry* (2011)].

Thus, ultimately, translational research describes a continuum of research in which basic science discoveries are utilized to prevent or treat human disease and, conversely, clinical observations are used to generate research foci for basic science: the "bench to bedside and back to bench" approach. In a review of translational literature, one can find disagreements about definition as well as multiple conflicting models in translational research.[11] Although multidisciplinary in nature, translational medicine does not strictly refer to the collaboration of physician specialists, nurses and care givers. More importantly, it demands participation and parallel communication from experts at all scientific levels. This also implies cooperation between these entities in an ethical and proactive manner with a focus on progress and application of state-of-the-art knowledge. Translational medicine is evidenced-based medicine taken to the next level. It is not pathognomonically bound to the notions of translational science and interdisciplinary research.

Current trends in the practice of medicine are shifting from systems-based medicine to even more personalized care. Combining all available resources — including biomarkers, genome sequences and molecular profiling — enables the modern clinician to best predict and manage complex diseases and guide patient-specific therapies. The pinnacle of the "medical pyramid" has its foundation in basic science and clinical knowledge, and through geno- and phenotyping can be focused towards so-called P4 medicine (Fig. 4).

This entails a convergence of modalities that are aimed at predictive, preventative, personalized and participatory (P4) medicine. Inclusion of diverse stake holders in this process is mandatory, as is the communication amongst them. This strategy demands creativity and adaptation in current thought processes and modification of traditionally inefficient management of knowledge. Full implementation of this strategy requires marrying basic and clinical research through advanced systems thinking and the employment of high-throughput technologies in genomics, proteomics, nanofluids, single-cell analysis and computation strategies in a highly orchestrated discipline we term translational systems medicine.[12]

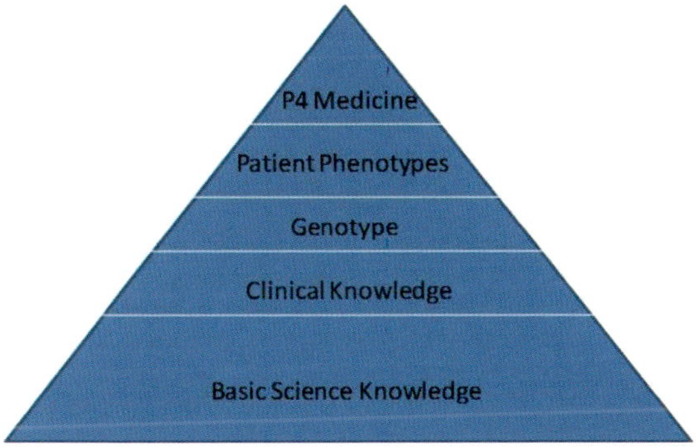

Fig. 4. P4 medicine pyramid: Predictive, Preventative, Personalized and Participatory Medicine.

3.3. TRANSLATIONAL TRIALS

In this era of instant gratification, many therapeutic ideas will prove worthless during the laboratory to clinical translation. The path from a promising discovery to an effective treatment may often consume a decade or more. It is important to point out that translational studies can sometimes be part of later developmental trials, provided that the subjects and the questions are compatible with them. Currently, almost every new therapeutic intervention will depend intrinsically upon a transition from laboratory to clinic. However, despite the tremendous growth of scientific information, only a small portion of therapeutic ideas progresses to developmental clinical trials.[13] Indeed, the interface between laboratory research and clinical development is dependent upon translational clinical trials. Although there is an enormous quantity and quality of basic science and accompanying translational science, knowledge about translational trials and their outcomes and translational medicine is less apparent.

Figure 5 lists several elements that must characterize a translational trial. Based on these assumptions, the same author suggests that the translational trial is:

"*. . . a clinical trial where the primary outcome: (1) is a biological measurement (target) derived from a well established paradigm of disease,*

Important Elements of a Translational Trial
Clinical need generates momentum from promising preclinical undertakings
The modality of treatment remains flexible, adaptive, and open to further investigation
Methodologies are formally and clearly recorded and maintained
The paradigm of disease includes one or more distinct biologic entity for evaluation
Outcomes are confidently and easily measured in a reasonable time period
Large effects upon outcomes are emphasized
The must be an unambiguous definition of the effects of therapy upon the target or a lack thereof
The next stage of experimentation is clearly known in the case of success or failure
Statistical significance is a secondary motive to results which provide sufficient evidence to continue
Studies are undertaken by small groups of investigators with limited access to resources

Fig. 5. Characteristics of translational trials (Based on Ref. 13).

and (2) represents an irrefutable signal regarding the intended therapeutic effect. The design and purposes of the trial are to guide further experiments in the laboratory or clinic, inform treatment modifications, and validate the target, but not necessarily to provide reliable evidence regarding clinical outcomes."

Translational trials have continued experimentation as the primary context. Such trials have the inherent potential to provide evidence or to demonstrate the utility of more than one outcome.

3.4. CLINICAL APPLICATIONS

The objective of this review is to illustrate, with some examples of preclinical and clinical applications, some modern diagnostic and therapeutic approaches integrated into translational research. Certainly, this review cannot be comprehensive and will focus on some very recent advances, addressing mainly molecular biology discoveries helping with diagnosis or treatment of selected known diseases.

Each biological process exhibits a preclinical phase that provides a window for interventions. These interventions may act to prevent overt disease by slowing or halting progression of metabolic dysfunction. Therefore, scientific discoveries might be translated into practical applications to reduce disease risk. A bench-to-bedside approach to translational research requires that basic scientists provide clinical researchers with new tools for use with patients to assess the impact of genetic risk factors. Simultaneously, clinical researchers will make novel observations about the nature and progression of treatments to stimulate basic research.[14]

It cannot be overemphasized that the path from a promising discovery to an effective treatment may often take a decade or more. Below are a few examples of emerging discoveries that have been recently translated into clinical practice.

3.4.1. Oncology

A major report published recently found reductions in cancer incidence and death rates, in part as a result of improvements in prevention and early detection.[15,16] The addition of neoadjuvant therapies has been found to improve outcomes.[17] Translational neoadjuvant therapy studies generally have the following aims: (i) predicting response/resistance to treatment, (ii) identifying response to particular treatments with the intention of employing them adjuvantly, and (iii) prediction of long-term outcome. Adjuvant therapy and long-term outcome are determined by micrometastatic disease, which may have different behavior and response to therapy to the primary tumor as assessed in neoadjuvant protocols.

3.4.2. Translational Genomics (Genome Medicine and Genome Biology)

Just a few years ago, the Human Genome Project sparked optimism that cures for multiple diseases were just around the corner. Access to a steady stream of knowledge was expected to provide data that enabled treatment of different problems. Given rapid technological advances, the potential effect on the lives of patients and the increasing use of genomic information in clinical care have provided bases for several areas of advancement in:

- growing artificial organs, including the heart;
- DNA sequencing for routine checkups;
- promoting the body's self-defense system to fight and counteract cancer;
- harnessing the body's own innate ability to heal and grow;

- matching drugs to tumors;
- personalizing treatment to specific a type and subtype of a cancer, in a specific patient;
- energizing naturally occurring genes (rejigging).

It is critically important to determine how genomic data can best be integrated with clinical practice so as to maximize patient benefit. Translational studies have allowed multiple genetic tests to be developed: identifying breast and ovarian cancers, diagnosing recessive diseases such as cystic fibrosis, determining drug dosages based on individual patient metabolism, and identifying therapeutic options for treating lung and breast tumors, melanoma, and leukemia.

3.4.3. Stem Cell Research and Therapy

Stem cells have transformed from political pawn into valuable tools in clinical practice and regenerative medicine. The utility of these cells has long been known, but social and political sentiments have retarded their experimentation and utilization for the last three decades.[18] Although cell therapy seems to be very promising, its application faces numerous challenges. This includes support for translational research due to the uncompetitive nature of required validation studies in cell therapy that, of necessity, are not hypothesis driven.[19] The ability to harvest stem cells from sources other than fetal tissue has thankfully allowed for better acceptance of this emerging technology. This newfound willingness to explore has promised radical discoveries and has been invigorated from the growing understanding of cell culture and biological mediums. Induced pluripotent stem cells exhibit characteristics and pluripotency similar to embryonic cells, even though they are generated from adult somatic cells.[20] This type of stem cell has been shown to have translational application in the regeneration of vascular tissue grafts. As with any other therapeutic technology, safety is always a concern. However, further translational research is warranted in order to be convinced that the cellular constructs maintain continued function *in vivo* without tumorgenicity or unwanted differentiation. The possibility of generating immune responses to the replaced cells is also a reason to be cautious. With clinical trials of pluripotent stem cell therapy on the horizon, the importance of understanding immunologic barriers and devising safe, effective strategies to bypass them is further underscored. This approach to overcoming immunologic barriers to stem cell therapy can take advantage of the validated knowledge acquired from decades of hematopoietic stem cell transplantation.[21]

3.4.4. Immunosuppression

Transplantation, whether in reference to cells, tissue or organs, has benefitted from frequent and significant advances in immunology. Complex transplants, e.g., hands and fingers, have a significant antigenicity involving the epidermis and other layers of the skin. This requires powerful immunosuppression, including the rapamycin (mTOR) pathway and monoclonal antibodies, or most recently, fusion proteins.[22] Currently, immunologics are costly, prone to serious side effects, and often ineffective. Generation of mixed hematopoietic chimerism by infusing the recipient with donor bone marrow cells has been shown to induce tolerance without chronic immunosuppression. Genetic matching of the donor and the recipient is another option for transplanting composite tissues with only an initial course of immunosuppression. Finally, new immunosuppressive agents with a more targeted action will reduce side effects and may prevent the development of chronic rejection.[23]

3.4.5. Pharmacogenomics

Personalized and individualized care has been established as an important element of future clinical standards. The abundance of phenotypes within the human population is matched with equally diverse genotypic characteristics. These differences not only provide for variation in one's physical appearance but determine the intricate function of the most basic chemical processes in the body. Metabolic, enzymatic and physiologic interactions in the body express a unique ability to achieve homeostasis, a feat that may be managed very differently from one person to another. Also, iatrogenic experience has shown that people do not tolerate given medications in a predictable manner. Adverse reactions can range from therapeutic failure to anaphylaxis to benign medication reactions. Pharmacogenomics has emerged as a field confronting this prevalent variability, down to the level of single-nucleotide polymorphism. Significant efforts to develop pharmacogenomic predictors have been made to guide more effective and safer chemotherapy. As a working example, cytochrome P450 is commonly held as a major player in drug metabolism, metabolism and hormone synthesis. Much is known about the mutational effects of the gene upon enzyme kinetics. The Human Genome Project found 57 genes that code for P450 among 18 subfamilies. These sequences range around 1,500 base pairs in length, representing a significant amount of potential variation in people. Although a considerable amount of data has been generated from numerous experimental and clinical studies, there is a large gap between pharmacogenomic knowledge and clinical application.[24] This discipline is also increasingly moving across the "translational interface" into the clinic and is being incorporated into the drug development process and governmental regulation of that process.[25]

3.4.6. Biomarkers

Basic science has been progressing dramatically since the induction of genetic techniques presented in the central dogma of molecular biology by Crick in 1957. Advances in the Human Genome Project seemingly dominated the literature for a decade in the 1990s.

Biochemistry soon became entwined with molecular protocols that began to describe pathophysiologic processes at the most basic level of understanding, and the advances were rapid. Antibody research has developed into a specialized field that has been able to detect the presence of specific antigens in tissue, serum and organs. These advances provided tools that could easily be applied in the screening, diagnosis and management of acute and chronic disease. The availability of molecular cloning techniques has enabled mass production of these protein based molecules for further use in the industry, with the limits of their introduction curtailed only by government safety regulations and a "cultural separation" between scientific disciplines. Fundamental issues related to tumor heterogeneity, cancer progression, natural history, and biomarker performance have provided challenges to biomarker development. Technical issues in biomarker assay detection limits, specificity, clinical deployment, and regulation have also slowed progress.[26] Additionally, the presence of potential "orphan" drugs, or compounds that may have potential use for off-label indications, has been suppressed by the same mechanism. The field of biomarker research requires extensive interactions between academic researchers and industrial developers, and clinicians are needed to help shape research directions that can be addressed only by a multidisciplinary, multi-institutional approach.[27]

3.4.7. The Breast

Breast cancer remains the most commonly diagnosed cancer for women in the United States. Extensive research has allowed significant progress to be made against the disease. The genomic profile, as opposed to histologic features seen under the microscope, allowed advancements in insights into the molecular pathways critical to the behaviors of specific breast cancers.

Genetic testing performed as part of a comprehensive risk reduction strategy has provided useful support for clinical decision-making in selected patients.[28] Molecular biology is now part of most translational research studies on breast cancer. Evolving new technologies has allowed profiling of tumor molecular characteristics, subsequently enabling biologists to produce more robust classifiers for prognosis. Personalization of treatment tailored to specific characteristics of the tumor allows more successful treatment outcomes.[29] A new genome-driven integrated classification of breast cancer may allow individualization of treatment approaches, bringing us a step closer to the realization of personalized management in breast cancer.[30]

The feasibility of characterizing and propagating human breast cancer "stem/progenitor cells" has been demonstrated. The group of investigators from MD Anderson Cancer Center characterized a number of mechanisms responsible for resistance of these cells.[31] Micro-array technology, specifically microRNAs assays, allows profiling of tumor molecular characteristics, leading to personalization of treatment according to molecular mapping of cancer in specific patients.[32] There is an exciting prospect of microarray-based tests that will allow multiple distinct predictions, including prognosis, ER and HER2 status, as well as sensitivity to various treatment approaches.[33,34]

In breast cancer, tumor biological markers are gaining impact and have become equal to traditional markers of pathology. Molecular expression profiling has led to new treatment modalities which have resulted from the incorporation of translational knowledge into immunochemical strategies used in routine pathology.[35] Although not always possible, biologists are close to constructing a gene expression profile predictive for local-regional failure after breast conservative treatment, which is characterized by genes involved in cell proliferation, but not a surrogate for high histologic grade.[36] The mechanisms underlying cancer cell growth and response of normal and malignant cells to radiation are being elucidated. New strategies aimed at enhancing the radio-sensitivity level of breast cancer cells are being developed. This research will undoubtedly pave the way for novel approaches directed at improving breast cancer therapy.[37]

There are ongoing trials of different medications to improve treatment outcomes for breast cancer. The term *SERMs* has been coined for selective estrogen receptor modulators. These are structurally different compounds that interact with intracellular estrogen receptors in target organs as estrogen receptor agonists or antagonists. The search for the "ideal" SERM is currently under way. As such, it would have the expected estrogenic effects on bone and serum lipids, neutral effects on the uterus, and antiestrogenic effects on breast tissue — but with none of the known adverse effects.[38]

3.4.8. Gastrointestinal/Colon Cancer

Translational research is critically needed to identify and evaluate potential treatment for different diseases at the bench before applying them at the bedside. Recently, preclinical evidence was presented regarding the efficacy of multiple molecules as potent radiosensitizers.[39] ATP citrate lyase (ACL or ACLY) is an extramitochondrial enzyme that is aberrantly expressed in many immortalized cells and tumors, such as breast, liver, colon, lung and prostate cancers. It is correlated inversely with tumor stage and differentiation, serving as a negative prognostic marker. ACL is a key enzyme of cellular lipogenesis and a potent target for cancer therapy. As a hypolipidemic strategy for metabolic syndrome and cancer treatment, many small chemicals targeting ACL have been designed and developed. They have proved promising as potential anticancer or cancer treatment modulating agents.[40]

Personalization of treatment has also impacted the field of colon cancer. Attempts have been made to reduce adverse events caused by chemotherapy, without interfering negatively with anticancer efficacy.[41] There is evidence from colon carcinoma cell culture studies that COX-2 activity may play an important role in regulating angiogenesis and apoptosis. Treatment of COX-2 expressing tumor cells with selective COX-2 inhibitors appears to reset the balance between cell proliferation and cell death such that there is no increase in tumor growth.[42] Mutations within the *KRAS* proto-oncogene have predictive value but are of uncertain prognostic value in the treatment of advanced colorectal cancer. In stage II–III colon cancer, the *KRAS* mutation status does not have major predictive value. *BRAF* is prognostic in older females with right-sided colon tumors characterized by high-grade features and microsatellite instability.[43]

3.4.9. The Heart

Pathophysiology of multiple diseases is very complex and is driven by multiple biologic processes, including inflammation, oxidative stress, neurohormonal activation, vascular remodeling, and myocyte injury.[44] The dramatic reduction in DNA sequencing costs allows us to delve deeper into the genomic alterations that increase susceptibility to many polygenic cardiovascular diseases. Marfan syndrome is an example of disease in which an *FBN1* mutation confers additional risk for many of the cardiovascular complications classically associated with the disease. Knowledge of an *FBN1* gene mutation may allow actionable interventions with an angiotensin receptor blocker earlier in the natural history of the condition.[45]

Multiple biomarkers integrating diverse biological pathways substantially improved prediction of adverse events in patients with chronic heart failure when compared to current metrics.[46] Addition of the multimarker score improved classification of patients into more appropriate, higher risk categories supporting the concept of a multimarker tool for prognosis in chronic human heart failure.

3.4.10. Critical Care

The practice of critical care has benefitted from the emergence of biomarkers from the laborious investigation of biochemistry, immunology and proteomics. The speculation of the past has been replaced with evidence-based truth that follows from specific, consistent quantification of biological molecules in the blood. Good examples of this would be cardiac troponins, which began very non-specifically with CPK and evolved into more specific targets such as troponin I and its isoforms. These compounds have enabled more timely and effective diagnosis of myocardial infarctions, cardiomyopathy and congestive heart failure.[47] Serum procalcitonin has also been demonstrated as a novel biomarker that can be a reliable predictor in the ICU. Using this sensitive modality, the likelihood of sepsis and subsequent mortality can be gaged preemptively in the critical care setting.[48]

3.4.11. Alzheimer's Research and Therapy

Demand for basic science knowledge often originates from common diseases. Alzheimer's dementia is a good example of a common affliction that touches innumerable families and care givers without warning. After decades of struggling with the difficult biology of Alzheimer disease, there has been a recent influx of information describing the nature and course of the cerebral atrophy. Therapeutics are presently aimed at balancing levels of neurotransmitters to maintain a higher standard of mental functioning, but little progress has been made in preventing, screening and eradicating the disability. Working backwards, investigators have made progress in their ability to diagnose the malady at an earlier stage using blood soluble proteins.[49] In the process of confronting this particular disease, timely diagnosis may prevent the onset of this rapidly progressing and prevalent condition by opening a wider window for therapeutic intervention.

3.4.12. Multiple Sclerosis

Much akin to Alzheimer disease is multiple sclerosis. Although two completely distinct entities affecting different parts of the nervous system, they are exquisitely debilitating and often strike younger patients in otherwise excellent states of health. Early detection of multiple sclerosis has become a focus due to the possibility of providing medical interventions to these patients. The course of multiple sclerosis is marked by rapid degeneration of oligodendrocytes and their protective myelin, and current therapies are targeted at modulating the immune response, or protection with monoclonal antibodies.[50] It is currently believed that an autoimmune dysfunction is the culprit in this degeneration. It cannot be stressed enough that the early detection of this pathology can potentiate greater longevity and less morbidity in the given patient population. Efforts are currently underway in this pursuit, investigating plausible biomarkers floating around in the bloodstream and cerebral spinal fluid.[51,52] Geneticists have also been busy confronting increasing public demand for new technology to combat neurodegenerative ailments. It is hoped that previous work concerning interferon and the positive outcomes for multiple sclerosis will enable reverse engineering of compounds capable of effecting proper gene expression of interferon-related cells and systems *in vivo*.[53]

3.4.13. Arthritis Research and Therapy

Rheumatoid arthritis management can be complicated and multifactorial. State-of-the-art computer modeling has enabled the advancement of many theoretical and practical medical investigations. Computational networks have enabled tissue-specific analysis of the therapeutics and their related molecules.Topological associations between the therapeutics, tissue composition, and outcomes has allowed for inadvertent data collection to participate in real-time analysis. Using these motifs, investigators have been able to predict mechanisms and postulate supplementary or unique solutions to treating rheumatoid arthritis. The current focus has been placed upon AKT2, IL6, MAPK1 and TP53 pathways.[54] Before the availability of disease-modifying antirheumatic drugs (DMARDS), cortisone, a "broad-spectrum" immunologic modifier, was the only effective treatment option. This clinical knowledge was an essential step in the translation of rheumatoid arthritis, initiating immunology as a practical discipline.[55] As an isolated event, discovery (1946), mass production, and implementation provided for utilization by rheumatologists and fuelled progress in the immunological realm that has not faltered with time. This reverse translation exemplifies the future of translational medicine — using the available evidence to stimulate further investigation. Returning to the bench with this knowledge spawned methotrexate and the use of monoclonal antibodies in the maintenance of individuals with rheumatoid arthritis.[56]

3.4.14. Cystic Fibrosis

Although cystic fibrosis was described many years ago, the understanding of this very common genetic condition gained much momentum with advances in genomic testing. Attempts have been made to initiate gene therapy through aerosol inhalation, using the cystic fibrosis transmembrane conductance regulator (CFTR). Knowing the specific target for the syndrome has potentiated much activity in this research.[57,58] The cystic fibrosis gene codes for a cAMP/PKA-dependent, ATP-requiring, membrane chloride ion channel, generally found in the apical membranes of many secreting epithelia and known as CFTR. There are currently over 1,700 known mutations affecting CFTR, many of which give rise to a disease phenotype. Around 75 percent of CF alleles contain the DeltaF508 mutation. Ongoing clinical trials where the mutant CFTR gene is spliced in the place of the wild type CFTR functional frame have produced fascinating results in which clinical benefit appears to have been achieved. Translational research feeding from this is now yielding compounds that provide tangible prospects for a pharmacotherapy for this disease.[59] Approximately 4 to 5 percent of cystic fibrosis patients have the G441D-CFTR mutation that is a target of recently approved "orphan drug," ivacaflor. Recent clinical studies showed that such genomically guided therapies herald a new era in the management of cystic fibrosis.[60–62]

3.5. THE FUTURE

Integrated knowledge translation is a different way of doing research. It meaningfully engages knowledge-users in the research process, from determining the research question, deciding on the methodology, being involved in data collection or tools development, interpreting the findings, and helping disseminate the research results.[63] This approach, also known by such terms as "mode 2" knowledge production, collaborative research, action-oriented research, and co-production of knowledge, is intended to produce research findings that are more likely to be relevant to and used by the end-users.[64]

Translational medicine is not limited to wet-lab science. Advances in computational biology and molecular modeling have enabled the establishment of dry-labs that are not subject to the strict regulations involved with handling tissues and biological specimens. There has also been a deluge of information involving discharge records, electronic health records, and adverse event reporting, all of which facilitate epidemiological research. Utilization of observational data has also enabled the establishment of phenotypic data sources that, when integrated properly, have the potential to facilitate cross-institutional and cross-population studies. Using genetic data in combination with electronic health records and expanding the continuity of care records have enabled a repository for this wealth of information. Technology of this kind will serve to streamline access and utilization of patient-specific phenotypes and treatment strategies. Not only does this organize information for the clinical care team, it makes available a raft of factors that may exhibit significance when combined with greater numbers of subjects. Social media and self reporting can also be utilized to reach the multitudes in a manner not previously possible with traditional surveys, thus enhancing the power of cohort and prospective studies. These methods have been validated in health-surveillance projects that have shown proof of concept.[65] Integration of population data and genomic data may soon facilitate screening of patients for clinical trials, which may benefit their specific conditions and help to identify drug safety signals. It is expected that large-scale genomic information will soon be integrated more fully into clinical practice. This also means that issues related to implementing the change need to be addressed. Large observational databases are a rich resource in support of translational research. From these observations, key clinically relevant issues can be identified and form the basis for further clinical studies. The ability to identify patterns of behavior and gaps in available data translates into new experiments but also impacts development of public policy and reveals patterns of clinical reality.[66]

The convergence of the aforementioned data sources has been a challenge both financially and logistically. In the US, electronic medical records will be required for all Medicare providers beginning from 2014. This infrastructure will expedite the process of reporting, organizing and centralizing data. In tandem with this, several organizations have established their own warehouses for clinically relevant information. These may include pharmacogenomics, proteomics and genomic information. When integrated, these disciplines will help to create a more uniform and cohesive framework for knowledge and its specifically tailored clinical significance.

Biobanks may include data resources from diverse forms of research. Pharmacogenomics research is translational in nature and ranges from discovery of genotype–phenotype relationships to clinical trials that can provide proof of clinical impact. Advances in pharmacogenomics offer significant potential for subsequent clinical application in individual patients; however, the translation of pharmacogenomics research findings into clinical practice has been slow.[67] It is presumed that these barriers to translation can be rectified by promoting regular and uniform reporting schemes, increasing widespread availability of data, and providing knowledge based support systems that offer clinical guides to therapy based upon these test results.

Different approaches are being developed to address future translational research. The Vanderbilt Institute for Clinical and Translational Research implemented the "Studio Program" in 2007 to bring together experts to provide free, structured, project-specific feedback for medical researchers. "Studios" are a series of integrated, dynamic and interactive roundtable discussions that bring together relevant research experts from diverse academic disciplines to focus on a specific research project at a specific stage.[67] It is programs such as this that will potentiate and organize the knowledge base, an essential requirement for the success of translational science and medicine.

Another concept includes an integrated informative technology infrastructure framework based on the single source concept, where data from electronic medical records are reused for clinical and translational research projects.[68] It might be expected that regulatory institutions will partner with academia and potentially industry to conduct meaningful clinical research. Translational projects have been developed between FDA and Duke University for the Clinical Trials Transformation Initiative, which will conduct research projects on design principles, data quality and quantity, including monitoring, study start-up, and adverse event reporting.[69] There is also growing evidence that collaborative research partnerships between academic centers and community-based practitioners can promote innovations in high quality and efficacious patient care.[70]

The evolution of evidence-based medicine and communication modalities has provided hope that the future will be successful in streamlining development of new clinical protocols based on laboratory experimentation, modeling, and accrued observational data. Within this framework, the safety of the study participants and potential treatment-associated risks must be delicately balanced. Clinical research is not without danger, and the overemphasis of new advances in knowledge has the potential to overshadow possible negative outcomes. These imminent confrontations will include basic scientists, clinicians, and bioethicists, who will together share the responsibility of formulating guidelines for the safest utilization of these technologies and their application on the individual level. It is expected that advances in treatment options will be provided through comparative effectiveness research, clinical trials, evidenced-based medicine, and basic biomedical investigations.[71]

Translational research of the future will undoubtedly rely upon the expansion of innovative electronic and computer-based technologies at every phase of the research process (Fig. 6).

These ideas may be better represented with an excerpt from one of Dr. Hood's editorials:

> "*We predict that this transition will occur through seamless exploitation, integration and modeling of a wealth of data collected regularly on each individual across all levels of biological organization in relation to environmental changes, using non-invasive measurements and advanced information and communication technologies. We expect that this will reverse the non-sustainable trend in escalating costs in diagnostics, drug development and healthcare. We are thus in the middle of a revolution (not simply an incremental evolution) in medical practice,*

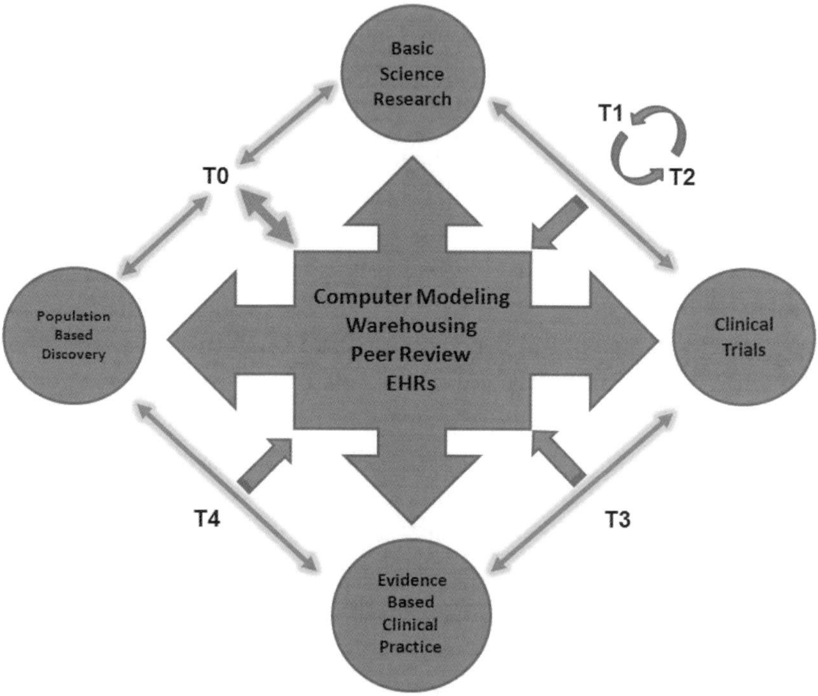

Fig. 6. Translational research algorithm (Adapted from Ref. 7).

acting as a community to catalyze a profound change with systems biology approaches."[72]

3.6. CONCLUSIONS

There is a growing emphasis on moving basic biomedical research laboratory findings into clinical patient-related applications to realize health benefits derived from such research findings. Ultimately, new approaches to diagnose, treat and prevent disease will be available and represent the translation of the valuable scientific evidence into clinical applications.

There is much concern that outsourcing of clinical trials and scientific research may compromise the inherent quality of results. In recent years, the global pharmaceutical industry has been facing challenges of increasing costs and delays in drug development. These substantial challenges — the saving of cost and time — has resulted in the globalization of clinical trials, with developing countries showing a rise in registered clinical trials. However, the differences between developed and developing countries in terms of regulatory processes, ethical issues, medical expertise, clinical practice, and health infrastructure has made the third objective — compliance with global quality — difficult and demanding.

It has become an intrinsic fact that the capacities to automate, organize and model human disease and conditions can be facilitated by modern information systems. Once known as computers, these machines are capable of integrating distant arms of the translational process. Not only do they simplify the flow of information, but they provide substantial transparency that can be utilized on a global scale. Centralization of data stores and integration of electronic medical records into a network provides this infrastructure, albeit complicated by politics and policy concerning patient rights and privacy issues. Other stakeholders may impose barriers that interrupt the flow and translation of knowledge. Although there is a consensus among scientists and clinicians that translational research will serve to advance medical knowledge, there are many obstacles that can disrupt the pathway to better medicine. Nothing is perfect.

REFERENCES

1. Sussman S. (2006) The transdisciplinary-translation revolution: Final thoughts. *Eval Health Prof* **29**: 348–352.
2. Sussman S, Valente TW, Rohrbach LA, *et al.* (2006) Translation in the health professions: Converting science into action. *Eval Health Prof* **29**: 7–32.
3. Glasgow RE, Lichtenstein E, Marcus AC. (2003) Why don't we see more translation of health promotion research to practice? Rethinking the efficacy-to-effectiveness transition. *Am J Public Health* **93**: 1261–1267.
4. Glasgow RE, Chambers D. (2012) Developing robust, sustainable, implementation systems using rigorous, rapid and relevant science. *Clin Transl Sci* **5**: 48–55.
5. Kerner JF. (2006) Knowledge translation versus knowledge integration: A "funder's" perspective. *J Contin Educ Health Prof* **26**: 72–80.

6. Glasgow RE, Klesges LM, Dzewaltowski DA, *et al.* (2004) The future of health behavior change research: What is needed to improve translation of research into health promotion practice? *Ann Behav Med* **27**: 3–12.
7. Glasgow RE, Vinson C, Chambers D, *et al.* (2012). National Institutes of Health approaches to dissemination and implementation science: Current and future directions. *Am J Public Health* **102**: 1274–1281.
8. NIH PHS Grants. (2012) US Department of Health and Human Services, Public Health Service, Grant Application (PHS 398).
9. Rubio DM, Schoenbaum EE, Lee LS, *et al.* (2010). Defining translational research: Implications for training. *Acad Med* **85**: 470–475.
10. Minna JD, Gazdar AF. (1996) Translational research comes of age. *Nat Med* **2**: 974–975.
11. Trochim W, Kane C, Graham MJ, Pincus HA. (2011) Evaluating translational research: A process marker model. *Clin Transl Sci* **4**: 153–162.
12. Hood L, Tian Q. (2012) Systems approaches to biology and disease enable translational systems medicine. *Genom Proteom Bioinform* **10**: 181–185.
13. Piantadosi S. (2005) Translational clinical trials: An entropy-based approach to sample size. *Clin Trials* **2**: 182–192.
14. Taal MW, Chertow GM, Marsden PA, *et al.*, eds. (2011) Brenner and Rector's The Kidney. E-book.
15. Kris MG, Benowitz SI, Adams S, *et al.* (2010) Clinical cancer advances 2010: Annual report on progress against cancer from the American Society of Clinical Oncology. *J Clin Oncol* **28**: 5327–5347.
16. Vogelzang NJ, Benowitz SI, Adams S, *et al.* (2012) Clinical cancer advances 2011: Annual report on progress against cancer from the American Society of Clinical Oncology. *J Clin Oncol* **30**: 88–109.
17. Dent S, Oyan B, Honig A, *et al.* (2013) HER2-targeted therapy in breast cancer: A systematic review of neoadjuvant trials. *Cancer Treat Rev* **39**: 622–631.
18. McAllister TN, Audley D, L'Heureux N. (2012) Autologous cell therapies: Challenges in U.S. FDA regulation. *Regen Med* **7**: 94–97.
19. Viswanathan S, Keating A. (2011) Overcoming the challenges of conducting translational research in cell therapy. *Front Med* **5**: 333–335.
20. Sone M, Nakao K. (2013) Vascular research using human pluripotent stem cells and humoral factors (Review). *Endocr J* **60**: 397–402.
21. de Almeida PE, Ransohoff JD, Nahid A, Wu JC. (2013) Immunogenicity of pluripotent stem cells and their derivatives. *Circ Res* **112**: 549–561.
22. Grinyo JM, Cruzado JM, Bestard O, *et al.* (2012) Immunosuppression in the era of biological agents. *Adv Exp Med Biol* **741**: 60–72.

23. Petit F, Lantieri L, Randolph MA, Lee WP. (2006) Future research in immunology for composite tissue allotransplantation. *Ann Chir Plast Esthet* **51**: 11–17.
24. Lee SY, McLeod HL. (2011) Pharmacogenetic tests in cancer chemotherapy: What physicians should know for clinical application. *J Pathol* **223**: 15–27.
25. Wang L. (2010) Pharmacogenomics: A systems approach. *Wiley Interdiscip RevSystBiol Med* **2**: 3–22.
26. Brooks JD. (2012) Translational genomics: The challenge of developing cancer biomarkers. *Genome Res* **22**: 183–187.
27. Wagner PD, Srivastava S. (2012) New paradigms in translational science research in cancer biomarkers. *Transl Res* **159**: 343–353.
28. van der Merwe N, Bouwens CS, Pienaar R, *et al.* (2012) CYP2D6 genotyping and use of antidepressants in breast cancer patients: Test development for clinical application. *Metab Brain Dis* **27**: 319–326.
29. Benowitz S. (2012) Personalized-medicine trials on the rise. *J Natl Cancer Inst* **104**: 1425–1426.
30. Dawson SJ, Rueda OM, Aparicio S, Caldas C. (2013) A new genome-driven integrated classification of breast cancer and its implications. *EMBO J* **32**: 617–628.
31. Woodward WA. (2011) Breast cancer stem cell targets. *Oncology (Williston Park)* **25**: 34, 36.
32. Liu H. (2012) MicroRNAs in breast cancer initiation and progression. *Cell Mol Life Sci* **69**: 3587–3599.
33. Sotiriou C, Pusztai L. (2009) Gene-expression signatures in breast cancer. *N Engl J Med* **360**: 790–800.
34. Sotiriou C, Wirapati P, Loi S, *et al.* (2006). Gene expression profiling in breast cancer: Understanding the molecular basis of histologic grade to improve prognosis. *J Natl Cancer Inst* **98**: 262–272.
35. Kreipe HH. (2012) Translational research and diagnostics for breast cancer. *Pathologe* **33**(Suppl 2): 282–290.
36. Kreike B, Halfwerk H, Armstrong N, *et al.* (2009). Local recurrence after breast-conserving therapy in relation to gene expression patterns in a large series of patients. *Clin Cancer Res* **15**: 4181–4190.
37. Bernier J. (2010) Translational breast cancer research: Recent advances through the lens of experimental radiotherapy. *Breast* **19**. 23–27.
38. Maximov PY, Lee TM, Jordan VC. (2012) The discovery and development of selective estrogen receptor modulators (SERMs) for clinical practice. *Curr Clin Pharmacol* **8**: 135–155.
39. Strimpakos AS, Syrigos KN, Saif MW. (2011) Translational research in pancreatic cancer. Highlights from the "2011 ASCO Gastrointestinal Cancers

Symposium". San Francisco, CA, USA. January 20–22, 2011. *J Oncol Prac* **12**: 120–122.
40. Zu XY, Zhang QH, Liu JH, *et al.* (2012). ATP citrate lyase inhibitors as novel cancer therapeutic agents. *Recent Pat Anticancer Drug Discov* **7**: 154–167.
41. Karlsson JO, Adolfsson K, Thelin B, *et al.* (2012). First clinical experience with the magnetic resonance imaging contrast agent and superoxide dismutase mimetic mangafodipir as an adjunct in cancer chemotherapy — A translational study. *Transl Oncol* **5**: 32–38.
42. Iimuro S, Shindo T, Moriyama N, *et al.* (2004). Angiogenic effects of adrenomedullin in ischemia and tumor growth. *Circ Res* **95**: 415–423.
43. Roth AD, Tejpar S, Delorenzi M, *et al.* (2010). Prognostic role of KRAS and BRAF in stage II and III resected colon cancer: Results of the translational study on the PETACC-3, EORTC 40993, SAKK 60-00 trial. *J Clin Oncol* **28**: 466–474.
44. Braunwald E. (2008) Biomarkers in heart failure. *N Engl J Med* **358**: 2148–2159.
45. Barrett PM, Topol EJ. (2013) The fibrillin-1 gene: Unlocking new therapeutic pathways in cardiovascular disease. *Heart* **99**: 83–90.
46. Ky B, French B, Levy WC, *et al.* (2012) Multiple biomarkers for risk prediction in chronic heart failure. *Circ Heart Fail* **5**: 183–190.
47. de Tombe PP, Solaro RJ. (2000) Integration of cardiac myofilament activity and regulation with pathways signaling hypertrophy and failure. *Ann Biomed Eng* **28**: 991–1001.
48. Russwurm S, Wiederhold M, Oberhoffer M, *et al.* (1999) Molecular aspects and natural source of procalcitonin. *Clin Chem Lab Med* **37**: 789–797.
49. Guo LH, Alexopoulos P, Wagenpfeil S, *et al.* (2013) Plasma proteomics for the identification of Alzheimer disease. *Alzheimer Dis Assoc Disord.* Epub ahead of print.
50. Fontoura P. (2010) Monoclonal antibody therapy in multiple sclerosis: Paradigm shifts and emerging challenges. *MAbs* **2**: 670–681.
51. Flood DG, Marek GJ, Williams M. (2011) Developing predictive CSF biomarkers — A challenge critical to success in Alzheimer's disease and neuropsychiatric translational medicine. *Biochem Pharmacol* **81**: 1422–1434.
52. Borovecki F, Habek M. (2010) Development of novel genomic blood biomarkers for neurodegenerative diseases. *CNS Neurol Disord Drug Targets* **9**: 669–678.
53. Croze E. (2010) Differential gene expression and translational approaches to identify biomarkers of interferon beta activity in multiple sclerosis. *J Interferon Cytokine Res* **30**: 743–749.

54. Wu G, Zhu L, Dent JE, Nardini C. (2010) A comprehensive molecular interaction map for rheumatoid arthritis. *PLoS One* **5**: e10137.
55. Hillier SG. (2007) Diamonds are forever: The cortisone legacy. *J Endocrinol* **195**: 1–6.
56. Chu CR, Beynnon BD, Buckwalter JA, *et al.* (2011) Closing the gap between bench and bedside research for early arthritis therapies (EARTH): Report from the AOSSM/NIH U-13 Post-Joint Injury Osteoarthritis Conference II. *Am J Sports Med* **39**: 1569–1578.
57. Sloane PA, Rowe SM. (2010) Cystic fibrosis transmembrane conductance regulator protein repair as a therapeutic strategy in cystic fibrosis. *Curr Opin Pulm Med* **16**: 591–597.
58. Castaldo G, Lembo F, Tomaiuolo R. (2010) Molecular diagnostics: Between chips and customized medicine. *Clin Chem Lab Med* **48**: 973–982.
59. Cuthbert AW. (2011) New horizons in the treatment of cystic fibrosis. *Br J Pharmacol* **163**: 173–183.
60. Ramsey BW, Davies J, McElvaney NG, *et al.* (2011) A CFTR potentiator in patients with cystic fibrosis and the G551D mutation. *N Engl J Med* **365**: 1663–1672.
61. Barrett PM, Alagely A, Topol EJ. (2012) Cystic fibrosis in an era of genomically guided therapy. *Hum Mol Genet* **21**: R66–R71.
62. Jing X, Kay S, Marley T, *et al.* (2012) Incorporating personalized gene sequence variants, molecular genetics knowledge, and health knowledge into an EHR prototype based on the Continuity of Care Record standard. *J Biomed Inform* **45**: 82–92.
63. Sargeant J, Hurley KF, Duffy J, *et al.* (2008) Lost in translation or just lost? *Ann Emerg Med* **52**: 575–576.
64. Graham ID, Tetroe J, Gagnon M. (2009) Lost in translation: Just lost or beginning to find our way? *Ann Emerg Med* **54**: 313–314.
65. Yip YL. (2012) Unlocking the potential of electronic health records for translational research. Findings from the section on bioinformatics and translational informatics. *Yearb Med Inform* **7**: 135–138.
66. Siciliano V, Pitino A, Gori M, *et al.* (2012) The application of observational data in translational medicine: Analyzing tobacco-use behaviors of adolescents. *J Transl Med* **10**: 89.
67. Byrne DW, Biaggioni I, Bernard GR, *et al.* (2012). Clinical and translational research studios: A multidisciplinary internal support program. *Acad Med* **87**: 1052–1059.
68. Prokosch HU, Ries M, Beyer A, *et al.* (2011). IT infrastructure components to support clinical care and translational research projects in a comprehensive cancer center. *Stud Health Technol Inform* **169**: 892–896.

69. Bhatt A. (2011) Quality of clinical trials: A moving target. *Perspect Clin Res* **2**: 124–128.
70. Carpenter WR, Meyer AM, Wu Y, *et al.* (2012) Translating research into practice: The role of provider-based research networks in the diffusion of an evidence-based colon cancer treatment innovation. *Med Care* **50**: 737–748.
71. Petrini C. (2011) From bench to bedside and to health policies: Ethics in translational research. *Clin Ter* **162**: 51–59.
72. Auffray C, Hood L. (2012) Editorial: Systems biology and personalized medicine — The future is now. *Biotechnol J* **7**: 938–939.

CHAPTER 4

Clinical Implications of miRNAs in Human Diseases

*Narinder K. Sharma**, *Sharmila Shankar*†,‡
*and Rakesh K. Srivastava**,§

4.1. INTRODUCTION

MicroRNAs (miRNAs) are a recently discovered class of non-coding RNAs that function as regulators of gene expression.[1,2] Many miRNAs are conserved in distant species, indicating their evolutionary selection and importance as modulators of biological pathways. miRNAs may regulate a particular gene, gene networks or pathways to control biological functions. In animals, miRNAs bind to partially complementary binding sites usually localized in the 3′ untranslated regions (3′-UTRs)of mRNAs and repress their expression. Repression is achieved by interfering at the translation level and causing degradation of the target, which involves deadenylation and decapping of the mRNAs.[3] miRNAs play regulatory roles in many cellular processes, such as differentiation, proliferation and apoptosis.

*Department of Pharmacology, Toxicology and Therapeutics, and Medicine, The University of Kansas Medical Center, Kansas City, Kansas, USA

†Department of Pathology and Laboratory Medicine, The University of Kansas Medical Center, 3901 Rainbow Boulevard, Kansas City, Kansas, USA

‡Corresponding author: Sharmila Shankar, Department of Pathology and Laboratory Medicine, The University of Kansas Medical Center, 3901 Rainbow Boulevard, Kansas City, KS, 66160, USA; E-mail: *sshankar@kumc.edu*

§Corresponding author: Rakesh K. Srivastava, Department of Pharmacology, Toxicology and Therapeutics, and Medicine, The University of Kansas Medical Center, 3901 Rainbow Boulevard, Kansas City, KS, 66160, USA; E-mail: *rsrivastava@kumc.edu*

Furthermore, they are key regulators in many diseases, including neurological disorders, heart disease, kidney disease and cancer.[4,5] The frequent irregular expression of miRNAs in various human diseases has led to their branding as preferred drug targets. In particular, in cancer, certain miRNAs meet the criteria for becoming ideal therapeutic targets by functioning as authentic oncogenes or tumor suppressors.[6,7]

Endogenous miRNA comprises a 15–22 nucleotide long single-stranded RNA that enters the multiprotein complex in the cytoplasm called RNA-induced silencing complex (RISC) to pair with mRNAs having complementary sequences and subsequently repress gene expression. In animals, miRNAs bind to complementary sites of mRNA typically localized in their 3′ untranslated regions. A particular miRNA can control multiple genes by imperfect base-pairing between miRNAs and mRNAs, though only certain given sets of mRNA are regulated.[1] The first miRNA assigned was *lin-4*, which mediated regulation of gene expression in the *Caenorhabditis elegans* heterochronic gene *lin-14*.[8] Thereafter, RNA interference (RNAi) gained immense interest as a post-transcriptional gene regulatory mechanism. There are two main types of short RNA molecule, small interfering RNA (siRNA) and miRNA, which have been identified as post-transcriptional regulators of gene expression. siRNAs are 21–23-nucleotide fully base-paired duplexes that interact with messenger RNAs (mRNAs) and trigger sequence specific degradation of the target via the activity of the Argonaute 2 protein, a part of the complex of proteins designated as RISC. miRNAs are 21–24-nucleotide duplexes with the Argonaute 2 and RISC usually incompletely based-paired and form partial duplexes within the 3′-UTR of targeted transcripts via an association with RISC.[2]

Although the biological functions of miRNAs are not completely understood, increasing evidence implies that the miRNA pathway is a new mechanism of gene regulation in both normal and diseased conditions. Therefore, investigation of miRNA in various diseases can yield new tools for gene functional study and drug development.

4.2. BIOGENESIS OF miRNA

The biogenesis of miRNAs involves a series of post-transcriptional steps (Fig. 1). Their maturation pathway, similar to protein-coding genes, is

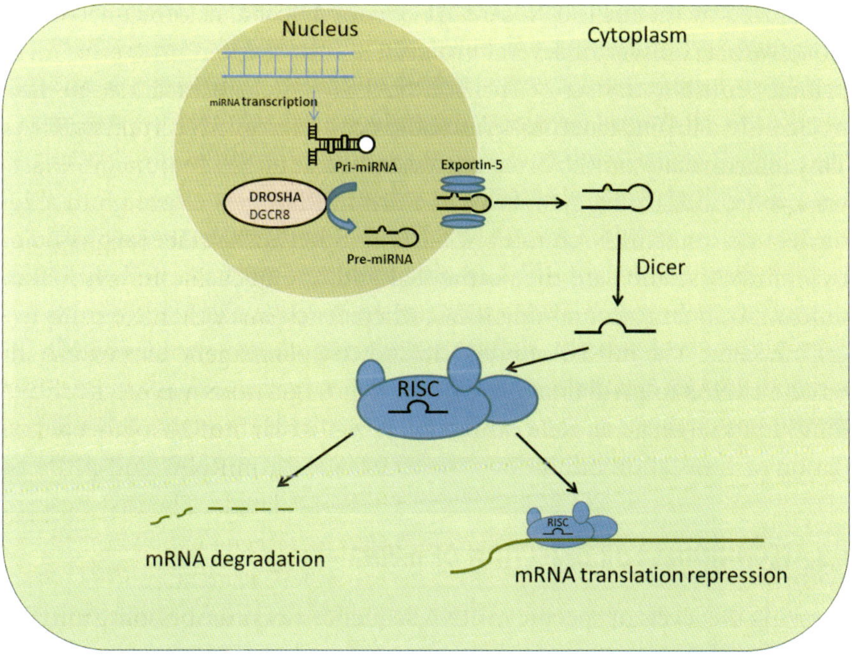

Fig. 1. The miRNA biogenesis pathway and mechanism of miRNA mediated gene repression: Primary miRNAs (pri-miRNA) are transcribed from DNA sequences by RNA polymerase II. In the nucleus, the pri-miRNA is excised by the microprocessor complex (Drosha/DGCR8), which generates the precursor miRNA (pre-miRNA). After export into the cytoplasm, the pre-miRNA is cleaved by a ribonuclease Dicer to produce RNA duplex. A single strand is incorporated into miRNA-induced silencing complex (RISC). Thereafter, the mature miRNA strand induces mRNA degradation and/or translational repression, causing inhibition of protein synthesis.

initiated at transcription (mostly by RNA polymerase II). The location of miRNA in the genome can be intergenic or intragenic. Intergenic miRNA is usually expressed with other miRNAs in clusters,[9] while intragenic miRNA, i.e., within the protein-coding gene (mostly in the introns), is often expressed from the same coding strand as for mRNA expression. miRNAs transcription by RNA polymerase II generates a primary miRNA (pri-miRNA) transcript that consists of a hairpin structure with a stem and loop. Pri miRNAs undergo post-transcriptional modifications with capping at the 5′ terminal, splicing, and polyadenylation at the 3′-end. These Pri-mRNA often produce more than one miRNA.[10] The pri-miRNA is recognized by the nuclear RNAse-III enzyme Drosha, its cofactor DGCR8 along with a complex of several proteins, known as Microprocessor.[11] The primary miRNA transcript (pri-miRNA) is processed into a ~60–100-nucleotide hairpin structure termed the precursor-miRNA (pre-miRNA). This intermediate miRNA is exported from the nucleus to the cytoplasm via Exportin-5. In the cytoplasm, the pre-miRNA gets cleaved into a 22-nucleotide-long miRNA duplex by Dicer, another RNAse III enzyme.[11] The two miRNA strands are then separated and one of the strands is loaded onto an Argonaute-containing RISC, where it acts as a guide to repress target messages. The miRNA guides RISC to complementary sites within the target mRNAs to mediate repression of that target message. After miRNA binds to its target gene, gene expression is regulated through mRNA degradation or translation inhibition.

4.3. TECHNIQUES FOR DETECTION OF miRNA

Assaying the levels of specific miRNA sequences was cumbersome initially. Northern blot analyses provided information about the various forms of miRNA, but the method was considered to have an insufficient throughput. With increasing numbers of miRNA characterized in various databases, microarray technology has been used for simultaneous screening of thousands of miRNAs in one RNA sample.[12,13] In solid-phase microarrays, oligonucleotides bound to sequences complementary to the target miRNA are used to detect cDNA in a sample. The cDNA is produced via reverse transcription reaction from an RNA sample using labeled primers. Once loaded onto a chip, the labeled cDNA samples containing complementary DNA hybridize with the probes. After subsequent steps to wash away any unhybridized DNA, the fluorescence intensity is measured. Alongside microarrays, which is a solid-phase method, there are also some solution-phase methods being developed for the detection of miRNA. Another commonly used method for the detection of miRNA in the biomedical field is reverse transcriptase polymerase chain reaction (RT-PCR), which can detect miRNA in real time. In RT-PCR, the miRNA is first modified with a polyadenylated tail. Thereafter, primer is added, which anneals to the miRNA target and forms cDNA via reverse transcription. Forward and reverse primers are added to the reaction once the cDNA is synthesized;

these primers anneal to the cDNA and produce multiple copies of the cDNA. Different approaches can be used for real-time monitoring of PCR amplification. For example, a fluorescent intercalator such as SYBR Green can be used. It is also possible to use a dual-labeled probe, with a fluorophore and quencher. The probe is cleaved by polymerase, which results in separation of the fluorophore from the quencher, thereby increasing the fluorescence. In both methods, RT-PCR can be used to quantitatively detect small amounts of miRNA.[12] Multiplex PCR can be performed if pooled samples from a homogeneous patient population are available, followed by analyses of individual samples. Conventional RT-PCR and microfluidic RT-PCR platforms both have better limits of detection and dynamic ranges than gene expression microarrays but cannot compete with the ability of these assays to analyze thousands of targets.

In some cases, results on miRNA profiles from samples vary despite analyses having been done under similar conditions. Many factors may be responsible for these differences, including gender, race, age, etc. In addition, lifestyle factors such as nutrition, alcohol or narcotic consumption, disorders such as obesity, or sampling differences could also contribute to the ambiguity in the results. Moreover, different methods are used for miRNA isolation. Other parameters such as epigenetic factors, copy number variations, and polymorphisms in the regulatory elements of genes that encode miRNAs could also be considered.[14]

4.4. ASSOCIATION OF miRNA WITH DISEASES

Although hundreds of miRNAs have been identified in humans, very few specific targets have been experimentally validated. A single miRNA can potentially target various mRNAs through complete or partial base complementarity, as predicted by bioinformatics analysis. The highly conserved sequences of many miRNAs among various organisms suggest strong evolutionary selection and role of miRNAs in important physiological processes.

miRNA expression abnormalities (excess or deficiency) have been associated with various human diseases, including Alzheimer's disease, Parkinson's disease, various cancers, and kidney and cardiovascular disorders (Table 1). The continuous discovery of new miRNAs suggests that the

Table 1 Illustrative List of miRNAs Involved in Various Human Diseases

Disease	miRNA Involved	miRNA Expression	Reference(s)
Alzheimer's disease	miR-34a, miR-34c	Increases with age in human hippocampus, and AD patients	15, 59
	miRNA-29	Down-regulated AD patients with high BACE1 expression, which is involved in amyloid formation	22, 23
	miR-107miR-103, miR-23b	Down-regulated	25, 26
	miR-9, miR- 125b and miR-128	Increased in the hippocampal region	27
Parkinson's disease	miR-34b and miR-34c	Down-regulated in the frontal cortex, cerebellum	17, 18
	miR-133b	Down-regulated	60, 61
	pre-let7a-1, pre-miR7-2, miR-99a	Enriched in midbrain	60
	miR-7 and miR-153	Regulates levels of synuclein, which is involved in Parkinson's disease	20, 21
	pre-miR-218-2, miR-101-1, miR-107, miR-335	Down-regulated in midbrain	60
Cancer	miR-21	Overexpressed in breast carcinoma	62, 63
	miR-10b	Up-regulated	33, 64
	miR-125a and b and miR-205	Down-regulated	65, 66
	miR-126 and miR-335	Down-regulated in breast cancer metastasis	64, 67
	miR-15, miR-16	Deletions in prostate cancer	68, 69
	miR-155	Up-regulated in various cancers	70, 71
	miR-372 and miR-373	Up-regulated, oncogenic miRNAs, which promote cell proliferation and tumor development	72
	miR-16	Down-regulated in tumor cells of the prostate	69, 73
	miR-34a	Down-regulated in various cancers	74, 75
	let-7	Down-regulated in various cancers	76–78
	miR-205	Down-regulated	79, 80

(*Continued*)

Table 1 (*Continued*)

Disease	miRNA Involved	miRNA Expression	Reference(s)
Kidney disease	miR-192	Up-regulated, highly expressed in renal cortex	43, 81
	miR-15a	Down-regulated	44
	miR-200 family and miR-205	Up-regulated in hypertensive nephrosclerosis	82, 83
	miR-377	Up-regulated in diabetic nephropathy	84
	miR-21	Up-regulated in diabetic conditions; involved in renal fibrosis	50, 51
	miR-10a, miR-106b, and miR-17–5p,	Down-regulated during nephrogenesis	85
	miR-29b	Up-regulated in rat models	86
Cardiovascular diseases	miR-1, miR-30, miR-133, and miR-150	Down-regulated in cardiac hypertrophy	47, 48
	miR-21, miR-23a, miR-125	Up-regulated in hypertrophy	48, 87, 88
	miR-1	Up-regulated in coronary artery disease	46, 55
	miR-195	Up-regulated	52
	miR-199b	Up-regulated in human heart failure	89, 90

present collection of miRNAs implicated in human disease is likely to be incomplete. Initial evidence of the role of miRNAs in cancer came from a study on chronic lymphocytic leukemia. Table 1 details the miRNAs involved in various human diseases, and the mechanisms of action of some well-studied miRNAs are explained below.

4.4.1. Neurodegenerative Diseases

The deregulation of miRNA expression has been reported in neurodegenerative diseases such as Alzheimer's and Parkinson's. For example, miR-34a has been found to be enriched in the adult mouse nervous system, in spinal cord and brainstem regions, and levels further increase with age in the cortex and hippocampus. miR-34a is enriched in the cerebral cortex in an

Alzheimer's mouse model, and miR-34c increases with age in the human hippocampus in Alzheimer's patients, as well as in mouse models.[15] miR-34c is associated with regulation of targets involved in memory impairment in mice. In patients with Parkinson's disease, miR-34b/c is downregulated in brain samples. Deficiency in miR-34b/c may promote mitochondrial dysfunction, concomitant with a decrease in Parkin and DJ-1, two genetic loci associated with Parkinson's disease. Based on disease-associated changes in miR-34 family miRNA levels, one could potentially use changes in miRNA expression as biomarkers of age-associated processes such as neurodegenerative disease.[16–18] α-synuclein is a neuronal protein that is linked to Parkinson's disease. Although point mutations in this protein are related to Parkinson's disease, higher levels of synuclein lead to the development of Parkinson's disease.[19] Two miRNAs, miR-7 and miR-153, have been found to be involved in regulating endogenous levels of synuclein.[20,21] These miRNAs could be potential candidates for therapeutics for modulating the levels of synuclein in Parkinson's patients.

In Alzheimer's patients, expression of miRNA-29 family has been found to decrease. miR-29a and miRNA-29b-1 can decrease the expression of β-amyloid cleavage enzyme 1 (BACE-1), which is required for the cleavage of amyloid precursor protein and the generation of toxic species.[22,23] It was found that the expression of miR-29a and miRNA-29b-1 was significantly decreased in a group of Alzheimer's patients with high levels of BACE-1 protein, while mRNA levels of this enzyme were unaffected.[24] Expression of another miRNA, miR-107, was also found to be decreased in the brains of Alzheimer's patients at the earliest stages with increased BACE-1 mRNA levels.[25] The predicted miR-107 binding sites were found in the 3′-UTR of human BACE-1 mRNA. miRNA profiling, *in situ* hybridization and biochemical experiments suggest that miR-107 may be involved in Alzheimer's progression through the regulation of BACE-1 expression.[25,26] Therefore, miRNA-107 could be potential candidate as a therapeutic agent. Another miRNA profiling study reported that miR-9, miR-125b and miR-128 were increased in the hippocampal region of Alzheimer's affected brains.[27] Despite the variety of different studies undertaken, there has been little overlap in miRNA profiles, with small sample sizes, differences in experimental approaches, and assay sensitivities likely accounting for these disparate results. However, with the increasing size of our database of miRNAs, good candidates that may be used in therapeutics will eventually emerge.

4.4.2. Cancer

One of the most attractive properties of miRNAs as therapeutic agents is their ability to target multiple molecules, frequently in the context of a network, making them extremely efficient in regulating distinct biological cell processes relevant to normal and malignant cell biology. Initial studies of high-throughput miRNA expression analysis in human disease were mostly focused on cancer. With different high-throughput methods to measure global miRNA levels in multiple tumor types, various reports suggested the differential expression of miRNAs in different tumor samples. Some miRNAs, such as miR-21, miR-17-5p and miR-191, were found to be overexpressed in tumors of different embryonic origin. miR-21, one of the first cancer microRNAs described, has been found to be overexpressed in a variety of malignancies, including glioblastomas and cancer of the ovary and lung.[62,63] In addition, miR-21 overexpression is also associated with poor survival and poor therapeutic outcome in colorectal and pancreatic cancer.[28] Further, miR-21 has been found to mediate cell survival and proliferation directly targeting the tumor suppressor genes PTEN, PDCD4 and TPM1, and it has been associated with advanced clinical stage, lymph node metastasis.[29] In the context of therapeutic uses of miRNAs, preliminary indications from preclinical experimental models aimed to understand the biological roles of specific miRNAs.[69] For example, reintroduction of miR-15a/16-1 induces apoptosis in leukemic MEG01 cells and inhibits tumor growth *in vivo* in a xenograft model, while silencing oncogenic miR-21 with antisense oligonucleotides generates a pro-apoptotic and anti proliferative response *in vitro* in different cell lines, and reduced tumor development *in vivo.*[30]

Other miRNAs, such as miR-10b and miR-16, have also been tested as therapeutic agents in cancer models.[31] miR-10b is transcriptionally induced by a transcription factor that contributes to epithelial–mesenchymal transitions known as TWIST 1.[32] In various metastatic cancer cells and tumor tissues, miR-10b has been found to be highly expressed. Further, miR-10b can induce the metastatic phenotype in cells that otherwise lack metastatic potential. The use of miR-10b as a therapeutic agent in breast cancer has been illustrated by the fact that the systemic treatment of tumor-bearing mice with miR-10b suppresses breast cancer metastasis.[33]

As reported by Tazawa and co-workers,[34] miR-34a transiently inhibits human colon cancer tumor progression when administered subcutaneously in complexes with atelocollagen, which was recently shown to be a very powerful system for efficient *in vivo* delivery of small interfering RNA molecules into tumors. Chen and colleagues have developed a liposome-polycation-hyaluronic acid(LPH) nanoparticle formulation modified with tumor-targeting single chain antibody fragment for systemic delivery of miR-34a to lung metastasis of murine melanoma cells.[35] In 2009, Kota *et al.*,[36] used a systemic administration of miR-26a in a mouse model of HCC using adeno-associated virus to inhibit cancer cell proliferation and induction of tumor-specific apoptosis. These results are consistent with previous findings made by the same group demonstrating that MYC induced liver tumors result in concomitant down-regulation of various miRNAs.[37]

let-7, initially discovered in *C. elegans*, was found to be involved in cell cycle exit and terminal differentiation. It has emerged as a tumor suppressor microRNA that regulates self-renewal and tumorigenicity of breast cancer cells, targeting molecules originally described in lung cancer: RAS37 as well as the oncogene HMGA2. Overexpression of the let-7 miRNA family can suppress tumor development in mouse models of breast and lung cancer.[38,39] In a study using a conditional mouse lung cancer model, Esquela-Kerscher *et al.* showed that the intranasal administration of an adenovirus expressing let-7a RNA hairpin reduced tumor formation *in vivo*.[40]

MicroRNAs involved in specific networks, such as the apoptotic or proliferation networks, could influence the response to targeted therapy or chemotherapy. For example, inhibition of miR-21 and miR-200b enhances sensitivity to the drug gemcitabine in cholangiocytes.[41] Slack's group has suggested a potential therapeutic use for anti-miR-34 as a radiosensitizing agent in p53-mutant breast cancer in radiotherapy.[42] Nevertheless, effective delivery into target tissues remains a major hurdle for microRNA-based therapy, including the applications of antagomirs and synthetic microRNA duplexes.

miRNAs involved in the regulation of apoptosis, proliferation or receptor-driven pathways could likely affect the results of chemotherapy, and therefore also their possible use as adjuvant tools. There are two main strategies to target miRNA expression in cancer. The first strategy involves the use of virus constructs or oligonucleotides to either lower the expression of an oncogenic miRNA or to reintroduce a tumor suppressor miRNA. Another strategy involves the use of drugs to modulate miRNA expression by targeting their transcription and their processing.[7]

4.4.3. Kidney Diseases

Studies of miRNA expression in kidney diseases have emerged predominantly from animal models. In one study, miR-192 levels were shown to be increased in glomeruli isolated from diabetic mice.[43] miR-192 was shown to regulate some repressors that are responsible for controlling the expression of extracellular matrix proteins, collagen 1a1 and collagen 2 (Col1a1 and Col2). Col1a1 and Col2 were shown to accumulate during diabetic nephropathy, suggesting a potential role of miR-192 in this kidney disease.[43] Polycystic kidney disease is one of the most common inherited renal diseases. In a rat model of polycystic kidney disease, 30 differentially expressed miRNAs were identified in diseased kidney tissues compared with healthy rat, 29 of which were down-regulated. miR-15a has been reported to modulate the expression of cell cycle regulator Cdc25A. miR-15a was found to be down-regulated in liver tissues of patients with polycystic kidney disease, as well as rats with the disorder. Overexpression of miR-15a in cells derived from the polycystic kidney rat led to a decrease in Cdc25A protein, and a larger drop in cyst growth.[44] Dai and colleagues compared miRNA expression of IgA nephropathy biopsy samples from patients. They identified 132 miRNAs, of which 31 were down-regulated and up-regulated in diseased tissues. Another study has reported differential intrarenal expression of miR-200c, miR-141, miR-205 and miR-192 in IgA nephropathy and findings correlated with disease severity and progression.[45] The deregulated expression of miR-200c and miR-205 is of particular interest given their link with epithelial-to-mesenchymal transitions. Sixty-six miRNAs have also been found to be differentially expressed in a small number of human kidney tissues from patients with class II lupus nephritis as compared with healthy control subjects. Differential expression of 16 miRNAs (7 down-regulated and 9 up-regulated) in peripheral blood mononuclear cells has also been reported in patients with systemic lupus erythematosus.

4.4.4. Cardiovascular Diseases

Involvement of miRNAs in the pathological process of the cardiovascular system has recently been recognized, and research on miRNAs in relation to cardiovascular disease is growing rapidly.[46] miRNAs have been found to play various roles in cardiovascular development, cardiac fibrosis and arrhythmia. Recent studies show that miRNAs play important roles in cardiovascular systems and therefore could be part of future medical therapies for heart diseases. Two miRNAs, miR-1 and miR-133, are expressed in cardiac and skeletal muscles during development and in adults. Both miR-1 and miR-133 are found to be down-regulated in human heart disease, as well as in models of cardiac hypertrophy.[47,48] Further, knockdown of miR-133 in mice by infusion of an antisense RNA oligonucleotide induced significant hypertrophic growth of the heart. These studies suggest an active role for miR-133 in the inhibition of cardiac hypertrophy and suggest that modulation of miR-133 levels *in vivo* may serve as a therapy for modulating hypertrophic growth.[49]

Cardiac fibrosis, an inappropriate accumulation of extracellular matrix proteins in the heart, causes cardiac dysfunction in diverse pathological conditions, such as myocardial infarction, dilated and hypertrophic cardiomyopathies, and heart failure. Certain miRNAs, such as miR-21 and miR-29, are found to be enriched in cardiac fibroblasts. Since miR-21 functions as an oncogene and has a role in tumorigenesis by promoting cell proliferation, induction of miR-21 in fibroblasts might increase fibroblast proliferation.[50,51] Inhibition of miR-21 might in turn inhibit fibroblast proliferation and block cardiac fibrosis and could, therefore, be a potential therapeutic candidate. The miR-29 family targets mRNAs encoding extracellular matrix-related proteins involved in fibrosis, including collagens, fibrillins and elastin. Down-regulation of miR-29 is found to be responsible for the induction of collagens and additional extracellular matrix genes in myocardial infraction. These data suggest that therapeutic up-regulation of miR-29 in response to cardiac stress might prevent the onset of cardiac fibrosis and thereby maintain cardiac function.[52] Several miRNAs, including miR-1 and miR-133, have recently been implicated in electrophysiological abnormalities.[53] miR-1 appears to play a major role in cardiac development and conductance. Deletion of miR-1-2 in mice resulted in 50 per cent lethality due to ventricular septal defects in the heart.[54] Yang *et al.* further confirmed the involvement of miR-1 in cardiac conductance, where miR-1 expression was found to be up-regulated in humans with coronary artery disease.[55] With increasing reports of miRNA involvement and its mechanism of action in cardiovascular disorders, ideal therapeutic candidates should emerge very soon.

4.5. METHODS FOR miRNA DELIVERY

As with other nucleotides, there are many obstacles to developing miRNAs as therapeutics, including their instability, non-targeted delivery, and low cellular uptake. Since miRNAs are chemically similar to DNA, novel delivery strategies for DNA could be applied to miRNAs. These strategies include the use of polymeric carriers, micelles, nanoparticles and conjugation to a targeting ligand. Moreover, there is an intense effort to identify new agents capable of targeted delivery of nucleic acids or oligonucleotides including miRNA to tissues and cells.[4,7] Formulations or conjugation-based approaches are employed in nucleic acid delivery. Conjugation strategies include direct attachment of targeting and cell-penetrating peptides, antibodies, and other bioactive molecules to the oligonucleotide. Formulations consist of emulsions, liposomes, polymersor nanoparticles. In order to enter mammalian cells, the nucleic acid needs to cross the lipid bilayer of the cell membrane. This can be achieved by packaging the nucleic acid into liposomes or nanoparticles, which facilitate their endocytosis through the cell membrane. Alternatively, the oligonucleotide can be linked to a lipophilic moiety or receptor ligand.[7] There have been significant advances in the systemic delivery of nucleic acids, with most delivery agents developed showing good efficacy in delivery to the liver. The expansion of effective delivery approaches is a primary requirement for the use of synthetic nucleic acids as therapeutics for various human diseases. Most nucleic acid therapeutic approaches that target intracellular mechanisms (antisense, siRNA) are currently focused on local or compartmentalized delivery or disorders in which the target is in the liver. In ongoing research, specific targeting components, such as cell surface receptor ligands, are being added to nucleic acids, which can enhance target binding to the tissue or cell type of interest.

4.6. CHALLENGES FOR DEVELOPING miRNAs AS THERAPEUTICS

During the development of disease, miRNA expression profiles frequently change, as compared to normal tissue. Significant differences in miRNA expression compared with normal tissue have been found in a number of diseases, including cancer, diabetes, Alzheimer's, Parkinson's and cardiovascular disorders. While the extensive involvement of miRNAs in disease makes them suitable therapeutic candidates to cure such diseases, miRNA-based therapeutics pose various challenges that are different from classical drugs. On the other hand, miRNA-based therapeutics share the same problems as with other nucleic acid-based therapies. Firstly, nucleic acids are degraded by serum and tissue nucleases, and synthetic nucleotide derivatives require specific chemical modifications to alter their biophysical properties. Chemical modifications that increase the stability of the oligonucleotides, including phosphorothioate, 2-*O*-methyl, and 2-fluoro substitutions, among many others, may be useful for developing a particular therapeutic molecule.[56] However, stability and effective delivery of miRNAs into target tissues remain major hurdles for direct miRNA-based therapy. Moreover, the size of an unconjugated therapeutic RNA is 7–20 kDa, and these molecules are filtered by the kidneys and excreted. To avoid these issues, several modifications, some of which have already been developed for siRNAs, can be applied to miRNAs. Some miRNAs have been chemically modified, such as chemically modified antimiR oligonucleotides (AMOs), which have greater specificity and higher binding affinity to RNA. Some cells, like scavenging macrophages, can uptake these molecules in a nonspecific manner. Further, these molecules have limited passage through the extracellular matrix. Most miRNAs have numerous molecular targets, which raises the possibility that the targeting of an miRNA may perturb multiple cellular functions, some pathological and others beneficial. Issues of pharmacokinetics, biodistribution, and cell penetration also represent potential obstacles to therapeutic miRNA manipulation strategies using synthetic nucleic acids.[5,7] Given the huge potential of miRNAs in therapeutics, these are challenges being actively addressed by various research groups.

4.7. miRNA AS BIOMARKERS

The identification of stable miRNAs in body fluids has opened new avenues for their use as novel biomarkers in clinical diagnosis. miRNAs qualify as worthy biomarkers for diagnosis because they are chemically defined and stable in cells and in the circulation of human body. In addition, the simplicity of miRNA detection, as well as the observed specificity, has led many researchers to suggest that miRNAs are revolutionary in the field of biomarkers.[57] Although proteins are more diverse and therefore potentially more informative, the complex composition of protein in blood, post-translational modifications, sequence variations, and difficulties associated with the development of high-affinity detection agents present significant challenges in the discovery and development of new protein-based biomarkers.

The majority of miRNA sequences are conserved in distant species, and these are expressed in specific tissues or biological stages. Moreover, levels of miRNAs can be measured easily by quantitative PCR, allowing for high-precision signal amplification as compared to methods associated with proteins. Moreover, next-generation sequencing technologies have greatly enhanced the discovery of novel miRNAs that may potentially be used as biomarkers. As the detection of miRNAs is sensitive, specific, robust and noninvasive, miRNAs possess various characteristics of the ideal biomarker.[58]

However, a number of factors pose challenges in the successful application of circulating miRNAs as biomarkers. One major problem is the lack of standardized procedures, which can introduce bias in the interpretation of results. The variability in miRNA profiles could arise from differences in sample collection, storage, RNA isolation, accurate assessment of quantity and quality of an miRNA, and the size of the starting material. Further, microarrays, quantitative RT-PCR, and next-generation sequencing require data normalization to account for this variability. Endogenous control miRNAs may vary under different conditions. Thus, miRNAs that are minimally disturbed and most stable across all samples in a study can thus serve as endogenous controls.

Considering the critical role of miRNAs in gene regulation, any fluctuations, either epigenetically induced or via other factors such as ethnicity, age and gender, can influence miRNA expression levels. However, analysis of multiple miRNA profiles is extremely valuable because specific signatures of miRNA combinations unique to a normal or pathological state can serve as a useful reference. In addition, assigning rank order to miRNAs for biological relevance can address challenges associated with their use as biomarkers. Another challenge with the use of miRNAs as markers is that their mRNA targets are not easily identified by computational methods. Further, targets of miRNAs should be confirmed biochemically, such as via immunoprecipitation of argonaute–miRNA–mRNA complexes. Still, as the database of miRNAs involved in disease continues to expand, more specific miRNAs are certain to emerge as potential biomarkers.[58]

4.8. CONCLUSION

In recent years, there has been dramatic increase in research focused on the role of small non-coding miRNAs in various human diseases. From viruses to plants, to humans, miRNA-based regulation of gene expression has been shown to be involved in every biological system. With the interest in miRNAs now greater than ever, there are constant reports on novel miRNAs, their validated gene targets, and the development of miRNA-based therapeutics. Although there is no doubt about the therapeutic potential of miRNAs, the task remains to translate this potential into readily available treatments. The main challenge in bringing the power of miRNAs to bear on various human diseases is the enablement of pharmacological drug delivery, a job that has hindered the progress of related siRNA therapeutics. On the other hand, advances have been made in such delivery systems and the systemic administration of miRNA using adeno-associated virus has been tested in a preclinical model. Further, cationic liposomes or polymer-based nanoparticle formulations may be developed to achieve the goal of effective drug delivery. Given the obvious involvement of miRNAs in numerous human diseases, and consistent innovation in delivery techniques, miRNA-based therapies would seem to hold good prospects for the future.

ACKNOWLEDGMENTS

The authors would like to acknowledge all the members of their laboratory for their critical reading of the manuscript and suggestions in the preparation of this chapter.

REFERENCES

1. Rodriguez A, Griffiths-Jones S, Ashurst JL, Bradley A. (2004) Identification of mammalian microRNA host genes and transcription units. *Genome Res* **14**(10A): 1902–1910.
2. Kim DH, Sætrom P, Snøve O, Jr, Rossi JJ. (2008) MicroRNA-directed transcriptional gene silencing in mammalian cells. *Proc Natl Acad Sci USA* **105**(42): 16230–16235.
3. Farh KK-H, Grimson A, Jan C, *et al.* (2005) The widespread impact of mammalian MicroRNAs on mRNA repression and evolution. *Science* **310**(5755): 1817–1821.
4. Liu Z, Sall A, Yang DC. (2008) MicroRNA: An emerging therapeutic target and intervention tool. *Int J Mol Sci* **9**(6): 978–999.
5. Jackson AL, LevinAA. (2012) Developing microRNA therapeutics: Approaching the unique complexities. *Nucleic Acid Ther* **22**(4): 213–225.
6. Soifer HS, Rossi JJ, SaetromP. (2007) MicroRNAs in disease and potential therapeutic applications. *Mol Ther* **15**(12): 2070–2079.
7. Bader AG, Brown D, Stoudemire J, Lammers P. (2011) Developing therapeutic microRNAs for cancer. *Gene Ther* **18**(12): 1121–1126.
8. Fire A, Xu S, Montgomery MK, *et al.* (1998) Potent and specific genetic interference by double-stranded RNA in *Caenorhabditis elegans*. *Nature* **391**(6669): 806–811.
9. Bartel DP. (2004) MicroRNAs. Genomics, biogenesis, mechanism, and function. *Cell* **116**(2): 281–297.
10. Carthew RW, Sontheimer EJ. (2009) Origins and Mechanisms of miRNAs and siRNAs. *Cell* **136**(4): 642–655.
11. Chendrimada TP, Finn KJ, Ji X, *et al.* (2007) MicroRNA silencing through RISC recruitment of eIF6. *Nature* **447**(7146): 823–828.
12. Cissell KA, Deo SK. (2009) Trends in microRNA detection. *Anal Bioanal Chem* **394**(4): 1109–1116.
13. Van Wynsberghe PM, Chan SP, Slack FJ, Pasquinelli AE. (2011) Analysis of microRNA expression and function. *Methods Cell Biol* **106**: 219–252.

14. Cissell KA, Deo SK. (2009) Trends in microRNA detection. *Anal Bioanal Chem* **394**(4): 1109–1116.
15. Wang X, Liu P, Zhu H, *et al.* (2009) miR-34a, a microRNA up-regulated in a double transgenic mouse model of Alzheimer's disease, inhibits bcl2 translation. *Brain Res Bull* **80**(4–5): 268–273.
16. Abe M, BoniniNM. (2013)MicroRNAs and neurodegeneration: Role and impact. *Trends Cell Biol* **23**(1): 30–36.
17. Junn E, Mouradian MM. (2012) MicroRNAs in neurodegenerative diseases and their therapeutic potential. *Pharmacol Ther* **133**(2): 142–150.
18. Miñones-Moyano E, Porta S, Escaramís G, *et al.* (2011) MicroRNA profiling of Parkinson's disease brains identifies early downregulation of miR-34b/c which modulate mitochondrial function. *Hum Mol Genet* **20**(15): 3067–3078.
19. Singleton AB, Farrer M, Johnson J, *et al.* (2003) Alpha-synuclein locus triplication causes Parkinson's disease. *Science* **302**(5646): 841.
20. Junn E, Lee KW, Jeong BS, *et al.* (2009) Repression of alpha-synuclein expression and toxicity by microRNA-7. *Proc Natl Acad Sci USA* **106**(31): 13052–13057.
21. Doxakis E. (2010) Post-transcriptional regulation of alpha-synuclein expression by mir-7 and mir-153. *J Biol Chem* **285**(17): 12726–12734.
22. Vassar R, Kovacs DM, Yan R, Wong PC. (2009) The beta-secretase enzyme BACE in health and Alzheimer's disease: Regulation, cell biology, function, and therapeutic potential. *J Neurosci* **29**(41): 12787–12794.
23. Hébert SS, Horré K, Nicolaï L, *et al.* (2008) Loss of microRNA cluster miR-29a/b-1 in sporadic Alzheimer's disease correlates with increased BACE1/beta-secretase expression. *Proc Natl Acad Sci USA* **105**(17): 6415–6420.
24. Hébert SS, Horré K, Nicolaï L, *et al.* (2008) Loss of microRNA cluster miR-29a/b-1 in sporadic Alzheimer's disease correlates with increased BACE1/beta-secretase expression. *Proc Natl Acad Sci USA* **105**(17): 6415–6420.
25. Wang WX, Rajeev BW, Stromberg AJ, *et al.* (2008) The expression of microRNA miR-107 decreases early in Alzheimer's disease and may accelerate disease progression through regulation of beta-site amyloid precursor protein-cleaving enzyme 1. *J Neurosci* **28**(5): 1213–1223.
26. Nelson PT, Wang WX. (2010) MiR-107 is reduced in Alzheimer's disease brain neocortex: Validation study. *J Alzheimers Dis* **21**(1): 75–79.
27. Lukiw WJ. (2007) Micro-RNA speciation in fetal, adult and Alzheimer's disease hippocampus. *Neuroreport* **18**(3): 297–300.
28. Bloomston M, Frankel WL, Petrocca F, *et al.* (2007) MicroRNA expression patterns to differentiate pancreatic adenocarcinoma from normal pancreas and chronic pancreatitis. *J Am Med Assoc* **297**(17): 1901–1908.

29. Yan LX, Huang XF, Shao Q, *et al.* (2008) MicroRNA miR-21 overexpression in human breast cancer is associated with advanced clinical stage, lymph node metastasis and patient poor prognosis. *RNA* **14**(11): 2348–2360.
30. Si ML, Zhu S, Wu H, *et al.* (2007) miR-21-mediated tumor growth. *Oncogene* **26**(19): 2799–2803.
31. Iorio MV, CroceCM. (2012) MicroRNA dysregulation in cancer: Diagnostics, monitoring and therapeutics. A comprehensive review. *EMBO Mol Med* **4**(3): 143–159.
32. Gangaraju VK, Lin H. (2009) MicroRNAs: Key regulators of stem cells. *Nat Rev Mol Cell Biol* **10**(2): 116–125.
33. Ma L, Reinhardt F, Pan E, *et al.* (2010) Therapeutic silencing of miR-10b inhibits metastasis in a mouse mammary tumor model. *Nat Biotechnol* **28**(4): 341–347.
34. Tazawa H, Tsuchiya N, Izumiya M, Nakagama H. (2007) Tumor-suppressive miR-34a induces senescence like growth arrest through modulation of the E2F pathway in human colon cancer cells. *Proc Natl Acad Sci USA* **104**(39): 15472–15477.
35. Chen Y, Zhu X, Zhang X, Liu B, Huang L. (2010) Nanoparticles modified with tumor-targeting scFv deliver siRNA and miRNA for cancer therapy. *Mol Ther* **18**(9): 1650–1656.
36. Kota J, Chivukula RR, O'Donnell KA, *et al.* (2009) Therapeutic microRNA delivery suppresses tumorigenesis in a murine liver cancer model. *Cell* **137**(6): 1005–1017.
37. Chang TC, Yu D, Lee YS, Wentzel EA, *et al.* (2008) Widespread microRNA repression by Myc contributes to tumorigenesis. *Nat Genet* **40**(1): 43–50.
38. Yu F, Yao H, Zhu P, *et al.* (2007)let-7 regulates self renewal and tumorigenicity of breast cancer cells. *Cell* **131**(6): 1109–1123.
39. Kumar MS, Erkeland SJ, Pester RE, *et al.* (2008) Suppression of non-small cell lung tumor development by the let-7 microRNA family. *Proc Natl Acad Sci USA* **105**(10): 3903–3908.
40. Esquela-Kerscher A, Trang P, Wiggins JF, *et al.* (2008) The let-7 microRNA reduces tumor growth in mouse models of lung cancer. *Cell Cycle* **7**(6). 759–764.
41. Meng F, Henson R, Lang M, *et al.* (2006) Involvement of human micro-RNA in growth and response to chemotherapy in human cholangiocarcinoma cell lines. *Gastroenterology* **130**(7): 2113–2129.
42. Weidhaas JB, Babar I, Nallur SM, *et al.* (2007) MicroRNAs as potential agents to alter resistance to cytotoxic anticancer therapy. *Cancer Res* **67**(23): 11111–11116.

43. Kato M, Zhang J, Wang M, *et al.* (2007) MicroRNA-192 in diabetic kidney glomeruli and its function in TGF-beta-induced collagen expression via inhibition of E-box repressors. *Proc Natl Acad Sci USA* **104**(9): 3432–3437.
44. Lee SO, Masyuk T, Splinter P, *et al.* (2008) MicroRNA15a modulates expression of the cell-cycle regulator Cdc25A and affects hepatic cystogenesis in a rat model of polycystic kidney disease. *J Clin Invest* **118**(11): 3714–3724.
45. Dai Y, Sui W, Lan H, *et al.* (2008) Microarray analysis of micro-ribonucleic acid expression in primary immunoglobulin A nephropathy. *Saudi Med J* **29**(10): 1388–1393.
46. Chen JH, WangDZ. (2012) microRNAs in cardiovascular development. *J Mol Cell Cardiol* **52**(5): 949–957.
47. Carè A, Catalucci D, Felicetti F, *et al.* (2007) MicroRNA-133 controls cardiac hypertrophy. *NatMed* **13**(5): 613–618.
48. van Rooij E, Marshall WS, OlsonEN. (2008) Toward microRNA-based therapeutics for heart disease: The sense in antisense. *CircRes* **103**(9): 919–928.
49. Carè A, Catalucci D, Felicetti F, *et al.* (2007) MicroRNA-133 controls cardiac hypertrophy. *Nat Med* **13**(5): 613–618.
50. Dey N, Das F, Mariappan MM, *et al.* (2011) MicroRNA-21 orchestrates high glucose-induced signals to TOR complex 1, resulting in renal cell pathology in diabetes. *J Biol Chem* **286**(29): 25586–25603.
51. Zarjou A, Yang S, Abraham E, *et al.* (2011) Identification of a microRNA signature in renal fibrosis: Role of miR-21. *Am J Physiol Renal Physiol* **301**(4): F793–F801.
52. van Rooij E, Sutherland LB, Liu N, *et al.* (2006) A signature pattern of stress-responsive microRNAs that can evoke cardiac hypertrophy and heart failure. *Proc Natl Acad Sci USA* **103**(48): 18255–18260.
53. Thum T, Catalucci D, Bauersachs J. (2008) MicroRNAs: Novel regulators in cardiac development and disease. *Cardiovasc Res* **79**(4): 562–570.
54. Zhao Y, Ransom JF, Li A, *et al.* (2007) Dysregulation of cardiogenesis, cardiac conduction, and cell cycle in mice lacking miRNA-1-2. *Cell* **129**(2): 303–317.
55. Yang B, Lin H, Xiao J, *et al.* (2007) The muscle-specific microRNA miR-1 regulates cardiac arrhythmogenic potential by targeting GJA1 and KCNJ2. *Nat Med* **13**(4): 486–491.
56. Soifer HS, Rossi JJ, Saetrom P. (2007) MicroRNAs in disease and potential therapeutic applications. *Mol Ther* **15**(12): 2070–2079.
57. Jackson DB. (2009) Serum-based microRNAs: Are we blinded by potential? *Proc Natl Acad Sci USA* **106**(1): E5.

58. Etheridge A, Lee I, Hood L, *et al.* (2011) Extracellular microRNA: A new source of biomarkers. *Mutat Res* **717**(1–2): 85–90.
59. Zovoilis A, Agbemenyah HY, Agis-Balboa RC, *et al.* (2011) microRNA-34c is a novel target to treat dementias. *EMBO J* **30**(20): 4299–4308.
60. Kim J, Inoue K, Ishii J, *et al.* (2007) A microRNA feedback circuit in midbrain dopamine neurons. *Science* **317**(5842): 1220–1224.
61. de Mena L, Coto E, Cardo LF, *et al.* (2010) Analysis of the Micro-RNA-133 and PITX3 genes in Parkinson's disease. *Am J Med Gen B Neuropsychiatr Genet* **153B**(6): 1234–1239.
62. Volinia S, Calin GA, Liu CG, *et al.* (2006) A microRNA expression signature of human solid tumors defines cancer gene targets. *Proc Natl Acad Sci USA* **103**(7): 2257–2261.
63. Markou A, Tsaroucha EG, Kaklamanis L, *et al.* (2008) Prognostic value of mature microRNA-21 and microRNA-205 overexpression in non-small cell lung cancer by quantitative real-time RT-PCR. *Clin Chem* **54**(10): 1696–1704.
64. Png KJ, Yoshida M, Zhang XH, *et al.* (2011) MicroRNA-335 inhibits tumor reinitiation and is silenced through genetic and epigenetic mechanisms in human breast cancer. *Genes Dev* **25**(3): 226–231.
65. Meister G, Landthaler M, Dorsett Y, Tuschl T. (2004) Sequence-specific inhibition of microRNA- and siRNA-induced RNA silencing. *RNA* **10**(3): 544–550.
66. Hutvágner G, Simard MJ, Mello CC, Zamore PD. (2004) Sequence-specific inhibition of small RNA function. *PLoS Biol* **2**(4): E98.
67. Tavazoie SF, Alarcón C, Oskarsson T, *et al.* (2008) Endogenous human microRNAs that suppress breast cancer metastasis. *Nature* **451**(7175): 147–152.
68. Calin GA, Sevignani C, Dumitru CD, *et al.* (2004) Human microRNA genes are frequently located at fragile sites and genomic regions involved in cancers. *Proc Natl Acad Sci USA* **101**(9): 2999–3004.
69. Cimmino A, Calin GA, Fabbri M, *et al.* (2005) miR-15 and miR-16 induce apoptosis by targeting BCL2. *Proc Natl Acad Sci USA* **102**(39): 13944–13949.
70. Greither T, Grochola LF, Udelnow A, *et al.* (2010) Elevated expression of microRNAs 155, 203, 210 and 222 in pancreatic tumors is associated with poorer survival. *Int J Cancer* **126**(1): 73–80.
71. Gironella M, Seux M, Xie MJ, *et al.* (2007) Tumor protein 53-induced nuclear protein 1 expression is repressed by miR 155, and its restoration inhibits pancreatic tumor development. *Proc Natl Acad Sci USA* **104**(41): 16170–16175.
72. Voorhoeve PM, le Sage C, Schrier M, *et al.* (2006) A genetic screen implicates miRNA-372 and miRNA-373 as oncogenes in testicular germ cell tumors. *Cell* **124**(6): 1169–1181.

73. Takeshita F, Patrawala L, Osaki M, *et al.* (2010) Systemic delivery of synthetic microRNA-16 inhibits the growth of metastatic prostate tumors via downregulation of multiple cell-cycle genes. *Mol Ther* **18**(1): 181–187.
74. Wiggins JF, Ruffino L, Kelnar K, *et al.* (2010)Development of a lung cancer therapeutic based on the tumor suppressor microRNA-34. *Cancer Res* **70**(14): 5923–5930.
75. Watahiki A, Wang Y, Morris J, *et al.* (2011) MicroRNAs associated with metastatic prostate cancer. *PloS ONE* **6**(9): e24950.
76. Johnson SM, Grosshans H, Shingara J, *et al.* (2005) RAS is regulated by the let-7 microRNA family. *Cell* **120**(5): 635–647.
77. Zhang B, Pan X, Cobb GP, Anderson TA. (2007) microRNAs as oncogenes and tumor suppressors. *Dev Biol* **302**(1): 1–12.
78. Takamizawa J, Konishi H, Yanagisawa K, *et al.* (2004) Reduced expression of the let-7 microRNAs in human lung cancers in association with shortened postoperative survival. *Cancer Res* **64**(11): 3753–3756.
79. Gregory PA, Bracken CP, Bert AG, Goodall GJ. (2008) MicroRNAs as regulators of epithelial-mesenchymal transition. *Cell Cycle* 7(20): 3112–3117.
80. Iorio MV, Casalini P, Piovan C, *et al.* (2009) microRNA-205 regulates HER3 in human breast cancer. *Cancer Res* **69**(6): 2195–2200.
81. Chung AC, Huang XR, Meng X, Lan HY. (2010) miR-192 mediates TGF-beta/Smad3-driven renal fibrosis. *J Am Soc Nephrol* **21**(8): 1317–1325.
82. Wang G, Kwan BC, Lai FM, *et al.* (2010) Intrarenal expression of miRNAs in patients with hypertensive nephrosclerosis. *Am J Hypertens* **23**(1): 78–84.
83. Oba S, Kumano S, Suzuki E, *et al.* (2010) miR-200b precursor can ameliorate renal tubulointerstitial fibrosis. *PloS ONE* 5(10): e13614.
84. Wang Q, Wang Y, Minto AW, *et al.* (2008) MicroRNA-377 is up-regulated and can lead to increased fibronectin production in diabetic nephropathy. *FASEB J* **22**(12): 4126–4135.
85. Ho J, Pandey P, Schatton T, *et al.* (2011) The pro-apoptotic protein Bim is a microRNA target in kidney progenitors. *J Am Soc Nephrol* **22**(6): 1053–1063.
86. Liu Y, Taylor NE, Lu L, *et al.* (2010) Renal medullary microRNAs in Dahl salt-sensitive rats miR-29b regulates several collagens and related genes. *Hypertension* **55**(4): 974–982.
87. Cheng Y, Zhu P, Yang J, *et al.* (2010) Ischaemic preconditioning-regulated miR-21 protects heart against ischaemia/reperfusion injury via anti-apoptosis through its target PDCD4. *Cardiovasc Res* **87**(3): 431–439.
88. Lin Z, Murtaza I, Wang K, *et al.* (2009) miR-23a functions downstream of NFATc3 to regulate cardiac hypertrophy. *Proc Natl Acad Sci USA* **106**(29): 12103–12108.

89. da Costa Martins PA, Salic K, Gladka MM, *et al.* (2010) MicroRNA-199b targets the nuclear kinase Dyrk1a in an auto-amplification loop promoting calcineurin/NFAT signalling. *Nat Cell Biol* **12**(12): 1220–1227.
90. Kuhn C, Frank D, Will R, *et al.* (2009) DYRK1A is a novel negative regulator of cardiomyocyte hypertrophy. *J Biol Chem* **284**(25): 17320–17327.

CHAPTER 5

Integrating Emerging Science into Clinical Practice: Targeting Androgen Signaling in Castration Resistant Metastatic Prostate Cancer

Sri Lakshmi S. Kollepara[*], *Srinivas K. Tantravahi*[†], *Julia Batten*[†] *and Neeraj Agarwal*[†,‡]

5.1. INTRODUCTION

Prostate cancer is the second most common cancer and one of the major causes of death in men.[1,2] In 2012, an estimated 242,000 men will be diagnosed with prostate cancer and 28,000 deaths will occur due to metastatic disease in the US.[2] About one-third of men with localized prostate cancer will eventually develop metastatic disease with approximately five per cent of men having metastatic disease at the time of initial presentation. Over 70 years ago, it was recognized that prostate cancer was an androgen

*Department of Internal Medicine, DMC-Sinai Grace Hospital, Detroit, Michigan, USA
†Department of Internal Medicine, Division of Medical Oncology, University of Utah Huntsman Cancer Institute, Salt Lake City, Utah, USA
‡Corresponding author: Neeraj Agarwal, MD, Assistant Professor of Medicine, Co-leader, Genitourinary Oncology Multidisciplinary Program, Huntsman Cancer Institute, University of Utah, 2000 Circle of Hope, Ste 2123, Salt Lake City, UT 84112, USA; E-mail: *neeraj.agarwal@hci.utah.edu*; Tel: +1-801-585-0255; Fax: +1-801-585-0124

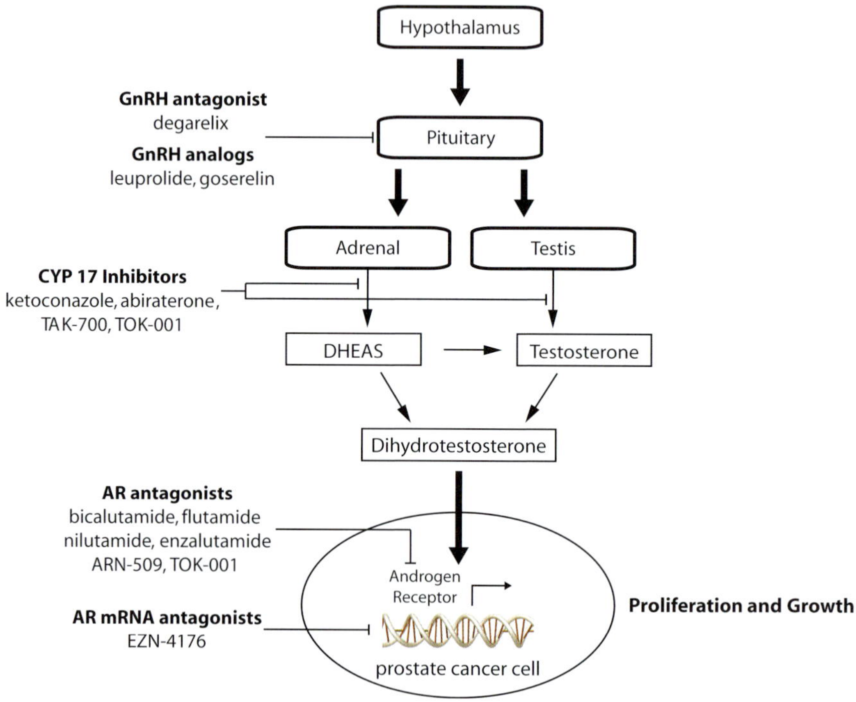

Fig. 1. Androgen dependent signaling of the prostate cancer cell, and drugs inhibiting along the hypothalamic-pituitary-adrenal and testicular axis, and androgen signaling. Thick arrows indicate stimulation; thin arrows indicate synthesis; flat lines indicate inhibition.

dependent disease and the blockade of testicular androgen production by surgical or medical castration has been the standard of care ever since.[3] Medical castration is achieved with either gonadotrophin releasing hormone (GnRH) agonists (such as leuprolide or goserelin), or GnRH antagonist (degarelix) (Fig. 1). Despite a high initial response rate to castration, the majority of patients develop disease progression by ~18 months,[3] a state known as castration refractory prostate cancer (CRPC). Over the last decade, it has been recognized that despite castration, most prostate tumors maintain some dependence on androgen and/or androgen receptor (AR) signaling for proliferation.[4]

5.2. MOLECULAR MECHANISMS UNDERLYING PROGRESSION OF CASTRATION RESISTANT PROSTATE CANCER

Although androgen deprivation therapy (ADT) reduces the serum level of androgens to castrate levels, it does not eliminate them completely. In a castrate state, the adrenal glands are the major source of androgens. Prostate cancer cells are also capable of initiating aberrant androgen signaling and can synthesize sufficient amounts of intratumoral androgens to allow continued androgen signaling and tumor growth during castration.[5] This helps to explain why the concentration of intratumoral testosterone in metastatic prostate tumors in men with CRPC is two to three times higher than in men who have never received ADT, despite the fact that those not receiving ADT have much higher serum testosterone levels.[6,7] In addition, many enzymes involved in androgen synthesis are highly up-regulated in CRPC, compared to those with androgen sensitive prostate cancer.[7] Notably, castrate resistant cell lines have been shown to synthesize much higher level of androgens than androgen dependent cell lines and are capable of directly converting radioactive cholesterol into testosterone *in vitro*.[8] Other mechanisms underlying CRPC include increased AR gene expression, either due to AR gene amplification and increased rate of transcription of the AR gene, or from the increased stability of the AR transcript.[8,9] The somatic mutation of the AR gene, resulting in promiscuous ARs, which are activated by antiandrogens (such as bicalutamide) and other endogenous steroids (such as progesterone or deoxycorticosterone), are also known to drive prostate cancer progression in many individuals.[4,10] One recently reported mechanism is AR gene rearrangement, resulting in constitutively active truncated AR splice variants that lack the AR ligand binding domain.[11] Many novel agents targeting these pathways have been successfully developed and have either been granted approval or are in late phases of development, and are reviewed here.

5.3. DRUGS TARGETING ANDROGEN BIOSYNTHESIS

Ketoconazole: Ketoconazole, a cytochrome P-450 inhibitor, is an imidazole antifungal agent that non-specifically inhibits several enzymes in androgen

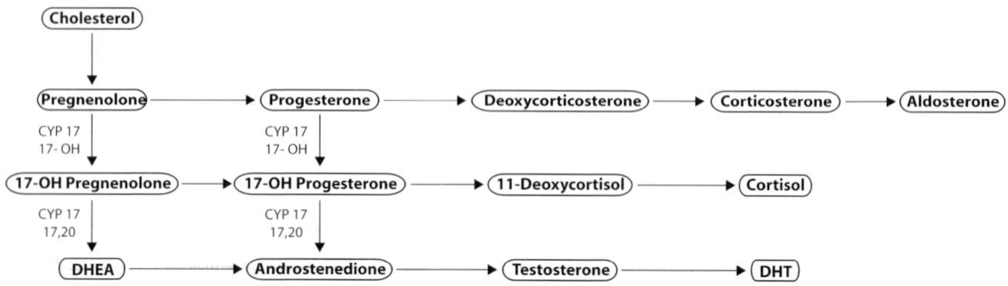

Fig. 2. A simplified version of the steroid synthesis, and mechanism of action of abiraterone and TAK-700. Arrows indicate synthesis; flat lines indicate inhibition. CYP 17: cytochrome p450 17; 17-OH: 17-hydroxylase; 17–20: 17,20-lyase; DHEA: dihydroepiandrostenedione; DHT: dihydrotestosterone.

biosynthesis. Although ketoconazole has never been shown to improve survival, it has been frequently used in the past, as a part of secondary hormonal manipulation after onset of CRPC.[12] However, the use of ketoconazole is associated with drug interactions, as well as significant toxicities due to non-specific inhibition of cytochrome P-450. The advent of more specific and effective novel CYP17 inhibitors has led to ketoconazole becoming a suboptimal treatment option.[13]

Abiraterone acetate: Abiraterone acetate, a pregnenolone analog and its metabolite abiraterone, is a selective irreversible inhibitor of CYP17 α-hydroxylase and C(17,20)-lyase, which are required for androgen biosynthesis (Fig. 2). *In vitro* studies have demonstrated that abiraterone is a more potent inhibitor of the CYP-17 when compared to ketoconazole.[14]

To evaluate the safety and establish the maximum tolerated dose of oral abiraterone acetate in patients with and without prior ketoconazole therapy, 33 men with chemotherapy-naive progressive CRPC were enrolled in a phase I clinical trial.[15] Abiraterone acetate was administered in escalated dosing cohorts of 250, 500, 750 and 1000 mg with non-fasting and fasting cohorts enrolled at each dose. Abiraterone acetate, at a dose of 1000 mg daily, was well tolerated irrespective of prior ketoconazole usage. In addition, there were no differences observed in toxicity or PSA declines between the fasting and non-fasting cohorts. The most frequent and serious toxicities were hypertension and hypokalemia, which were attributable to secondary mineralocorticoid excess, and which responded to medical management.

In a phase II study, the efficacy and safety of abiraterone acetate in combination with prednisone was studied in 58 men with progressive CRPC who experienced a prior treatment failure to docetaxel-based chemotherapy.[15] Patients received abiraterone acetate at a dose of 1000 mg daily, along with prednisone, 5 mg twice a day, to reduce secondary hyperaldosteronism with abiraterone monotherapy. The primary outcome was a 50 per cent or greater decline in PSA and was achieved in 36 per cent of patients. The addition of prednisone reduced the incidence of mineralocorticoid-related toxicity. This was followed by phase III studies in patients with CRPC in the post- and pre-docetaxel settings, respectively (Table 1). One phase III trial enrolled 1,195 patients with metastatic CRPC with a history of prior docetaxel chemotherapy. Patients were randomized in a 2:1 fashion to receive 5 mg of prednisone twice daily, with either 1000 mg of abiraterone acetate (797 patients) or placebo (398 patients).[16] A pre-specified interim analysis demonstrated a survival benefit of abiraterone acetate over placebo [14.8 months versus 10.9 months; hazard ratio (HR), 0.65; 95 per cent confidence interval (CI), 0.54 to 0.77; $p < 0.001$), resulting in crossover of all eligible patients in the placebo group to receive abiraterone. The final analysis before the crossover demonstrated that at a median follow-up of 20.2 months, overall survival with abiraterone acetate was significantly better than that with placebo (15.8 months versus 11.2 months; HR, 0.74; 95 per cent CI, 0.64–0.86; $p < 0 \cdot 0001$). In addition, a survival benefit was observed across all subgroups.[17] Another phase III study evaluated 1,088 men with CRPC who had never received chemotherapy. Patients were randomized in 1:1 fashion to receive either abiraterone with prednisone or placebo with prednisone.[18] The co-primary endpoints were radiographic progression-free survival and overall survival. At the planned interim analysis, the study was unblinded after 43 per cent of the expected deaths had occurred. The median radiographic progression-free survival was significantly improved with abiraterone–prednisone compared to placebo–prednisone (16.5 months versus 8.3 months; HR, 0.53; 95 per cent CI, 0.45–0.62; $p < 0.001$). Overall survival was also improved

Table 1 Phase III Clinical Trials of Abiraterone, Enzalutamide, and TAK-700. CRPC: Castration Resistant Prostate Cancer

Intervention	Number of Patients	Primary Question	Primary Endpoint(s)	Outcome	Identifier (*clinicaltrials.gov*)
Abiraterone acetate + predisone versus placebo + prednisone	1,088	To compare the clinical benefit of abiraterone acetate plus prednisone in asymptomatic or mildly symptomatic patients with CRPC	OS, R-PFS	Improved OS (median not reached, versus 27.2 months; $p = 0.01$) and improved R-PFS (16.5 months versus 8.3 months; $p < 0.001$)	NCT00887198
Abiraterone + prednisone versus placebo + prednisone	1,197	To compare the clinical benefit of abiraterone plus prednisone with placebo plus prednisone in patients with metastatic CRPC who were previously treated with docetaxel-based chemotherapy	OS	Improved OS (15.8 months versus 11.2 months; $p < 0.0001$)	NCT00638690
Enzalutamide versus placebo	1,199	To compare the clinical benefit of MDV3100 versus placebo in patients with CRPC who have been previously treated with docetaxel-based chemotherapy (AFFIRM trial)	OS	Improved OS (18.4 months versus 13.6 months; $p < 0.001$)	NCT00974311

(*Continued*)

Table 1 (Continued)

Intervention	Number of Patients	Primary Question	Primary Endpoint(s)	Outcome	Identifier (*clinicaltrials.gov*)
Enzalutamide versus placebo	1,680	To study the efficacy and safety of oral enzalutamide in chemotherapy-naive patients with metastatic prostate cancer who have failed ADT (PREVAIL trial)	OS PFS	Ongoing (enrolling)	NCT01212991
TAK-700 + prednisone versus placebo + prednisone	1,083	To evaluate the the effect of TAK-700 plus prednisone compared with placebo plus prednisone in metastatic CRPC patients who have progressed following docetaxel therapy	OS	Ongoing (completed enrollment in 2012)	NCT01193257
TAK-700 + prednisone versus placebo + prednisone	1,454	To evaluate the efficacy TAK-700 plus prednisone compared with placebo plus prednisone in chemo-naive metastatic CRPC	OS R-PFS	Ongoing (completed enrollment in 2012)	NCT01193244

NCT: *clinicaltrials.gov* indentifier. (OS overall survival; PFS: progression-free survival; R-PFS: radiographic progression-free survival; ADT: androgen deprivation therapy) with abiraterone–prednisone (median not reached, versus 27.2 months for placebo–prednisone; HR, 0.75; 95 per cent CI, 0.61–0.93; $p = 0.01$), but did not cross the efficacy boundary. Notably, all secondary endpoints, including the time to initiation of cytotoxic chemotherapy, opiate use for cancer-related pain, prostate-specific antigen (PSA) progression, and decline in performance status, were improved with abiraterone–prednisone compared to placebo–prednisone. These data led to the regulatory approval of abiraterone acetate in the treatment of metastatic CRPC in the pre- and post-chemotherapy setting.

TAK 700: TAK-700 (orteronel), a novel naphthyl methylimidazole derivative, is a highly selective inhibitor of 17,20-lyase activity of CYP17, and has been demonstrated to potently reduce serum testosterone and dehydroepiandosterone (DHEA-S) levels in animal models (Fig. 2).[19] The data from a phase II study of TAK 700 in chemo-naive patients were presented at the 2012 Genitourinary Cancers Symposium.[20] Ninety-seven patients were treated with TAK-700 in four different dose cohorts: 300 mg BID ($n = 23$), 400 mg BID + prednisone 5 mg BID ($n = 24$), 600 mg BID + prednisone ($n = 26$), or 600 mg QD ($n = 24$). Sixty-two percent of patients withdrew from the study, including 19 per cent due to secondary adverse effects and 19 per cent due to disease progression. At a 12-week follow-up analysis, the median levels of testosterone, DHEA-S, as well as the mean circulating tumor cell numbers, were decreased in all groups. The PSA response rates (50 per cent or greater) at 12 weeks were 63 per cent, 50 per cent, 41 per cent, and 60 per cent in the 300 mg BID, 400 mg BID + prednisone, 600 mg BID + prednisone, and 600 mg QD groups, respectively. The most common grade 3 or greater adverse effects were fatigue (12 per cent) and hypokalemia (8 per cent). Another phase II trial evaluated TAK 700 in 38 patients with non-metastatic CRPC with biochemical recurrence and demonstrated that treatment was achievable with minimal toxicities.[22] Patients were treated with TAK 700 at a dose of 300 mg twice daily and after three months of treatment, nearly 76 per cent of men achieved a 50 per cent or greater decrease in PSA levels. Currently, two phase III randomized, placebo controlled trials are ongoing comparing the efficacy of TAK-700, 400 mg orally BID with placebo in chemotherapy-naive patients, and in patients who have previously progressed on docetaxel (Table 1).

5.4. DRUGS TARGETING THE ANDROGEN RECEPTOR

Enzalutamide: Enzalutamide, formerly referred to as MDV3100, is a novel a thiohydantoin androgen receptor antagonist that binds to the androgen binding site of the androgen receptor with a greater relative affinity than the clinically used antiandrogen bicalutamide. Enzalutamide reduces the efficiency of the nuclear translocation androgen receptor, DNA binding to androgen response elements and recruitment of co-activators by the androgen receptor.[21]

In a phase I–II trial to assess the safety and antitumor activity of enzalutamide in progressive metastatic CRPC, 140 patients were treated with enzalutamide at doses ranging from 30 mg to 600 mg daily.[22] Once the safety of a dose was established, cohorts were expanded to include at least 12 chemotherapy-naive and 12 post-chemotherapy treated patients. The maximum tolerated dose was determined to be 240 mg once daily. Antitumor effects were seen at all doses, including decreases in serum PSA of 50 per cent or greater in 56 per cent of patients, soft tissue responses in 22 per cent of patients, stabilization of bone disease in 56 per cent of patients, and conversion from unfavorable to favorable circulating tumor cell counts in 49 per cent of patients. Enzalutamide was generally well tolerated, with fatigue as the most common dose-dependent grade 3–4 side effect.

In the phase III double-blind, placebo-controlled AFFIRM trial, 1,199 men with CRPC following chemotherapy were randomized in a 2:1 ratio to receive either enzalutamide at a dose of 160 mg per day (800 patients) or placebo (399 patients)[23] (Table 1). The study was stopped following the planned interim analysis after 520 deaths had occurred. Due to the superior results seen with enzalutamide, the study was unblinded and patients were allowed to crossover to the enzalutamide arm. Results from the interim analysis demonstrated that survival was significantly better in all the subgroups who received enzalutamide over placebo (18.4 months versus 13.6 months; HR, 0.63; 95 per cent CI, 0.53–0.75; $p < 0.001$). Enzalutamide was also superior to placebo with respect to all secondary endpoints including 50 per cent or greater reduction in PSA levels (54 per cent versus 2 per cent; $p < 0.001$), soft tissue response (29 per cent versus 4 per cent; $p < 0.001$), quality of life response (43 percent versus 18 per cent; $p < 0.001$), time to PSA progression (8.3 months versus 3 months; $p < 0.001$), radiographic progression free survival (8.3 months versus 2.9 months; HR, 0.40; $p < 0.001$) and time to the first skeletal related event (16.7 versus 13.3 months; HR, 0.69; $p < 0.001$). Rates of fatigue, diarrhea and hot flashes were higher in the enzalutamide group. In addition, the risk of seizure was higher in the enzalutamide treated group, with 0.9 per cent of patients experiencing a seizure. There are two ongoing studies evaluating the role of enzalutamide prior to cytotoxic chemotherapy in men with prostate cancer after failure of primary ADT, both in metastatic and non-metastatic settings. Safety and Efficacy Study of Enzalutamide Versus Bicalutamide in Men With Prostate Cancer (STRIVE) is a phase-II study (*clinicaltrials.gov* ID: NCT01664923) comparing the efficacy and safety of oral enzalutamide (160 mg/day) with oralbicalutamide (50 mg/day) in men with prostate cancer who have failed primary androgen deprivation therapy (Table 1). The STRIVE trial is scheduled to be completed by July 2014 with an estimated enrollment of 400 patients. The primary outcome is progression-free survival at 24 months and the secondary outcomes are PSA response, time to PSA progression, time to radiographic progression, safety, and Functional Assessment of Cancer Therapy-Prostate (FACT-P). The second study, PREVAIL, is a phase-III multinational, randomized, double-blind, placebo-controlled trial to assess the safety and efficacy of oral MDV3100 in chemotherapy-naive patients with progressive metastatic prostate cancer who have failed androgen deprivation therapy (Table 1). The goal is to accrue 1,680 patients with an estimated study completion date of September 2014. The primary outcomes are overall and progression-free survival and the secondary outcomes are time to initiation of cytotoxic chemotherapy and first skeletal related event.

ARN-509: ARN-509 is a novel small molecule AR antagonist, which is structurally and mechanistically similar to enzalutamide. ARN-509 impairs AR nuclear translocation, as well as AR binding to DNA, thereby inhibiting tumor growth and promoting apoptosis. In prostate cancer cell line models with AR over expression, ARN-509 ($IC50 = 16$ nmol/L) was 7 to 10 times more potent than the clinically approved bicalutamide ($IC50 = 160$ nmol/L).[24] Similarly, in a murine xenograft model of CRPC, ARN-509 inhibited tumor growth more effectively than enzalutamide at a lower optimal biological dose and at a steady state plasma level.[24] These findings led to the development of phase I clinical trials with encouraging results. In a dose-escalated phase I study of 33 men with metastatic CRPC, ARN-509 was found to be safe and well tolerated and with pharmacodynamic evidence of AR antagonism with promising clinical activity, with 42 per cent of patients demonstrating a 50 per cent or greater PSA decline. The most common treatment related grade 1–2 side effects were fatigue (38 per cent), nausea (29 per cent), and pain (24 per cent), with one patient developing grade 3 abdominal pain at a dose of 300 mg. A dose of 240 mg daily was established for further phase II studies.[25] One phase II study is currently enrolling patients to one the following three cohorts: (i) non-metastatic treatment-naive CRPC; (ii) chemotherapy-naive metastatic (m) CRPC and (iii) chemotherapy-naive, post-abirateronem CRPC. The primary study objective is to determine the PSA response at 12 weeks (Table 1). Overall, given its significantly high potency, ARN-509 has potential for use in the setting of "combined androgen blockade" in men with hormone sensitive prostate cancer.

TOK-001: TOK-001 (galeterone) is a rationally designed inhibitor of androgen biosynthesis that is structurally similar to abiraterone. Like abiraterone, TOK-001 directly inhibits CYP17, as well as androgen receptor, but TOK-001 has the additional unique ability to down-regulate AR expression.[26] In mouse xenograft models, TOK-001 reduced tumor growth more effectively than castration and bicalutamide.[26] In a phase I dose-escalated study of 49 patients with chemotherapy-naive CRPC, TOK-001 was well tolerated, and the maximal tolerated dose was not reached. TOK-001 demonstrated clinical activity with 11 (22 per cent) patients demonstrating a 50 per cent or greater PSA decline and an additional 13 patients (26 per cent) with 30–50 per cent declines.[27] Additional pharmacokinetic and phase II studies are currently being planned.

EPI-001: The androgen receptor (AR) consists of three distinct functional domains, a C-terminal ligand-binding domain (LBD), DNA-binding domain (DBD), and an amino-terminal domain (NTD). The NTD of the AR plays an important role in the transcriptional activity of the androgen bound AR, and is also activated by several ligand independent mechanisms.[28] Targeting the NTD of the AR with small molecule inhibitors has recently gained much-needed attention. EPI-001 is the lead compound that inhibits AR, regardless of the presence of ligand. Treatment with EPI-001 reduced the size of the prostate in intact mice compared with control treated animals, and also reduced tumor growth in mouse xenograft models.[29] Unlike traditional antiandrogens that target the LBD, EPI-001 has the unique ability to overcome castration resistance associated with gain of function mutations of the LBD, and expression of constitutionally active splice variants. However, EPI-001 is yet to enter clinical trials in men.

EZN-4176: Targeting AR mRNA is a novel therapeutic strategy in prostate cancer. EZN-4176 is a locked nucleic acid-based antisense oligonucleotide (LNA-ASO) that specifically binds within exon 4 of the AR mRNA and down-modulates AR expression.[30] EZN-4176 was also shown to reduce AR mediated transcriptional activity and cell growth in prostate cancer cell line models and inhibit tumor growth in mouse xenograft models in both androgen sensitive and castration resistant settings. This data led to an ongoing phase I study of EZN-4176 in men with CRPC (*clinicaltrials.gov* ID: NCT01337518).

5.5. CONCLUSIONS

Improved understanding in the molecular biology underlying progression of CRPC over the last two decades has led to unraveling of novel molecular targets. This has led to a revolution in the development of drugs designed for these targets. Many drugs have been approved by the regulatory bodies and are already in clinical use. Many others are either at the verge of approval or in advanced phases of development. Within a short span of three years, these exciting developments have fundamentally changed the paradigm of treatment of CRPC. These developments have also established CRPC as a poster child for the application of bench research and emerging science to clinical practice, with the hopes that similar developments will also continue to improve treatment outcomes in other types of cancer.

REFERENCES

1. Jemal A, Bray F, Center MM, *et al.* (2011) Global cancer statistics. *CA Cancer J Clin* **61**: 69–90.

2. Siegel R, Naishadham D, Jemal A. (2012) Cancer statistics, 2012. *CA Cancer J Clin* **62**: 10–29.
3. Crawford ED, Eisenberger MA, McLeod DG, *et al.* (1989) A controlled trial of leuprolide with and without flutamide in prostatic carcinoma. *N Engl J Med* **321**: 419–424.
4. Taplin ME, Rajeshkumar B, Halabi S, *et al.* (2003) Androgen receptor mutations in androgen-independent prostate cancer: Cancer and Leukemia Group B Study 9663. *J Clin Oncol* **21**: 2673–2678.
5. Titus MA, Schell MJ, Lih FB, *et al.* (2005) Testosterone and dihydrotestosterone tissue levels in recurrent prostate cancer. *Clin Cancer Res* **11**: 4653–4657.
6. Chen Y, Clegg NJ, Scher HI. (2009) Anti-androgens and androgen-depleting therapies in prostate cancer: New agents for an established target. *Lancet Oncol* **10**: 981–991.
7. Montgomery RB. (2008) Maintenance of intratumoral androgens in metastatic prostate cancer: A mechanism for castration-resistant tumor growth. *Cancer Res* **68**: 4447–4454.
8. Dillard PR, Lin MF, Khan SA. (2008) Androgen-independent prostate cancer cells acquire the complete steroidogenic potential of synthesizing testosterone from cholesterol. *Mol Cell Endocrinol* **295**: 115–120.
9. Edwards J, Krishna NS, Grigor KM, *et al.* (2003) Androgen receptor gene amplification and protein expression in hormone refractory prostate cancer. *Br J Cancer* **89**: 552–556.
10. Steinkamp MP, O'Mahony OA, Brogley M, *et al.* (2009) Treatment-dependent androgen receptor mutations in prostate cancer exploit multiple mechanisms to evade therapy. *Cancer Res* **69**: 4434–4442.
11. Li Y, Chan SC, Brand LJ, *et al.* (2013) Androgen receptor splice variants mediate enzalutamide resistance in castration-resistant prostate cancer cell lines. *Cancer Res* **73**: 483–489.
12. Small EJ, Halabi S, Dawson NA, *et al.* (2004) Antiandrogen withdrawal alone or in combination with ketoconazole in androgen-independent prostate cancer patients: A phase III trial (CALGB 9583). *J Clin Oncol* **22**: 1025–1033.
13. Small EJ, Vogelzang NJ. (1997) Second-line hormonal therapy for advanced prostate cancer: A shifting paradigm. *J Clin Oncol* **15**: 382–388.
14. Haidar S, Ehmer PB, Barassin S, *et al.* (2003) Effects of novel 17 alpha-hydroxylase/C17, 20-lyase (P450 17, CYP 17) inhibitors on androgen biosynthesis *in vitro* and *in vivo*. *J Steroid Biochem Mol Biol* **84**: 555–562.
15. Danila DC, Morris MJ, de Bono JS, *et al.* (2010). Phase II multicenter study of abiraterone acetate plus prednisone therapy in patients with docetaxel-treated castration-resistant prostate cancer. *J Clin Oncol* **28**: 1496–1501.

16. de Bono JS, Logothetis CJ, Molina A, *et al.* (2011) Abiraterone and increased survival in metastatic prostate cancer. *N Engl J Med* **364**: 1995–2005.
17. Fizazi K, Scher HI, Molina A, *et al.* (2012) Abiraterone acetate for treatment of metastatic castration-resistant prostate cancer: Final overall survival analysis of the COU-AA-301 randomised, double-blind, placebo-controlled phase 3 study. *Lancet Oncol* **13**: 983–992.
18. Ryan CJ, Smith MR, de Bono JS, *et al.* (2013) Abiraterone in metastatic prostate cancer without previous chemotherapy. *N Engl J Med* **368**: 138–148.
19. Kaku T, Hitaka T, Ojida A, *et al.* (2011) Discovery of orteronel (TAK-700), a naphthyl methylimidazole derivative, as a highly selective 17,20-lyase inhibitor with potential utility in the treatment of prostate cancer. *Bioorg Med Chem* **19**: 6383–6399.
20. Agus DA, Stadler WM, Shevrin DH, *et al.* (2012) Safety, efficacy, and pharmacodynamics of the investigational agent orteronel (TAK-700) in metastatic castration-resistant prostate cancer (mCRPC): Updated data from a phase I/II study. *J Clin Oncol* **30**: abstract 98.
21. Tran C, Ouk S, Clegg NJ, *et al.* (2009) Development of a second-generation antiandrogen for treatment of advanced prostate cancer. *Science* **324**: 787–790.
22. Scher HI, Beer TM, Higano CS, *et al.* (2010) Antitumour activity of MDV3100 in castration-resistant prostate cancer: A phase 1–2 study. *Lancet* **375**: 1437–1446.
23. Scher HI, Fizazi K, Saad F, *et al.* (2012) Increased survival with enzalutamide in prostate cancer after chemotherapy. *N Engl J Med* **367**: 1187–1197.
24. Clegg NJ, Wongvipat J, Joseph JD, *et al.* (2012) ARN-509: A novel antiandrogen for prostate cancer treatment. *Cancer Res* **72**: 1494–1503.
25. Rathkopf DE, Danila DC, Slovin SF, *et al.* (2012) A phase I study of the androgen signaling inhibitor ARN-509 in patients with metastatic castration-resistant prostate cancer (mCRPC). *J Clin Oncol* **30**(suppl): abstract 4548.
26. Vasaitis T, Belosay A, Schayowitz A, *et al.* (2008) Androgen receptor inactivation contributes to antitumor efficacy of 17{alpha}-hydroxylase/17,20-lyase inhibitor 3 beta-hydroxy-17-(1H-benzimidazole-1-yl)androsta-5,16-diene in prostate cancer. *Mol Cancer Ther* **7**: 2348–2357.
27. Montgomery RB, Eisenberger MA, Rettig M, *et al.* (2012) Phase I clinical trial of galeterone (TOK-001), a multifunctional antiandrogen and CYP17 inhibitor in castration resistant prostate cancer (CRPC). *J Clin Oncol* **30**(suppl): abstract 4665.
28. Quayle SN, Mawji NR, Wang J, *et al.* (2007) Androgen receptor decoy molecules block the growth of prostate cancer. *Proc Natl Acad Sci USA* **104**: 1331–1336.

29. Andersen RJ, Mawji NR, Wang J, *et al.* (2010) Regression of castrate-recurrent prostate cancer by a small-molecule inhibitor of the amino-terminus domain of the androgen receptor. *Cancer Cell* 17: 535–546.
30. Zhang Y, Castaneda S, Dumble M, *et al.* (2011) Reduced expression of the androgen receptor by third generation of antisense shows antitumor activity in models of prostate cancer. *Mol Cancer Ther* **10**: 2309–2319.

CHAPTER 6

Recruitment to Early Phase Cancer Clinical Trials: Barriers and Opportunities

Izabella Zandberg[*,†] *and Colleen R. Leonard*[*]

6.1. INTRODUCTION

Clinical trials are a crucial component in the research, development and evaluation of disease treatment strategies. However, clinicians and researchers have historically experienced problems in recruiting adequate numbers of participants to clinical trials. In fact, patient recruitment is one of the most significant bottlenecks in treatment development; many patients who would be eligible to participate never have the opportunity to do so, and most potential patients do not know that a clinical trial might be a treatment option for them. In addition, various barriers prevent many physicians from participating in clinical research, thereby making it less likely that their patients will participate. Slow or insufficient patient enrollment in clinical trials contributes significantly to the slow rate of completion and occasional failure of some trials. The costs of failed or delayed trials include not only wasted resources that were allocated to them, but also the costs of participants' time and discouragement of primary care professionals from cooperating with further research. There is a critical need to increase the number of adult patients with cancer who participate

[*]Independent Consultant, Research Solutions International, LLC, Rockville, Maryland, USA
[†]Corresponding author: Izabella Zandberg, PhD, Research Solutions International, LLC, 1142 Regal Oak Drive, Rockville, MD 20852, USA; E-mail: *izandberg@rsi-research.com*, *izandberg@aol.com*; Tel: +1-301-545-0083
Large parts of the original research for this article were conducted by the authors at Westat, under contract to the National Cancer Institute. Carl Setzer contributed to this research.

in clinical trials. This chapter broadly reviews the issues concerning patient participation in cancer clinical trials and explores the structural and individual determinants of patient recruitment.

6.2. FACTORS THAT INFLUENCE PATIENT PARTICIPATION IN EARLY PHASE CANCER CLINICAL TRIALS

6.2.1. Public Attitudes and Knowledge toward Participation in Clinical Trials

When analyzing factors that may influence participation in early phase cancer clinical trials, one must consider that patients eligible for such trials are facing death from an incurable cancer and therefore represent an audience that is very different from the general population. Thus, the decision-making context for these patients is particularly complex and difficult, and the extent to which public attitudes and knowledge about clinical trials influence accrual to early phase cancer clinical trials is not at all clear. However, current public sentiment and knowledge are a part of the environment in which patients are recruited to early phase trials.

In 2000, the Coalition of National Cancer Cooperative Groups in collaboration with Harris Interactive fielded surveys on the subject of cancer clinical trials with American adults (without cancer), cancer patients, and physicians (both oncologists and primary care physicians). A large proportion of adults surveyed indicated positive attitudes towards cancer clinical trials, with 80 percent saying that they would consider a clinical trial if faced with cancer. Also, 80 percent of the respondents believed that patients who participate in clinical trials benefit themselves and others[1]; however, it is unclear to what extent these findings can be extrapolated to the early phase cancer clinical trials. There is also evidence that public perception of clinical trials still has strong negative overtones of medical experimentation, and public knowledge about clinical research in general seems limited.[1–3]

6.2.2. Patients' Barriers and Motivators for Participation in Early Phase Cancer Clinical Trials

Many researchers have sought to illuminate the factors that influence whether a person with cancer decides to participate in an early phase clinical trial. While there is convergence in the literature about the role of some factors (e.g., hope), there is less agreement about others (e.g., the role and importance of altruism as a motivator). There is still more scholarly discussion in related areas, such as the extent to which terminally ill cancer patients are a vulnerable population, the extent to which patients understand the objectives of early phase trials, and how facing death may redefine patients' thinking about their treatment. In their examination of arguments for patient participation in phase I trials, Agrawal and Emanuel[4] suggested that advanced cancer patients' values may be profoundly changed by their poor prognoses, and those values may in turn affect how phase I trial enrollees view the risks and benefits of participation. That is, a risk–benefit ratio that might appear unacceptable to anyone else (e.g., physicians) may be acceptable to a patient with advanced cancer. Consequently, the authors suggest, any analysis of factors motivating terminally ill patients to participate in early phase cancer trials should be conducted from the patients' perspective, taking into consideration both the complexity of the decision-making context of a person facing mortality and resulting from it possible change in values of the person making the decision.

6.2.3. Awareness of Clinical Trials among Patients with Cancer

In order to make a judgment about participating in a clinical trial, a patient must first be aware that the option exists. The Harris survey of the general public, cancer patients, and primary care physicians conducted in 2000 found that lack of awareness about clinical trials was a major factor inhibiting patient accrual to cancer clinical trials in general. In fact, 85 percent of the cancer patients surveyed said they were not aware of clinical trials, while most of these patients (about 75 percent) said they would be willing to enroll, had they known it was possible.[5] Although physicians appeared to be the leading source of awareness, patients also indicated that they learned of clinical trials through other sources such as the Internet, news media, and advocacy organizations. With a growing number of Internet resources that provide information about cancer clinical trials, access to information has become easier over time, and studies suggest that improved written information increases participation in clinical trials.[6] The extent to which these findings can be extrapolated to the early phase cancer clinical trials is not clear.

6.2.4. Patients' Understanding of the Objectives of Early Phase Clinical Trials

Patients who enroll in early phase clinical trials harbor considerable hope of receiving significant therapeutic benefit or being among the "lucky few" who experience tumor reduction.[7,8] Yet the purpose and procedures of early phase trials mean that each patient's chance of tumor reduction is exceedingly slim.[9] This tension between the staying power of seemingly unrealistic high hopes and the reality that informed consent procedures seek to convey is at the center of some debate.[4,10,11] At its heart, the unresolved question is whether patients can hold out such hope while also completely understanding that the study itself is not specifically intended to make them well, nor is it likely that it will. One perspective is that hope and such understanding cannot truly coexist, and that even the most well-intentioned doctors may unknowingly allow patients to maintain some positive misconceptions about a trial.[10] Meropol *et al.*[12] explored the discrepancy between patients' and physicians' expectations and concluded that patients rated their chances of benefit higher than did their physicians. The authors thus posited that the communication between physicians and patients on the purpose of trials and likelihood of benefit may be flawed.

However, other researchers argue that while there are paradoxes in patients' experiences, patients can and do find ways to resolve them — including understanding the reality of their disease while also hoping for miracles.[11] In a re-examination of the arguments and data surrounding the ethics of phase I cancer studies, Agrawal and Emanuel[4] concluded that most patients understand that they may not directly benefit from participation even when they hope to. Additionally, Weinfurt *et al.*[13] suggested that by reporting their high expectations for a positive outcome of a trial, patients may in fact be reporting their belief about the future, reassuring their family members, and/or trying to improve the potential outcome by publicly expressing their optimism.

Although the apparent disconnect between physicians and patients on the matter of early phase trials' reality versus hope is clear, its meaning for recruitment is not as obvious. In some cases, authors have pointed to potentially negative consequences for recruiting. For example, the fact that patients often either misrepresent the purpose of early phase trials or have unrealistic expectations may lead to strained patient–physician relationships.[8] Yet hope remains one of the strongest motivators for phase I and II trial participants.

6.2.5. Factors that May Motivate Patients to Participate in Early Phase Clinical Trials

Researchers' findings were clear that hope for a therapeutic benefit, and even for a cure, is a strong and abiding motivator among those who opt to participate in early phase trials.[7,8,14] In one of the few studies to explore the differences between cancer patients who decline to participate and those who accept, Meropol *et al.*[12] found that those who joined a phase I trial believed themselves more likely to benefit from experimental therapy than did those who did not join. Conversely, those who declined had higher expectations for standard treatment than those who accepted.

For early phase cancer clinical trial participants, altruism — specifically, the desire to help future cancer patients by advancing research — is said to play a role in decision-making. However, the extent to which it is a motivator is less clear. In some cases, altruism was said to be present but *not* a motivating factor for phase I trial participants.[14,15] Moore[11] integrated this lack of consensus by characterizing the role of altruism as "receiving and giving," whereby patients feel that they are both receiving the best treatment and also helping future cancer patients.

Other people, most importantly doctors, were found to play a role in patients' decisions about whether or not to join a trial. For example, Daugherty *et al.*[15] found that the physician–patient relationship played a major role in decision-making for approximately two-thirds of the surveyed phase I patients. Also, the Harris poll, conducted in 2000, found that most patients in clinical trials said that a doctor had a great deal of influence on their decision to participate. Respondents in this poll were cancer patients participating in trials, yet it is not known how many (if any) of them were phase I or II participants. Nonetheless, trial participants were far more likely than non-participants to have a doctor who helped them understand the benefits and drawbacks of participating, and helped them find an appropriate trial.[1] Relevant details of doctor–patient communication and doctors' motivators are described below. Furthermore, family members also played a role, with early phase trial patients in one study saying that they felt more support than they ever expected.[8]

Expectations about the trial itself were found to facilitate participation. For example, phase I patients expected and often received support and positive interaction with the trials' doctors and nurses. Interacting with clinical trial staff may offer a special kind of relief and comfort that is difficult to find in day-to-day life, as the staff members are uniquely familiar with cancer and cancer patients' experiences. Trial participation also had other documented benefits such as providing a meaningful cadence to day-to-day life. Finally, those who joined clinical trials had strong expectations that the care they would receive would be better in the trial.[8]

Some factors were less thoroughly described, but suggest promising avenues for future study. Specifically, Moore[11] illuminated the culturally embedded refusal to "give up" (i.e., to stop seeking and using treatment options), and early phase clinical trial patients' fears about facing cancer "unarmed" when treatment options have been exhausted. In Moore's qualitative study of the experiences of these clinical trial participants, patients expressed a need to try anything and everything, and even described themselves as feeling lucky or honored to have been offered another treatment opportunity through the trial. Moore went on to describe a "paradox of hope," in which phase I and II clinical trial patients fully grasp the reality of their situation and the fact that their clinical trial participation is not likely to result in being cured, but embrace and benefit from participation because it means "trying everything" and not giving up hope.

6.2.6. Factors that May Prevent Patients with Cancer from Participating in a Clinical Trial

The reasons that cancer patients choose *not* to participate in trials have been explored less than the reasons that they do. Writing about patients in all phases of cancer clinical trials, Cox and McGarry[16] speculated that so few studies have addressed these barriers owing to challenges associated with finding patients who have opted out, because researchers may lack interest in those who are not participating, and because refusing to participate may cause internal turmoil for patients (e.g., feeling they have chosen death over prolonged life), thereby making them reluctant to answer questions about their decision.

Research suggests that concerns about quality of life, and whether the potential improvement is worth the possibly acute side effects, are an important factor in patients' decision to enroll in an early phase clinical trial.[17] A study of 30 cancer patients participating in a phase I trial by Cheng *et al.*[18] found that quality of life may be an important determinant of patients' expectations regarding the potential benefit of experimental therapy and, ultimately, their choice of treatment. The authors conclude that better understanding of the interactions between quality of life and patients' perceptions of potential benefit should inform the informed-consent process in the future.

Furthermore, for prospective trial participants who are aware of clinical trials in general or have been invited to participate in a specific trial, a handful of known key factors may tip the scales against participation. Specifically, practical matters such as work obligations and logistical matters such as travel difficulties might have deterred potential participants.[1,19,20] NCI's *Cancer Clinical Trials: A Resource Guide for Outreach, Education, and Advocacy*[21] pointed specifically to the time commitment, travel issues, and indirect costs of being away from work and family as barriers to participation for adults with cancer. These factors are known to be related to trial participation in general, but are not well explored for phase I and II trials in particular.

Some patients do not enroll in trials because of fears related to experimentation. In 1999, Klabunde *et al.*[22] reported that 15 percent of the 407 clinically eligible patients who did not enroll in cancer treatment trials of a large Community Clinical Oncology Program (CCOP) cited such fears. In the 2002 Harris poll,[2] 22 percent of non-participating patients feared such treatment. In addition to fearing experimentation, patients also were concerned about receiving a placebo rather than a medication they need or expect to receive. In one study unrelated to cancer treatment, both the assumption that a new treatment is better than placebo and the fear of receiving a placebo were found to diminish the possibility that a patient will elect to participate in a trial.[23] While this concern is less an issue for early phase trials, which do not typically include a placebo arm, the existing concern among patients and the public is a part of the milieu in which early phase trials must recruit patients.

Although it is less pertinent to the clinical trials conducted in the Warren Grant Magnuson Clinical Center, which are free, it is important to note that until the year 2000, phase I, II and III clinical trials were considered by the Centers for Medicare & Medicaid Services as "experimental" and therefore not eligible for coverage. Concerns about health insurance (e.g., potential denial of coverage, increased out-of-pocket costs) are other known deterrents to participation in cancer treatment trials, particularly for minority and other under served groups, as will be discussed below.[1] In general, the literature provides some understanding of how health insurance status can influence patient accrual to cancer treatment trials, but does not focus specifically on phase I and II trials. A 1999 US General Accounting Office (GAO) report[24] indicated that "as a general rule," health insurance policies do not cover clinical trials, although most say that they will consider particular treatments or activities case by case. While health insurance matters are mitigated at NCI because public monies, rather than patients, pay for trial treatments, potential enrollees may not be aware of this fact and may remain deterred by their insurance concerns. Two studies of enrollees in NCI cancer treatment trials considered how health insurance may influence enrollment by exploring the insurance status of enrolled patients. Sateren *et al.*[25] found patients in NCI phase I, II, and III clinical trials were significantly less likely to be *un*insured than the US population in general. These patients were also significantly more likely to have Medicare. A study of patients who were evaluated for enrollment in NCI-sponsored trials at 15 medical facilities in the Southeast[22] found that patients with fee-for-service insurance coverage were more than twice as likely to become enrolled as patients with HMO/PPO, Medicare, Medicaid, self-pay, or other coverage. On the other hand, a recent study of the effects of state-mandated insurance coverage on accrual to community cancer clinical trials[26] found that the state mandate does not appear to increase patient accrual to NCI Community Clinical Oncology Program (CCOP) clinical trials. It is unclear to what extent these findings apply to patient accrual to early phase cancer clinical trials.

6.2.7. Participation in Cancer Clinical Trials among Racial/Ethnic Minorities

Historically, minority groups have been under represented in clinical research in general. This low participation has been the subject of numerous research studies, and the reasons for it vary among populations. For example, for the African American population, distrust and suspicion are cited as one of the most important factors obstructing participation[27,28] For the Native American patients, distrust of research as well as practices of folk medicine might constitute a barrier.[29,30] Asian and Pacific Islander patients, as well as doctors and family members, might react to various cultural stigma associated with illness[31,32]

It is important to note that while differences exist within racial/ethnic groups, some themes about how various populations relate to clinical trial participation are common.[33] The single factor that applies across the board is that past and current stereotyping of minority patients as "difficult to reach," "noncompliant," or "unwilling" exists and is glaringly unhelpful in the effort to ensure that cancer research includes and benefits all.[34–36] In addition, issues related to social and economic difficulties among patients may be particularly relevant among minority populations, who are poor in disproportionate numbers. Such issues have included lack of access to health care in general, poor quality of available health services, transportation barriers and costs, time away from work and family, and health insurance concerns.[25,37,38] Additional barriers for minority women to participate in cancer trials were thought to include poor physical functioning, as well as advanced disease and comorbidities.[39] Also, low participation of minority physicians in clinical trials, lack of provider awareness about clinical trials, as well as attitudinal barriers among physicians related to their perceptions of patient adherence to the study protocol, patient cost and data collection cost, were proposed as possible additional barriers to the accrual of minority patients.[28,38] The fact that no consistent measurement approach has been developed to compare the outcomes of various recruitment strategies for minority populations across trials was suggested as impending "equity in distribution of benefits and burdens of cancer-related trials."[40] In addition, differential access to medical facilities with unequal research infrastructures has been identified as a systemic barrier to the equitable inclusion of minorities in clinical research.[41] The following factors have been identified in the literature as affecting participation in clinical trials among specific racial/ethnic minorities:

African Americans: Shavers, Lynch and Burmeister[27] argued that lack of trust in medical research is the most critical impediment to African American participation (see also Ref. 42). This premise is borne out across the literature on this subject, with the issue described in terms ranging from "fear and suspicion" to "longstanding mistrust."[21,43] Specifically, the impact of the legacy of the Tuskegee Syphilis Study, in which African American men were studied but not given needed treatment for syphilis, was undeniable in a variety of studies. Studies both suggested and empirically demonstrated that high levels of awareness of the wrongdoing at Tuskegee exist among African Americans and directly influence feelings and attitudes about participation in medical research studies.[27,38] Among others, Shavers, Lynch and Burmeister[27] proposed that openness, genuineness and trust building — on the part of society as a whole and medical science in particular — are the most promising avenues to increased participation. Other barriers noted in the literature for African Americans in particular included fear of being used as guinea pigs, economic barriers, hidden illiteracy, the failure to actively recruit African Americans for studies, and cultural matters such as fatalistic attitudes about serious diseases like cancer.[30,33,44,45] Additional barriers for minority women to participate in cancer trials were thought to include poor physical functioning, as well as advanced disease and comorbidities.[39] Research also suggests that African American patients were less likely than white patients to be approached by their physicians to participate in a clinical trial.[39]

Native American Indians and Alaska Natives: Within the Native American and Alaska Native populations, there are more than 500 separate tribes and hundreds of languages. Themes in the literature relevant to recruiting for clinical trials include the existence of distrust of research, based upon negative experiences with researchers who have collected information from this population and given little or nothing in return.[29] Further, communication preferences of Native populations may vary from others in ways that can affect doctor–patient communication. For example, there exists a cultural preference for a reserved approach to communication that includes slower speaking patterns and important strictures against interrupting others. Another key factor is that many in this population integrate traditional medical practices and beliefs into their overall health care, which may have prevented them from participating in clinical trials.[30] With regard to the health care system, most Native American Indians are eligible for health care services provided by the Indian Health Service (USDHHS, 2002), and many tribes have their own Internal Review Boards, which must be consulted about clinical trials recruiting. Hodge *et al.*[29] offered the overarching recommendation that tribal governments and local health program administrators be involved in trials, and that researchers actively learn about their subjects' culture, demonstrate respect by sharing findings, and understand the complexities for patients of the health care delivery system unique to Native Americans.

Asian Americans/Pacific Islanders: Very little data exist on knowledge, attitudes and barriers to participation in clinical trials among Asian Americans.[31] However, some studies illuminate differences between the cultural values and practices of many Asian Americans and those most prominent in the general population and among medical scientists, which may play a role. For example, Guo *et al.*[32] pointed to the importance of cultural norms and taboos, including social stigma associated with illness, that need to be taken into consideration in planning recruitment efforts targeting Chinese American patients and their caretakers and health care providers (see also Ref. 46). Other possible factors included the use of traditional medicine, the relatively greater importance of the welfare of the group rather than the individual, the importance of face saving, and the challenges inherent in immigration and acculturation (e.g., language barriers and difficulties with access to services).[21] Noting, however, that Asian American children have significantly greater participation in treatment trials than the oldest Asian Americans (65+ years), Alexander *et al.*[31] suggested that there may be some generational changes within this diverse population such that parents of young children are more informed or positively disposed toward clinical trials. These authors were careful to point out the wide ethnic, cultural, linguistic and socioeconomic variations that exist among this population.

Latinos/Hispanic Americans: Although Latinos/Hispanic Americans are the largest and fastest-growing minority population in the US, their participation in clinical trials has been far below their representation in the population.[47,48] Among issues that may have affected patient accrual are cultural factors such as fatalism, use of traditional medicines, and machismo, or the feeling that men should not show weakness.[21] Research showed that family members play a strong role in Hispanic Americans' decision to participate in clinical research, especially husbands' influence on their wives' participation. Also, caretaking responsibilities for grandchildren may have been important in decision-making by older potential participants.[49,50] Additionally, language and acculturation barriers existed for this population.[30] As Hazuda *et al.*[50] pointed out, awareness of the cultural background and ability to adapt recruitment approaches to match the life context of Latinos/Hispanic Americans are preconditions to a successful recruitment of clinical research participants from this population.

6.2.8. Participation in Clinical Trials among the Elderly

Elderly patients have scarcely been represented in cancer clinical trials, including early phase trials, in spite of the high frequency of cancer in this age group.[51–54] A host of age-related factors that can impede recruitment includes the reality that older patients often present at a later stage of disease and may have a history of prior malignancy, as well as more frequent and serious comorbid conditions.[55] Lewis *et al.*[56] found that protocol exclusions due to functional status limitations and organ-system abnormalities were a major factor limiting participation of the elderly in NCI-sponsored clinical trials. Other barriers to accrual are thought to include lower levels of scientific education (which puts elderly patients at a disadvantage for understanding trials and medical developments), general mistrust of health research projects, caring for a spouse or grandchildren, transportation difficulties (which may be exacerbated by inability or reluctance to drive to some study sites, such as those in congested areas), and the perceived additional time that participation in a trial would require.[21,57–59] However, Kemeny *et al.*,[60] in their pilot study of older women's participation in breast cancer trials, contended that while older patients with stage I or II disease were significantly less likely than younger patients to be offered a trial, age was not a significant predictor as to whether women would participate in a treatment clinical trial, once they had been offered a trial by their oncologists. A number of studies have also shown that elderly patients tolerated standard regimens almost as well as younger ones.[61,62] These findings suggest that besides unjustified, exclusive protocol eligibility criteria,[63] lack of physicians' referrals might pose a major barrier to the accrual of elderly patients for clinical trials.[28,60,64,65] Barriers that physicians perceive to accruing older patients might include significant comorbid conditions that are not excluded by the protocol, difficulty of older patients' understanding and complying with the trial, worries about undue hardships for the patients, and treatment toxicity.[66]

6.3. PHYSICIAN-RELATED BARRIERS TO AND MOTIVATORS FOR PARTICIPATION

A review of the literature shows that there have been far fewer research articles published on early phase trials compared to phase III randomized clinical trials. Consequently, little is known about the role that oncologists and other physicians play in referring patients to phase I and II trials. As shown in the following paragraphs, most research into the role of oncologists and physicians has been performed with phase III and randomized control trials in mind. Nonetheless, it is likely that some findings of the research on phase III trials can be extrapolated to earlier phase trials.

Perhaps one of the more widely researched topics concerning early phase trials and the role of oncologists and other physicians includes the perception of the ethical nature of phase I and II cancer trials. Critics of early phase trials believe that patients' cost-to-benefit ratio is too high. Costs may include slight risk of death, side effects, and time commitment, while there is only a slight chance of therapeutic benefit to the patient. An article by Agrawal and Emanuel[4] provides a good review of these arguments, in addition to counter-arguments that favor early phase trials. The authors claim that the data that critics often used to make these arguments are outdated and even sometimes misinterpreted. They also argue that critics do not take into account the psychological and social benefits of participation, and add that there are indeed cases where an oncological trial resulted in large clinical benefits to its participants.

Other ethical imperatives related to human experimentation may also play a role, including the fact that phase I trials, to a certain degree, call into question a number of requirements specified by the Nuremberg Codes (i.e., that the research design assures acquiring the sought information in the least onerous way possible, that unnecessary suffering and injury are avoided and that death or disability injury are not anticipated, that risks never exceed benefits, and that the experiment will be stopped if it becomes likely that injury, disability, or death will result).[10]

Although most of the literature on early phase trials that is relevant to physicians focuses on ethics and communication, there has been much more research into the role physicians and oncologists play in patient accrual for phase III and randomized clinical trials. The following paragraphs are a brief review of many of the issues raised. Despite the fact that early phase trials have different goals than phase III or higher, it may be possible to extrapolate many of the issues raised with later phase trials to early phase trials.

Ideally, all patients who are fighting cancer would receive an opportunity to join clinical trials, including phase I and II trials. When patients are diagnosed, their physicians would introduce these opportunities and together a decision would be made about whether or not the patient should participate in clinical trials. This would assume that physicians are knowledgeable of available trials and willing to refer their patients to appropriate ones. Otherwise, physicians would refer patients to oncologists who would be able to make additional recommendations. The study by Daugherty *et al.*[15] provides evidence that research oncologists are an important factor in patients' decisions to participate in early phase trials. Because of their influence, it is important to investigate what influences an oncologist to refer (or not refer) a patient to a phase I or II trial.

6.3.1. Awareness of Clinical Trials among Oncologists and Primary Care Physicians

Referral patterns for phase I and II cancer clinical trials are not clear, although it is generally assumed that the last point of care, i.e., oncologists, play a major role in patient accrual. There is also no systematic understanding of the role of primary care providers in patient referrals, although it is speculated that introduction of the idea of clinical trials by primary care providers early during cancer diagnosis and treatment might positively impact patient accrual.[67] However, before any oncologist or other physician can refer (or not refer) a patient to a clinical trial, he or she must know about available trials, and the specific types of cancer the trials address. Research has suggested that primary care physicians in general do not have sufficient information on clinical trials or knowledge about specific trials, and they often leave discussion of clinical research to patients' oncologists.[68] Also, Kemeny *et al.*[60] found that a large percentage of oncologists treating stage I and II breast cancer patients, who do not refer their eligible patients to a clinical trial, were unaware of the fact that a trial was available. These results suggest that community physicians' as well as oncologists' limited awareness of clinical trials, especially those at the clinical center, both early phase as well as phase III, might constitute a serious barrier to patient recruitment and accrual.

6.3.2. Facilitators of Patient Participation

There is some literature on phase III trials that reveals factors correlating with patient accrual. In particular, several studies provided evidence that characteristics specific to the physician or oncologist correlate with a patient's likelihood of joining a clinical trial. For example, Spaight, Nash, Finison *et al.*, as cited in Ref. 69, found that certain types of medical practices, such as hospital clinics and group practices, correlated higher with patient accrual than oncologists in private practices. Additionally, McCusker *et al.*[70] found some evidence that physicians who had trained at or near a cancer center (such as at a university) may correlate positively with patient accrual in randomized clinical trials.[1] According to Feigl, Diehr, Allison *et al.*, as cited in Ref. 69, physicians who had participated in the NCI's Community Clinical Oncology Program also correlated positively with patient accrual. Oncologists who are board certified or specialize in treating patients with cancer also may have more influence on their patients' enrollment in clinical trials (Spaight, Nash, Finison *et al.*, as cited in Ref. 69).

[1] As McCusker *et al.* pointed out, their results are not generalizable due to the sample selection methods.

Critics of early phase trials often cite ethical reasons for not referring patients[4] (also see Refs. 17 and 70), claiming that there is little chance of benefit to the patient while risks are high. Protocol eligibility also plays a major role in deciding whether to refer patients to randomized clinical trials, especially for medical oncologists.[71,72] Patient's financial status, occupational status, and other sociodemographic factors have shown a mixed influence on patient accrual to randomized control trials.[22,25,70] Stage of patient's disease also plays a role in the physician's decision to refer. NCI's study of primary care physicians[68] found that a higher percentage of physicians were likely to discuss clinical trials with patients who had advanced stages of disease. Furthermore, those patients who had higher education levels were more likely to be referred to phase III clinical trials. Other factors leading to referrals were optimistic attitudes and patients' ages; specifically, middle-aged or very young patients were more likely to be referred.

6.3.3. Why Physicians Do Not Refer Patients to Cancer Clinical Trials

Research suggests that oncologists and other physicians are the most important persons with whom patients discuss their decision to enroll in clinical trials. As mentioned, early phase cancer trial participants feel that the relationship between patient and physician plays a large role in the decision-making process. In fact, for all trial phases, patients relatively often leave it to their oncologists to decide whether they should participate in a trial or not.[15,73] Consequently, research suggests that patients often do not enroll in phase III or higher cancer research protocols because of their oncologists' reluctance.[70,71,74,75] Many oncologists often do not make options available to patients and cite a number of reasons for withholding information on clinical trials. One study found that oncologists' reasons were evenly split between patient protocol entry, patients' concerns, and practices' concerns.[76] Other studies, however, found the most-cited reason for not recruiting patients was design protocols that are too rigid.[70,71,74,75]

Communication with patients about clinical trials, including issues surrounding informed consent and complex protocol information, was also listed as one of the major concerns.[77] Primary care physicians have reported reservations about conversations with patients concerning clinical trials, which may have occurred when they felt inadequately prepared to talk about the trials and did not want to be perceived as being uninformed or uncertain.[68] Also, oncologists might be reluctant to convey complex information on study design to their patients. Especially for phase I trials, there are two particular areas of concern: toxicity and its potential harm to the patient, and the scientific — that is, the nonmedical — nature of the trial's goals.[10,78]

Although research has suggested that various practice- and business-related reasons can also impede patient recruitment by their primary care providers, it is unclear to what extent these factors play a role in patient accrual to phase I and II cancer clinical trials. Potential cost implications of being involved in clinical trials might include lack of compensation to the physician for time spent evaluating the patient prior to trial enrollment, laboratory fees and diagnostic tests (that might not be covered by insurance), additional staff involvement, as well as increased paper work (perceived or actual). In addition, monetary loss might occur when physicians lose their patients to trials.[79]

Several other practical reasons for physicians to choose not to participate in clinical trials have been proposed, including conflicts of interest, tight trial deadlines, and fear of having inadequate protection from patients who claim mistreatment.[68] This latter reason may be accompanied by concerns about being punished by fines, barred from research, or imprisoned. Furthermore, oncologists may object to what they perceive as excessive amounts of testing and subsequent follow-up, which may become burdensome to both the physician and the ailing patient.[71] Again, the extent to which these factors impact patient accrual to early phase cancer clinical trials is unknown.

Aside from making practical business decisions, oncologists and other physicians frequently have different philosophies about their practices and clinical trials. For example, the conflict between playing the role of clinician versus that of scientist may lead to non-participation.[30,77] Additionally, distrust of academic medicine might play a role in minority physicians' decision to abstain from referring their patients to clinical trials,[38] as might culturally based stigma associated with illness.[32]

6.3.4. Role of Clinical Research Associates and Clinical Nurses

Relatively few studies have investigated the role of clinical research associates (CRAs) and clinical nurses in patient accrual to clinical trials in general. CRAs and clinical nurses assess patients' understanding of the clinical trial, review trial-specific information with the patients, discuss issues related to informed consent, and formally enroll patients into the clinical trial. They also mediate the flow of information between physicians and patients and collaborate with trial staff members on other aspects of the clinical trial process. Consequently, it makes sense to investigate how CRAs influence patient accrual.[8,38,80–82]

Findings from Wright's study[81] to elicit CRAs' opinions on the relationship of physicians, CRAs and patient accrual to phase III cancer trials suggest that the relationship formed between the CRA and patient often influenced the patient's decision to participate in clinical trials. The manner in which CRAs approach eligible patients seems to be especially influential. As Morse *et al.*[34] pointed out, this relationship might be of particular importance when eligible patients need to overcome additional barriers to research participation, and the CRA helps to find possible solutions to the problem.

Wright's findings also provided evidence that CRAs view themselves as informers. Thus, the content and style of their delivery can influence patients' decisions. CRAs contended that communication about the pros and cons of the clinical trial could resolve patients' reluctance to participate (i.e., allowing patients who are entering investigational therapy to maintain a level of hope, while realistically counseling them about the objectives of early phase trials, may foster a bond of trust with the CRA and can, in turn, influence the patient's decision to enroll). This point may be significant, given that the CRA or clinical nurse who is trying to recruit the patient often is the person who cares for the patient during the trial. Wright's findings suggest that the CRAs often had preconceived ideas about the patient, as well as impressions of the specific trial, both of which may have influenced their effort to recruit that patient. In addition, as Ulrich *et al.*'s[82] study indicates, CRAs might have ethical concerns about clinical trials, particularly related to issues of randomization, informed consent and patient burden, that might prevent them from bringing up clinical trials with their patients.

6.4. RECRUITMENT METHODS TO PHASE I AND II CANCER CLINICAL TRIALS

Cancer patients participating in phase I and II clinical trials are usually referred to clinical research by their physicians, although an unknown percentage of participating patients are self-referred. Anecdotal and unpublished reports suggest that interpersonal relationships and outreach among medical professionals are also important to recruiting, but the topic is not addressed in the literature. A number of additional strategies may be employed by investigators to recruit participants, although it is unknown how it differs among different phases of cancer clinical trials. Among them are mass mailings to patients and physician practices; study notices and bulletins; radio, television and newspaper ads; public service announcements; fliers; and websites. In some cases, those recruitment strategies may be supplemented with public relations campaigns to help increase awareness of the project in the communities studied. Such outreach strategies might include media-related activities, such as placement of news stories, or community presentations as forums for key opinion leaders in the communities to endorse the study among their constituents.[83–85] The strategy or combination of recruitment strategies employed is influenced by available funds, the nature of the targeted patient population, the trial's timeframe, and the number of required subjects.[86]

Little systematic research exists on the effectiveness of various recruitment methods to cancer clinical trials in general, and to early phase trials in particular. In most instances when such information is provided, it is anecdotal rather than systematic, and/or pertains to phase III clinical trials. Also, although such analysis is not available for the early phase cancer trial reports, a review of general randomized trials reports[87] suggested that investigators rarely documented how many people were identified as eligible for enrollment, and the number of potential participants that needed to be screened to identify one enrollee. Furthermore, a study of methods utilized in patient recruitment to the randomized controlled trials[88] found that the recruitment methods used by the investigators were not evidence based, and that organizational characteristics, such as previous research experience or patient eligibility criteria, could be more influential in trial recruitment than the use of specific interventions. No similar analysis has been conducted for the phase I or II cancer clinical trials, and these gaps in the literature clearly suggest that further research is necessary to discern the effectiveness of various recruitment methods for the early phase clinical trials.

6.5. POTENTIAL APPROACHES TO IMPROVEMENT OF ACCRUAL TO EARLY PHASE CANCER CLINICAL TRIALS

The reviewed literature suggested that clinical trials recruitment in general, and early phase cancer clinical trials recruitment in particular, is not satisfactorily efficient, and numerous efforts will be required to address the known barriers to patient participation. As the authors detailed the barriers and obstacles to patient accrual, they also suggested a number of strategies to overcome these barriers. While most of the articles speculated on possible approaches to improve patient recruitment based on the perceived barriers, a limited number of preliminary studies attempted to verify some of the proposed strategies. An even more limited number of articles pertained to phase I or II cancer clinical trials. The following section discusses potential strategies to target the recruitment barriers and enhance recruitment rates to early phase clinical trials identified in the literature. These strategies can be grouped into two categories: strategies to enhance clinical trials literacy among patients, and protocol-related strategies that would make the accrual to early phase trials more likely. The section concludes with a discussion of strategies and tools to improve the process of general patient recruitment in the future.

6.5.1. General Enhancement of Clinical Trials Literacy among Patients

Improvement of Communication to Patients about Clinical Trials: General enhancement of clinical trials literacy among cancer patients is considered one of the most important strategies to improve patient accrual.

Tomamichel *et al.*[89] found that providing cancer patients with information on the option of participation in phase I trials can be done in a way felt to be appropriate by patients and relatives, as well as nurses and investigators. The authors also found that providing information in an appropriate manner does not increase patients' anxiety and depression. A study of cancer patients participating in a phase II trial[90] suggested that such appropriate physician–patient communication needs to involve not only explanation of a clinical trial, but also feedback about trial processes and results. Also, communication between physicians and patients regarding informed consent needs to be improved, to make sure that patients easily recall and fully comprehend the information provided to them, and fully comprehend the purpose of early phase clinical trials.[12,15,91] Authors suggested research to define strategies that can improve patients' recall and understanding, and meet their preference for simplified material.[91] Lengacher *et al.*'s model for successful clinical trial participation summarizes timing, readability and the complexity of consent forms as areas for improvement. Specifically, the researchers state that it may be advantageous not to present trials as an option at the stressful time of diagnosis, but to suggest trials during presentation of treatment options. Also, less-complex consent forms with higher readability levels may help to fulfill the informative purpose of the forms and to meet patients' needs.[92]

Additionally, general literature on clinical trials suggests, as Welton *et al.*[23] concludes,"that including potential benefits for other people in patient information, as well as personal benefits and risks, may increase recruitment." Collyar[93] proposed that changing terminology may also help cancer patients consider participation as an option, since the term "clinical trial" might bring connotations of something sterile and beyond patients' control, while terms like "new treatment options" might sound less intimidating and, research shows, would not endanger patients' preference for it over a standard treatment.[94] Clinical trial participants have been shown to use the Internet to seek clinical trial information as well as general disease related information and for psychosocial support.[95] Making information on clinical trials and other learning resources easily available on the Internet, and via other multimedia resources, may increase patients' understanding of their conditions, help them identify which questions to ask their health care providers, and encourage consideration of participation in clinical trials.[96] In addition, providing ongoing "communicative support" to trial participants has been proposed as a way to ensure continuing participation and lower drop-out rates.[97]

Involvement of Patient Advocacy and Support Groups in Patient Recruitment: General trial literature suggests that advocacy groups can be strong partners for clinical researchers. Advocacy groups connect with their audiences through multiple channels and keep them updated on clinical trials through direct contact, newsletters and/or website listings. They also know their constituents and understand their needs. Collyar[93] suggested that cancer patient advocates can be helpful in eliminating accrual barriers by explaining individual clinical trials to their constituents in a way that potential participants would find easy to comprehend. Patient advocates have been also found to provide valuable contribution to optimizing cancer trials' information materials.[98] Additionally, Krueger[99] recommended involvement of advocacy groups in devising exclusion criteria and clinical endpoints that are acceptable to potential participants. Further involvement of patient advocates in the National Cancer Clinical Trials System is strongly supported by the American Society of Clinical Oncology and Institute of Medicine.[100]

Improvement of Public Attitudes and Knowledge about Clinical Trials: The improvement of general public literacy regarding the importance and benefits of clinical trials may help to increase patient accrual, since adults who report a high level of understanding of clinical trials are more positively inclined toward participation than adults who lack such understanding.[2,76,101] For example, although it is not clear to what extent this may pertain to the early phase cancer trials, Grilli, Ramsay and Minozzi[102] and Pentz *et al.*[82] found that mass media communications, both planned campaigns and unplanned coverage, can encourage the use of health services and improve prospective participants' understanding and interest in trials without increasing their hope for personal benefit. Also, NIH/NCI[103] found that positive media attention might be an essential source of information, as well as a possible motivator, of prospective trial participants. Mackenzie *et al.*[104] found that a well-designed media campaign can contribute to the improvement of public awareness of clinical research in general; however, they concluded that further research is needed to ascertain whether improved public awareness leads to increased participation in clinical trials.

6.5.2. Improvement of Communication to Oncologists and Other Physicians about Clinical Trials

Since community physicians and primary care physicians are usually the first to deliver a diagnosis to patients, they must be made aware of clinical trials to be able to introduce the concept of a clinical trial early during the treatment. Sufficient information will make them more comfortable and confident in discussing the trials with their patients. The primary care physicians also need to be reassured that they will not lose control of their referred patients.[79] Establishment of research networks of physicians and oncologists can promote greater participation in clinical research.[88] Such networks could work to provide physicians, both primary care specialists and oncologists, with the information and materials they need to feel confident talking about clinical research and facilitate their patients' participation in clinical trials. Interactive approaches, such as workshops at existing national, regional, and local meetings, and Internet-delivered activities, were found to be physicians' preferred methods for delivery of continuing education,[105] and health-related websites, including the flagship site *www.cancer.gov*, are a potentially effective vehicle for reaching both professionals and the general public with information about NCI-sponsored clinical trials.[106] Other technological approaches that have shown some promise in facilitating recruitment to clinical trials in general include the Electronic Health Record (EHR)-based approaches.[107] Additionally, printed educational materials, although they have little or no effect on professional behavior, may still raise awareness, potentially enhancing effectiveness of other interventions targeting physicians.[88]

Improvement of Education Communication to Clinical Nurses: Clinical nurses oftentimes mediate the flow of information between physicians and patients and are in a position to bring up and educate patients on clinical research, and refer patients to clinical trials. As reported by Ulrich *et al.*,[82] nurse practitioners might be more likely to bring up clinical trials if they are comfortable discussing treatment options and options of entering clinical trial with their patients, as well as have sufficient time during patients' visits to discuss and explain those options. At the same time, it has been found that nurse practitioners report ethical concerns about clinical trials related to issues such as randomization, informed consent and patient burden. Providing more education and communication to clinical nurses on the benefits and burdens of clinical research might alleviate the above concerns and contribute to improved communication with patients about clinical trials.

6.5.3. Increased Participation of Underserved Populations

The literature lacks a discussion of the best practices for accrual of minority patients into the early phase cancer clinical trials. However, it has been found that most successful strategies to recruit minority patients to clinical trials in general involve opportunities to build trust, and optimal recruitment response among those populations has been achieved by strategies involving face-to-face contact with potential participants. Community outreach, education and involvement of patients' families in the decision-making process are suggested as ways to reduce suspicion and distrust of clinical research among those populations.[38,45,108] Including racial/ethnic minorities among the research staff was found to be necessary in studies that specifically target racial/ethnic minorities.[27,37,108] Additionally, involving social workers in patient accrual and retention, as well as maximizing study staff access, availability and rapport with participants may improve patient recruitment from underserved populations.[109–111] Other possible strategies to increase participation of underserved populations include establishing cancer centers in institutions that directly serve these populations, conducting outreach through community members, and improving access and availability of services (e.g., provide stipends, transportation to research facilities).[38,108,112–114] For elderly populations, making personnel available to explain clinical trials to patients and their families, and providing oncologists with educational materials on treatment toxicity in the elderly have been suggested.[115] The program on Enhancing Minority Participation in Clinical Trials (EMPaCT), funded in 2010 by the National Institutes of Health's National Center on Minority Health and Health Disparities (NCMHD), is the latest major initiative aiming to systematize the insights on the barriers and facilitators to minority patient participation in clinical research (*www.empactconsortium.com*).

6.5.4. Protocol-related Strategies/Justification and Monitoring of Complex Protocol Designs

Critical Assessment of Eligibility Criteria and Protocol Design: Rather than planning protocol design and patient recruitment as separate steps, all planning should be done concurrently. Criteria for clinical trial eligibility, which are among the key barriers to trial accrual, should be explicitly justified and continuously assessed from trial to trial, and made as inclusive as possible to reflect the whole population to whom the new treatment will be offered.[116] Involvement of referring physicians and CRAs early in the process of protocol development may provide additional insights into the likelihood of patient accrual to the study and help avoid the necessity of amending difficult-to-recruit protocols and resulting delays.[61,72,70] In addition, protocols should be monitored to assure that the required complex procedures are justified and that any unessential protocol requirements are eliminated.[76,92]

Development of Innovative Protocol Designs: Concerns related to early phase protocol design range from the fact that the scientific objectives of phase I trials are nonmedical and do not include patient benefit, to selection of starting dose and rapidity of dose escalation. In order to address these concerns, some investigators have proposed novel design strategies that would allow more patients to be treated at biologically active doses.[117] The new designs would allow for intra-patient dose escalation, increasing the chances for a positive therapeutic response.[118–120] Additionally, suggested modifications of the traditional phase I include providing patients with an opportunity to choose the starting dose of the treatment under study, and involving patients in direct decisions on dose escalation. The proposed modifications aim at giving patients some control of their care and alleviating feelings of vulnerability during the trial.[7]

6.5.5. Additional Strategies and Tools to Improve General Process of Patient Accrual in the Long Term

Applying Principles of Market Research to Patient Recruitment Planning: Literature referring to the late stage clinical trials suggests use of marketing research principles that may prove to be effective in identifying the best and the most efficacious approaches to patient recruitment.[121,122] Audience research involving focus groups or one-on-one telephone or in-person interviews is considered a cost-effective way to identify those strategies, especially for trials with very restricting eligibility criteria. Patient database searches may give insight into disease prevalence in various geographic areas, as well as help researchers learn whether enough patients exist to fulfill their study. Protocol feasibility studies may determine the likelihood of reaching enrollment targets as well as help identify the key problems in the inclusion/exclusion criteria that are making recruitment difficult. A business model has been developed to plan and manage randomized clinical trials, and consequently improve recruitment.[123,124] It is unclear, however, to what extent utilization of market research techniques may be useful in planning for patient recruitment to early phase cancer clinical trials.

Keeping and Sharing a History of Patient Accrual-Related Experiences within and among Research Groups: Careful documentation of recruiting strategies, along with supporting quantitative data, should be kept within research groups. These data could be used to drive the use of appropriate recruiting strategies in future clinical trials, since, as Foy *et al.*[88] pointed out, skills used to recruit patients often have to be "relearned" with each new clinical trial. Coupled with staff turnover, this lack of historical experience may act as a barrier to successful recruitment since each new trial may essentially be starting from scratch. Other strategies related to the improvement of the process of patient accrual could include maintaining logs of callers interested in being involved with a particular clinical trial but screened out due to particular eligibility requirements, as well as training all trial staff, including receptionists and nurses, so that every person who has contact with patients could explain the trial and obtain basic information from the caller.[125] Setting *a priori* recruitment goals and developing consistent measures of "success" in recruitment of under-represented populations might also help to compare effectiveness of various recruitment strategies across trials.[40] In addition, using strategies such as regular meetings by the research team and transparent communication on the subject of recruitment can enhance patient accrual to cancer trials.[57] The extent to which implementation of these strategies would impact patient accrual to phase I and II cancer clinical trials needs to be further investigated.

Development and Utilization of Tools in Planning and Evaluating Patient Recruitment Strategies: Patient recruitment approaches should allow for systematic recording and analysis of recruitment experiences from each trial, including assessment of effectiveness and cost efficiency of different methods.[126] Utilization of statistical tools such as metrics or surveys for recording and analyzing accrual data can provide very precise, objective information and help identify appropriate recruitment strategies. Information contained in such metrics would allow researchers to plan for the numbers of patients they will need to screen, the types of recruitment strategies that could be successful with the targeted populations, and the budget for those efforts. It is suggested that, with time, as the use of metrics becomes more systematic, the tool may also serve to identify differences among various types of patients that enter the trial, such as self-referred versus physician-referred patients.[121,127] The extent to which such tools might prove useful in planning and evaluation of recruitment strategies to early phase cancer trials is unclear.

Systematic Research to Validate Various Recruitment Methods: Investigators need research-based guidance on how to identify potential facilitators and how to approach potential barriers to patient accrual. Their detailed understanding of the nature of recruitment interventions required for particular types of conditions and particular patient populations would lead to the improved efficacy of recruitment efforts. Given that the improvement of recruitment methods has the potential to enhance participation to all potential subjects, further hypothesis-driven empirical research is necessary to validate the various recruitment methods that have been used, as well as those that are being put forward as potentially enhancing patient participation in clinical research.[38,88,92]

6.6. CONCLUSIONS

The comprehensive literature review identified a rich body of research related to patient recruitment to clinical trials, providing valuable information on barriers and motivators to patient accrual. However, there are also significant gaps and limitations in the literature, which are important to keep in mind when drawing broader conclusions. Many of the studies mentioned above relied on research techniques such as case studies, convenience samples, focus groups and exploratory analyses that make generalizations to a wider population difficult. Although many of the results of these studies ultimately converge and support one another, it is clear that more scientific, hypothesis-driven analyses are needed.

Studies that focus on phases I and II are also particularly few in number. Although many of the studies mentioned in the above review could be extrapolated to include early phase trials, one should be cautious when drawing such conclusions. Patients targeted for phase I and II cancer treatment trials may be a special population that warrants a different set of outreach strategies from those in later trial phases or in trials researching other types of conditions (e.g., chronic illness). The only way to determine this is to continue researching and detecting, using scientific methods, covariates of patient participation in phase I and II trials.

In particular, the review of the literature concerning clinical trials demonstrates that more information is needed on recruitment strategies that result in higher patient accrual. Additionally, data are needed to determine which strategies work best with certain populations, including minority patients and those traditionally underserved. For example, questions such as the following remain: Which strategies are appropriate for increasing physicians' and patients' awareness of clinical trials? How can researchers increase patients' understanding of early phase trials? Which strategies are cost effective, and which are not? In order to increase the effectiveness and sophistication of patient recruiting — and ultimately benefit cancer treatment research — all of these questions and doubtless others should be addressed in a new wave of early phase clinical trial recruitment research.

REFERENCES

1. Comis RL, Aldigé CR, Stovall EL, *et al.* (2000) A quantitative survey of public attitudes towards cancer clinical trials [online], Coalition of National Cancer Cooperative Groups, Cancer Research Foundation of America, Cancer Leadership Council, and Oncology Nursing Society. *www.cancertrialshelp.org/static_ binary/308-9.pdf*
2. Comis RL, Miller JD, Aldigé CR, *et al.* (2003) Public attitudes toward participation in cancer clinical trials. *J Clin Oncol* **21**(5): 830–835.
3. Campbell HM, Raisch DW, Sather MR, *et al.* (2008) Impact of a clinical trials information booklet on patient knowledge, perceptions, and likelihood of participation. *IRB* **30**(1): 6–14.
4. Agrawal M, Emanuel EJ. (2003) Ethics of phase 1 oncology studies: Reexamining the arguments and data. *J Am Med Assoc* **290**: 1075–1082.
5. Harris Interactive. (2001) Misconceptions and lack of awareness greatly reduce recruitment for cancer clinical trials. *Health Care News* **1**(3). *www. harrisinteractive.com/news/newsletters/healthnews/HI_ HealthCareNews2001-Vol1_ iss3.pdf*
6. Flory J, Emanuel E. (2004) Interventions to improve research participants' understanding in informed consent for research: A systematic review. *J Am Med Assoc* **292**(13): 1593–1601.
7. Daugherty CK, Ratain MI, Minami H, *et al.* (1998) Study of cohort-specific consent and patient control in phase I cancer trials. *J Clin Oncol* **16**(7): 2305–2312.
8. Yoder LH, O'Rourke TJ, Etnyre A, *et al.* (1997) Expectations and experiences of patients with cancer participating in phase I clinical trials. *Oncol Nursing Forum* **24**(5): 891–896.
9. Von Hoff DD, Turner J. (1991) Response rates, duration of response, and dose response effects in phase I studies of antineoplastics. *Invest New Drugs* **9**: 115–122.
10. Miller M. (2000) Phase I cancer trials: A collusion of misunderstanding. *Hastings Center Rep* **30**(4): 34–42.
11. Moore S. (2001) A need to try everything: Patient participation in phase I trials. *J Adv Nursing* **33**(6): 738–747.
12. Meropol NJ, Weinfurt KP, Burnett CB, *et al.* (2003) Perceptions of patients and physicians regarding phase I cancer clinical trials: Implications for physician-patient communication. *J Clin Oncol* **21**(13): 2589–2596.

13. Weinfurt KP, Sulmasy DP, Schulman KA, Meropol NJ. (2003) Patient expectations of benefit from phase I clinical trials: Linguistic considerations in diagnosing a therapeutic misconception. *Theory Med Bioethics* **24**(4): 329–344.
14. Schutta KM, Burnett CB. (2000) Factors that influence a patient's decision to participate in a phase I clinical trial. *Oncol Nursing Forum* **27**(9): 1435–1438.
15. Daugherty CK, Ratain MJ, Grochowski E, *et al.* (1995) Perceptions of cancer patients and their physicians involved in phase I trials. *J Clin Oncol* **13**(5): 1062–1072.
16. Cox K, McGarry J. (2002) Why patients don't take part in cancer clinical trials: An overview of the literature. *Eur J Cancer Care* **12**: 114–122.
17. Lawrence W. (1993) Patient selection for clinical trials: Risks versus benefits and quality of life issues. *Cancer* **72**(Suppl 9): 2798–2800.
18. Cheng JD, Hitt J, Koczwara B, *et al.* (2000) Impact of quality of life on patient expectations regarding phase I clinical trials. *J Oncol* **18**(2): 421–428.
19. Cunny KA, Miller HW. (1994) Participation in clinical drug studies: Motivations and barriers. *Clin Ther* **16**: 273–282.
20. Richardson M, Post-White J, Singletary S, Justice B. (1998) Recruitment for complementary/alternative medical trials: Who participates after breast cancer. *Ann Behav Med* **20**: 190–198.
21. National Institutes of Health, National Cancer Institute. (2002) Cancer clinical trials: A resource guide for outreach, education, and advocacy [online]. *www.cancer.gov/clinicaltrials/resources/outreach-education-advocacy*
22. Klabunde CN, Springer BC, Butler B, *et al.* (1999) Factors influencing enrollment in clinical trials for cancer treatment. *South Med J* **92**(12): 1189–1193.
23. Welton AJ, Vickers MR, Cooper JA, *et al.* (1999) Is recruitment more difficult with a placebo arm in randomised controlled trials? A quasirandomised, interview based study. *Br Med J* **318**: 1114–1117.
24. US General Accounting Office. (1999) *NIH Clinical Trials: Various Factors Affect Patient Participation.* Report to Congressional Requestors, GAO/HEHS 99–182. Washington, DC.
25. Sateren WB, Trimble EL, Abrams J, *et al.* (2002) How sociodemographics, presence of oncology specialists, and hospital cancer programs affect accrual to cancer treatment trials. *J Clin Oncol* **20**(8): 2109–2117.
26. Ellis SD, Carpenter WR, Minasian LM, Weiner BJ. (2012) Effects of state-mandated insurance coverage on accrual to community cancer clinical trials. *Contemp Clin Trials* **33**(5): 933–941.
27. Shavers VL, Lynch CF, Burmeister LF. (2002) Racial differences in factors that influence the willingness to participate in medical research studies. *Ann Epidemiol* **12**: 248–256.

28. Howerton MW, Gibbons MC, Baffi CR, *et al.* (2007) Provider roles in the recruitment of underrepresented populations to cancer clinical trials. *Cancer* **103**(3): 465–476.
29. Hodge FS, Weinmann S, Roubideaux Y. (2000) Recruitment of American Indians and Alaska Natives into clinical trials. *Ann Epidemiol* **10**(Suppl 8): S41–S48.
30. Roberson NL. (1994) Clinical trial participation: Viewpoints from racial/ethnic groups. *Cancer* **74**: 2687–2691.
31. Alexander GA, Chu KC, Ho RCS. (2000) Representation of Asian Americans in clinical cancer trials. *Ann Epidemiol* **10**(Suppl 8): S61–S67.
32. Guo Z, Levy BR, Hinton WL, *et al.* (2000) The power of labels: Recruiting dementia-affected Chinese American elders and their caregivers. In: SE Levkoff, TR Prohaska, P Flynn Weitzman, MG Ory (eds.), *Recruitment and Retention in Minority Populations.* Springer, New York, pp. 103–112.
33. Giuliano AR, Mokuau N, Hughes C, *et al.* (2000) Participation of minorities in cancer research: The influence of structural, cultural, and linguistic factors. *Ann Epidemiol* **10**(Suppl 8): S22–S34.
34. Morse EV, Simon PM, Besch CL, Walker J. (1995) Issues of recruitment, retention, and compliance in community-based clinical trials with traditionally underserved populations. *Appl Nursing Res* **8**(1): 8–14.
35. Underwood SM. (2000) Minorities, women, and clinical cancer research: The charge, promise, and challenge. *Ann Epidemiol* **10**(Suppl 8): S3–S12.
36. Durant RW, Davis RB, St. George DM, *et al.* (2007) Participation in research studies: Factors associated with failing to meet minority recruitment goals. *Ann Epidemiol* **17**(8): 634–642.
37. Stark N, Paskett E, Bell R, *et al.* (2002) Increasing participation of minorities in cancer clinical trials: Summary of the "Moving Beyond the Barriers" conference in North Carolina. *J Natl Med Assoc* **94**(1): 31–39.
38. Swanson MG, Ward A. (1995) Recruiting minorities into clinical trials: Toward a participant friendly system. *J Natl Cancer Inst* **87**(23): 1747–1759.
39. Brown DR, Fouad MN, Basen-Engquist K, Tortolero Luna G. (2000) Recruitment and retention of minority women in cancer screening, prevention, and treatment trials. *Ann Epidemiol* **10**(Suppl 8): S13–S21.
40. Bolen S, Tilburt J, Baffi C, *et al.* (2006) Defining "success" in recruitment of underrepresented populations to cancer clinical trials: Moving toward a more consistent approach. *Cancer* **106**(6): 1197–1204.
41. Joseph G, Dohan D. (2012) Recruitment practices and the politics of inclusion in cancer clinical trials. *Med Anthropol Quart* **26**(3): 338–360.

42. Corbie-Smith G, Thomas SB, St. George DM. (2002) Distrust, race, and research. *Arch Intern Med* **162**: 2458–2462.
43. Royal C, Baffoe-Bonnie A, Kittles R, *et al.* (2000) Recruitment experience in the first phase of the African American Hereditary Prostate Cancer (AAHPC) Study. *Ann Epidemiol* **10**(Suppl 8): S68–S77.
44. Harris Y, Gorelick PB, Samuels P, Bempong I. (1996) Why African Americans may not be participating in clinical trials. *J Natl Med Assoc* **88**: 630–634.
45. Holcombe RF, Jacobson J, Li A, Moinpour CM. (1998) Inclusion of Black Americans in oncology clinical trials. *Am J Oncol* **22**(2): 18–21.
46. Levkoff SE, Prohaska TT, Flynn Weitzman P,Ory MG (eds.). (2000) *Recruitment and Retention in Minority Populations.* Springer, New York.
47. US Census Bureau. (2003) Hispanic population reaches all-time high of 38.8 million, new Census Bureau estimates show (press release) [online]. *www.census.gov/Press-Release/www/releases/archives/hispanic_origin_population/001130.html*
48. Evelyn B, Tolgo T, Banks D, *et al.* (2001) Participation of racial/ethnic groups in clinical trials and race-related labeling: A review of new molecular entities approved 1995–1999. *J Natl Med Assoc* **92**(Suppl 12): S18–S24.
49. Naranjo LE, Dirksen SE. (1998) The recruitment and participation of Hispanic women in nursing research: A learning process. *Public Health Nursing* **15**(1): 25–29.
50. Hazuda HP, Gerety M, Williams JW Jr, *et al.* (2000) Health promotion research with Mexican American elders: Matching approaches to settings at the mediator- and micro-levels of recruitment. In: SE Levkoff, TR Prohaska, P Flynn Weitzman, MG Ory (eds.), *Recruitment and Retention in Minority Populations.* Springer, New York, pp. 79–90.
51. Cope DG, Reb AM (eds.). (2006) *An Evidence-Based Approach to the Treatment and Care of the Older Adult with Cancer.* Oncology Nursing Society, Pittsburgh, PA.
52. Talarico L, Chen G, Pazdur R. (2003) Elderly patients in trials for cancer drug registration: A 7-year experience by the Food and Drug Administration (FDA). Presented at: *2003 ASCO Annual Meeting*, Chicago, IL. *www.asco.org*
53. Lai G, Gary T, Tilburt J, *et al.* (2006) Effectiveness of strategies to recruit underrepresented populations into cancer clinical trials. *Soc Clin Trials* **3**: 133–141.
54. Meropol N, Buzaglo J, Millard J, *et al.* (2007). Barriers to clinical trial participation as perceived by oncologists and patients. *J Natl Compr Cancer Netw* 5(8): 655–664.

55. Ford J, Howerton M, Lai G, *et al.* (2007) Barriers to recruiting underrepresented populations to cancer clinical trials: A systematic review. *Cancer* **112**(2): 228–242.
56. Lewis JH, Kilgore ML, Goldman DP, *et al.* (2003) Participation of patients 65 years of age and older in cancer clinical trials. *J Clin Oncol* **21**(7): 1383–1389.
57. Payne J. (2006) Research issues and priorities. In: DG Cope, AM Reb (eds.), *An Evidence-Based Approach to the Treatment and Care of the Older Adult with Cancer.* Oncology Nursing Society, Pittsburgh, pp. 13–40.
58. Payne J, Hendrix CC. (2010) Clinical trial recruitment challenges with older adults with cancer. *Appl Nursing Res* **23**: 233–237.
59. Trimble EL, Carter CL, Cain D, *et al.* (1994) Representation of older patients in cancer treatment trials. *Cancer* **74**(Suppl 7): 2208–2214.
60. Kemeny MM, Peterson BL, Kornblith AB, *et al.* (2003) Barriers to clinical trial participation by older women with breast cancer. *J Clin Oncol* **21**(15): 2268–2275.
61. Balducci L, Carreca I. (2002) The role of myelopoietic growth factors in managing cancer in the elderly (Review). *Drugs* **62**(Suppl 1): 47–63.
62. Giovanazzi-Bannon S, Rademaker A, Lai G. (1994) Treatment tolerance of elderly cancer patients entered into phase II clinical trials: An Illinois Cancer Center study. *J Clin Oncol* **12**: 2447–2452.
63. Cherubini A, Oristell J, Pla X, *et al.* (2007) The persistent exclusion of older patients from ongoing trials regarding heart failure. *Arch Intern Med* **28**(171): 550–556.
64. National Institutes of Health, National Cancer Institute. (2000) Lack of older patients in cancer studies a problem, report warns [online]. *www.cancer.gov/clinicaltrials/developments/older-patients0200*
65. National Institutes of Health, National Cancer Institute. (2001) Cancer trial barriers falling for people over 65 [online]. *www.cancer.gov/clinicaltrials/developments/barriers-falling0101*
66. Townsley C, Selby R, Siu L. (2005) Systematic review of barriers to the recruitment of older patients with cancer onto clinical trials. *J Clin Oncol* **23**(13): 3112–3124.
67. Schilsky RL (2003) Meeting the challenges of clinical trial enrollment. In: *Conversation in Care* [Web-book]. *www.conversationsincare.org*
68. CODA. (2000). *Primary Care Physicians' Attitudes, Knowledge, and Practices Related to Cancer Clinical Trials: Final Study Results.* Silver Spring, MD.
69. Gotay CC. (1991) Accrual to cancer clinical trials: Directions from the research literature. *Soc Sci Med* **33**(5): 569–577.

70. McCusker J, Wax A, Bennett JM. (1982) Cancer patient accessions into clinical trials: A pilot investigation into some patient and physician determinants of entry. *Am J Clin Oncol* **5**: 227–236.
71. Benson AB III, Prokop-Pregler JP, Bean JA, *et al.* (1991) Oncologists' reluctance to accrue patients onto clinical trials: An Illinois Cancer Center study. *J Clin Oncol* **9**(11): 2067–2075.
72. Fuks A, Weijer C, Freedman B, *et al.* (1998) A study in contrast: Eligibility criteria in a twenty-year sample of NSABP and POG clinical trials. *J Clin Epidemiol* **51**(2): 69–79.
73. Lynoe N, Sandlund M, Jacobsson L. (1996) Clinical cancer research: Some aspects on doctors' attitudes to informing participants. *Acta Oncologica* **35**(6): 749–754.
74. Begg CB. (1983) Cooperative groups and community hospitals: Measurement of impact in the community hospitals. *Cancer* **52**(9): 1760–1767.
75. Hunter CP, Frelick RW, Feldman AR, *et al.* (1987) Selection factors in clinical trials: Results from the Community Clinical Oncology Program Physician's Patient Log. *Cancer Treat Rep* **71**(6): 559–565.
76. Foley JF, Moertel CG. (1991) Improving accrual into cancer clinical trials. *J Cancer Educ* **6**(3): 165–173.
77. Fallowfield L, Ratcliffe D, Souhami R. (1997) Clinicians' attitudes to clinical trials of cancer therapy. *Eur J Cancer* **33**(13): 2221–2229.
78. Degos L. (2000) Phase I trials in cancer treatment. The maximum tolerated dose: A barbarian guideline. *Hematol J* **1**(4): 219.
79. Mansour EG. (1994) Barriers to clinical trials. Part III: Knowledge and attitudes of health care providers. *Cancer* **74**(9): 2672–2675.
80. Melink TJ. (1989) Phase I trials: Role of nurse investigator. *Cancer Treat Res* **42**: 105–124.
81. Wright JR, Crooks D, Ellis PM, *et al.* (2002) Factors that influence the recruitment of patients to phase III studies in oncology: The perspective of the clinical research associate. *Cancer* **95**(7): 1584–1591.
82. Ulrich CM, Zhou Q, Ratcliffe SJ, *et al.* (2012) Nurse Practitioners' attitudes about cancer clinical trials and willingness to recommend participation. *Contemp Clin Trials* **33**(1): 76–84.
83. Lewis CE, Fouad M, Bowen C, Urban N. (1998) Recruitment strategies in the Women's Health Trial: Feasibility study in minority populations. *Control Clin Trials* **19**: 461–467.
84. Pentz RD, Flamm AL, Sugarman J, *et al.* (2002) Study of the media's potential influence on prospective research participants' understanding of and

motivations for participation in a high-profile phase I trial. *J Clin Oncol* **20**(18): 3785–3791.

85. Schoen L. (1999) Clinical trials black eye: Can public relations provide a makeover? *Pharm Exec* **19**(12): 50–56.
86. Spilker B, Cramer JA. (1992) *Patient Recruitment in Clinical Trials.* Raven Press, New York.
87. Gross C, Raburn M, Heiat A, Krumholtz HM. (2002) Reporting the recruitment process in clinical trials: Who are these patients and how did they get there? *Ann Intern Med* **137**(1): 10–16.
88. Foy R, Parry J, Duggan A, *et al.* (2002) How evidence based are recruitment strategies to randomized controlled trials in primary care? Experience from seven studies. *Fam Pract* **20**(1): 83–92.
89. Tomamichel M, Jaime H, Degrate A, *et al.* (2000) Aproposing phase I studies: Patients', relatives', nurses' and specialists' perceptions. *Ann Oncol* **11**(3): 289–294.
90. Partridge AH, Burstein HJ, Gelman RS, *et al.* (2003) Do patients participating in clinical trials want to know study results? *J Natl Cancer Inst* **95**(6): 491–492.
91. Ellis PM. (2000) Attitudes towards and participation in randomized clinical trials in oncology: A review of the literature. *Ann Oncol* **11**: 939–945.
92. Lengacher CA, Gonzalez LL, Giuliano R, *et al.* (2001) The process of clinical trials: A model for successful clinical trial participation. *Oncol Nursing Forum* **28**(7): 1115–1120.
93. Collyar DE. (2000) The value of clinical trials from a patient perspective. *Breast J* **6**(5): 310–314.
94. Kerr CEP, Robinson EJ, Lilford RJ, *et al.* (2004). The impact of describing clinical trial treatments as new or standard. *Patient Educ Couns* **53**(1): 107–113.
95. Ehrenberger HE. (2001) Cancer clinical trial patients in the information age. *Cancer Pract* **9**(4): 191–197.
96. Shneerson C, Windle R, Cox K. (2013) Innovating information-delivery for potential clinical trials participants. What do patients want from multi-media resources? *Patient Educ Couns* **90**(1): 111–117.
97. Gillies K, Entwistle VA. (2012) Supporting positive experiences and sustained participation in clinical trials: Looking beyond information provision. *J Med Ethics* **38**(12): 751–756.
98. Dellson P, Nilbert M, Bendhal P-O, *et al.* (2011) Towards optimised information about clinical trials: Identification and validation of key issues

in collaboration with cancer patient advocates. *Eur J Cancer Care* **20**: 445–454.

99. Krueger M. (2001) Common ground: A collaborative approach to clinical trial recruitment. *Pharm Exec* **21**(5): 114–120.
100. IOM (Institute of Medicine). (2011) *Implementing a National Cancer Clinical Trials System for the 21st Century: Workshop Summary.* The National Academies Press, Washington, DC.
101. Morrow, GR, Hickok JT, Burish TG. (1994) Behavioral aspects of clinical trials. *Cancer* **74**(Suppl 9): 2676–2682.
102. Grilli R, Ramsay GR, Minozzi S. (2003) Mass media interventions: Effects on health services utilization. In: The Cochrane Library, Issue 3. John Wiley & Sons, Chichester, UK. *www.update-software.com/abstracts/AB000389.htm*
103. National Institutes of Health, National Cancer Institute, National Action Plan on Breast Cancer. (1999) *Developing a Marketing Communication Campaign to Increase Enrollment in Clinical Trials. Focus Groups Report.* Balch Associates, Oak Park, IL.
104. Mackenzie IS, Wei L, Rutheford D, *et al.* (2010) Promoting public awareness of randomised clinical trials using the media: the "Get Randomised" campaign. *Br J Clin Pharmacol* **69**(2): 128–135.
105. National Institutes of Health, National Cancer Institute, Office of Education & Special Initiatives. (2000) *Healthcare Providers' Wants and Needs in Continuing Medical Education on Clinical Trials: A Focus Group Study.* Bethesda, MD.
106. National Institutes of Health, National Cancer Institute, Office of Communication. (undated) *Colorectal Cancer Trial Web Site Promotion Evaluation. Findings from a Study.* Bethesda, MD.
107. Embi PJ, Jain A, Martin Harris C. (2008) Physicians' perceptions of an electronic health record-based clinical alert approach to subject recruitment: A survey. *BMC Med Inform Decision Making* **8**(13). *www.biomedcentral.com/1472-6947/8/13*
108. Sinclair S, Myers HF, Hawes-Dawson J, Kington R. (2000) Recruiting African Americans for health studies. In: SE Levkoff, TR Prohaska, P Flynn Weitzman, MG Ory (eds), *Recruitment and Retention in Minority Populations.* Springer, New York, pp. 39–52.
109. Barnett J, Aguilar S, Brittner M, Bonuck K. (2012) Recruiting and retaining low-income, multi-ethnic women into randomized controlled trials: Successful strategies and staffing. *Contemp Clin Trials* **33**(5): 925–932.
110. Kadushin G. (2001) Clinical trials: A wider lens 2. *Health Soc Work* **26**(3): 203–206.

111. Robins Sadler G. (2001) A call to action: Patients' access to clinical trials. *Health Soc Work* **26**(3): 196–200.
112. Freeman H. (1993) The impact of clinical trial protocols on patient care systems in a large city hospital. Access for the socially disadvantaged. *Cancer* **72**(Suppl 9): 2834–2838.
113. Gomez VM. (1997) Effective strategies in recruiting special populations: Rural residents, migrants, older adults, and people with disabilities. Presented at: *Midwest Regional Conference on Recruitment and Retention of Minorities and Women in Cancer Clinical Research*, University of Illinois, Chicago, IL.
114. McCabe M, Varricchio CG, Padberg RM. (1994) Efforts to recruit the economically disadvantaged to national clinical trials. *Sem Oncol Nursing* **10**(2): 123–129.
115. Kornblith AB, Kemeny M, Peterson BL, *et al.* (2002) Survey of oncologists' perceptions of barriers to accrual of older patients with breast carcinoma to clinical trials. *Cancer* **95**(5): 989–996.
116. Fillion M, Forget G, Brochu O, *et al.* (2012) Eligibility criteria in randomized phase II and III adjuvant and nonadjuvant breast cancer trials: Not a significant barrier to enrollment. *Clin Trials* **9**(5): 652–659.
117. Dent SF, Eisenhauer EA. (1996) Phase I trial design: Are new methodologies being put into practice? *Ann Oncol* **7**(6): 561–566.
118. Dillman RO, Koziol JA. (1992) Phase I cancer trials: Limitations and implications. *Mol Bio Ther* **4**(3): 117–121.
119. Mathé G, Reizenstein P. (1986) Ethics and errors of clinical trials and the role and place of different types of trial. *Drugs Under Exp Clin Res* **12**(1–3): 1–9.
120. Ratain MJ, Mick R, Schilsky RL, Siegler M. (1993) Statistical and ethical issues in the design and conduct of phase I and II clinical trials of new anticancer agents. *J Natl Cancer Inst* **85**: 1637–1643.
121. Anderson DL. (2001) The importance of market research in patient recruitment. In: DL Anderson (eds), *A Guide to Patient Recruitment.* Center Watch, Boston, MA.
122. National Institutes of Health, National Cancer Institute, National Action Plan on Breast Cancer. (1999) *Developing a Marketing Communication Campaign to Increase Enrollment in Clinical Trials. Focus Groups Report.* Balch Associates, Oak Park, IL.
123. McDonald AM, Treweek S, Shakur H, *et al.* (2011) Using a business model approach and marketing techniques for recruitment to clinical trials. *Trials* **12**: 74.
124. Francis D, Roberts I, Elbourne DR, *et al.* (2007) Marketing and clinical trials: A case study. *Trials* **8**: 37.

125. Cramer JA. (1998) *Improving and Supporting Patient Recruitment in Clinical Trials Conducted by Academic Medical Centers.* University Health System Consortium, Oak Brook, IL.
126. Kumar N, Crocker T, Smith T, *et al.* (2012) Challenges and potential solutions to meeting accrual goals in a Phase II chemoprevention trial for prostate cancer. *Contemp Clin Trials* **33**(2): 279–285.
127. Kaur G., Smyth RL, Williamson P. (2012) Developing a survey of barriers and facilitators to recruitment in randomized controlled trials. *Trials* **13**: 218.

III. Organization, Prioritization, Review and Funding for the Translational Research

CHAPTER 7

Sport Programs and Transcational Research in Cancer

*Peter Ujhazy**, *Andrew M. Hruszkewycz and Toby T. Hecht*

7.1. INTRODUCTION

Since 1992, the Specialized Programs of Research Excellence (SPOREs) has been the U.S. National Cancer Institute's premier translational cancer research grants program. SPOREs support multi-project, interdisciplinary research that uses knowledge of human biology to develop and test the feasibility of cancer-relevant interventions in humans. These grants use a team science approach — basic and applied scientists in each project — to develop innovative and diverse approaches to the prevention, early detection, diagnosis and treatment of human cancers. For more than 20 years, the program contributed to the successful movement of many cancer-related discoveries to clinical testing and further — to integration into cancer patient care.

7.2. HISTORY OF TRANSLATIONAL SCIENCE RESEARCH SUPPORT AT THE NATIONAL CANCER INSTITUTE

Before 1992, when SPOREs were initiated, the National Cancer Institute (NCI) had tried various experiments to put serious effort into creating

*National Cancer Institute, Rockville, Maryland, USA

Corresponding author: Peter Ujhazy, MD, PhD, Translational Research Program, Division of Cancer Treatment and Diagnosis, National Cancer Institute, 9609 Medical Center Drive, Room 3W106 MSC 9726, Rockville, MD 20892-9702, USA; Tel: +1-240-276-5730; Fax: +1-240-276-5826; E-mail: ujhazyp@mail.nih.gov.

a funding mechanism by which investigators could translate novel basic science findings into clinical testing for the benefit of patients.

As a result of the passage of the National Cancer Act in 1971 that would "ascertain the causes and develop means for the treatment, cure and elimination of cancer," the NCI's budget grew, with many resources given initially to the discovery of retroviral oncogenes and the study of lymphomas and leukemias. During the 1970s, the NCI established the Organ Site Cancer Program to provide emphasis and funding for four solid tumors: large bowel, bladder, prostate and pancreas, diseases that accounted for much of the cancer incidence and mortality in the U.S. An unusual aspect of this organ site program was the location of the governance of the program: at headquarter sites outside the NCI, by committees with responsibilities for both programmatic oversight *and* review. The underlying philosophy was that "active scientists in the field are also those best suited to organize and implement national programs aimed at the full scope of problems of cancer in specific organ sites." This novel approach to the development and implementation of programs outside the NCI was subject to criticism, mainly in the area of peer review, conflicts of interest, and the role of basic research in a targeted cancer program. Yet, by 1976, 53 projects were supported by the National Bladder Cancer Project, one of the four components of the Organ Site Cancer Program.[1]

By the early 1980s, new resources for funding the program rapidly disappeared and transparency about the manner in which decisions were made and priorities set was demanded by the public. Divisional Boards of Scientific Counselors were established, and they and the National Cancer Advisory Board's meetings had open forum sessions. Based on advice from these advisory bodies, the Organ Site Cancer Program was converted to a new format and called The Organ Systems Program. This new program would reside in the Organ Systems Branch in the NCI Division of Resources, Centers and Community Activities. The program consolidated the four original headquarter sites and established, through a cooperative agreement, the Organ Systems Coordinating Center (OSCC) at Roswell Park Memorial Institute, whose function was to "scan the entire scientific horizon for research advances ready for clinical application in the common tumors"[2] with the goal of reducing cancer incidence, morbidity and/or mortality. The responsibility of peer review returned to the National Institutes of Health, and later to the NCI.

The NCI also recognized that other organ sites required attention and funding and so the Breast Cancer Task Force was integrated into the new Organ Systems Program. Previously, this body, which was established in the 1960s, was governed entirely within the NCI. The OSCC would now concentrate on breast, large bowel, pancreas, prostate and urinary bladder cancers and would form working groups for program planning, conducting workshops and identifying areas for emphasis and de-emphasis.[3] Approval by the NCI Boards of Scientific Counselors would be required for these activities.

By the end of the decade, Dr. Samuel Broder, the director of the NCI, saw the need for research, not only in the basic science of organ-specific cancers, but also in the translation of the cancer biology advances to human testing, a concept that required a multi-discipline team approach. In developing this vision, he was supported by investigators who felt the time had come to span the *discovery to clinic* funding chasm, and by the enthusiasm of patient advocates.

In 1989, Dr. Broder detailed a new plan for the operations of the Organ Systems Program in order to create a mechanism to "stimulate investigator-initiated research ideas across a broad range of basic and clinical solid tumor research."[4] The Organ Systems Program would now become a branch led by Dr. Andrew Chiarodo in NCI's Division of Cancer Biology and Diagnosis under Dr. Brian Kimes, the Associate Director for Extramural Programs.

In 1991, Congress urged the NCI to establish the Specialized Programs of Research Excellence (SPOREs) with U.S.$20 million using the P50 grant mechanism, a mechanism that had not been used by the NCI in the previous 20 years. The Board of Scientific Counselors of the Division of Cancer Biology, Diagnosis and Centers approved the concept in June of 1991 and the NCI director expressed a hope that new money from Congress would be forthcoming for this program, and in any case, the funding would not come out of the research grants pool or from the existing Cancer Centers (*The Cancer Letter*, Vol. 17, No. 27, 1991). Later that year, the NCI released three Requests for Applications (RFAs) for SPOREs in breast, lung, and prostate cancer for translational studies in patients and in populations at risk for cancer (RFAs CA-91-33; CA-91-34; CA-91-35).

Initially, eight fully funded SPOREs (four in breast cancer, two in prostate cancer, and two in lung cancer) were awarded for three years only to seven different institutions. In addition, 12 feasibility grants were awarded at a reduced annual funding level to allow these institutions to develop their programs in order to reapply. A ninth fully funded SPORE in gastrointestinal cancers was added in 1993 as a result of a new RFA (CA-93-16). The plan was to be able to fund successful competitive renewal grants in future years for five years. In 1999, ovarian cancer was added to the list of SPOREs for which institutions could apply.

In 2000, under Dr. Jorge Gomez, chief of the Organ Systems Branch, the SPOREs were converted from an RFA-enabled program to an investigator-initiated program enabled by a Program Announcement. This move provided investigators the possibility to apply for amended application in a timely manner and allowed for greater scientific opportunity in translational cancer research. Competition was opened up to additional organ sites and over the years, first 14, then 16, and finally all organ sites were permitted. Pancreatic cancer became a separate SPORE category, apart from gastrointestinal SPOREs, in 2003. In 2010 there were 17 organ site funded SPOREs. A change in philosophy was partly responsible for this evolution: it was now thought the SPOREs should study not only the major incident malignancies, but also the rarer cancers and highly related groups of cancers, such as sarcoma.

With the conversion to a Program Announcement as the funding opportunity, the SPORE program established other changes: (a) five years of funding became the standard, (b) a minimum of four translational projects that must reach a human endpoint within the funding period was required, and (c) a funding cap of U.S.$1.5 million direct cost and later a cap of U.S.$2.5 million total cost was instituted. One of the biggest changes came in 2007 when the NCI leadership announced that SPOREs for any organ site may be submitted for any receipt date. Earlier, applications were restricted in their receipt dates and years by their organ site focus. Now applicants who applied in January and were not successful might amend their applications and reapply in the same fiscal year.

However, the key features of the SPOREs have remained constant and set the program apart from other NCI funding mechanisms:

- the translational requirement of all scientific projects;
- a team science approach, requiring a basic and an applied or clinical investigator co-leading each project;
- a biospecimen/pathology resource CORE (COmmonREsource) that acts as a resource not only for the SPORE, but for other researchers as well;
- flexibility to advance new promising projects by replacing projects that were either successfully completed early in the funding period or were failing to meet translational goals;
- a developmental research program that serves as a proving ground for high risk, high payoff projects, or for new collaborative projects;
- a career development program that supports budding careers or refocused careers in organ site translational science;
- a required research project in early detection, prevention or population science studies for SPOREs in the major incidence malignancies;
- the requirement for both inter-SPORE collaboration and collaboration with other research groups that facilitate movement along the translational/clinical research continuum;
- the requirement for substantial access to cancer patient populations;
- institutional involvement and commitment.

In addition, the advice of patient advocates is strongly encouraged for each SPORE.

Over the years, each new NCI Director has sought to establish his imprint on the program. In the late 1990s, the Organ Systems Branch was moved to the Office of Centers, Training, and Resources in the Office of NCI director. In 2008, the branch was renamed the Translational Research Program and became one of the six programs in the Division of Cancer Treatment and Diagnosis in order for it, according to Dr. John Niederhuber, "to gain greater prominence and integration within NCI's translational research and laboratory science portfolio."[5] Dr. Toby T. Hecht became the Associate Director of the program.

In 2012, there were 53 fully funded SPOREs in 17 organ sites from 31 institutions in 21 states.[a] There is also one SPORE from a non-profit

[a]Available from: http://trp.cancer.gov.

consortium of multiple institutions. In the future, depending upon the level of funding received, the SPORE program is considering including applications in viral-related malignancies, neuroendocrine tumors, pediatric cancers, as well as other areas (such as hepatocellular carcinoma) where there are gaps in the NCI translational research portfolio.

The most current Program Announcement (PAR-12-296) was approved by the NIH in September 2012 together with updated SPORE guidelines.

7.3. PROGRAM RULES

The following two sections discuss the current rules of the program. The rules evolved over the years and are a result of ongoing adjustments to new challenges in translational research and of the experience drawn from the management of the program, while observing existing U.S. federal grant laws and regulations.

7.3.1. SPORE Eligibility

Many kinds of institutions in the U.S. are eligible for an NCI SPORE. These include domestic for-profit and not-for profit organizations, either public of private, including universities, colleges, hospitals, laboratories, units of state and local governments, units of tribal governments, certain agencies of the federal government, as well as faith-based and other community-based organizations. To be eligible, institutions must demonstrate strong institutional commitment to the SPORE, and they must have access to the appropriate cancer patient populations. Currently, most NCI Specialized Programs of Research Excellence are at academic medical institutions with NCI-designated Cancer Centers.

Although foreign institutions are not eligible to apply for a SPORE, the U.S. institution may propose a scientific collaboration or a consortium agreement with the foreign institution. The foreign activities may not exceed 49 percent of the direct costs of the budget and these allocations must be approved by the U.S. State Department. The foreign institutions must also have appropriate federal-wide assurances for the protection of human subjects and animals. SPORE investigators currently work with researchers in Canada, Europe and Asia, and some SPOREs have incorporated foreign activities as key components of their team research, though the budgetary commitments by the SPOREs are relatively small at this time.

SPORE guidelines[b] allow multiple SPORE applications from the same institution as long as the proposals are from different organ sites and are to be led by different principal investigators. The program encourages applications from investigators that are frequently under-represented among scientific leadership, including minority individuals, women, and persons with disabilities.

7.3.2. SPORE Requirements

The SPORE program endeavors to assemble strong multidisciplinary scientific teams with extensive depth and breadth of expertise in the types of cancers to be investigated. A SPORE must include among its scientific leadership at least four investigators that are acknowledged experts in the cancer-specific science being addressed by the SPORE. This required minimum research base may include individuals that are independently funded through peer-reviewed grants, or they may be chairpersons on active NCI cooperative group clinical trials focused on the cancer type(s) to be studied through the SPORE. It is important that parent institutions incorporate the SPORE within their institutional priorities, integrate SPORE activities within its Cancer Center activities, and provide resources that promote the scientific progress. Matching funds are usually provided by the institution, particularly in support of the SPORE's Developmental Projects.

SPORE directors should be leaders in the field and commit at least 20 per cent of their professional time to the SPORE. The director should be prominent within the lines of authority of the institution. While overseeing and planning the translational research activities of the SPORE, the SPORE director often serves as a leading investigator on research projects within the SPORE.

Each SPORE should have a minimum of four major projects. Multidisciplinary leadership is a central feature of each project, and each major

[b]Available from: http://trp.cancer.gov/investigator_resources/docs/spore_ guidelines_ 2013.pdf.

project is required to have co-leadership by a basic scientist and an applied scientist. The applied investigator may be a physician-scientist or, in the case of a population study, an epidemiologist. The projects are to be planned and executed through strong collaboration of these equal and complementary partners.

Each project should test novel translational ideas with high potential impact on human cancer intervention(s). These projects must meet the definition of translational research as defined for the SPORE program: ***Translational research uses knowledge of human biology to develop and test the feasibility of cancer-relevant interventions in humans AND/OR determines the biological basis for observations made in individuals with cancer or in populations at risk for cancer***. The term *interventions* is used in its broadest sense to include molecular assays, imaging techniques, drugs, biological agents, and/or other methodologies applicable to the prevention, early detection, diagnosis, prognosis, and/or treatment of cancer.

Each project must be centered on the biology of human cancer, have a laboratory component, and perform an investigation that will include a human endpoint within the five-year period of the SPORE grant. The human endpoint may be achieved by performing analysis with human biospecimens to test hypotheses or to generate new hypothesis. The human endpoint may also be realized through the conduct of an early phase clinical trial. In cases where a project is developing an investigational new drug, IND-directed toxicology studies utilizing U.S. Food and Drug Administration (FDA)-approved protocols may be considered translational.

Since the beginning of the SPORE program there has been a requirement that SPOREs in cancers of the breast, prostate, lung, and gastrointestinal tract include at least one project in early detection, prevention or population science.With the expansion of the program to all organ sites, this additional requirement has remained in place for the four organ sites with the highest cancer death rates.

All SPORE applications must include COREs that provide biospecimen and pathology resources, and they are also required to have an administrative CORE. The SPORE may opt to include other shared resource COREs, such as a biostatistics CORE, clinical CORE or informatics CORE. All proposed COREs should provide support for at least one project, and SPORE COREs should not duplicate existing CORE resources within the institution. Shared resource COREs may include non-hypothesis-driven research activities designed to improve CORE services for the SPORE.

The SPORE Biospecimen/Pathology CORE has always been a requirement of the SPORE program because the availability and analysis of biospecimens are key conditions to acquiring requisite good data for the translational science of the SPORE. This CORE is essential not only to the research activities of the individual SPORE but also to serve scientists outside the parent institution who are invested in translation research. Each SPORE must have a plan for prioritizing the distribution of biospecimens to SPORE scientists and other members of the cancer research community, based on the merit of the translational cancer research activity. This CORE is expected to be able to provide service beyond conventional pathology specimen banking activities. Human specimens should be annotated with clinical information and there should be careful attention to pre-analytical parameters that may confound the analyses to be conducted for the SPORE's research. In many cases, this CORE is directed by experts in laboratory medicine and academic pathology. This CORE often provides a range of analytic services, including histologic evaluation, immunohistochemistry, laser-capture microdissection, tissue array preparation, as well as proteomic analyses and nucleic-acid-based analyses. Given the ever-increasing amount of data generated by new analytic technologies, such as high throughput sequencing of DNA, this CORE frequently includes a bioinformatics component. The Biospecimen/Pathology CORE is becoming the keystone for biomarker driven development of precision medicine.

The Administrative CORE has long been included by investigators as part of their SPORE infrastructure, and this CORE has recently become a required component of the SPORE. This CORE facilitates the identification of new research opportunities and is required to include an External Advisory Board. The CORE is responsible for appropriate fiscal and data management, coordination of collaborations, sharing of new ideas, sharing of resources, involvement of patient advocates, and the potential succession for the SPORE director. This CORE also stewards funds that support investigator participation in NCI sponsored meetings/workshops, and it is responsible for the allocation of discretionary funds in support of the SPORE.

Each SPORE program is required to conduct a Developmental Research Program (DRP) and a Career Development Program (CDP). These developmental programs are the SPORE's research engines for expediting the exploration of new research opportunities and for the mentoring of clinicians and scientists interested in translational cancer research. Each SPORE is required to allocate significant fiscal support of these programs. The SPORE is required to have a formal administrative process for the solicitation, review and award of DRPs and candidates for the CDP. These programs must be maintained throughout the entire term of the funding period.

The DRP explores innovative ideas by funding pilot projects in basic research and/or early phase clinical research related to the organ site(s) that are the focus of the SPORE. A human endpoint is not required for a DRP project. These pilot projects may be collaborative and offer an opportunity to pursue high risk/high payoff research. With the approval of the SPORE's External Advisory Board and the NCI Translational Research Program, the DRP studies may become full projects that are to achieve new translational goals for the SPORE. The CDP supports both established investigators as well as basic or clinical scientists that are about to become faculty. This is not a training program but a mentored opportunity to conduct research that will enable career transition toward translational cancer research.

With the growing recognition that the success of translational cancer research is increasingly dependent on a team science approach, each SPORE must demonstrate a commitment to collaborations. These may be "horizontal" collaborations in which there are plans, logistics, timelines and formal agreements for groups to work together to accomplish a set of translational research aims. Collaborative plans should also promote the "vertical" transition of scientific achievements from the SPORE to other government or non-government mechanisms that will further advance the accomplishments in translational science toward patient care.

7.4. SPORE COLLABORATIONS

The program is distinct from many other NCI grant funding mechanisms by its collaborative nature. With time, collaborations have proven to strengthen the program's quality and productivity. Most of translational research requires constant interaction among investigators or teams with diverse expertise. Critical is the dialogue between basic scientists on one side and applied or clinical investigators on the other. The structure of SPORE projects with the co-leadership of basic scientists and clinicians provides an environment with ongoing information exchange between laboratories and the clinic. Support services from SPORE COREs secure additional expertise and help to individual projects. The result is a culture of interaction and constant cross-pollination between teams and their members. Sometimes, limited resources in one institution (e.g., for rare specimens) compel investigators to reach out for collaborative partners elsewhere. Program guidelines encourage and rules of SPORE grant review reward collaborations with other institutes, government programs, industry, and non-profit organizations. The creation of such a collaborative culture among SPOREs led to many successful accomplishments. From a simple exchange of specimens, experimental models or agents, through more complex collaborations on early phase clinical trials and population studies, to highly demanding phase II clinical studies with genomic, proteomic, imaging and clinical analysis, SPOREs have documented hundreds of collaborations and some of their results are highlighted here.

7.4.1. The Cancer Genome Atlas (TCGA) and Other Genomic Projects

The Cancer Genome Atlas is the NCI's comprehensive and coordinated effort to accelerate understanding of the molecular basis of cancer through genome analysis.[c] SPOREs contributed with expertise and with more than 1,600 specimens to TCGA studies in glioblastoma, ovarian, breast, colon, and rectal cancers, squamous cell carcinoma, and others.[6–8]

As investigator-initiated programs, SPOREs also spearheaded several independent genomic collaborative projects that led to authoritative publications. In small-cell lung cancer (SCLC), three lung cancer SPOREs teamed up with the company Genentech to sequence 53 samples containing human primary tumors and cell lines.[9] The study revealed mutated

[c]Available from: http://cancergenome.nih.gov.

and amplified members of the SOX family in tumor specimens. Moreover, RNA sequencing identified multiple fusion transcripts and a recurrent RLF-MYCL1 fusion.

Another multi-institutional study in lung adenocarcinoma was partly funded through a SPORE Career Development Award.[10] Using massively parallel sequencing, the authors found, besides previously known mutations, recurrent splicing factor U2AF1 mutations and truncating mutations affecting RBM10 and ARID1A genes.

In head and neck cancer, the University of Pittsburgh, MD Anderson Cancer Center, and Johns Hopkins University SPOREs in collaboration with the Broad Institute published two seminal genomic papers. The first provided an analysis of whole-exome sequencing data from 74 head and neck squamous cell carcinomas. Besides the detection of a tobacco exposure mutational profile and a profile linked to the presence of papillomavirus in infected tumors, data revealed known (e.g.,TP53, CDKN2A, PTEN) and previously unknown HNSCC-associated genes (NOTCH, IRF1 and TP63).[11] The second study identified inactivating mutations of NOTCH1.[12]

The IDH1 and IDH2 mutations in glioblastoma were described in a collaborative paper with the participation of the Duke University Brain Tumor SPORE.[13] Finally, a seminal paper that studied consensus coding sequences of human breast and colorectal cancers involved multiple institutions and grants including the Johns Hopkins University Gastrointestinal Cancer SPORE.[14]

7.4.2. Prostate Cancer Clinical Trials Consortium (PCCTC)

The partnership between Prostate Cancer SPOREs and the PCCTC dwells on the design and implementation of hypothesis-driven phase I and II clinical trials of novel agents and combination treatments with the aim of prolonging lives of prostate cancer patients. The NCI SPORE program collaborates with the Prostate Cancer Foundation and the Department of Defense, which funds the PCCTC. Many of the PCCTC principal investigators are also project leaders in Prostate Cancer SPOREs and many of the SPORE trials are conducted through the PCCTC infrastructure. From this partnership, eight agents have already reached the phase III clinical trial testing including drugs such as MDV3100 (enzalutamide) and abiraterone (Zytiga), which were approved by the FDA for clinical use.

7.5. SPORE ACHIEVEMENTS

Equipped with the right translational research philosophy and infrastructure, shortly after its establishment, the SPORE program generated several outstanding discoveries and clinically applicable tools that placed it in the forefront of NCI's successful initiatives.

In the 1990s, while still focused on the four major disease/organ sites (breast, prostate, lung and gastrointestinal cancers), SPOREs critically contributed to the discovery of new tumor suppressor genes (DPC4/SMAD4 in pancreatic cancer,[15] FUS1 in lung cancer,[16]) metastasis suppressor genes (e.g., KAI1/CD82 in prostate cancer[17]), oncogenes (ZABC1/ZNF217 in breast cancer[18]), and several tumor susceptibility genes.[19,20] In pancreatic cancer, the Johns Hopkins GI SPORE, led by Dr. Scott Kern, identified the most commonly mutated gene (p16/MTS1[21]) and described the location and mutation of the BRCA2 gene.[22] Another group of SPORE investigators at Johns Hopkins University under the leadership of Dr. Stephen Baylin opened an entire new field of DNA methylation alterations in neoplasia and pioneered the use of demethylation agents in the clinic.[23,24] The Breast Cancer SPORE led by Dr. C. Kent Osborne showed that breast cancer in African American women occurs at a younger age and is associated with estrogen receptor-negativity and higher tumor cell proliferation rates[25] compared with Caucasian women. The Prostate Cancer SPORE at Baylor developed the first transgenic mouse model for prostate cancer and pioneered the first attempt of gene therapy of the same disease.[26,27]

In this period, the first major contribution of SPOREs toward clinical applications was the development and introduction of nomograms for prediction of five-year probability of progression, first in prostate cancer, later in other areas of oncology.[28,29] Nomograms have since then been integrated into every phase of patient management and have fundamentally changed the way clinicians predict outcomes and establish prognosis for their patients.

With the expansion of the program in the first decade of the 21st century, SPORE support of translational research rapidly made its impact on other diseases such as myeloma, leukemia, skin, head and neck cancers, and continued producing major advances in the original four disease sites. Within the following pages some of the most relevant stories will demonstrate how the SPOREs transformed, in many cases, the clinical conduct of cancer diagnosis and treatment, how carefully designed preclinical studies facilitated a rapid translation into successful early phase clinical testing, and how paradigm-shifting discoveries changed the way we look at prediction of response to cancer treatment today.

7.5.1. Lenalidomide in Myeloma Therapy

In 2003, when Ken Anderson and his team at Dana Farber/Harvard Cancer Center received the first Myeloma SPORE award, they were already an established prominent myeloma research group. Besides other discoveries, their laboratory data contributed to a major accomplishment: the approval in 2003 by the Food and Drug Administration (FDA) of a new proteasome inhibitor, bortezomib (Velcade), for the treatment of recurrent refractory multiple myeloma, and in 2005 for recurrent disease.[30] This work created a solid basis for SPORE explorations of bortezomib in combination with other promising compounds and for the search for new active drugs against myeloma. Along those lines, SPORE investigators validated the anti-myeloma activity of lenalidomide (Revlimid), a derivative of thalidomide, with multiple mechanisms of action. They identified its effects against tumor cells in their micro environment, described molecular mechanisms of drug sensitivity and resistance, proved the benefit of its combination with other anti-myeloma agents, and rapidly translated the findings to phase I trials and to a multicenter phase II trial that confirmed both anti-myeloma activity and a favorable side effect profile.[31,32] Based upon these results two phase III trials confirmed superiority of lenalidomide/dexamethasone over dexamethasone alone as treatment for recurrent multiple myeloma, results that led to the FDA approval of lenalidomide for relapsed multiple myeloma in 2006. In 2010, bortezomib, lenalidomide and dexamethasone combination was found to be highly effective in newly diagnosed multiple myeloma with 74 per cent progression-free survival and 97 per cent overall survival within 18 months.[33] Thus myeloma, while still incurable, has become a chronic condition with multiple options for treatment.

Remarkably, the Dana Farber Cancer Institute Myeloma SPORE team proved that sometimes moving scientific concepts to FDA-approved clinical application may take only a few years instead of decades. Doctor Anderson likes to refer to the collaborative spirit between government, academic institutes, industry, and non-profit organizations as "the United Nations against myeloma."

7.5.2. Epidermal Growth Factor Receptor Mutations in Lung Cancer

Until the early years of the 21st century, most lung cancer patients were treated either by surgery, radiation, or with standard doublet chemotherapy (usually a combination of cis-platinum and taxol). In most cases, the disease was diagnosed at later stages and the treatment secured a five-year survival to only a small fraction of patients. With the advent of a molecular rather than a histological definition of cancer, the scientific community and the pharmaceutical industry directed their attention to potential druggable molecular targets for agent design. One of them was the epidermal growth factor receptor (EGFR), which was present in the majority of patients with lung adenocarcinoma. In 2003, there were already reports on the clinical response of patients with this disease to the tyrosine kinase inhibitor (TKI) gefitinib (Iressa). However, when a single agent phase II clinical trial (IDEAL) was performed, only about 12 per cent of the U.S. patients responded to the treatment.[34,35] This finding prompted several Lung Cancer SPORE groups at Dana Farber/Harvard Cancer Center led by Bruce Johnson plus Thomas Lynch and at Vanderbilt University led by David Carbone to investigate the reason. The responding patients' tumors were studied and specific mutations of the EGFR were identified in those patients that responded to therapy.[36–38] This paradigm-changing discovery was then validated by several clinical trials and by additional evidence in lung cancer cell line models. It meant that lung cancer could be now divided into molecularly defined entities that exhibit a certain clinical response to targeted therapy. Tyrosine kinase inhibitors (TKIs) soon became agents of choice in patients bearing EGFR mutations (present in about 10–15 per cent in Western European populations, but up to 30 per cent in Asian lung adenocarcinoma patients). In parallel, new prediction markers based on EGFR gene amplification were developed by the Colorado Lung Cancer SPORE.[39]

As with chemotherapy and other targeted therapy drugs, the responses to TKIs turned out to be temporary and within a year from treatment start drug-resistant clones emerged in patients. Even here, SPORE investigators contributed to the field by discovering the first resistance mutation to TKIs, T790M,[40] and by describing Met-based mechanisms of resistance to EGFR-targeted therapies.[41] Moreover, they found novel mutant-selective EGFR kinase inhibitors against EGFR T790M in functional pharmacological screens against clinically important mutant kinases. They developed a powerful strategy to identify new classes of mutant-selective kinase inhibitors.[42] More recently, genotypic and histological evolution of lung cancers acquiring resistance to EGFR inhibitors showed that some resistant non-SCLCs transform into SCLC and are sensitive to standard SCLC therapies. In the absence of the selective pressure of EGFR inhibitor treatment, resistant cancers may become sensitive to a second round of treatment with EGFR inhibitors.[43]

It is fair to conclude that SPORE investigators made a decisive imprint with this major shift in lung cancer standard of care and they have changed the direction in the development of predictive tests. By joining forces with other centers through a unique grant as a result of the American Recovery and Reinvestment Act and by further support from the National Lung Cancer Partnership foundation, SPORE investigators have created the Lung Cancer Mutation Consortium to prospectively examine non-small cell lung cancer tumors for more than 10 genomic changes and match patients to the appropriate targeted therapies. The initiative was led by SPORE Principal Investigators Paul Bunn, Bruce Johnson, John Minna; and by Mark Kris from the Memorial Sloan Kettering Cancer Center.

7.5.3. Molecular Classification of Breast Cancer

The following story changed the way we look at breast cancer today. The University of North Carolina Breast Cancer SPORE under the leadership of Drs. Shelton Earp, Chuck Perou, Lisa Carey and the late Bob Millikan is one of the longest funded programs of its kind. In collaboration with the Lineberger Comprehensive Cancer Center and the Gillings School of Global Public Health, SPORE investigators established the Carolina

Breast Cancer Study to examine the causes of breast cancer in African American and Caucasian women. By 2001, they accrued 2,311 cases, of which 894 were African American, and 2,022 controls, of which 788 were African American. This cohort served, in 2006, for validation of a new molecular classification that divided breast cancer into four major subtypes: basal-like, luminal A, luminal B, and HER2-positive.[44] Furthermore, it was shown that microarray-based classification of breast cancers provided one explanation for the disparity in cancer mortality rates between African American and Caucasian women.[45] Basal-like breast tumors with worse prognosis occurred at a higher incidence among premenopausal African American patients compared with postmenopausal African American and non-African American patients. In turn, luminal A type, with the best prognosis, was more common in non-African Americans. In 2010, after collection of more cases and further analysis, SPORE investigators confirmed the association of basal-like breast cancer with poor prognosis and suggested that basal-like breast cancer was not an inherently more aggressive disease in African American women compared with Caucasians.[46] They also showed that African American women had a higher death rate from luminal A and B cancers perhaps indicating socioeconomic and health services access issues as additional causes of disparity in outcome. The UNC SPORE has launched the Carolina Breast Cancer Study (CBCS) phase III now accruing 3,000 new cases (50 per cent African American) with detailed treatment and follow-up data as well as biospecimens and tumor samples. CBCS III will provide more definitive data on the contribution of biologic factors and health services access to the disparities in breast cancer outcomes.

7.5.4. Recurrent Fusion of Transcription Factor Genes in Prostate Cancer

Prostate cancer incidence and death toll make it one of the most studied malignancies. Several SPOREs were created since the early 1990s to study this group of diseases. The University of Michigan Prostate Cancer SPORE under Dr. Kenneth Pienta achieved one of the major advances in epithelial cancers in general, and in prostate cancer in particular, with the discovery of the recurrent fusion of TMPRSS2 and ETS transcription factor genes. In 2005, this became the first known fusion gene related to epithelial cancers.

The seeds of the study were planted by SPORE Career Development and Developmental Research projects awarded to a young rising scientific star, Dr. Arul Chinnaiyan. He and his team developed a method called Cancer Outlier Profile Analysis (COPA) that sought to identify outlier profiles by applying a simple numerical transformation based on the median and median absolute deviation of a gene expression profile.[47] Two years later, the ETS gene fusions were proposed to mediate the transition from prostate cells with pre-existing lesions to carcinoma.[48] The clinical relevance of these findings became more apparent in 2009 by a study from the Memorial Sloan Kettering Prostate SPORE led by Dr. Peter Scardino, when TMPRSS2-ERG gene rearrangement alone was shown to be associated with a lower grade while copy number increase with a higher grade, i.e., more advanced stage prostate cancer.[49] Rearrangements were not associated with the clinical outcome in these patients. In 2010, two more gene fusions were discovered by SPORE investigators (SLC45A3-BRAF and ESRP1-RAF1), indicating a phenotype sensitive to RAF and MAP2K1 inhibitors.[50] The Michigan group identified the first oncogenic mutant KRAS gene fusion (UBE2L3-KRAS) in prostate cancer,[51] and in 2011 it introduced the therapeutic targeting of SPINK1-positive/ETS fusion negative prostate cancer.[52]

Altogether, gene fusion discoveries in prostate cancer by the SPOREs opened a new window of opportunity for the design of precision medicine interventions for different types of cancers where actionable molecular aberrations are identified. While serving as potential therapeutic targets, gene fusions are also becoming a new means for cancer detection.

Some of the other significant accomplishments of the Program are listed in Table 1.

It is beyond the scope of this chapter to list all discoveries, successful early phase clinical trials, biomarker validations, and population-based findings produced by the SPOREs. Each year about 800 papers acknowledge the SPORE granting mechanism, many of them in top ranked scientific journals (see Table 2). At the end of 2012, SPORE grants were credited in more than 8,000 scientific publications.

In any given year, more than 100 active early phase clinical trials are associated with the SPORE program either by direct funding from the grant or by complementing trials run by other programs or industry with clinical research studies.

Table 1 Additional Selected SPORE Accomplishments

Accomplishment	SPORE
Screening and monitoring in endometrial cancer and hereditary non-polyposis colorectal cancer (HNPCC)/Lynch syndrome	Johns Hopkins University, University of Texas MD Anderson Cancer Center[53,54]
Genes expressed in human tumor endothelium are different from those expressed in normal endothelium	Johns Hopkins University[55]
Difluoromethylornithine (DFMO) and sulindac for prevention of colorectal cancer	University of Arizona, University of California Irvine, Johns Hopkins University[56–59]
Chromosomal 1p/19q deletion as an oligodendroglioma prognostic/predictive marker	Mayo Clinic Rochester, University of Texas MD Anderson Cancer Center[60,61]
Diagnostic test for EML4-ALK translocation in non-small cell lung cancer (NSCLC) patients	University of Colorado, Dana Farber Harvard Cancer Center[62,63]
BRAF mutation detection and prognostic value in papillary thyroid cancer	Johns Hopkins University, University of Texas MD Anderson Cancer Center[64–66]
Enzalutamide (MDV3100) for late-stage prostate cancer	Memorial Sloan Kettering Cancer Center, Fred Hutchinson Cancer Center[67]
Heat shock protein peptide complex (HSPPC) 96 vaccine for brain cancer	University of California San Francisco[68]
Brentuximab for Hodgkin's lymphoma and T-cell lymphoma	Beckman Research Institute[69]

Table 2 Number of SPORE Publications in High Impact Journals in Years 1993–2012

High Impact Journal	Number of Articles by SPOREs
Blood	175
Cancer Research	766
Cell	19
Clinical Cancer Research	584
Journal of Biological Chemistry	136
Journal of Clinical Investigations	53
Journal of Clinical Oncology	188
Journal of the National Cancer Institute	119
Lancet	13
Nature	201
New England Journal of Medicine	30
Proceedings of the National Academy of Sciences	160
Science	74

7.6. CONCLUSION

Over the years the SPORE program has proven its unequivocal role in the movement of discoveries to the clinic and in explaining clinical observations by experimental findings. This was achieved by the visionary foresight in the original design of the program and by constant programmatic adjustments to new needs in translational cancer research driven by periodic rigorous reviews and evaluations by the NCI. Throughout 20-plus years of its existence, the SPORE program developed into a dynamic and productive scientific endeavor ultimately serving patients and people at risk for cancer.

ACKNOWLEDGMENTS

The authors wish to thank Drs. Kenneth Anderson, Shelton Earp and Bruce Johnson for their helpful suggestions.

AUTHORS' DISCLAIMER

Drs. Hecht, Hruszkewycz and Ujhazy contributed to this article in their personal capacity. The views expressed in this chapter do not necessarily represent the views of the National Institutes of Health or the U.S. Government.

REFERENCES

1. King TJ. (1977) The Organ Site Programs and the National Cancer Program. *Cancer Res* **37**(8 Pt 2): 2743–2744.
2. DeVita VT, Jr. (1983) The governance of science at the National Cancer Institute: A perspective on misperceptions. *Cancer Res* **43**(8): 3969–3973.
3. Boyd JD. (1982) NCI implementing changes in organ, site program, directing grant applications to NIH study sections. *Cancer Lett* **8**(40): 1–6.
4. Broder S. (1989) *JNCI J Natl Cancer Inst* **81**(12): 899. Available from: http://jnci.oxfordjournals.org/content/81/12/899.extract.
5. Niederhuber J. (2008) SPOREs move to strengthen program, vision. *NCI Cancer Bull* 5(4).

6. Cancer Genome Atlas Network. (2012) Comprehensive molecular portraits of human breast tumours. *Nature* **490**(7418): 61–70.
7. Yang D, Khan S, Sun Y, *et al.* (2011) Association of BRCA1 and BRCA2 mutations with survival, chemotherapy sensitivity, and gene mutator phenotype in patients with ovarian cancer. *J Am Med Assoc* **306**(14): 1557–1565.
8. Noushmehr H, Weisenberger DJ, Diefes K, *et al.* (2010) Identification of a CpG island methylator phenotype that defines a distinct subgroup of glioma. *Cancer Cell* **17**(5): 510–522.
9. Rudin CM, Durinck S, Stawiski EW, *et al.* (2012) Comprehensive genomic analysis identifies SOX2 as a frequently amplified gene in small-cell lung cancer. *Nat Genet* **44**(10): 1111–1116.
10. Imielinski M, Berger AH, Hammerman PS, *et al.* (2012) Mapping the hallmarks of lung adenocarcinoma with massively parallel sequencing. *Cell* **150**(6): 1107–1120.
11. Stransky N, Egloff AM, Tward AD, *et al.* (2011) The mutational landscape of head and neck squamous cell carcinoma. *Science* **333**(6046): 1157–1160.
12. Agrawal N, Frederick MJ, Pickering CR, *et al.* (2011) Exome sequencing of head and neck squamous cell carcinoma reveals inactivating mutations in NOTCH1. *Science* **333**(6046): 1154–1157.
13. Yan H, Parsons DW, Jin G, *et al.* (2009) IDH1 and IDH2 mutations in gliomas. *N Engl J Med* **360**(8): 765–773.
14. Sjöblom T, Jones S, Wood LD, *et al.* (2006) The consensus coding sequences of human breast and colorectal cancers. *Science* **314**(5797): 268–274.
15. Hahn SA, Schutte M, Hoque AT, *et al.* (1996) DPC4, a candidate tumor suppressor gene at human chromosome 18q21.1. *Science* **271**(5247): 350–353.
16. Kondo M, Ji L, Kamibayashi C, *et al.* (2001) Overexpression of candidate tumor suppressor gene FUS1 isolated from the 3p21.3 homozygous deletion region leads to G1 arrest and growth inhibition of lung cancer cells. *Oncogene* **20**(43): 6258–6262.
17. Dong JT, Lamb PW, Rinker-Schaeffer CW, *et al.* (1995) KAI1, a metastasis suppressor gene for prostate cancer on human chromosome 11p11.2. *Science* **268**(5212): 884–886.
18. Collins C, Rommens JM, Kowbel D, *et al.* (1998) Positional cloning of ZNF217 and NABC1: Genes amplified at 20q13.2 and overexpressed in breast carcinoma. *Proc Natl Acad Sci USA* **95**(15): 8703–8708.
19. Smith JR, Freije D, Carpten JD, *et al.* (1996) Major susceptibility locus for prostate cancer on chromosome 1 suggested by a genome-wide search. *Science* **274**(5291): 1371–1374.

20. Wooster R, Bignell G, Lancaster J, *et al.* (1995) Identification of the breast cancer susceptibility gene BRCA2. *Nature* **378**(6559): 789–792.
21. Caldas C, Hahn SA, da Costa LT, *et al.* (1994) Frequent somatic mutations and homozygous deletions of the p16 (MTS1) gene in pancreatic adenocarcinoma. *Nat Genet* **8**(1): 27–32.
22. Schutte M, da Costa LT, Hahn SA, *et al.* (1995) Identification by representational difference analysis of a homozygous deletion in pancreatic carcinoma that lies within the BRCA2 region. *Proc Natl Acad Sci USA* **92**(13): 5950–5954.
23. Baylin SB, Herman JG, Graff JR, *et al.* (1998) Alterations in DNA methylation: A fundamental aspect of neoplasia. *Adv Cancer Res* **72**: 141–196.
24. Merlo A, Herman JG, Mao L, *et al.* (1995) 5' CpG island methylation is associated with transcriptional silencing of the tumour suppressor p16/CDKN2/MTS1 in human cancers. *Nat Med* **1**(7): 686–692.
25. Elledge RM, Clark GM, Chamness GC, Kent Osborne C. (1994) Tumor biologic factors and breast cancer prognosis among white, Hispanic, and black women in the United States. *J Natl Cancer Inst* **86**(9): 705–712.
26. Eastham JA, Hall SJ, Sehgal I, *et al.* (1995) *In vivo* gene therapy with p53 or p21 adenovirus for prostate cancer. *Cancer Res* **55**(22): 5151–5155.
27. Greenberg NM, DeMayo F, Finegold MJ, *et al.* (1995) Prostate cancer in a transgenic mouse. *Proc Natl Acad Sci USA* **92**(8): 3439–3443.
28. Kattan MW, Eastham JA, Stapleton AM, *et al.* (1998) A preoperative nomogram for disease recurrence following radical prostatectomy for prostate cancer. *J Natl Cancer Inst* **90**(10): 766–771.
29. Kattan MW, Stapleton AM, Wheeler TM, Scardino PT. (1997) Evaluation of a nomogram used to predict the pathologic stage of clinically localized prostate carcinoma. *Cancer* **79**(3): 528–537.
30. Chauhan D, Hideshima T, Mitsiades C, *et al.* (2005) Proteasome inhibitor therapy in multiple myeloma. *Mol Cancer Ther* **4**(4): 686–692.
31. Richardson PG, Blood E, Mitsiades CS, *et al.* (2006) A randomized phase 2 study of lenalidomide therapy for patients with relapsed or relapsed and refractory multiple myeloma. *Blood* **108**(10): 3458–3464.
32. Vallet S, Palumbo A, Raje N, *et al.* (2008) Thalidomide and lenalidomide: Mechanism-based potential drug combinations. *Leuk Lymphoma* **49**(7): 1238–1245.
33. Richardson PG, Weller E, Lonial S, *et al.* (2010) Lenalidomide, bortezomib, and dexamethasone combination therapy in patients with newly diagnosed multiple myeloma. *Blood* **116**(5): 679–686.
34. Kris MG, Natale RB, Herbst RS, *et al.* (2003) Efficacy of gefitinib, an inhibitor of the epidermal growth factor receptor tyrosine kinase, in symptomatic patients

with non-small cell lung cancer: A randomized trial. *J Am Med Assoc* **290**(16): 2149–2158.

35. Fukuoka M, Yano S, Giaccone G, *et al.* (2003) Multi-institutional randomized phase II trial of gefitinib for previously treated patients with advanced non-small-cell lung cancer (The IDEAL 1 Trial) [corrected]. *J Clin Oncol* **21**(12): 2237–2246.
36. Lynch TJ, Bell DW, Sordella R, *et al.* (2004) Activating mutations in the epidermal growth factor receptor underlying responsiveness of non-small-cell lung cancer to gefitinib. *N Engl J Med* **350**(21): 2129–2139.
37. Ohm JE, Amann JM, Carbone DP. (2004) Acquired EGFr TKI resistance associated with mutation of the EGFr. *AACR Meeting Abstracts* (1): 570-b.
38. Paez JG, Jänne PA, Lee JC, *et al.* (2004) EGFR mutations in lung cancer: Correlation with clinical response to gefitinib therapy. *Science* **304**(5676): 1497–1500.
39. Cappuzzo F, Hirsch FR, Rossi E, *et al.* (2005) Epidermal growth factor receptor gene and protein and gefitinib sensitivity in non-small-cell lung cancer. *J Natl Cancer Inst* **97**(9): 643–655.
40. Kobayashi S, Boggon TJ, Dayaram T, *et al.* (2005) EGFR mutation and resistance of non-small-cell lung cancer to gefitinib. *N Engl J Med* **352**(8): 786–792.
41. Engelman JA, Zejnullahu K, Mitsudomi T, *et al.* (2007) MET amplification leads to gefitinib resistance in lung cancer by activating ERBB3 signaling. *Science* **316**(5827): 1039–1043.
42. Zhou W, Ercan D, Chen L, *et al.* (2009) Novel mutant-selective EGFR kinase inhibitors against EGFR T790M. *Nature* **462**(7276). 1070–1074.
43. Sequist LV, Waltman BA, Dias-Santagata D, *et al.* (2011) Genotypic and histological evolution of lung cancers acquiring resistance to EGFR inhibitors. *Sci Transl Med* **3**(75): 75ra26.
44. Hu Z, Fan C, Oh DS, *et al.* (2006) The molecular portraits of breast tumors are conserved across microarray platforms. *BMC Genomics* **7**: 96.
45. Carey LA, Perou CM, Livasy CA, *et al.* (2006) Race, breast cancer subtypes, and survival in the Carolina Breast Cancer Study. *J Am Med Assoc* **295**(21): 2492–2502.
46. O'Brien KM, Cole SR, Tse CK, *et al.* (2010) Intrinsic breast tumor subtypes, race, and long-term survival in the Carolina Breast Cancer Study. *Clin Cancer Res* **16**(24): 6100–6110.
47. Tomlins SA, Rhodes DR, Perner S, *et al.* (2005) Recurrent fusion of TMPRSS2 and ETS transcription factor genes in prostate cancer. *Science* **310**(5748): 644–648.

48. Tomlins SA, Laxman B, Dhanasekaran SM, *et al.* (2007) Distinct classes of chromosomal rearrangements create oncogenic ETS gene fusions in prostate cancer. *Nature* **448**(7153): 595–599.
49. Gopalan A, Leversha MA, Satagopan JM, *et al.* (2009) TMPRSS2-ERG gene fusion is not associated with outcome in patients treated by prostatectomy. *Cancer Res* **69**(4): 1400–1406.
50. Palanisamy N, Ateeq B, Kalyana-Sundaram S, *et al.* (2010) Rearrangements of the RAF kinase pathway in prostate cancer, gastric cancer and melanoma. *Nat Med* **16**(7): 793–798.
51. Wang XS, Shankar S, Dhanasekaran SM, *et al.* (2011) Characterization of KRAS rearrangements in metastatic prostate cancer. *Cancer Discov* **1**(1): 35–43.
52. Ateeq B, Tomlins SA, Laxman B, *et al.* (2011) Therapeutic targeting of SPINK1-positive prostate cancer. *Sci Transl Med* **3**(72): 72ra17.
53. Liu B, Parsons R, Papadopoulos N, *et al.* (1996) Analysis of mismatch repair genes in hereditary non-polyposis colorectal cancer patients. *Nat Med* **2**(2): 169–174.
54. Soliman PT, Broaddus RR, Schmeler KM, *et al.* (2005) Women with synchronous primary cancers of the endometrium and ovary: Do they have Lynch syndrome? *J Clin Oncol* **23**(36): 9344–9350.
55. St Croix B, Rago C, Velculescu V, *et al.* (2000) Genes expressed in human tumor endothelium. *Science* **289**(5482): 1197–1202.
56. Giardiello FM, Yang VW, Hylind LM, *et al.* (2002) Primary chemoprevention of familial adenomatous polyposis with sulindac. *N Engl J Med* **346**(14): 1054–1059.
57. Meyskens FL Jr, McLaren CE, Pelot D, *et al.* (2008) Difluoromethylornithine plus sulindac for the prevention of sporadic colorectal adenomas: A randomized placebo-controlled, double-blind trial. *Cancer Prev Res* (*Phila*) **1**(1): 32–38.
58. McLaren CE, Fujikawa-Brooks S, Chen WP, *et al.* (2008) Longitudinal assessment of air conduction audiograms in a phase III clinical trial of difluoromethylornithine and sulindac for prevention of sporadic colorectal adenomas. *Cancer Prev Res* (*Phila*) **1**(7): 514–521.
59. Zell JA, Pelot D, Chen W-P, *et al.* (2009) Risk of cardiovascular events in a randomized placebo-controlled, double-blind trial of difluoromethylornithine plus sulindac for the prevention of sporadic colorectal adenomas. *Cancer Prev Res* (*Phila*) **2**(3): 209–212.

60. Jenkins RB, Blair H, Ballman KV, *et al.* (2006) A t(1;19)(q10;p10) mediates the combined deletions of 1p and 19q and predicts a better prognosis of patients with oligodendroglioma. *Cancer Res* **66**(20): 9852–9861.
61. Wu A, Aldape K, Lang FF. (2010) High rate of deletion of chromosomes 1p and 19q in insular oligodendroglial tumors. *J Neurooncol* **99**(1): 57–64.
62. Shaw AT, Yeap BY, Solomon BJ, *et al.* (2011) Effect of crizotinib on overall survival in patients with advanced non-small-cell lung cancer harbouring ALK gene rearrangement: A retrospective analysis. *Lancet Oncol* **12**(11): 1004–1012.
63. Shaw AT, Yeap BY, Mino-Kenudson M, *et al.* (2009) Clinical features and outcome of patients with non-small-cell lung cancer who harbor EML4-ALK. *J Clin Oncol* **27**(26): 4247–4253.
64. Henderson YC, Fredrick MJ, Clayman GL. (2007) Differential responses of human papillary thyroid cancer cell lines carrying the RET/PTC1 rearrangement or a BRAF mutation to MEK1/2 inhibitors. *Arch Otolaryngol Head Neck Surg* **133**(8): 810–815.
65. Henderson YC, Shellenberger TD, Williams MD, *et al.* (2009) High rate of BRAF and RET/PTC dual mutations associated with recurrent papillary thyroid carcinoma. *Clin Cancer Res* **15**(2): 485–491.
66. Brait M, Loyo M, Rosenbaum E, *et al.* (2012) Correlation between BRAF mutation and promoter methylation of TIMP3, RARbeta2 and RASSF1A in thyroid cancer. *Epigenetics* **7**(7): 710–719.
67. Scher HI, Beer TM, Higano CS, *et al.* (2010) Antitumour activity of MDV 3100 in castration-resistant prostate cancer: A phase 1–2 study. *Lancet* **375**(9724): 1437–1446.
68. Crane CA, Han SJ, Ahn B, *et al.* (2012) Individual patient-specific immunity against high-grade glioma after vaccination with autologous tumor derived peptides bound to the 96 KD chaperone protein. *Clin Cancer Res* **19**(1): 205–214.
69. Chen R, Palmer JM, Thomas SH, *et al.* (2012) Brentuximab vedotin enables successful reduced-intensity allogeneic hematopoietic cell transplantation in patients with relapsed or refractory Hodgkin lymphoma. *Blood* **119**(26): 6379–6381.

CHAPTER 8

Challenges in the Peer Review Process for Applications to Conduct Translational Research in Biomedical Sciences

Brian Wojcik, Yvonne Lau† and Wlodek Lopaczynski*

8.1. INTRODUCTION

Public and private organizations that support biomedical research and clinical trials need to insure that their funding decisions are fair, unbiased, and support the goals and program objectives of the organization. To insure this, most agencies use a system of expert or peer review. Translational research, which can be broadly defined as taking discoveries from the laboratory into the clinic and *vice versa*, is usually broader in scope than basic laboratory research. This presents certain challenges for the peer review of translational research. The purpose of this chapter is to provide an overview of the peer review process with a focus on the review of translational research. Examples from the National Institutes of Health (NIH) system will be cited as the NIH funds most studies conducted at research centers and academic institutions in the US.

In general, all peer review systems involve the receipt of applications, an administrative review of the applications, assignment to a peer review

*Corresponding author: Brian Wojcik, PhD. E-mail: *wojcikb@comcast.net*

†NIH Extramural Research Integrity Officer OD/OER/OEP, Bethesda, Maryland, USA

group with specific expertise (in the case of large numbers of applications from diverse fields of science), recruitment of independent peer review experts, a review meeting, generation of peer review reports and funding priority scores, and a final funding decision by the agency. These will be discussed below with an emphasis on the challenges presented by translational science.

8.2. PROCEDURES AND HOW TRANSLATIONAL RESEARCH IS REVIEWED

8.2.1. Specific Policies

8.2.1.1. *Conflict of Interest (COI)*

The review of translational research (programs/applications) is governed by the two essential underlying principles of peer review — freedom from conflict of interest and confidentiality. A conflict of interest (COI) is defined as the ability of outside considerations (personal, financial, academic) to potentially influence or bias an individual playing a role in the peer review process such that the outcome of the review is compromised. It is vitally important to avoid COIs in order to uphold the integrity of the review. It is also important to identify COIs as early in the review process as possible. The person in charge of the review is usually the one to vet these conflicts. In the federal government, this individual is the Designated Federal Official (DFO). At the level of National Institutes of Health extramural grants, this person is also known as the Scientific Review Officer (SRO). It is important to note that all peer review systems define, identify and vet COIs in order to assure an unbiased review.

COIs, either real or perceived, can be roughly divided into three categories: personal, academic and financial. A personal conflict can be difficult to identify and usually depends on the honesty and integrity of the individuals involved. Personal conflicts are defined as any friendship or familial relationship between an applicant and a reviewer or the DFO. It could also involve personal animosity. There are often strong perceptions of personal conflicts in review. For example, a person who criticizes a speaker's work at a scientific meeting may be identified as having personal animosity toward the speaker and thus having a personal conflict with the speaker's grant application. It is up to the DFO to investigate and determine if the conflict is real or just a perception.

Academic COIs relate to an expert's affiliations, research collaborations, joint publications, or previous supervisory roles. For example, potential reviewers from an applicant's institution are considered to be in conflict by almost every reviewing agency. Being at the same institution has the potential to introduce bias into a review, as the reviewer and the applicant may have past or current interactions that can bias the reviewer. Current collaborators of an applicant are considered in conflict as reviewers since they are not sufficiently independent of the applicant. Most academic COIs can be identified through a search. However, these COIs are not always apparent (i.e., current collaborations) and depend on the applicant and/or potential reviewer to self identify, as there may not yet be a record of joint publications. Former collaborators are also considered to be in conflict. However, the degree of conflict is considered to reduce with time. There are also practical considerations, as the field of potential reviewers would be greatly restricted if COIs due to joint publication/collaboration were maintained over time. At the NIH, the practice is that three years after a joint publication is a sufficient amount of time for such a conflict to be resolved.

Translational and clinical research presents a unique circumstance in that large clinical trials often involve multiple sites, with one serving as the coordinating site. This results in publications with many co-authors, many of whom may never have been in direct contact during the conduct of the trial. If all of these co-authors were considered in conflict with the review of an application from one of the co-authors, there may not be sufficient experts available to adequately review the application. To resolve this situation, review policy has been modified over time to consider only those co-authors who had a direct intellectual collaboration (i.e., trial design, data analysis, etc.) to be in conflict. Co-authors who only supplied reagents, patients, patient data, and so on are not considered to have a true COI. This is the current practice at the NIH, with the SRO rendering the final decision on which co-authors have valid COIs and which co-authors can review an application without compromising the integrity of the review. A COI that may not be immediately apparent occurs when the potential reviewer serves on an advisory board for the applicant. These COIs can be discovered by requesting a list of advisors to the applicant. Reviewers who recently mentored an applicant have a COI as they can be considered to be invested in the success of the applicant. Similarly, potential reviewers who have been mentored by an applicant have a COI. Additionally, reviewers should be viewed as independent of one another. For that reason, NIH policy only allows for up to two reviewers from a single institution as long as they are in different academic departments. If a review panel has more than one member from a particular department, those reviewers could exert, or be perceived as exerting, an undue influence over the course of the review. It is especially important that a subordinate relationship (i.e., department chair and member of that department) be avoided as the reviewer in the superior position could exert an influence on a reviewer who is his subordinate.

The strongest COIs involve financial relationships. These could be related to industry ties (i.e., paid consultants) or grants (paid advisor or collaborator). Examples include a reviewer who is co-holder of a grant with an applicant, as the reviewer could be seen to benefit from the applicant receiving additional funds, or a paid advisor to an applicant. For translational research, many potential reviewers could have financial ties to an applicant through industry-linked drug development, clinical trials, or business relationships. For example, a potential reviewer could be an investor in research that is being moved from the laboratory into clinical testing. In this case, the potential reviewer stands to gain from a favorable review of the application. Conversely, if the investment is in a rival treatment, then the potential reviewer could benefit from a peer review outcome that inhibits funding of the application.

For all three categories of COI listed above, there is the potential for the perception of a conflict when a true conflict does not exist. One example, cited above, is co-authorship on a publication in which there was not a true intellectual exchange between the parties. Others can be the result of past relationships, public criticism of another's work, or a perceived financial relationship. In these cases, it is up to the SRO to obtain the information necessary to determine if there is a true COI or not. In some cases, for example, where there are other experts available, it can be beneficial to avoid even the perception of a COI. The degree to which perceived COIs are allowed is a judgment of the SRO based on the nature of the research under review. In almost every case, a COI can be identified and resolved or mitigated. For example, during the review of single project applications (i.e., NIH R01), a reviewer can be asked to leave the room during the discussion of an application for which he/she is in conflict and return to review those applications for which he/she is not in conflict. For contract mechanisms, COIs are more critical and more closely monitored; even the perception of a COI could jeopardize the review.

Several multi-project/-component funding mechanisms exist [e.g., Specialized Programs of Research Excellence (P50) and Program Project Grants (P01) at the NIH]. In addition to a Principal Investigator of the entire application, multi-project/-component applications involve different Project Leaders/Component Directors, even those from outside institutions. These applications can be an effective way to fund translational research as the different projects can be working on various aspects of translational research (laboratory, animal testing, clinical). For this type of application a reviewer's COI with one of the projects means that the reviewer is in conflict with the entire application. For example, a reviewer from institution B is in conflict with an application from institution A, if one of the components is being conducted at institution B, as funding the application may indirectly benefit the reviewer at institution B.

On occasion, however, the specialized expertise of a reviewer with a potential COI cannot be excluded from the review of an application, as it would mean that a reviewer would not be present to cover an area of expertise required for the proper review of the application. Some agencies issue a waiver in these cases. The potential COI is declared and recorded, the review proceeds, and the funding agency then takes the potential COI into account when making its final funding decision. In all cases, funding agencies require a COI form signed by the reviewer attesting to his/her COIs, or lack thereof. No system is foolproof, however, and it always comes down to trust in the diligence of the SRO and the honesty and integrity of the reviewers and applicants.

8.2.1.2. *Confidentiality*

The second fundamental principle of peer review is confidentiality. The review of proposed research involves confidential and/or proprietary information. In the case of translational research, applications can involve the use of patient data and samples, as well as potential commercial applications. It is vitally important to the integrity of the review that all applicant materials and deliberations of the peer review panel are kept confidential. All reviewers are asked to maintain confidentiality; most funding agencies require reviewers to sign a confidentiality agreement, depending on the sensitivity of the application topics. Review materials are distributed in a confidential manner; the most commonly used system today is a secure IT system, such as password (or even biometric) protected website or email. Peer reviews can be conducted as double blind, in which the identities of the applicants and reviewers are not revealed to each other; single blind, in which the identity of the reviewers are not known to the applicants (in some cases, the reverse may apply); and open review, in which the identities of the applicants and reviewers are known to each other. The NIH employs an open review system. Usually, multiple applications are reviewed at a single review session. The NIH will release the full roster of reviewers prior to the review meeting, although the specific reviewer assignments are not revealed. At many funding agencies, applicants have the opportunity to challenge the roster. It is the SRO, or equivalent, who renders the final decision on the composition of the roster.

8.3. REVIEW REQUIREMENTS AND FORMAT

8.3.1. Quality, Structure and Representation

Quality assurance of the review process is maintained through an effective structure of governance. Most funding organizations assure the quality and integrity of peer review by adopting set policies and procedures for conducting peer review. Staff, whether in-house or contracted, are trained in and expected to maintain these policies and procedures. As DFOs for the peer review process, SROs at the NIH are primarily responsible for clearly conveying these policies and procedures to peer reviewers. Their presence during the actual review meetings is required by regulation to ensure that grant applications receive a fair, thorough and objective review.

Most agencies involve a dedicated office for the conduct of peer review. NIH has a fully trained staff with a clear mandate for conducting peer review. Additionally, an advisory or oversight board, with members from outside of the funding organization, is delegated to insure that peer review is held to the highest standards. For example, the NIH has a two-tiered process of peer review with Boards at each of the Institutes/Centers (I/Cs) comprised of outside experts to conduct a second level of review. For the peer review of intramural research programs at the NCI, a panel of outside experts in the field conducts an initial review via a site visit. The Board of Scientific Counselors (BSC) then reviews the site visit report. The BSC is comprised of experts in the major areas of research conducted by the intramural research program. This second level of review serves as a check of the peer review process of the site visit as well as providing a more global perspective in advising the NCI on investing its funds in the most deserving research. The National Cancer Advisory Board performs a similar role in the review of extramural grant applications for the NCI. It should be noted that many of the smaller I/Cs at the NIH have streamlined this process with a simultaneous meeting of the panel of outside experts and the I/C's Board.

8.4. APPLICATION PROCESS

8.4.1. Submission, Receipt and Referral

When all of the above pillars are in place, a methodology for conducting peer review can be developed. In general, such a methodology starts with the receipt of applications. Applications for research funding usually involve a specific proposed research project or program of research projects that the submitting Principal Investigator intends to pursue during the funding period (usually five years). For larger funding agencies, such as the NIH, the receipt of applications also entails the referral of the applications received to the appropriate NIH institute or Study Section of the Center for Scientific Review (CSR). Applications to the NIH can be submitted independently or in response to a specific Request for Applications (RFA). An RFA is issued to strengthen a specific portfolio of research or to exploit a new opportunity or technology. An RFA can be designed to specifically fund translational research. To insure equitable peer review, study sections and/or ad hoc review groups or Special Emphasis Panels (SEPs) are set up around specific areas of research or types of research. Multi-component applications, like all other Public Health Service (PHS) grant applications, are received and processed initially by the NIH CSR and assigned to an appropriate NIH institute, which subsequently assigns the application to the appropriate program area.

In addition to grants, the NIH uses cooperative agreements and contracts as mechanisms to support extramural research and technology development. Cooperative agreements are similar to grants; however, there is a substantial scientific and technical role provided by NIH staff. Cooperative agreement applications are usually solicited via a specific RFA, which addresses a well-defined area of research and set-aside budget. In contrast, Program Announcements (PAs) generally address a relatively broad scope of the proposed research and not a detailed set-aside budget. The NIH uses contract proposals to purchase a service or product, which are almost always solicited through specific Requests for Proposals (RFP). The NIH may invite submission of grant applications or proposals to address areas of special interest or priorities issuing an RFA, PA or RFP in the NIH Guide for Grants and Contracts. In practice, each of these mechanisms may specifically support translational studies, although most grants are investigator initiated. Translational research is usually broader in scope than laboratory basic research, but most basic as well as clinical scientists do not receive adequate training in applying for a grant to support translational research. This is reflected in recent studies at the NIH which showed that the overall success rate of applications proposing clinical research and clinical trials is somewhat lower than the success rate for applications for basic research.[1]

For the review of the intramural research programs at the NIH, applications are not received. Rather, each Principal Investigator is subject to a peer review of his/her entire research portfolio every four years in order to receive funding for the next four years. The Principal Investigator prepares a written overview of his/her major accomplishments over the past four years, as well as a summary of the major projects he/she intends to pursue in the coming four years. During a site visit, the Principal Investigator makes an oral presentation and the site visit team has the opportunity to question the Principal Investigator directly. The site visit team then drafts a site visit report, which is in turn reviewed by the BSC at the NIH institute funding the research. The BSC may review the Principal Investigator's work, not only on its scientific merits, but also on the basis of how it fits the goals and programmatic objectives of that institute. All of the principles and practices of peer review described in this article are applicable to the NIH intramural peer review system.

8.4.2. Administrative Review of Applications

The administrative review of grant applications can vary from funding agency to funding agency, depending on their priorities and procedures. At the NIH, applications are received at a central Office of Receipt and Referral. This office sorts the applications and refers them to the appropriate CSR Study Section or the I/C review entity. Applications proposing translational research, like all other PHS grant applications, are received and processed initially by the NIH CSR and are assigned to appropriate Study Section or the NIH institute. Upon receipt of an application, the SRO reviews the application for conformance to NIH policies and guidelines. If there are administrative or policy deficiencies that can be resolved easily post-submission, the SRO will contact the Principal Investigator with the remedial action necessary. If there are extensive deficiencies in the structure, organization or format of the application, or the application fails to address required NIH policies in ways that cannot be resolved quickly, the application will be returned to the applicant without further consideration. The applicant may then submit a complete application for a later receipt date.

8.4.3. Communications with Applicants and NIH Program Staff During the Review Process

Prior to a review meeting, the SRO will contact the Principal Investigator to obtain background information relevant to the application and names of investigators collaborating with the members of the applicant group and other investigators who may be in conflict with the group. Applicants may suggest types of expertise that are required to review the application. Program Officers can also be consulted for lists of potential expert reviewers.

Shortly after receipt of the applications, the SRO contacts appropriate NIH program staff to discuss programmatic issues related to the review of submitted applications and for recommendations for prospective reviewers, where appropriate. However, all review-related communications with actual or potential reviewers are only conducted through the SRO. Applicants and program staff are forbidden from contacting reviewers, or potential reviewers. The size and composition of each SEP review panel will be determined by the particular details of the applications to be reviewed. It is the responsibility of the SRO to make these determinations based upon thorough understanding of the work proposed in the applications and consultation with NIH program staff and other review staff, as appropriate. Also, the SRO can provide a deadline for submission of a small amount of supplemental data that can be forwarded to the reviewers. This deadline generally is set up several weeks prior to the review so that all reviewers have adequate time to study and evaluate the information. Any changes in the scope of the projects or other program components cannot be accepted after submission of the application.

8.4.4. Selection of Reviewers

One of the most important parts of the peer review process is the selection of reviewers. Qualified reviewers must have the requisite expertise to review the science contained in the applications and they must be free from COIs. This is particularly important in the case of translational research, where expertise should cover the entire process. As translational research often comprises a range of scientific endeavors, from basic science research to animal models to clinical trials, recruiting and assigning reviewers can present a challenge. It is the role of the SRO to select and vet the review team members.

The characteristics of the reviewers can vary according to the type of review. However, the primary criterion should be scientific excellence in the field under review as demonstrated by a successful history of contributions to the field. Common measures of this are a record of independent funding and a record of publication in the field. Prior participation on peer review panels is also a strong indicator of a qualified reviewer. Reviewers are required to work effectively in a group, facilitate balanced discussion of potentially differing perspectives, complete well-written review assignments, and express independent viewpoints. Reviewers who have served on multiple past reviews can be considered to exhibit these qualities. Many panels also recruit reviewers on the basis of minority, gender, and geographic balance; this is a requirement for study sections and boards at the NIH. An additional consideration that factors into some reviews is a need to match reviewers to applicants at a similar stage in their careers.

The number of reviewers on a particular review panel will vary based on the number of applications and the diversity of the science represented in the applications. For single project applications that focus on a relatively narrow window of science, two reviewers may possess the requisite expertise to provide a thorough and comprehensive review. To evaluate proposed translational research, reviewers who are conversant in the full spectrum of translational science are not always available. Thus, it will often be necessary to recruit reviewers who are expert in specific aspects of the proposed research to adequately review an application in translational research. This can result in more than two reviewers assigned to an application with the final evaluation resulting from a merger of diverse viewpoints. Whenever possible, it is best to form review panels composed of more-senior investigators, who can provide a broader overview of the field, as well as investigators with expertise in specific aspects of the application. This should result in the breadth and depth required of the review. As translational research often involves clinical applications, patient advocates should be included on the review panel. Advocates are well versed in the impact of disease on patients and their families as well as more practical aspects of which strategies are likely to result in good patient participation and compliance with clinical procedures. For two-tiered reviews, such as those conducted at the NIH, an initial review panel may be comprised of reviewers with specific expertise in a field. The second tier reviewers (e.g., NCI BSC) are more-senior investigators who have been active in a field for sufficiently long duration such that they can provide a more global view of the proposed research, its level of innovation, and likely contribution to advancing the field. Reviewers matching these criteria can be found through investigation of databases on grant application history and publication records, as well as recommendations from scientific officers at the funding agency and the recommendations of other reviewers.

8.4.5. Role and Responsibilities of a Chair and Discussion Leader

A key part of the peer review is the Chair of the review meeting, an experienced reviewer with broad expertise in the field capable of leading reviewers efficiently through the agenda. He/she announces the application to be discussed, including the specific nature of the application (i.e., new or competing renewal). The SRO does not usually lead the discussion during a review meeting, but serves to observe that all review policies and procedures are maintained. The role of the Chair is to:

- insure that the review is free from any bias;
- see that there is a fair and equitable review of each application;
- insure all review criteria (e.g., at the NIH: significance, investigators, innovation, approach, environment) are addressed in each application/project/component discussion;
- moderate differences of opinion, call for scoring of the applications and/or its different components, and assess the potential overall impact of the application.

In addition, Discussion Leaders may be designated on multi-component applications to introduce the application and also take detailed notes during the discussion as they formulate the overall critique, summarizing the strengths and weaknesses prior to final scoring.

8.4.6. Role and Responsibilities of the SRO in the Handling of Allegations of Scientific Misconduct

Concerns with scientific misconduct are serious and arise infrequently during the review process. As scientific experts in areas similar to the applicants, peer reviewers are in an excellent position to identify irregularities in the research process. Many of these concerns are likely to relate to flaws or inadequacies in the scientific process described in the application. These are not considered research misconduct. Rarely, concerns may fall within the rubric of research misconduct. At the NIH, research misconduct is defined according to the code of federal regulation 42 C.F.R. Part 93 as fabrication, falsification or plagiarism in proposing, performing or reviewing research, or in reporting research results. It does not include honest errors or differences of opinion. For findings of research misconduct to be made, it is necessary to show intention, and there must also be the presence of a preponderance of evidence. At the time of review, it is vital to insure fair and objective reviews and that applications will not be tainted by mere suspicions of research misconduct. Therefore, specific policies and procedures are involved in the handling of allegations of research misconduct discovered during the review process. SROs are charged with briefing and reminding reviewers of these policies and procedures. Essentially, reviewers are instructed that (a) they should only direct their suspicions of research misconduct to the SROs in private; (b) to insure confidentiality, they should never discuss their concerns in the context of potential scientific misconduct openly during the review meeting or in their review reports; and (c) they should not talk about these suspicions with anyone else. At the NIH, there is a close network of Research Integrity Officers (RIOs) from each IC. SROs are directed to refer allegations of research misconduct promptly to their IC RIOs for review. Ultimately, allegations that fit the criteria for research misconduct will be forwarded to the Department of Health and Human Services (HHS) Office of Research Integrity (ORI) for review and oversight. Everyone is considered innocent until proven otherwise. Thus, before the ORI can confirm any findings of research misconduct, the sanctity of peer review must be protected and the process must be allowed to take its natural course.

Allegations of research misconduct are taken very seriously at the NIH. All allegations are appropriately reviewed and handled according to a clear set of procedures. Reviewers who bring forth allegations of research misconduct can be assured that their concerns are duly processed. This kind of active engagement is essential to insure the integrity of the scientific process and public confidence.

8.5. SPECIFIC REVIEW PROCESS

8.5.1. Review Policies and Procedures

Applications, along with the review criteria, are distributed to the reviewers prior to the review meeting. The reviewers are expected to write independent critiques for each of the applications to which they have been assigned.

After submission of their critiques, the reviewer may view the critiques of the other reviewers so that they may be better prepared for the discussion at the meeting.

During a review panel meeting, each application is reviewed via the same process — an open discussion of its strengths and weaknesses by panel members. The final assessment of merit should be based on the balance of strengths and weaknesses of the application, addressing each of the review criteria used. In addition to scientific criteria, there are additional practical criteria that need to be considered, including human subjects, vertebrate animals, biohazards, and comments on renewal and resubmission, if applicable. Also, each funding agency or mechanism may specify additional criteria or comments on evaluation specific to the proposed programs.

In multi-component applications (i.e., NCI SPORE or P01), each individual research project score as well the overall impact of the proposed program are based on the NIH review criteria. Review criteria for other components, i.e., shared resource cores, program integration (in P01), developmental programs, program organization and capabilities or scientific collaborations, are provided individually according to the specific funding mechanism.

Perhaps the best way to illustrate the review process is to discuss a specific example. For SPORE projects, reviewers need to assess the importance of the translational research objective to human cancer and its likelihood of completion within the proposed project period. Within the SPORE concept of translational research, the five NIH core review criteria are evaluated: Significance, Investigators, Innovation, Approach, and Environment. For Significance, it needs to be assessed whether the studies take an observation from the laboratory to the clinic or from the clinic to the laboratory in a manner that will significantly impact the disease. For Investigators, reviewers have to answer the question: Are the basic and more applied co-leaders of the project appropriately qualified and is their expertise integrated? For Innovation, novelty in concept, design or approach needs to be assessed, remembering that not all translational research is innovative but rather often takes what is innovative into a clinical setting. For Approach, the adequacy of the experimental design and methods needs to be evaluated, remembering that every detail of the research plan does not need to be in the application and, in fact, cannot be given the application page limits; it only needs to be described in such a manner that leads the assigned reviewers to believe that it can be completed successfully by the investigative team. For the Environment, reviewers need to assess whether the investigators, both basic and clinical, are making full use of the available resources (i.e. cores, clinical and laboratory facilities, collaborative opportunities, etc.)

Also, it is important that translational research includes hypothesis-generating projects, not only hypothesis-driven projects, as long as they have a human endpoint, and have potential for translational impact. In addition, a project does not need to be strong in all five NIH review criteria in order to be viewed as highly meritorious. For competing renewal applications, progress during the current funding period needs to be addressed. Any difficulties in achieving the prior goals should be addressed in the application, and if a project has changed direction, it is important to assess whether there is sufficient rationale provided for the new approach or direction. SPORE projects do not have to interact with one another as they do for other mechanisms such as P01 program projects. Thus, integration of the projects is not a review criterion for SPOREs as it is for other mechanisms and is not considered during review panel discussions. However, sometimes synergy between projects can be viewed as beneficial as it can advance the science more rapidly or innovatively than if the projects don't interact.

Many multi-project application mechanisms involve required elements: for SPORE applications, Specimen and Administrative Cores are now required components. For the Specimen Core, it is important to evaluate the proposed plan to develop, annotate, and maintain a human cancer site-specific specimen resource and adequacy of the proposed plan to prioritize distribution of specimens within and outside the SPORE; and if applicable, to perform analyses on specimens. For the required Administrative Core, the proposed plans for administratively managing fiscal and data operations and communication need to be evaluated, especially if more than one institution is involved. Are the qualifications, experience and commitment of the Core Directors adequate? Finally, for renewal applications, has disposition of any discretionary funds been adequately addressed? In all other cores, the overall merit is discussed by describing major strengths and weaknesses, focusing on the review criteria of Approach, Investigators and Environment.

Two hallmarks of a successful SPORE program are component programs in developing new avenues of research and careers in translational research. The reviewers need to consider the SPORE Developmental Research Program in terms of the appropriateness of the process for attracting new ideas and pilot studies within and outside of the SPORE institution, and for reviewing and monitoring progress. For competing renewal applications, this program should also be evaluated on the ability to promote outstanding pilot projects to full projects and/or demonstrate the successful competition of these projects for outside funds. Reviewers need to consider the Career Development Program in terms of the adequacy of the process for selecting promising candidates for independent careers in translational cancer research, including qualified women and minorities. For competing renewal applications, this should include the current status and research activities of individuals who have been supported by the Career Development Program. In both developmental programs, the proposed processes are only evaluated, using any projects or candidates listed as a means to see how well the process is constructed, but without considering the science.

Scientific Collaborations are a new component of the SPORE application. Horizontal Collaborations present the plans for or evidence of scientific collaborations with other SPOREs, other NIH/NCI programs or other government or non-government organizations that will enhance the likelihood of more rapidly and efficiently completing the translational goals. Vertical Collaborations include the plans for potential collaborative agreements in developing cancer therapeutics or biomarkers, or for expanding population and cancer prevention studies beyond the limits of the SPORE.

In Program Organization and Capabilities, the following six review criteria are evaluated: (i) Leadership, (ii) Institutional Commitment, (iii) Integration within the SPORE and the Institution, (iv) Adequacy of the Cancer Patient Population, (v) Data Management, and (vi) Planning and Evaluation of Activities. Thus, one can see the complexity in the evaluation of translational research within this funding mechanism facing reviewers. It is the responsibility of the SRO, Meeting Chair, and Discussion Leaders to insure that the review criteria are understood and followed.

8.5.2. Flow of a Typical SPORE Review for Scientific Merit of Multi-Component Applications

At the start of the discussion of each SPORE application, the Discussion Leader gives a brief overview of the proposed program. Then, the assigned reviewers state their preliminary impact scores (SPOREs follows the NIH scoring of assigning a single-digit whole number, between 1 and 9, with 1 being the best. Other funding mechanisms and agencies may use different scoring critieria, e.g. different numeric range, letter grades or merit descriptors). The primary reviewer gives a very brief introduction to the project, highlighting the significance of the project relative to the state-of-the-art for that disease, and summarizes its strengths and weaknesses according to appropriate review criteria. Following the primary reviewer, other assigned reviewers add only new points or indicate areas of agreement or disagreement. If there is agreement in the scores, little discussion is required: the written critiques will be incorporated into the final summary statements. Thus, reviewers do not need to repeat all points, and if minor points are not discussed, the applicant will still have the benefit of the full critique. Thereafter, the application's components are open for a full panel discussion and other panel members may add additional points or request clarification. Then, human subjects and animal welfare concerns can be addressed. Next, all the panel members score the component. Budgetary and other administrative issues, such as a resource-sharing plan, are discussed following scoring. In a multi-component application, projects are discussed first, followed by other components (shared resource cores, developmental programs, program organization and capabilities or program integration), concluded with a discussion and evaluation of the application as a whole.

8.5.3. Scoring Multi-Component Applications involving Translational Research

When considering significance or innovation and their impacts on the translational research project, reviewers are asked to keep in mind "broad fields" such as gene therapy, tumor biology, cancer therapy, chemopreven tion, early detection, epidemiology, and so on. A project does not have to be strong in all categories in order to be judged likely to have major scientific and potential clinical impact.

During the review meeting, the scoring guidelines are always available to the reviewer, and the assigned merit scores are based on the five NIH criteria and the other component criteria are provided. The guidelines are used by reviewers to determine the impact score for each of the projects, considering the balance of strengths and weaknesses, including its translational value. It is important that they include all of the review criteria when deciding on project impact. The individual review criteria are not pre-weighted: the SRO relies upon each reviewer to decide how the strengths and weaknesses contribute to overall impact. In addition, in considering strengths and weaknesses, the reviewer should consider their relative importance and the likelihood that the project will have a sustained, powerful impact on the broad research involved, or clinical practice, and then decide which of the scores (ranging from 1 to 9 for most NIH reviews) best reflects the reviewer's determination of the level of impact. A score of 1 indicates that a project is exceptionally strong in all review criteria with essentially no weaknesses and that it will have a very high impact. A score of 9 indicates a project with serious and substantial weaknesses with very few strengths. Generally, reviewers are advised to suggest a range of scores; the SROs provide the characteristics for different scoring ranges from 1 to 9. Using this scoring guide, review staff can be assured that all review panels use the same standard criteria. Also, each application in the same review panel is evaluated as a single application and cannot be compared with other applications in the cluster. Usually, the 1–2 scoring range is assigned for a "perfect" application. In a program project (P01) or SPORE, such perfection is very unusual, but it is easy to identify programs that are uniformly well balanced in all review criteria, corresponding to the 2–3 range. Such programs have some minor flaws, but are highly meritorious overall.

In addition, reviewers may be asked to evaluate progress in the current funding period (e.g. for a competing renewal application, or a review of NIH Intramural Research Programs). For an amended (resubmitted) application, the proposed research is evaluated as newly submitted in light of recent scientific advancement, although applicants' responses are taken into consideration. However, reviewers cannot use the old scores as the starting point. The review of NIH intramural research is weighted toward achievement and productivity during the prior four year funding period.

Each application is scored not only by the assigned reviewers but also by the entire review panel. Scoring outside the range specifically suggested by the assigned reviewers is allowed for every panel member as long as a reviewer shares his/her views and opinions with the committee. Finally, the preliminary scores given before the review meeting can be modified at any time during this meeting. For SPOREs the assigned reviewers post individual scores for each of the "core" review criteria in their preliminary critiques before the review meeting, but they do not give these scores during the review meeting. Although these are not discussed, they are included in the individual critiques that become a part of the final written report (at the NIH, this is called the summary statement) sent to the applicants. Therefore, reviewers are requested to revise their criteria scores if their opinions change following discussion at the review meeting. But the criteria scores and evaluation of strengths and weaknesses need to be consistent, so that applicants can understand the summary statement and the basis for the scores. Many reviews do not include the preliminary scores as part of the final review report; they only provide the final consensus score.

For a SPORE, all other components of the proposed application are also scored using the numerical range 1–9. In contrast, for a P01, the following descriptors are used to rate the shared resource cores: Superior (for only the best, most well-planned components with remarkable services to the program); Satisfactory (a broad range of quality evident across the components); Minimally Satisfactory (with some significant weaknesses but still potential to provide the required services); Unsatisfactory (formerly "Not Recommended for Further Consideration"; with fatal flaws, such as having human or animal welfare issues, being poorly described, proposing services unlikely to be provided, having unqualified leaders or serving for only one project). Evaluation of the Program as an Integrated Effort for P01 is a part of the round table discussion, with each review panel member making a statement and providing his/her merit rating using the following descriptors: Highly Integrated, Integrated, and Not Integrated. Considerations include quality of interaction between the projects and cores, scientific integration (which can include, but is not limited to, strategic and intellectual integration), programmatic integration/management, and synergy.

It should be noted that a program rated "Highly Integrated" is one having both integrated and synergistic relationships among the majority of projects and cores.

Finally, Overall Program Evaluation is assessed based on the following review criteria:

- Overall Significance, in terms of potential to advance knowledge in a global scientific area;
- Overall Investigators;
- Overall Innovation;
- Overall Approach;
- Overall Scientific, Organizational and Administrative Environment (if multi-institutional, this refers to the communication between institutions).

At the end of review, all panel members are asked to assign the overall impact score (again in 1–9 range) based on previous discussion. In some cases, the reviewers may not be able to reach consensus on a score. Some funding agencies (e.g. review of NIH Intramural Research Programs) a minority opinion is drafted to explain the reason(s) for this difference for inclusion in the written report.

8.6. COMMUNICATING THE RESULTS OF THE REVIEW AND THE FUNDING DECISION

After the review meeting, the SRO prepares a written report (summary statement) for each reviewed application to document the deliberation of the review panel. The summary statement is the official record from the review meeting and includes the assigned reviewers' written critiques and final scores. The SRO also provides a summary of the discussion. Summary statements may also include budget recommendations and administrative notes with potential concerns about research involving human subjects or animals, or potential overlap with other ongoing projects. The second-level review for grant applications is done by each NIH I/C's advisory council or board, which assesses the quality of the review panel's scientific merit review and considers the relevance of the proposed research to the institute's programs and priorities.[1]

Overall, awards are made based on the scientific and technical merit of the application as reflected by its impact/priority score, the relevance of the application to the mission and programs of the NIH, and the availability of funds. The award and administration of translational research grants are subject to the same policies and procedures as other research grants. These policies and cost principles are set forth in the current PHS Grants Policy Statement, other NIH issuances, and federal legislation and regulations.

8.7. CONCLUSION

Translational research is usually broader in scope than laboratory basic research, and most basic and clinical scientists do not receive adequate training in applying for a grant to support translational research. Examples from the NIH system are cited in this chapter, as the NIH funds most studies conducted at research centers and academic institutions in the US. The review of translational research (programs/applications) is governed by the two main underlying principles of peer review: confidentiality and freedom from conflict of interest. Most funding organizations assure the quality and integrity of peer review by adopting set policies and procedures. For larger funding agencies such as the NIH, the receipt of applications also entails the referral of the applications received to the appropriate NIH institute or Study Section of the Center for Scientific Review (CSR). Although the specifics may vary between funding agencies, each application is reviewed via the same process: an open discussion of its merit and weaknesses by a panel of experts. The final assessment of merit should be based on the balance of strengths and weaknesses of the application, addressing each of the review criteria used, with consideration of its translational/clinical impact. After the review, a summary statement is prepared for each reviewed application, which is the official record that includes the assigned reviewers' written critiques and final scores.

AUTHORS' DISCLAIMER

Drs. Wojcik and Lopaczynski contributed to this article in their personal capacity. The views expressed in this chapter do not necessarily represent the views of the National Institutes of Health or the US Government.

REFERENCE

1. Bartlett OT. (2012) Getting the funding you need to support your research: navigating the National Institutes of Health peer review process. In: Gallin JI, Ognibene FP (eds), *Principles and Practice of Clinical Research*, Academic Press (Elsevier), New York, pp. 519–538.

IV. Translational Sciences in Cancer Research

Insights into the Process of Translating Emerging Immunologic Paradigms to Clinical Trial in Patients with Cancer

Theresa L. Whiteside[*,‡], *Lisa H. Butterfield*[*] *and Edward P. Cohen*[†]

9.1. INTRODUCTION

This is a story of the discovery, development, and preclinical and translational efforts to bring a new and potentially promising anti-tumor vaccine for patients with non-small cell lung cancer (NSCLC) to the clinic. This is a true story. It goes back about 20 years, and it has not ended. The reader will be taken through the years of work invested by numerous basic scientists, laboratory workers, physician-scientists and clinicians to create and prepare for safe delivery an FDA-approved cellular vaccine for patients with lung cancer. The vaccine has been developed in their laboratories, and although it is fully approved for phase I clinical trials, it is yet to accrue patients. Its development involved academicians, clinicians, government officials and industrial partners, all eager to succeed in offering this immune therapy to patients with NSCLC. The patients that are eligible for the vaccine have failed conventional therapies or become resistant to them and desperately

[*]University of Pittsburgh Cancer Institute, Pittsburgh, Pennsylvania, USA
[†]University of Illinois, College of Medicine, Chicago, Illinois, USA
[‡]Corresponding author: Theresa L. Whiteside, PhD, University of Pittsburgh Cancer Institute, Hillman Cancer Center, 5117 Centre Avenue, Pittsburgh, PA 15213, USA; E-mail: *whitesidetl@upmc.edu*; Tel: +1-412-624-0096; Fax: +1-412-624-0264

need an alternative. After some 20 years of trying and considerable financial investment, the vaccine seems to be on the brink of being "lost in translation," but for reasons that are identifiable and perhaps avoidable. The issues addressed in this chapter deal not so much with whether the vaccine is truly "lost in translation" or not, but rather with obstacles that have prevented and/or retarded the translation of potentially promising biologic therapies to clinical trials that are ultimately necessary for testing efficacy.

9.2. WHY AN ANTI-TUMOR VACCINE?

The story starts in late 1990s when the idea of immunizing a cancer patient with a vaccine specific for his/her own tumor was broadly embraced by the immunotherapy community. The enthusiasm was largely based on the results emanating from a previous decade of experiments aimed at the discovery of tumor antigens.[1–3] As the identity and number of well-characterized tumor-associated antigens (TAA) expanded throughout the 1990s, so did the efforts to create the most effective anti-cancer vaccines. In principle, and similar to anti-bacterial or anti-viral vaccines, the delivery of an anti-cancer vaccine was expected to result in tumor-specific immune responses that would not only lead to elimination of the tumor but also protect the patient from relapse for years to come. The development of immunologic memory specifically activated to prevent the tumor recurrence was an important objective. The notion that such a vaccine could have therapeutic effects in patients bearing established tumors galvanized basic scientists throughout the world to initiate *in vivo* vaccination studies in various murine models of tumor growth.[4,5] The objective was to test the hypothesis that immunization with a vaccine targeting TAAs indeed leads to tumor rejection and the establishment of immunologic memory. Results of these *in vivo* experiments largely confirmed the validity of the hypothesis for experimental murine tumor models[6,7] and were accepted by the scientific community as a rationale for translation.

9.3. TUMOR DNA CAN BE A SOURCE OF TAAs FOR VACCINATION

The basis for Edward Cohen's initial experiments that ultimately led to the NSCLC vaccine development was an observation that tumor DNA can be a source of tumor antigens, and that an effective vaccine can be prepared by transfer of genomic DNA from the tumor to a highly immunogenic foreign (allogeneic) nonmalignant cell. Genes coding for TAAs would be expressed by the cells that took up tumor-derived DNA. It was well known at the time that the transfer of DNA from one cell type to another would result in the stable alteration of the genome of the recipient cell.[8] In fact, this approach was used in the classic studies that resulted in the identification of oncogenes in 1979.[9] It was also known that the transfer of genomic DNA from cells expressing an enzyme such as adenine phosphoribosyl transferase or unique membrane-associated determinants such as the major histocompatibility complex (MHC) molecules to a recipient cell which is genetically deficient in these determinants results in their stable expression in the recipient cells.[10–12]

Genetic instability is a well-known characteristic of human tumors, including NSCLC[13–15] and is considered to be responsible for emergence of multiple TAAs. These antigens are products of dysregulated or mutated genes in cancer cells[16,17] that differ from the homologous genes expressed in nonmalignant cells of the cancer patient. In consequence, within the same individual, the malignant cell population is characterized by expression of numerous TAAs, some of which are unique (i.e., due to mutations) and others which are normal but differentially expressed or overrepresented (e.g., due to gene amplifications or dysregulation). As the number of TAAs within a tumor cell population is likely to be large, successful immunization will require the vaccine capable of inducing immunity to a broad array of TAAs characterizing the patient's cancer. This perception has been more recently confirmed by results showing that multi-epitope cancer vaccines are more efficacious than single-epitope vaccines.[18]

Human tumor cells are generally weakly immunogenic or non-immunogenic, presumably due to immunoinhibitory factors they release,[19] down modulated MHC antigens,[20] lack of co-stimulatory signals,[20] dysregulated antigen-presenting machinery[21] or a loss from the tumor cell surface of TAAs recognized by immune cells.[22] To bypass these obstacles to effective immunization, anti-tumor vaccines have been generally designed to depend on the TAA cross-presentation by autologous dendritic cells (DCs) considered to be the best antigen presenting cells.[23]

Cohen's laboratory has provided ample, convincing evidence in mouse models that transfer of DNA from tumor cells to semi-allogeneic fibroblasts, which are able to process and express transferred TAAs, can induce potent anti-tumor immunity in tumor-bearing mice.[8,24–29] Expression of "foreign" MHC determinants by allogeneic fibroblasts, which are the recipients of transferred tumor DNA, was shown to stimulate their uptake by DCs and subsequent TAA presentation to immune cells.[30,31] In tumor-bearing mice, immunization with tumor DNA-transfected allogeneic fibroblasts resulted in the development of robust anti-tumor immune responses and immunologic memory, leading to tumor regression.[8,24–29] In Cohen's *in vivo* experiments, tumor-bearing mice treated solely by immunization with a vaccine prepared by transfection of unfractionated and sheared genomic DNA from mouse melanoma, lymphoma, breast carcinoma or squamous cell carcinoma cells into a semi-allogeneic mouse fibroblast cell line survived significantly longer than mice in control groups.[8,24–29] In some instances, the immunized animals survived indefinitely without any evidence of toxic effects.[8]

The major advantage of this vaccination approach is that the transferred DNA is integrated into the genome of the recipient cells and replicated as these cells divide. The number of cells available for the vaccine can thus be conveniently expanded for multiple rounds of immunotherapy. This vaccination strategy, aside from its therapeutic efficacy documented in several mouse tumor models, offered a number of advantages over the DC-based therapies being widely developed at that time. The major advantages are: (i) no identification or isolation of TAAs is necessary, as the tumor-derived DNA includes a full array of mutant/dysregulated genes that code for an array of TAAs, and thus is an equivalent of multi-epitope vaccines; (ii) the MHC alloantigens constitutively expressed by fibroblasts serve as powerful immune adjuvants; (iii) the fibroblasts can be further modified in advance to secrete immune-augmenting cytokines and these fibroblasts can proliferate to provide a large number of immunizing cells without procedures such as the leukapheresis required for the autologous DC preparation. While these advantages of the tumor DNA transfection to fibroblasts were being evaluated in several mouse tumor models with favorable results,[32–37] the question arose as to whether and how a process that worked well in mouse tumor models could be translated to human cells.

9.4. TUMOR-DERIVED DNA TRANSFECTION INTO HUMAN RECIPIENT CELLS

In a logical course of events, the next developmental step was to perform a series of *in vitro* studies with human tumor-derived DNA and human recipient cells to confirm the validity of the process established in mice. The choice of a human recipient cell that could be readily transfected and then given as a vaccine had to be made. At the time, human monocyte-derived dendritic cells were widely used as cancer vaccine components,[38] and so the decision was made to experiment with immature human DCs. At that time, transfection of human DCs had been attempted but with little success.[39] The Economou group at the University of California, Los Angeles tested calcium phosphate precipitation, lipofection and electroporation of plasmid DNA to transfect DCs or tumor cells. While tumor cells were relatively easily transfected by these methods, DCs were resistant. In contrast, transduction with adenoviral vectors into DCs was very efficient, allowing high levels of transgene production.[40] Subsequently, the electroporation-related technique of nucleofection was developed and optimized for DCs.[30,41] Numerous transfers of native tumor-derived DNA into the nucleus of DCs were performed by nucleofection with an objective to induce the presentation by DCs of TAAs encoded in the donor DNA and to elicit tumor-specific T-cell responses. The *in vitro* readout for these experiments was initially the detection of transfected DNA in the recipient cells, then a more important immunologic readout, an ELISPOT assay.[30,31] The model system used consisted of an HLA-A2+ gp-100+ melanoma cell line that was genetically modified to express enhanced green fluorescent protein (EGFP) and served as a DNA donor. Genomic tumor DNA was sheared by gentle sonication and electroporated into human immature DCs, which were then matured in a mix of cytokines. In ELISPOT assays, interferon-gamma (IFN-γ) production by a gp$100_{209-217}$ peptide-specific, HLA-A2-restricted T-cell line co-incubated with the DCs was measured. The experiments showed that transfection of total genomic DNA from tumor to DCs had led to successful expression and presentation of the gp-100 protein by DCs to T cells.[30] The spot formation was inhibited by anti-MHC class I antigen-specific and HLA-A2-specific antibodies but not by antibodies specific for the MHC class II antigens. Additional experiments showed that the transfected DCs co-incubated with peripheral blood mononuclear cells (PBMCs) of normal donors were able to prime naive T cells in culture to proliferate and develop into melanoma-specific effector T cells.[30,31] These *in vitro* experiments with human tumor-derived DNA and DCs documented the feasibility and specificity of the process.

Based on the results of successful *in vivo* experiments in tumor-bearing mice, the lack of toxicity in these murine models and subsequent *in vitro* immune responses observed with DNA-transfected human DCs, an IND application was submitted to the FDA for approval of the procedure to generate the DC-based DNA vaccine for clinical use. The accompanying clinical protocol proposed immunizing patients with advanced-stage of head and neck squamous cell carcinoma (HNSCC) with a vaccine containing DCs transfected with autologous tumor-derived DNA. Not unexpectedly, in getting approval for the clinical-grade vaccine production, a number of issues had to be resolved. Specifically, the FDA required documentation that tumor-derived DNA was sterile, that autologous DCs could be generated from PBMCs of patients with advanced oral carcinoma, and that transfection efficiency was adequate to ensure antigen presentation. While these requests were rational and fair, they required extensive preclinical studies and, in order to perform them, financial support had to be obtained. This was secured via a research grant from the NIH, which, of course, involved a competitive peer review and consumed almost two years. With the funds available, the recommended preclinical laboratory studies commenced.

In the course of these feasibility studies, a significant amount of information was gained about the processes of human DC generation for therapy and DC transfection with tumor-derived genomic DNA. The studies resulted in significant improvements of the transfection process by: (a) defining the phenotype and quality of human DCs that are most receptive to DNA transfers; (b) establishing methods for DNA fragmentation prior to nucleofection; (c) introducing nucleofection as a reliable means of DNA electroporation into human DCs; (d) defining optimal conditions for DC nucleofection and establishing its efficiency; and (e) establishing an *in vitro* model in which nucleofection of a plasmid encoding EGFP together with tumor-derived DNA could be used to test nucleofection efficiency. The generation of tumor-specific T-cell lines from

PBMCs primed with nucleofected DNA could also be tested in this *in vitro* model.

It took almost four years to complete the optimization studies and prepare the amended FDA application. Admittedly, the studies were very useful for establishing the vaccine production, and they resulted in several peer-reviewed publications.[32,42–45] While numerous regulatory issues were successfully resolved in this instance, the investment in time and effort has been extraordinary and perhaps not entirely justified given the overwhelming evidence for the safety of DC-based vaccines in patients with cancer. The next step in the approval process was to submit the clinical protocol for review by the institutional review board (IRB). The IRB approval was obtained after four months, and the clinical trial was opened for accrual in February 2006.

9.5. DC-BASED PHASE I CLINICAL TRIAL IN PATIENTS WITH HNSCC

The clinical trial entitled "Active Immunization of Patients with Carcinoma of Oral Cavity or Oropharynx with Autologous Dendritic Cells Transfected with DNA from Autologous Tumor (Phase I/II Study)" was designed as an uncontrolled, non-randomized trial to evaluate safety, immunogenicity and feasibility of the new vaccine, consisting of autologous monocyte-derived DCs transfected with autologous tumor-derived DNA (BB-IND-12198). Briefly, the plan was to use a two-stage trial design and to initially enroll 17 subjects with primary advanced carcinoma of the oral cavity or oropharynx over a period of two years. The subjects were to undergo surgery, and a portion of the primary tumor specimen not necessary for the pathologic diagnosis was to serve as a source of tumor DNA. Each DC-based vaccine was expected to contain 1×10^7 DNA-transfected DCs, which were to be administered intranodally under ultrasound guidance. Given there was no evidence of toxicity, and more than three subjects showed immunologic response, the second stage of the study would be opened for accrual of 22 subjects. All subjects were to be immunologically monitored by IFN-γ secretion in ELISPOT assays prior to and after vaccination for the frequency of T cells responsive to autologous tumor and to the vaccine.

The clinical trial opened for accrual in March 2006. Almost immediately it became apparent that there was a problem with patient eligibility, which was based in part on the ability to mount a positive delayed-type hypersensitivity (DTH) response to one of three recall antigens. Because the patients had advanced disease, most did not meet this requirement, and we were obliged to ask the IRB for modification in the eligibility criteria, namely, the permission to remove the DTH test as a requirement for trial entry, although we required that the DTH be measured and response be recorded. Modifications in the clinical protocol were approved in April 2007. Nevertheless, the accrual to the trial did not improve, largely due to demands on patients for a three- to four-hour long leukapheresis, intranodal vaccine delivery requiring special visits to the radiology suite and the frequent follow-up. While the trial remained open for another three years, only one patient was treated, and we were obliged to close the trial. The funding available for DC generation had expired. Some valuable lessons were learned from this experience, especially with regard to the feasibility issues for the autologous DC-based vaccine generation in patients with advanced disease. Unfortunately, the opportunity for testing the well developed and preclinically promising vaccine in patients with cancer was lost.

9.6. HUMAN MRC-5 FIBROBLASTS AS RECIPIENTS OF TUMOR-DERIVED DNA

The story now takes on a new twist brought about by a decision to drastically alter and simplify the vaccine production by introducing a universal allogeneic recipient cell line instead of autologous DCs. This change also represented a return to Cohen's original studies in animal tumor models, which provided the rationale for the development of this vaccine. Tumor-derived DNA was now to be nucleofected into semi-allogeneic MRC-5 cells. This HLA-A2+ human fibroblast cell line had been previously approved by the FDA for use in clinical trials. A working bank of MRC-5 fibro-blasts was created in a c-GMP facility, and a series of new preclinical experiments was conducted to show that following successful DNA nucleofection, MRC-5 cells express the transferred genes and that the cell number could be expanded as needed for the entire immunization protocol required for an individual patient (approximately 5×10^7 cells). The vaccine consisted of lethally-irradiated semi-allogeneic MRC-5 fibroblasts transfected with genomic tumor-derived DNA and expanded in culture. This strategy for vaccine production was judged meritorious by an NIH program (Production Assistance for Cellular Therapies, or PACT), which was specifically interested in the use of cells for human therapies. Funding for the vaccine production was provided, and the c-GMP facility, successfully working with nucleofection of MRC-5 cells, generated new data that made it once again possible to apply to the FDA for the permission to conduct a phase IB clinical trial, this time in patients with NSCLC, where a therapeutic vaccine would provide a badly needed option for relapsed disease. The process was made easier by the option to cross-file on the original protocol (BB-IND-12198), since the isolation of genomic DNA, nucleofection and vaccine preparation remained the same, and the process for the vaccine production had been previously approved.

9.7. WHY IS THE DNA-BASED VACCINE FOR CANCER PATIENTS NOT IN CLINICAL TRIALS?

We are now approaching the final stage of this long story. A few years ago, Dr. Cohen, capitalizing on the promising preclinical *in vivo* data and the available IND for the clinical application of the vaccine, decided to establish a private company in order to facilitate and promote its transfer to clinical trials. The rationale to provide corporate funding for these trials in addition to the support available from hard-won NIH grants and limited PACT program support was considered to be an essential component of the development program if the vaccine was to progress to clinical trials. Clearly, at this stage, the objective of implementing the vaccination protocol in the clinic became a priority. A phase I/II clinical protocol for immunotherapy of patients with an early stage of NSCLC was prepared, discussed with clinical personnel and plans were made for the corporate support of the clinical trial. The method for vaccine production was provided to an external cGMP facility in anticipation of vaccine production and delivery for a multi-institutional trial. However, the university-based c-GMP facility was prevented from distributing cellular products it generated to external clinical sites by the existing liability and oversight issues. The institution that makes the cellular vaccine is concerned about the liability for potentially serious adverse events that might occur in patients treated at a distant site. This policy makes it difficult to contemplate a multi-institutional vaccination protocol. Nevertheless, the process of securing IRB approvals at more than one institution is ongoing, and an option to contract the vaccine production to a commercial laboratory is being explored. Meanwhile, it is expected that the vaccine will soon be tested in an IRB-approved clinical trial for patients with NSCLC at the original institution in which the cGMP facility able to make the vaccine is located.

Almost 20 years have passed since Cohen's initial successful *in vivo* experiments in mice, and this potentially promising therapeutic vaccine still lingers somewhere between the lab and the clinic. It is therefore, important to consider the reasons for the slow progress in moving the vaccine to clinical trials.

9.8. REASONS FOR THE UNSATISFACTORY FATE OF THE NSCLC VACCINE

The 20-year long and tortuous translational pathway from *in vivo* studies in tumor-bearing mice to as-yet uninitiated phase I/II clinical trials in patients with NSCLC offers a valuable lesson to investigators embarking on the vaccine development journey. The unsatisfactory state of affairs surrounding the development of this and probably many other anti-tumor vaccines appears even worse when investments in labor, money and infrastructure are added to the equation. The fact that this DNA-based vaccine was successful in therapy of several different animal tumor models as well as in *in vitro* studies with human cells leaves no doubt that the decision to undertake its translation was correct. The requirement for the patient's own tumor for vaccine production is not difficult to fulfill when surgeons and pathologists are aware of the therapeutic protocol goals and surgery is already part of standard clinical management for the target patient population. The technical and laboratory aspects of DNA isolation from the tumor, transfection and gene expression analyses in recipient cells, while not trivial, are readily accomplished in the today's cGMP facilities. The selection of the DNA recipient cell, which serves as expression and delivery vehicle and as a semi-allogeneic immune adjuvant in this vaccine is probably the most critical aspect of the production process. As indicated above, autologous DCs, despite their superior antigen presenting capability, cannot proliferate, have no adjuvant-like effects and are more resistant to nucleofection than fibroblasts. The shift from autologous DCs as a DNA carrier to semi-allogeneic fibroblasts prolonged the preclinical feasibility studies by nearly four years, and the clinical protocol writing and the IRB approval added another two. Thus, in retrospect, the departure from Cohen's original protocol to incorporate human DCs into the vaccine was probably a mistake made because of the then-prevalent view that DCs were superior to fibroblasts as antigen presenting cells.

The production of any vaccine is costly, and the unending efforts to obtain funding for various aspects of the translation were time-consuming and disruptive. After the FDA approval was secured and the clinical protocol developed, a lack of interest and cooperation by the oncologists proved to be the biggest and most serious obstacle to translation. Despite considerable efforts of the development team to communicate potential advantages of this immune therapy, and despite the initial enthusiasm for the vaccine from many laboratory and clinical investigators, the prospect of the vaccine preparation, administration and required correlative studies as well as complex regulatory oversight had a significant negative impact on clinicians' willingness to participate in the trial. Without clinicians who are dedicated to immune therapies and willing to embrace translation with all its difficult and challenging aspects, this anti-tumor vaccine, like so many others, will likely be "lost in translation." This is a sad and depressing conclusion for those of us who have expected to make a difference in cancer therapy and have spent over 20 years in the pursuit of this elusive goal. For the reader, the saga of this vaccine serves an example of a tremendous effort facing investigators who attempt to translate a novel concept for therapy of cancer from murine studies to the clinic.

REFERENCES

1. van der Bruggen P, Traversari C, Chomez P, *et al.* (2007) A gene encoding an antigen recognized by cytolytic T lymphocytes on a human melanoma. *J Immunol* 178: 2617–2621.

2. Boon T, Cerottini J-C, van den Eynde B, *et al.* (1994) Tumor antigens recognized by T lymphocytes. *Ann Rev Immunol* **12**: 337–365.
3. Boon T, Coulie PG, van der Bruggen P. (1997) T-cell defined tumor antigens. *Curr Opin Immunol* **9**: 684–693.
4. Cavallo F, Pierro FD, Giovarelli M, *et al.* (1993) Protective and curative potential of vaccination with interleukin-2-gene-transfected cells from a spontaneous mouse mammary adenocarcinoma. *Cancer Res* **53**: 5067–5070.
5. Connor J, Bannerji R, Saito S, *et al.* (1993) Regression of bladder tumors in mice treated with interleukin 2 gene-modified tumor cells. *J Exp Med* **177**: 1127–1134.
6. Golumbek PT, Lazenby AJ, Levitsky HI, *et al.* (1991) Treatment of established renal cancer by tumor cells engineered to secrete interleukin-4. *Science* **254**: 713–716.
7. Mullen CA, Coale MM, Levy AT, *et al.* (1992) Fibrosarcoma cells transduced with the IL-6 gene exhibit reduced tumorigenicity, increased immunogenicity, and decreased metastatic potential. *Cancer Res* **52**: 6020–6024.
8. de Zoeten B, Carr-Brendel V, Markovic D, *et al.* (1999) Immunity to breast cancer in mice immunized with semi-allogeneic fibroblasts transfected with DNA from breast cancer cells. *J Immunol* **162**: 6934–6941.
9. Shih C, Shilo B-Z, Goldfarb MP, *et al.* (1979) Passage of phenotypes of chemically transformed cells via transfection of DNA and chromatin. *Proc Natl Acad Sci USA* **76**: 5714–5718.
10. Kavathas P, Herzenberg LA. (1983) Stable transformation of mouse LM cells (a transformed fibroblast cell line) for human membrane T-cell differentiation antigens, HLA and B2 microglobulin: Selection by fluorescence-activated cell sorting. *Proc Natl Acad Sci USA* **80**: 524–528.
11. Wigler M, Pellicer A, Silverstein S, *et al.* (1979) DNA-mediated transfer of the adenine phosphoribosyltransferase locus into mammalian cells. *Proc Natl Acad Sci USA* **76**: 1373–1376.
12. Hsu C, Kavathas P, Herzenberg LA. (1984) Cell surface antigens expressed on L cells transfected with whole DNA from non-expressing and expressing cells. *Nature* **312**: 68–69.
13. Peltomaki P, Lothe RA, Aaltonen LA, *et al.* (1993) Microsatellite instability is associated with tumors that characterize the hereditary non-polyposis colorectal carcinoma syndrome. *Cancer Res* **53**: 5853–5855.
14. Gonzalez-Zulueta M, Ruppert JM, Tokino K, *et al.* (1993) Microsatellite instability in bladder cancer. *Cancer Res* **53**: 5620–5623.
15. Woenckhaus M, Stoehr R, Dietmaier W, *et al.* (2003) Microsatellite instability at chromosome 8p in non-small cell lung cancer is associated with

lymph node metastasis and squamous differentiation. *Int J Oncol* **23**: 1357–1363.
16. Peoples GE, Goedegebuure PS, Smith R, *et al.* (1995) Breast and ovarian-cancer specific cytotoxic T lymphocytes recognize the same HER2/neu-derived peptide. *Proc Natl Acad Sci USA* **92**: 432.
17. de Vries TJ, Fourkour A, Wobbes T, *et al.* (1997) Heterologous expression of immunotherapy candidate proteins gp100, MART-1 and tyrosinase in human melanoma cell lines and in human melanocytic lesions. *Cancer Res* **57**: 3223–3229.
18. Quakkelaar ED, Melief CJ. (2012) Experience with synthetic vaccines for cancer persistent virus infections in nonhuman primates and patients. *Adv Immunol* **114**: 77–106.
19. Whiteside TL. (2010) Inhibiting the inhibitors: Evaluating agents targeting cancer immunosuppression. *Expert Opin Biol Ther* **10**: 1019–1035.
20. Ferrone S, Whiteside TL. (2007) Tumor microenvironment and immune escape. *Surg Oncol Clin N Am* **16**: 755–774.
21. Ferris RL, Whiteside TL, Ferrone S. (2006) Immune escape associated with functional defects in antigen-processing machinery in head and neck cancer *Clin Cancer Res* **12**: 3890–3895.
22. Campoli M, Ferrone S. (2011) HLA antigen and NK cell activating ligand expression in malignant cells: A story of loss or acquisition. *Semin Immunopathol* **33**: 321–334.
23. Steinman RM, Pope M. (2002) Exploiting dendritic cells to improve vaccine efficacy. *J Clin Invest* **109**: 1519–1526.
24. Kim TS, Cohen EP. (1994) Interleukin-2-secreting mouse fibroblasts transfected with genomic DNA from murine melanoma cells prolong the survival of mice with melanoma. *Cancer Res* **54**: 2531–2535.
25. Kim TS, Cohen EP. (1994) MHC antigen expression by melanomas recovered from mice treated with allogeneic mouse fibroblasts genetically modified for interleukin-2 secretion and the expression of melanoma-associated antigens. *Cancer Immunol Immunother* **38**: 185–193.
26. Sun T, Kim TS, Waltz MR, Cohen EP. (1995) Interleukin-2-secreting mouse fibroblasts transfected with genomic DNA from murine neoplasms induce tumor-specific immune responses that prolong the lives of tumor-bearing mice. *Cancer Gene Ther* **2**: 183–190.
27. Sun T, de Zoeten BF, Carr-Brendel V, Cohen EP. (1998) Immunization with interleukin-2-secreting allogeneic cells transfected with DNA from mouse melanoma cells induces immune responses that prolong the lives of mice with melanoma. *Cancer Gene Ther* **5**: 110–118.

28. Kim TS, Cohen EP. (1994) MHC antigen expression by melanomas recovered from mice treated with allogeneic fibroblasts genetically modified for interleukin-2-secretion and the expression of melanoma associated antigens. *Cancer Immunol Immunother* **38**: 185–191.
29. de Zoeten BF, Carr-Brendel V, Cohen EP. (1998) Resistance to melanoma in mice immunized with semi-allogeneic fibroblasts transfected with genomic DNA from melanoma cells. *J Immunol* **160**: 2915–2922.
30. Artusio E, Hathaway B, Stanson J, Whiteside TL. (2006) Transfection of human monocyte-derived dendritic cells with native tumor DNA induces antigen-specific T cell responses *in vitro*. *Cancer Biol Ther* **5**: 1624–1631.
31. Whiteside TL, Gambotto A, Albers A, *et al.* (2002) Human tumor-derived genomic DNA transduced into a recipient cell induces tumor-specific immune responses *ex vivo*. *PNAS* **99**: 9415–9420.
32. O-Sullivan I, Ng LK, Martinez DM, *et al.* (2005) Immunity to squamous carcinoma in mice immunized with dendritic cells transfected with genomic DNA from squamous carcinoma cells. *Cancer Gene Ther* **12**: 825–834.
33. Cohen EP. (2001) DNA-based vaccines for the treatment of cancer — An experimental model. *Trends Mol Med* **7**: 175–179.
34. Lichtor T, Glick RP, O-Sullivan I, Cohen EP. (2005) Intratumoral injection of IL-2 secreting allogeneic fibroblasts transfected with DNA from breast cancer cells prolongs the survival of mice with intracerebral breast cancer. *Cancer Gene Ther* **12**: 708–714.
35. Liang W, Cohen EP. (1976) Resistance to murine leukemia in mice rejecting syngeneic somatic hybrid cells. *J Immunol* **116**: 623–628.
36. Lichtor T, Glick RP, Tarlock K, *et al.* (2002) Application of interleukin-2 secreting allogeneic fibroblasts in the treatment of primary and metastatic brain tumors. *Cancer Gene Ther* **9**: 464–469.
37. Lichtor T, Glick RP, Cohen EP. (2003) Approaches to the treatment of brain tumors using cytokine-secreting allogeneic fibroblasts. *Cancer Ther* **1**: 109–120.
38. Figdor CG, de Vries JM, Lesterhuis WJ, Melief CJM. (2004) Dendritic cell immunotherapy: Mapping the way. *Nat Med* **10**: 475–480.
39. Meng WS, Butterfield LH. (2005) Activation of antigen-presenting cells by DNA delivery vectors. *Expert Opin Biol Ther* **5**: 1019–1028.
40. Arthur JF, Butterfield LH, Roth MD, *et al.* (1997) A comparison of gene transfer methods in human dendritic cells. *Cancer Gene Ther* **4**: 17–25.
41. Lenz P, Bacot SM, Frazier-Jessen MR, Feldman GM. (2003) Nucleoporation of dendritic cells: Efficient gene transfer by electroporation into human monocyte-derived dendritic cells. *FEBS Lett* **538**: 149–154.

42. McCullough J, Key N, Gee A, *et al.* (2004) Production assistance for cellular therapies. *Transfusion* **44**: 1793–1795.
43. Tourkova IL, Shurin GV, Chatta GS, *et al.* (2005) Restoration by IL-15 of MHC class I antigen processing machinery in human dendritic cells inhibited by tumor-derived gangliosides. *J Immunol* **175**: 3045–3052.
44. Nicolette C, Healey D, Tcherepanova I, *et al.* (2007) Dendritic cells for active immunotherapy: Optimizing design and manufacture in order to develop commercially and clinically viable products. *Vaccine* **25S**: B47–B60.
45. Butterfield LH, Gooding W, Whiteside TL. (2008) Development of a potency assay for human dendritic cells: IL-12p70 production. *J Immunother* **31**: 89–100.

CHAPTER 10

Translational Research of Tyrosine Kinase Inhibitors in Cancer

Terry W. Moody[*,‡] *and Jill P. Smith*[†]

10.1. INTRODUCTION

Cancer is a serious public health problem with over 1,500,000 patients diagnosed with cancer in the US annually and over 560,000 deaths.[1] The most deaths per year occur in lung cancer patients (158,000), followed by colon, breast and prostate cancer patients (53,000, 40,000 and 29,000 deaths, respectively). Traditionally, cancer patients are treated with surgery, chemotherapy and/or radiation therapy, but in lung cancer these treatments are largely ineffective. As a result, the median survival time for lung cancer patients is less than one year.

A new approach to therapy is target-specific regimens with small molecules. One target is receptor tyrosine kinases (RTKs), which are large proteins that are embedded into the plasma membrane of specific cancer cells. At the cell surface, RTKs bind extracellular growth factors and the activated RTK causes the transient tyrosine phosphorylation of cellular protein substrates. RTKs are oncogenes in certain cancers resulting in

*National Cancer Institute, Center for Cancer Research, Office of the Director, Bethesda, Maryland, USA
†National Institute of Diabetes and Digestive and Kidney Diseases, Division of Digestive Diseases and Nutrition, Bethesda, Maryland, USA
‡Corresponding author. Dr. Terry Moody, NCI Office of the Director, CCR, Bldg. 31, Rm. 4A48, Bethesda, MD 20892, USA; Tel: +1 301 451 9451; Fax. +1-301-480-4323; E-mail: *moodyt@mail.nih.gov*

increased proliferation. Several RTKs are mutated in cancer, such as the epidermal growth factor receptor (EGFR), resulting in high tyrosine kinase activity. Tyrosine kinase inhibitors (TKIs) are small molecules that bind to the RTK and block the ATP binding site of the RTK, reducing tyrosine kinase activity.[2] For the EGFR, gefitinib and erlotinib are small molecules that act as TKIs in lung cancer patients. Thus, RTKs are molecular targets for the development of new drugs using translational research.

In the past decade, translational research has facilitated the development of numerous TKIs. For example, imatinib is a TKI used to treat patients with chronic myelogenous leukemia (CML). In CML, the RTK is constitutively active due to translocation of segments of chromosomes 9 and 22. The resulting fused chromosome 22 contains Bcr-Abl, which causes tyrosine phosphorylation of protein substrates. In a phase I clinical trial, imatinib was active when a dose of 300 mg or greater was administered into CML patients.[3] Dose-limiting toxicities in CML patients treated with imatinib included nausea, vomiting, edema and rash. In a phase II clinical trial, imatinib restored normal blood counts in 53 out of 54 chemotherapy-resistant CML patients. Subsequent studies showed that imatinib was effective at treating patients with gastrointestinal stromal tumors (GIST). Surprisingly, in GIST cells, imitinib blocks ATP binding in c-Kit and the platelet derived growth factor receptor (PDGF); Bcr-Abl is not abundant in GIST cells.[4] Thus, a barrier in using TKIs is their specificity. At low doses a TKI can be specific for a certain RTK, but using high doses of TKI, ATP binding sites can be blocked in multiple RTKs (Table 1).

During treatment with TKIs, additional mutations arise in RTKs. In CML patients, over a five-year period, 17 per cent of the CML patients

Table 1 TKIs in Cancer. The Drugs Used to Treat Cancer Patients are Indicated

Tumor Type	Mutated/Amplified Kinase	Drug
Breast cancer	HER2	Herceptin/lapatanib
CML	BCR-ABL	imatinib/dasatanib
GIST	c-KIT/PDGFR	imatinib/sunitinib
Melanoma	B-RAF	PLX4032
NSCLC	EGFR	gefitinib/erlotinib
NSCLC	Alk	crizotinib

became resistant to imatinib.[5] In these patients, BCR-ABL point mutations such as T315I occurred near the ATP binding site, resulting in impaired imatinib binding. Hence, a second generation of TKI, ponatinib was developed. Novel approaches to overcome drug resistance required bridging the knowledge derived from basic science research to patient care, e.g., translational research. This chapter will focus on an overview of the importance of translational research in the area of lung cancer TKIs and cancer therapeutics.

10.2. ONCOGENES AND TUMOR SUPPRESSOR GENES

10.2.1. TP53

In most adult human tumors, dozens of genes are altered during the process of carcinogenesis.[6] Analysis of over 13,000 genes indicated that 189 genes were frequently mutated in breast and colon cancer. *TP53*, a tumor suppressor gene, encodes for the protein p53, which is inactivated in approximately 90 percent of small-cell lung cancers (SCLC) and 50 percent of non-SCLC (NSCLC) patients. NSCLC is comprised of adenocarcinoma, squamous cell carcinoma and large cell carcinoma, and accounts for approximately 85 percent of lung cancer deaths. *TP53* is a tumor suppressor gene that mediates the G1- to S-phase checkpoint of the cell cycle. If DNA is damaged by carcinogen exposure, *TP53* mediates programmed cell death or apoptosis. When *TP53* is phosphorylated, expression of BAX (mediates apoptosis) and GADD45 (mediates DNA repair) is increased. Somatic and germ line mutations have been reported in *TP53*. In smokers, there is an increase in G-to-T transversion in *TP53* at CpG rich codons, including 153–158 (exon 5), 248 and 249 (exon 7), and 273 (exon 8). With *TP53* mutation and loss of heterozygosity, *TP53* is rendered inactive.[7] *TP53* mutations are driver and not passenger mutations in lung cancer patients.[8] An active area of research involves development of agents that recover or activate p53 function.

10.2.2. EGFR and HER2

The epidermal growth factor receptor (EGFR), or ErbB1, is an oncogene in NSCLC that is activated by endogenous transforming growth factor alpha

(TGF-α). The EGFR is amplified in approximately 30 percent of NSCLC patients.[9] Normally, co-expression of the EGFR and its ligand leads to an autocrine growth factor loop increasing cellular proliferation.[10] The EGFR is mutated in approximately 10 percent of US and European populations and 30 percent of Asian populations, especially in non-smoking women that have adenocarcinoma. The L858R mutation in exon 21 or short in-frame deletions (exon 19) lead to constitutive activation of the EGFR tyrosine kinase.[11] Gefitinib or erlotinib are TKIs that bind with high affinity to the mutant EGFR ATP binding site but not the wild-type EGFR.[12–14] Alternatively, the EGFR can be blocked with cetuximab, a chimeric immunoglobulin G that binds to the extracellular domain of the EGFR and affects ligand-induced tyrosine phosphorylation. While the EGFR is mutated in only 13 percent of NSCLC patients, treatment with TKIs can improve the lives of tens of thousands of lung cancer patients in the US.[15] Routinely, TKIs are administered to lung cancer patients with driver mutations of the EGFR around the ATP binding site who have failed chemotherapy.

The EGFR can form heterodimers with HER2/Neu (ErbB2). HER2 (1,233 amino acids) has a 580 amino acid intracellular domain with tyrosine kinase activity, but the extracellular domain of 630 amino acids does not bind TGF-α or any other known ligand with high affinity. HER2 is amplified in a small percentage of lung cancer patients but is amplified in 30 percent of breast cancer patients.[16,17] Anti-HER2 monoclonal antibodies (mAb) were developed and the mAb 4D5 was humanized (Herceptin) for clinical trials.[18] In breast cancer patients with amplified HER2, the addition of Herceptin to their chemotherapy regimens results in increased disease-free survival and decreased disease recurrence. In patients who develop resistance to Herceptin, use of the TKI dacomitinib, which inhibits HER2 tyrosine phosphorylation, may be beneficial.[19]

10.2.3. RAS, RAF, MEK and ERK

The activated RTK causes signal transduction involved in regulation of normal cellular processes and proliferative mechanisms in cancer cells. When the C-terminal of the EGFR becomes activated, it associates with a

Scr homology2 (SH2) domain adapter protein (Shc) and Grb-2.[20] Grb-2 has two SH3 domains which bind the guanine nucleotide exchange factor son of sevenless homolog (SOS). Activated SOS promotes the removal of GDP from RAS. RAS-GTP is biologically active, but it has GTPase activity, which metabolizes RAS-GTP to biologically inactive RAS-GDP. Mutation of RAS inhibits GTPase activity, resulting in increased levels of RAS-GTP. K-RAS is mutated in approximately 20 percent of NSCLC patients, especially those with adenocarcinoma; K-RAS is mutated in approximately 80 percent of patients with advanced pancreatic cancers.[21] Most of the K-RAS mutations are G-to-T transversions in codon 12. K-RAS mutations are independent of EGFR mutations and are associated with clinical resistance to TKIs.

RAS and RAF are oncogenes for certain cancers. Figure 1 shows that RAF is activated after RAS. RAF is a serine/threonine kinase that subsequently activates MEK. While RAF is mutated in only 1 percent of lung cancer patients, B-RAF-V600E mutations occur in approximately 60 percent of melanoma patients, resulting in a constituitively active kinase.[22] Numerous B-RAF inhibitors have been identified, such as PLX4032, which binds with high affinity to B-RAF-V600E (Ki = 44 nM). When PLX4032 (50 mg/kg) was orally administered to mice containing B-RAF-V600E melanoma xenografts, tumor regression was observed. PLX4032 showed an 81 percent response rate in patients with metastatic melanoma carrying B-RAF mutations.[23] RAS and B-RAF are driver mutations in several types of cancer.

RAF phosphorylates mitogen activated protein kinase (MAPK), or MEK. MEK1 and MEK2 are phosphorylated at serine residues by RAF. A MEK inhibitor (PD98059) is routinely used *in vitro* and prevents phosphorylation of tyrosine and threonine residues on extracellular signal-regulated kinases (ERK)1 and 2. Phosphorylated ERK goes from the cytoplasm into the nucleus, where it regulates expression of transcription factors such as fos or myc. These transcription factors bind to the promoters of many genes, increasing growth and preventing apoptosis. ERK is a gatekeeper gene in that it directly regulates cell growth. In melanoma patients, activated BRAF is associated with constitutive ERK activation.[24] In some melanoma patients, treatment with PLX4032

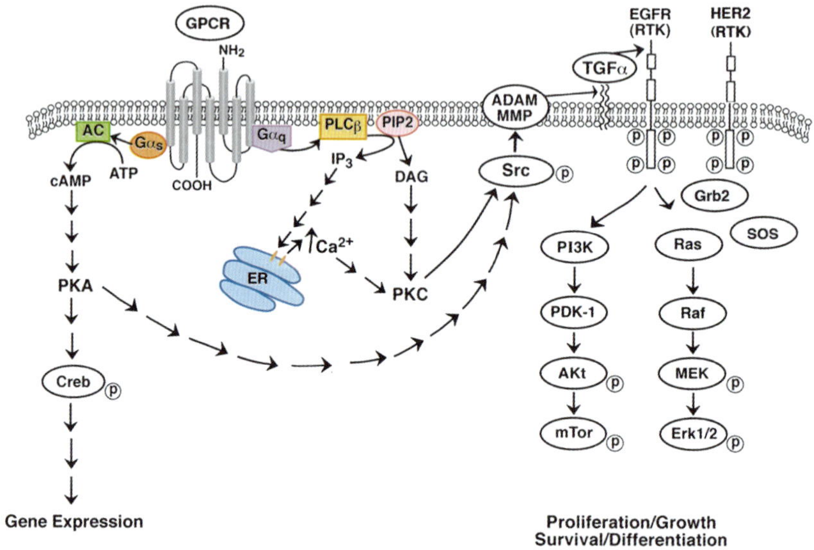

Fig. 1. EGFR transactivation. Some GPCRs interact with Gs, which increases adenylylcyclase (AC) activity, resulting in elevated cAMP. The cAMP activates protein kinase (PK) A, which causes Src phosphoryation and Creb phosphorylation, resulting in altered gene expression. Other GPCRs interact with Gq, leading to PLC activation and PIP_2 metabolism. The PIP_2 products include IP_3, which causes calcium release from the endoplasmic reticulum (ER), and DAG, which activates PKC, triggering Src phosphorylation. When Src is phosphorylated, it activates MMP, causing TGF-α release from lung cancer cells. The TGF-α activates RTK such as the EGFR, which can form heterodimers with HER2. The activated EGFR interacts with Grb2 and SOS, leading to Ras and Raf activation, followed by phosphorylation of MEK and ERK. The activated EGFR interacts with PI3K, leading to PIP_3 formation and subsequent activation of PDK-1, Akt and mTOR, leading to cancer cell survival and proliferation.

is associated with little tumor response and increased P-MEK as well as P-ERK. The MEK1/MEK2 inhibitor trametinib had significant clinical activity in B-RAF inhibitor-naive patients previously treated with chemotherapy and/or immunotherapy.[25] In contrast, trametinib had minimal clinical activity in patients previously treated with a B-RAF inhibitor. Also, the MEK1/MEK2 inhibitor selumetinib plus docetaxel had promising efficacy in KRAS-mutant NSCLC patients.[26] These studies warrant further clinical investigation of MEK1/MEK2 inhibitors in cancer patients.

10.2.4. PI3K, PKD, Akt and mTor

Phosphatidylinositol 3-kinase (PI3K) is a lipid kinase with a 110-kDa catalytic subunit and 85-kDa regulatory subunit causing PIP_2 to form phosphatidylinositol 3,4,5-trisphosphate (PIP_3). PI3K is activated by autophosphorylation of Tyr^{177}, which generates a docking site for the SH2 domain of the Grb2 adapter protein. PI3K is frequently mutated in breast (25 percent), brain (27 percent), colon (30 percent) and stomach (25 percent) cancer.[27] Mutations in the PI3K pathway may result in resistance to TKIs in lung cancer patients. The majority of the PI3K mutations occur at E542, E545 or H1047 of the kinase domain at the interface of the p110 and p85 resulting in gain of enzymatic function. Figure 1 shows that after PI3K activation, PDK1, which has a pleckstrin homology domain, is activated. PDK1 in turn phosphorylates T308 and S473 of Akt. PIP_3 binds to the PH domains of Akt and recruits Akt to the plasma membrane followed by phosphorylation by PKD. Akt promotes cellular survival by phosphorylating and inactivating BAD, which causes cellular apoptosis. Also, Akt causes phosphorylation of caspase-9, preventing apoptosis of cancer cells. Akt can be activated by genetic mutations, genome amplifications or mutations in upstream signaling components such as PI3K. AKT1 is mutated in 5 percent of breast, 6 percent of colorectal and 2 percent of ovarian cancers.[28] Akt promotes cellular growth by activating the serine/threonine kinase mTor (mammalian target of rapamycin). mTor is a 289-kDa kinase that has a catalytic domain, an FRB (FKBP12-rapamycin binding) domain, and a repressor domain near the C-terminal. Akt-dependent activation of mTor enhances the phosphorylation of p70S6 kinase and 4E-BP1, increasing protein translation and cell proliferation. mTor is the repressor of autophagy, a lysosome-dependent degradation pathway. The first agents developed to target Akt were rapamycin analogs. More selective agents such as the dual PI3K/mTor inhibitor XL765 are being tested.[29]

PI3K mutations involve chromosome 10q, which contains phosphatase and tensin homolog (PTEN). PTEN is a lipid and protein phosphatase that down-regulates phosphorylated Akt by suppression of PIP_3. PTEN degrades PIP_3 to PIP_2 in the phosphatase domain, whereas it binds to the phospholipid membrane through the C2 domain. PTEN is mutated[30] in breast cancer (13 percent) but loss of heterozygosity is more common (30 percent). PTEN is a driver mutation.

10.3. EGFR TKI

The EGFR is a subfamily of RTK with 1,186 amino acids including a 621 amino acid extracellular domain, a 24 amino acid transmembrane domain and a 541 intracellular domain with tyrosine kinase activity.[2] Upon activation by ligands such a EGF or TGF-α, Lys^{721} binds ATP, resulting in phosphorylation of protein substrates such as phospholipase C (PLC)γ or PI3K. In addition, the EGFR forms homodimers and phosphorylates itself at Tyr^{1068}, Tyr^{1086}, Tyr^{1148} and Tyr^{1174}. The tyrosine phosphorylation of protein substrates is transient and reversed by protein tyrosine phosphatases (PTP). Signaling through the EGFR can be blocked with TKIs such as erlotinib or gefitinib.

Figure 2 shows that within seconds after the addition of EGF to NSCLC cells, the 170-kDa EGFR is the major protein tyrosine phosphorylated. Also, the 145-kDa PLC and 110-kDa PI3K subunit is tyrosine phosphorylated. The tyrosine phosphorylation caused by EGF is reversed if gefitinib is present. The sensitivity of NSCLC cells to gefitinib varies dramatically, being 12.8 μM using NCI-H157 cells (squamous cell carcinoma) and 0.02 μM using NCI-H3255 cells.[31] Subsequent studies showed that NCI-H3225 had high levels of E-cadherin, which contributes to the epithelial phenotype,

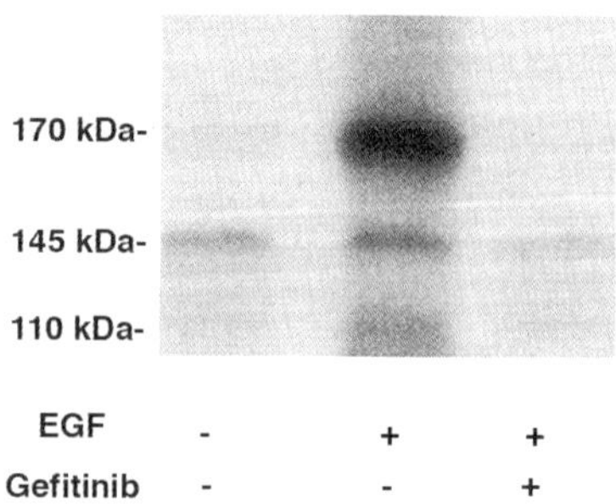

Fig. 2. Western blot of EGFR tyrosine kinase activity. After addition of 100 ng/ml of EGF to NCI-H727 cells, major phosphotyrosine bands were observed at 170, 145 and 110 kDa. Gefitinib (10 μg/ml) inhibited the increase in phosphotyrosine caused by EGF.

where NCI-H157 had low levels of E-cadherin, which contributes to the mesenchymal phenotype. EGFR TKIs are more potent in cancer cells that have not undergone epithelial-mesenchymal transitions.

Additional studies showed that NSCLC cell line NCI-H157 has wild-type EGFR whereas cell line NCI-H3255 has the L858R mutation. Eighty-five percent of the EGFR mutations are L858R point mutations (exon 21) or exon 19 deletions near the ATP binding site,[32–34] resulting in increased gefitinib sensitivity. When patients with EGFR mutations are treated with gefitinib or erlotinib, the time to disease progression is prolonged significantly.[35–37] Additional studies showed that treatment of NSCLC patients who have EGFR mutations with TKIs increased the response rate by 55–82 percent and the increased progression-free survival from 8.9 to 13.3 months.[38–39] Thus, gefitinib or erlotinib is useful for treating NSCLC patients with EGFR mutations.

Gefitinib (Iressa) is N-(3-chloro-4-fluorophenyl)-7-methoxy-6-(3-morpholin-4-ylpropoxy)quinazolin-4-amine, and it was approved by the US Food and Drug Administration (FDA) in 2003 for NSCLC. The FDA withdrew approval in new patients in 2004 due to lack of evidence that it extended patient life. Erlotinib hydrochloride (Tarceva) is N-(3-ethynylphenyl)-6,7-bis(2-metnosyethoxy)quinazolin-4-amine, and it was approved by the FDA for treatment of NSCLC patients who failed chemotherapy. Common side effects include rash that resembles acne and primarily involves the face and neck. Unfortunately, after 8 to 12 months of erlotinib treatment, patients develop resistance, primarily due to additional EGFR mutations, especially T790M. Subsequently, second-generation EGFR TKIs were developed. A major problem with use of TKIs in cancer patients is that resistance develops because cancers continue to mutate.

10.4. TKI RESISTANCE

Approximately 50 percent of lung cancer patients acquire resistance to gefitinib or eroltinib as a result of the T790M EGFR mutation. Dacomitinib (PF-00299804) was designed to inhibit HER2-amplified breast cancer that is resistant to trastuzumab (Herceptin) and lapatinib (Tykerb).[19]

Subsequent studies showed that dacomitinib is effective on NSCLC cells that have L858R and T790M EGFR mutations.[40] Clinical trials are being conducted with dacomitinib for NSCLC patients who fail erlotinib therapy. Lung cancers with resistance to EGFR TKIs occasionally harbor BRAF gene mutations,[41] and dasatinib is useful for some NSCLC patients with BRAF mutations.[42]

MET is an RTK that is amplified in approximately 20 percent of NSCLC patients that become resistant to gefitinib or erlotinib. MET binds hepatocyte growth factor (HGF) with high affinity, causing tyrosine phosphorylation of protein substrates. Trivantinib is a MET TKI that is being investigated in lung cancer clinical trials.[43] MET amplification leads to gefitinib resistance in lung cancer through activated ErbB3 signaling.[44] This results in activation of PI3K circumventing the effects of the EGFR TKI.

ALK translocates with echinoderm microtubule-associated protein-like 4 (EML4) in approximately 4 percent of NSCLC patients.[45] EML4-ALK translocations occur independently of KRAS or EGFR mutations. EML4-ALK binds PF-02341066 (crizotinib), a TKI, with high affinity.[46] EML4-ALK contains 1,620 amino acids with a single transmembrane region and a 254 amino acid intracellular kinase domain. Patients (57 percent) with ALK-positive NSCLC responded to crizotinib and many of the patients were Asians who did not smoke and had adenocarcinoma.[47]

For NSCLC, approximately 20 percent, 13 percent, 5 percent and 2 percent of the tumors have KRAS, EGFR, ALK and BRAF mutations, respectively. Genes that are extensively mutated in lung cancer include p53, KRAS and EGFR with 65, 60 and 35 mutations identified in adenocarcinoma of the lung, respectively.[48] Translational research has facilitated the age of molecular medicine whereby the genetic profile of the tumor dictates the patient treatment and makes cancer therapy "personalized."

10.5. CLINICAL TRIALS WITH TKIs

Several clinical trials tested the efficacy of TKIs for treatment of NSCLC patients. IDEAL 1 and IDEAL 2 were randomized, double-blind phase II multicenter trials which evaluated 250 mg or 500 mg of oral gefitinib in more than 400 patients.[49,50] A tumor objective response rate (ORR) was observed in 9–19 percent of the patients with a median survival of 6–8 months and improvement in lung cancer symptoms. There was no difference in the time to progression and median survival between the two doses, and the 500 mg dose was associated with more adverse effects. The INTACT 1 and INTACT 2 trials demonstrated no survival benefit when gefitinib was given in combination with cisplatin and gemcitabine compared to carboplatin and paclitaxel chemotherapy alone.[51,52] The results of these studies indicate that gefitinib therapy results in an ORR with improved symptoms in lung cancer patients but does not increase overall survival.

Subsequent studies showed that gefitinib demonstrated a superior ORR and progression free survival (PFS) in East Asian patients when compared with platinum based therapy.[53] Early trials indicated that females with adenocarcinoma, of East Asian descent and no history of smoking, had the best clinical response to TKIs. Additional research revealed that EGFR in-frame deletions of exon 19 or L858R mutations in exon 21 of the EGFR lead to excellent clinical response to TKI therapy.[54] There is little difference in the response rate whether gefitinib or erlotinib is used and both drugs have similar toxicity profiles.[55] The most common adverse reactions to EGFR TKIs include a papulopustular skin rash and diarrhea. These studies indicate that gefitinib or erlotinib can be used safely to treat NSCLC patients with EGFR mutations.

Resistance to TKIs in NSCLC primarily occurs because of T790M mutations of the EGFR. The gefitinib or erlotinib resistant patients can then be treated with alternative medications such as lapatinib (targets EGFR and HER2) or dacomitinib (irreversible pan ErbB inhibitor). NSCLC patients (57 percent) responded subsequently to dacomitinib and achieved a PFS of 9 months.[56] In approximately 20 percent of the cases, TKI resistance in NSCLC patients was associated with MET amplification. ARQ197, a MET inhibitor that impairs kinase activation allosterically, when given in combination with erlotinib improved PFS from 9.7 to 16.1 weeks.[57] Additional mechanisms of resistance to EGFR-TKI include PTEN mutations and epithelial-to-mesenchymal transitions of NSCLC cells.

Another RTK mutated in NSCLC is EML4-ALK. Crizotinib is an EML4-ALK TKI that is used to treat patients with ALK translocations. In NSCLC patients with ALK tranlocations, crizotinib increased the 1-year overall survival from 46 percent to 71 percent.[58] Unfortunately, with

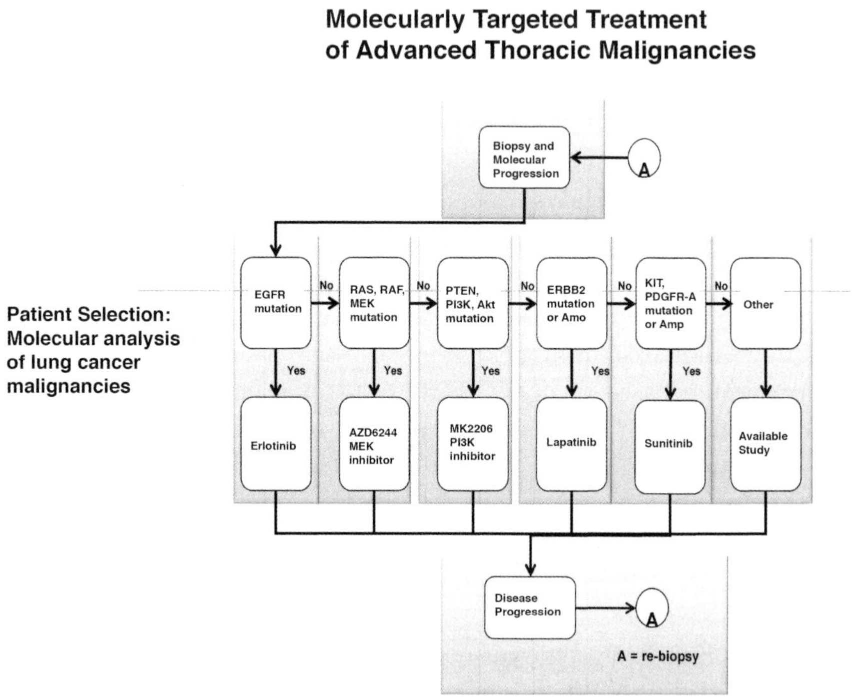

Fig. 3. NCI clinical protocol. A biopsy specimen is obtained from thoracic cancer patients and a molecular analysis is performed. Based on the mutation observed, patients are treated with the indicated drugs. At the end of therapy, a new biopsy specimen is obtained and another molecular analysis performed to determine if additional genetic mutations occurred during drug treatment.

continued drug administration ALK mutations occur, leading to crizotinib resistance.[59]

Figure 3 shows a clinical protocol for treatment of patients at the NCI with advanced thoracic malignancies. Initially, the molecular profile for each patient's tumor is determined. If EGFR mutations are detected, subjects are treated with erlotinib. Those with RAS RAF or MEK mutations are treated with AZD6244, a MEK inhibitor. MK2206, a PI3K inhibitor, is used in those with PTEN, PI3K or Akt mutations. Lastly, ErbB2, KIT or PDGFR-A mutations are treated with lapatinib, sunitinib or sunitinib, respectively. At the completion of the study, the molecular profiling is repeated to determine if additional gene mutations developed during the treatment. Thus far, 235 patients with NSCLC have enrolled, of which 77 were never smokers and 130 were former smokers. Of these patients, the following mutations were detected: EGFR (27 percent); RAS, RAF or MEK (26 percent); PTEN, PI3K or AKT (8 percent); ERBB2, KIT or PDGFR-A (4 percent). This illustrates how translational research may be employed in real time to investigate the utility of kinase inhibitors in patients with thoracic malignancies.

10.6. LUNG CANCER GROWTH FACTORS

One of the first autocrine growth factors identified in lung cancer was gastrin-releasing peptide (GRP). The 27-amino-acid GRP is present in high concentrations in SCLC.[60] SCLC cells have dense core neurosecretory vesicles that undergo exocytosis when the cAMP is elevated, increasing the GRP concentration in the extracellular fluids.[61] Initially, mAbs were developed that neutralize GRP,[62] and one mAb named 2A11 was found to inhibit the growth of SCLC cells and tumors in animal models. Unfortunately, 2A11 was found to have little effect on human subjects with SCLC.[63] Because GRP binds with high affinity to the bombesin (BB)R, antagonists were developed that block receptor binding. One particular antagonist named ($Psi^{13,14}$, Leu^{14})BN blocks BB_2Rs and inhibits the growth of lung cancer cells.[64] The BB_2R contains 384 amino acids[65] and interacts with a guanine nucleotide binding protein (Gq) resulting in PI turnover. PI-4,5,-bisphosphate is metabolized to inositol-1,4,5-trisphosphate (IP_3), which causes release of Ca^{2+} from the endoplasmic reticulum (ER). Figure 1 shows that diacylglycerol (DAG) is released, activating protein kinase (PK)C. PKC causes serine/threonine phosphorylation of protein substrates such as Src. Treatment of SCLC cells with GRP induced ERK tyrosine phosphorylation, leading to SCLC proliferation. ($Psi^{13,14}$, Leu^{14}) BB inhibited both basal proliferation of SCLC cells as well as that stimulated by exogenous GRP.[66] Clinical trials have not yet been conducted using BB_2R antagonists.

In addition to GRP, SCLC cells produce neuromedin (NM)B, which has seven of the 10 same amino acids residues as does GRP.[67] The BB_1R binds NMB and GRP with high and low affinity, respectively. The BB_1R is a GPCR that has 390 amino acids with 48 percent sequence homology to the BB_2R.[68] PD168368 is a nonpeptide antagonist that inhibits binding of NMB to the BB_1R and subsequent growth of lung cancer cells.[69] The BB_1R, similar to the BB_2R, interacts with Gq, causing PI turnover. Subsequent studies showed that the BB_1R and BB_2R are present on many SCLC and NSCLC cells and tumors.[70] An additional BB receptor subtype (BRS)-3 has been identified as an orphan receptor[71] for which no endogenous ligand is known. BRS-3 receptors are present in SCLC and NSCLC cells; however, no high affinity antagonists for BRS-3 are known.[72] These results indicate that multiple ligands and receptors of the BB family are present in lung cancer cells. BBRs may function as molecular targets that regulate SCLC proliferation (SCLC cells do not have high densities of EGFR). In NSCLC (100,000 EGFR/cell), however, BBRs regulate EGFR tyrosine phosphorylation.

10.7. EGFR TRANSACTIVATION

The EGFR can be transactivated by G protein-coupled receptors (GPCRs). GPCRs contain about 400 amino acids and cross the cellular plasma membrane seven times (Fig. 1). As a result, the N-terminal and extracellular domains 1, 2 and 3 are exposed to the extracellular fluids. The C-terminal and intracellular domains 1, 2 and 3 are exposed to the cytosol of the cell. Because GPCRs do not have enzymatic activity like RTK, they interact with G proteins to initiate signal transduction. Some of the GPCRs for prostaglandin (PG)E_2 or vasoactive intestinal peptide (VIP) activate a stimulatory guanine nucleotide binding protein (Gs), increasing adenylyl cyclase (AC) activity.[73] AC metabolizes ATP to cyclic AMP (cAMP) and the elevated cAMP activates protein kinase (PK)A. PKA causes the serine/threonine phosphorylation of the cAMP response element binding protein (CREB). Phosphorylated CREB diffuses to the nucleus wherein it binds to a cAMP response element (CRE) in certain genes such as vascular endothelial growth factor (VEGF), altering gene expression.[74] NSCLC has cyclooxygenase (COX) enzymes that convert the substrate arachidonic acid to PGE_2. Two types of COX enzymes are present in NSCLC cells: COX-1, which is inhibited by non-steroidal anti-inflammatory drugs (NSAIDs), and COX-2, which is inducible by EGF.[75] PGE_2 production in NSCLC cells

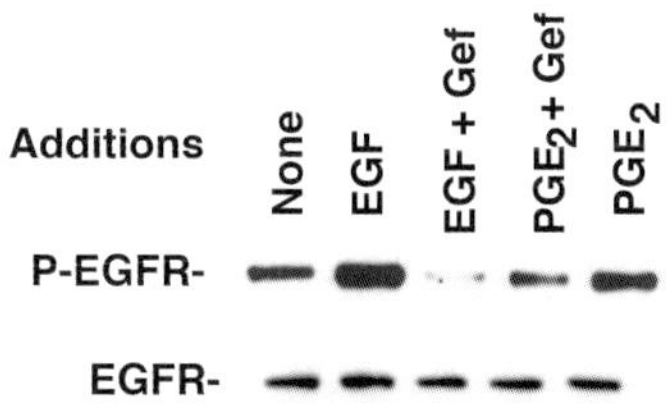

Fig. 4. EGFR transactivation. EGFR tyrosine phosphorylation was increased after addition of 100 ng/ml EGF or 1 μM PGE_2 to NCI-H1299 cells. Addition of 10 μg/ml gefitinib decreased the EGFR tyrosine phosphorylation caused by EGF or PGE_2. In contrast, EGF, PGE_2 or gefitinib had no effect on total EGFR. The Western blot was probed using anti-PY^{1068}-EGFR or anti-EGFR.

is inhibited by NSAIDs such as aspirin, S-valproate and S-sulindac as well as selective COX-2 blockers such as DuP-697 or celecoxib.[76] PGE_2 binds with high affinity to EP_2-Rs, which are present in NSCLC cells. PGE_2 addition to NSCLC cells increases the cAMP levels 10-fold, and this effect is blocked by AH6809, an EP_2-R antagonist.[77] PGE_2 increased VEGF in NSCLC cells which was blocked by H89, a PKA inhibitor. The proliferation of NSCLC cells was inhibited by NSAIDs as well as AH6809. In preclinical studies, the growth of NSCLC tumors was inhibited by NSAIDs. Because COX-2 is a molecular target in NSCLC, numerous clinical trials are being conducted using COX-2 inhibitors such as celecoxib.

Figure 4 shows that addition of PGE_2 to NSCLC cells increased Tyr^{1068}-EGFR phosphorylation. The mechanism of EGFR transactivation is complex and involves Src and matrix metallo proteases (MMP). GRP addition to squamous cell carcinoma of the head and neck(SCCHN) cell line PCI-37A increased association of Src with a TNF-α converting enzyme, a disintegrin and metalloproteinase (ADAM)-17. This reaction resulted in the phosphorylation of ADAM-17.[78] Amphiregulin and TGF-α release from PCI-37A cells was increased after the addition of GRP and this increase was suppressed if ADAM-17 was down-regulated.[79] EGFR ligand release was further suppressed by PP2, a Src inhibitor. Addition of exogenous PGE_2 or EGF to NSCLC cells increased the tyrosine phosphorylation of the EGFR which was inhibited by gefitinib. PGE_2 or EGF had no effect on total EGFR

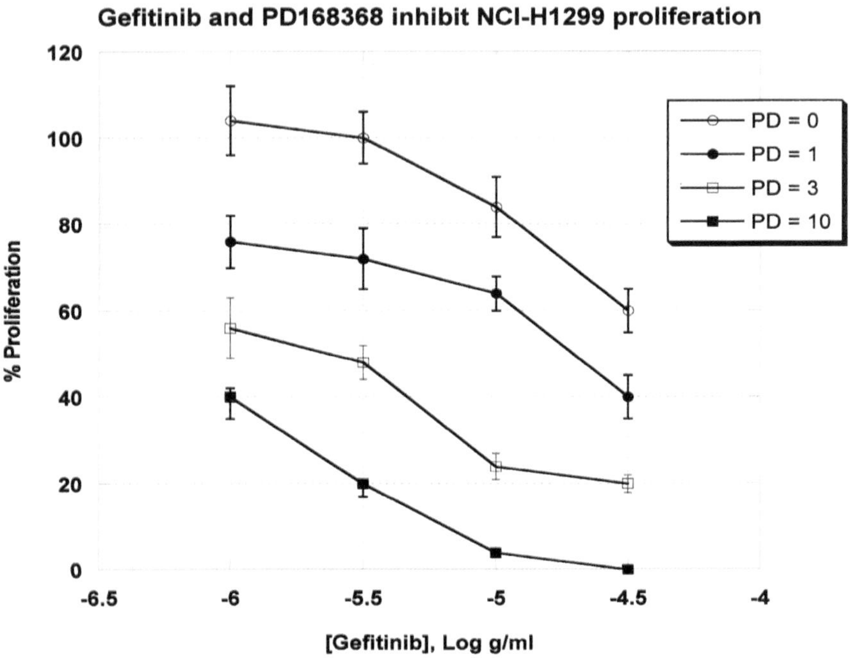

Fig. 5. NSCLC proliferation. The effects of increasing doses of PD168368 and gefitinib on NCI-H1299 cellular proliferation were investigated using the MTT assay. The results indicate that PD168368 shifts the gefitinib dose–response curve to the left. PD168368 and gefitinib were synergistic at inhibiting NSCLC proliferation. The mean value ±S.D. of eight determinations is indicated.

in NSCLC cells (Fig. 4). The ability of PGE_2 to cause EGFR transactivation in NSCLC cells was inhibited by addition of PP2 (Src inhibitor), GM6001 (MMP inhibitor) or AH6809 (EP_2-R antagonist). These results indicate that TKIs and GPCR antagonists can block EGFR transactivation in NSCLC cells.

GRP addition to head and neck cancer cells caused EGFR transactivation which was blocked by the BB_2R antagonist PD176252.[80] Subsequent studies showed that PD176252 inhibited the growth of SCCHN and potentiated the effects of gefitinib. Figure 5 shows that the BB_1R antagonist PD168368 and gefitinib inhibited the growth of lung cancer cells with IC_{50} values of 6 μg/ml and 50 μg/ml, respectively. Increasing amounts of PD168368 shifted the gefitinib dose–response curve to the left by approximately an order of magnitude.[81] The combination index (0.52 ± 0.11) indicated that PD168368 and gefitinib were synergistic at inhibiting NSCLC proliferation *in vitro*, and we are currently investigating these effects using animal models *in vivo*. These results indicate that GPCR antagonists potentiate the growth inhibitory effects of gefitinib using cancer cells that have wild-type EGFR. It is important to develop new therapies for the 87 percent of the NSCLC patients who have wild-type EGFR.

10.8. TRANSLATIONAL RESEARCH EDUCATION

New programs are needed that are dedicated to the education of postdoctoral and clinical fellows in translational research. At the NIH, there are approximately 3,600 postdoctoral and 700 clinical fellows who train for three to five years. In addition to learning new basic research and clinical techniques, these fellows need to learn how to implement translational research for development of new cancer drugs.

At NCI, a course in the Translational Research in Clinical Oncology (TRACO) was developed nine years ago. The course, which is offered each fall and occurs for two hours/week over a 13-week period, discusses basic and clinical cancer research from a viewpoint of the past, present and future. Molecular medicine is emphasized whereby patient treatment is dictated by the subtype of cancer that the patient has.

Each year the course has approximately 170 registrants. Registrants can watch the live lecture in the classroom or on videocast. In addition, videocasts are archived so that registrants can call up previous lectures at any time on their own computer. Handouts are provided in the classroom and posted on the course website so that registrants can print them out prior to watching the videocast. A certificate of completion of the class can be obtained by passing a computer graded final examination. Both clinical and basic concepts are emphasized because lectures are given by PhDs and/or MDs.

Lecture topics include cancer growth, angiogenesis and metastasis. It is emphasized that treatment is most effective when cancer is detected early, prior to metastasis. A lecture on imaging emphasizes how small tumors can be detected and surgically removed. For large tumors, chemo- and/or radiation therapy are traditionally employed. If this treatment fails then small molecules such as TKIs may be used. Organ specific lectures are given on lung, breast, prostate, colon, ovarian and pancreatic cancers. In addition, lectures are given on new treatment approaches such as small interfering RNA, micro RNAs, and nanotechnology.

In addition to a lecture component, registrants can sign up for visits to tumor boards and/or core facilities. At tumor boards, registrants learn about cancer patients and their treatment on an individual basis. At core facilities, registrants learn the latest techniques, including proteomics and genomics using next-generation sequencing. The goal of the TRACO course is to broaden fellows' knowledge about cancer research.

At NCI, a Translational Research Working Group (TRWG) was established in 2005 to review the NCI portfolio. Over a span of two years, the TRWG evaluated the intramural and extramural program and listed recommendations. In phase 1, ways to improve and enhance its focus, integration and effectiveness were provided. In phase 2, the TRWG interacted with the cancer community of invited public input. In phase 3, the recommendations were finalized to speed the development of new diagnostic tests, cancer treatments and other interventions that benefit people with and at high risk for cancer. In particular, NCI emphasizes basic science discovery, including promising molecule or gene targets, candidate protein biomarkers, and basic epidemiologic findings. Also NCI emphasizes early translation, including partnerships and collaborations (academia, government and industry), intervention development, and phase I and II clinical trials. For NIH, barriers in translational research include increased costs and complexity, a need for better information systems, increased regulatory burdens, low patient recruitment for clinical trials, and difficulties in recruiting, mentoring and retaining translational research investigators. Last year at NIH a new institute was formed to deal with these problems: the National Center for Advancing Translational Sciences (NCATS).

10.9. SUMMARY

In cancer, translational research has been embraced in the past decade, and this has resulted in the development of numerous TKIs to treat cancer patients. Patients with mutated RTK respond initially to TKIs. After a year of treatment with TKIs, many of the cancer patients become unresponsive due to further mutations of the RTK. A major problem to address in translational research is the development of drugs that will result in more effective therapy for cancers that continue to mutate. The development of TKIs has improved the quality of life and provides hope for cancer patients.

For lung cancer, only 13 percent of NSCLC patients have EGFR mutations. Patients with EGFR mutations respond to the TKI gefitinib or erlotinib, but there are side effects associated with TKI use, e.g., skin rashes and diarrhea. A goal in cancer research is to increase the sensitivity of NSCLC patients with wild-type EGFR to TKIs. One way to do this is to use GPCR antagonists. The BB_1R antagonist PD168368 increases the potency of gefitinib in NSCLC cells by approximately an order of magnitude. Also, PD168368 inhibits EGFR transactivation caused by addition of NMB to NSCLC cells. It is important to determine if stopping EGFR transactivation will make NSCLC patients with wild-type EGFR more sensitive to TKIs.

In an era of molecular medicine, cancer patient therapy will be dictated by a molecular analysis of the tumor. For NSCLC, approximately 20 percent, 13 percent, 5 percent and 2 percent of the tumors have KRAS, EGFR, ALK and BRAF mutations, respectively. While TKI inhibitors have been developed for the EGFR, ALK and BRAF, an effective therapy for patients with KRAS mutations remains to be elucidated. Cancer deaths in the US have leveled off and with the continued efforts of translational research, the number of cancer survivors should increase dramatically in the next decade.

10.10. ACKNOWLEDGMENTS

The authors thank Drs. R. Jensen, G. Giaccone and D. Wink for helpful discussions. This research is partially supported by the NCI and NIDDK, of NIH.

REFERENCES

1. Jermal A, Siegel R, Xu J, *et al.* (2010) Cancer statistics. *CA Cancer J Clin* **60**(5): 277–300.

2. Lemmon MA, Schlessinger J. (2010) Cell signaling by receptor tyrosine kinases. *Cell* **141**: 1117–1134.
3. Sawyers CL, Druker B. (1999) Tyrosine kinase inhibitors in chronic myeloid leukemia. *Cancer J Sci Am* **5**: 63–69.
4. Blay J-Y, Le Cesna A, Cassier PA, Ray-Coquard IL. (2012) Gastrointestinal stromal tumors (GIST): A rare entity, a tumor model for personalized therapy and ten different molecular subtypes. *Discov Med* **13**(72): 357–367.
5. O'Hare T, Deininger MW, Eide CA, *et al.* (2011) Targeting the BCR-ABL signaling pathway in therapy-resistant Philadelphia chromosome-positive leukemia. *Clin Cancer Res* **17**: 212–221.
6. Sjoblom T, Jones S, Wood LD, *et al.* (2006) The consensus coding sequences of human breast and colorectal cancers. *Science* **314**(5797): 268–274.
7. Schetter AJ, Harris CC. (2012) Tumor suppressor p53 (TP53) at the crossroads of the exposome and the cancer genome. *Proc Natl Acad Sci USA* **109**: 7955–7956.
8. Negrini S, Gorgoulis VG, Halazonetis TD. (2010) Genomic instability — An evolving hallmark of cancer. *Nat Rev Mol Cell Biol* **11**: 220–228.
9. Kaufman J, Horn L, Carbone D. (2011) Molecular biology of lung cancer. In: DeVita Jr. VT, Lawrence TS, Rosenberg SA. *Cancer: Principles and Practice of Oncology*, Lippincott, Williams & Wilkins, Philadelphia, pp. 789–798.
10. Moody TW, Lee M, Kris RM, *et al.* (1990) Lung carcinoid cell lines have bombesin-like peptides and EGF receptors. *J Cell Biochem* **43**: 139–147.
11. Shepherd FA, Rodrigues Pereira J, Ciuleanu T, *et al.* (2005) Erlotinib in previously treated non-small-cell lung cancer. *New Eng J Med* **353**(2): 123–132.
12. Lynch TJ, Bell DW, Sordella R, *et al.* (2004) Activating mutations in the epidermal growth factor receptor underlying responsiveness of non-small-cell lung cancer to gefitinib. *N Engl J Med* **350**(21): 2129–2139.
13. Paez JG, Janne PA, Lee JC, *et al.* (2004) EGFR mutations in lung cancer: Correlation with clinical response to gefitinib therapy. *Science* **304**: 1497–1500.
14. Helfrich BA, Raben D, Varella-Garcia M, *et al.* (2006) Antitumor activity of the epidermal growth factor receptor (EGFR) tyrosine kinase inhibitor gefitinib (ZD1839, Iressa) in non-small cell lung cancer cell lines correlates with gene copy number and EGFR mutations but not EGFR protein levels. *Clin Cancer Res* **12**: 7117–7125.
15. Sharma SV, Bell DW, Settleman J, Haber DA. (2007) Epidermal growth factor receptor mutations in lung cancer. *Nat Rev Cancer* **7**: 169–181.
16. Brabender J, Danenberg KD, Metzger R, *et al.* (2001) Epidermal growth factor receptor and HER2-neu mRNA expression in non-small cell lung cancer is correlated with survival. *Clin Cancer Res* **7**: 1850–1855.

17. Slamon DJ, Godolphin W, Jones LA, *et al.* (1989) Studies of the HER-2/neu proto-oncogene in human breast and ovarian cancer. *Science* **244**(4905): 707–712.
18. Park JW, Stagg R, Lewis GD, *et al.* (1992) Anti-p185HER2 monoclonal antibodies: Biological properties and potential for immunotherapy. *Cancer Treat Res* **61**: 193–211.
19. Kalous O, Conklin D, Desai AJ, *et al.* (2012) Dacomitinib (PF-00299804), an irreversible Pan-HER inhibitor, inhibits proliferation of HER2-amplified breast cancer cell lines resistant to trastuzumab and lapatinib. *Mol Cancer Ther* **11**: 1978–1987.
20. Cantley LC, Carpenter CL, Hahn WC, Meyerson M. (2011) Cell signaling, growth factors and their receptors. In: VT DeVita, Jr., TS Lawrence, SA Rosenberg. *Cancer: Principles and Practice of Oncology*. Lippincott, Williams & Wilkins, Philadelphia, pp. 57–67.
21. McCubrey JA, Steelman LS, Chappell WH, *et al.* (2012) Mutations and deregulation of Ras/Raf/MEK/ERK and PI3K/PTEN/Akt/mTOR cascades which alter therapy response. *Oncotarget* **3**: 954–987.
22. Davies H, Begnell GR, Cox C, *et al.* (2002) Mutations of the BRAF gene in human cancer. *Nature* **417**: 949–954.
23. Kim DH, Sim T. (2012) Novel small molecule Raf Kinase Inhibitors for targeted cancer therapeutics. *Arch Pharm Res* **35**(4): 605–615.
24. Hoeflich KP, Herter S, Tien J, *et al.* (2009) Antitumor efficacy of the novel RAF inhibitor GDC-0879 is predicted by BRAFV600E mutational status and sustained extracellular signal-regulated kinase/mitogen-activated protein kinase pathway suppression. *Cancer Res* **69**: 3042–3051.
25. Kim KB, Kefford R, Pavlick AC, *et al.* (2013) Phase II study of the MEK1/MEK2 inhibitor trametinib in patients with metastatic BRAF-mutant cutaneous melanoma previously treated with or without a BRAF inhibitor. *J Clin Oncol* **31**(4): 482–489.
26. Janne PA, Shaw AR, Oereira JR, *et al.* (2013) Selumctinib plus docetaxel for KRAS-mutant advanced non-small cell lung cancer: A randomized, multicentre, placebo-controlled, phase 2 study. *Lancet Oncol* **14**(1): 38–47.
27. Hafsi S, Pezzino FM, Candido S, *et al.* (2012) Gene alterations in the PI3K/PTEN/Akt pathway as a mechanism of drug resistance. *Int J Oncol* **40**: 639–644.
28. Carpten JD, Faber AL, Horn C, *et al.* (2007) A transforming mutation in the plckstin homology domain of Akt1 in cancer. *Nature* **448**: 439–444.
29. Prasad G, Sottero T, Yang X, *et al.* (2011) Inhibition of PI3K/mTOR pathways in glioblastoma and implications for combination therapy with temozolomide. *Neuro Oncol* **13**(4): 384–392.

30. Rhei E, Kang L, Bogomolniy F, *et al.* (1997) Mutation analysis of the putative tumor suppressor gene PTEN/MMAC1 in primary breast cancer. *Cancer Res* 57: 3657–3659.
31. Witta SE, Gemmill RM, Hirsch FR, *et al.* (2006) Restoring E-cadherin expression increases sensitivity to epidermal growth factor receptor inhibitors in lung cancer cell lines. *Cancer Res* **66**: 944–949.
32. Herbst RS, Heymach JV, Lippman SM (2008) Lung cancer. *N Eng J Med* **359**: 1367–1380.
33. Gazdar A. (2009) Personalized medicine and inhibition of EGFR signaling in lung cancer. *N Eng J Med* **361**: 1018–1020.
34. Carter CA, Giaccone G. (2012). Treatment of non-small cell lung cancer: Overcoming resistance to epidermal growth factor receptor inhibitors. *Curr Opin Oncol* **24**(2): 123–129.
35. Sequist LV, Martins RG, Spigel D, *et al.* (2008) First-line gefitinib in patients with advanced non-small cell lung cancer harboring somatic EGFR mutations. *J Clin Oncol* **26**: 2442–2449.
36. Jackman DM, Yeap BY, Sequist LV, *et al.* (2006) Exon 19 deletion mutations of epidermal growth factor receptor are associated with prolonged survival in non-small cell lung cancer patients treated with gefitinib or erlotinib. *Clin Cancer Res* **12**: 3908–3914.
37. Van Zandwick N, Mathy A, Boerrigter L, *et al.* (2007)EGFR and KRAS mutations as criteria for treatment with tyrosine kinase inhibitors: Retro- and prospective observations in non-small cell lung cancer. *Ann Oncol* **18**: 99–103.
38. Inoue A, Suzuki T, Fukuhara T, *et al.* (2006) Prospective phase II study of gefitinib for chemotherapy-naive patients with advanced non-small cell lung cancer with epidermal growth factor receptor gene mutations. *J Clin Oncol* **24**: 3340–3346.
39. Asahina H, Yamazaki K, Kinoshita I, *et al.* (2006) A phase II trial of gefitinib as first-line therapy for advanced non-small cell lung cancer with epidermal growth factor receptor mutations. *Br J Cancer* **95**: 998–1004.
40. Engelman JA, Zejnullahu K, Gale CM, *et al.* (2007) PF00299804, an irreversible pan-ERBB inhibitor, is effective in lung cancer models with EGFR and ERBB2 mutations that are resistant to gefitinib. *Cancer Res* **67**: 11924–11932.
41. Ohashi K, Sequisty LV, Arcila ME, *et al.* (2012) Lung cancers with acquired resistance to EGFR inhibitors occasionally harbor BRAF gene mutations but lack mutations in KRAS, NRAS, or MEK1. *Proc Natl Acad Sci USA* **109**(31): E2127–E2133.
42. Sen B, Peng S, Tang X, *et al.* (2012) Kinase-impaired BRAF mutations in lung cancer confer sensitivity to dasatinib. *Sci Trans Med* **4**: 136.

43. Peters S, Adjei AA. (2012) MET: A promising anticancer therapeutic target. *Nat Rev Clin Oncol* **9**: 314–326.
44. Engelman JA, Zejnullahu K, Mitsudomi R, *et al.* (2007) MET amplification leads to gefitinib resistance in lung cancer by activating ERBB3 signaling. *Science* **316**: 1039–1043.
45. Soda M, Choi YL, Enomoto M, *et al.* (2007) Identification of the transforming EML4-ALK fusion gene in non-small-cell lung cancer. *Nature* **448**(153): 561–566.
46. Ou S-HI, Huang Bartlett C, Mino-Kenudson M, *et al.* (2012) Crizotinib for the treatment of ALK-rearranged non-small cell lung cancer: A success story to usher in the second decade of molecular targeted therapy in oncology. *Oncologist* **17**: 1351–1375.
47. Kwak EL, Bang YJ, Camidge DR, *et al.* (2010) Anaplastic lymphoma kinase inhibition in non-small-cell lung cancer. *New Eng J Med* **363**: 1693–1703.
48. Ding L, Getz G, Wheeler DA, *et al.* (2008) Somatic mutations affect key pathways in lung adenocarcinoma. *Nature* **455**: 1069–1075.
49. Kris MG, Natale RB, Herbst RS, *et al.* (2003) Efficacy of gefitinib, an inhibitor of the epidermal growth factor receptor tyrosine kinase, in symptomatic patients with non-small cell lung cancer: A randomized trial. *J Am Med Assoc* **290**(16): 2149–2158.
50. Fukuoka M, Yano S, Giaccone G, *et al.* (2003) Multi-institutional randomized phase II trial of gefitinib for previously treated patients with advanced non-small-cell lung cancer. *J Clin Oncol* **21**(12): 2237–2246.
51. Giaccone G, Herbst RS, Manegold C, *et al.* (2004) Gefitinib in combination with gemcitabine and cisplatin in advanced non-small-cell lung cancer: A phase III trial — INTACT 1. *J Clin Oncol* **22**(5): 777–784.
52. Herbst RS, Giaccone G, Schiller JH, *et al.* (2004) Gefitinib in combination with paclitaxel and carboplatin in advanced non-small-cell lung cancer. *J Clin Oncol* **22**(5): 785–794.
53. Moemondo M, Inoue A, Kobayashi K, *et al.* (2010) Gefitinib or chemotherapy for non-small cell lung cancer with mutated EGFR. *N Engl J Med* **362**(25): 2380–2388.
54. Thomas A, Rajan A, Giaccone G. (2012) Tyrosine kinase inhibitors in lung cancer. *Hematol Oncol Clin N Am* **26**: 589–605.
55. Sequist LV, Lynch TJ. (2008) Epidermal growth factor receptor tyrosine kinase inhibitors in lung cancer. An evolving story. *Ann Rev Med* **59**: 429–442.
56. Boyer MJ, Blackhall GH, Park K, *et al.* (2010) Efficacy and safety of PF299804 versus erlotinib (D): A global randomized phase II trial in patients with advanced non-small cell lung cancer (NSCLC) after failure of chemotherapy. *J Clin Oncol* **28**: 18s.

57. Schiller JH, von Powell J, Garmey EG, *et al.* (2011) Randomized phase II study of erlotinib plus tivavtinib versus erlotinib plus placebo in previously treated non-small cell lung cancer. *J Clin Oncol* **29**: 3307–3315.
58. Shaw AT, Yeap BY, Solomon BJ, *et al.* (2011) Effect of crizotinib on overall survival in patients with advanced non-small cell lung cancer harbouring ALK gene rearrangement: A retrospective analysis. *Lancet Oncol* **12**(11): 1004–1012.
59. Voena C, Chiarle R. (2012)The battle against ALK resistance: Successes and setbacks. *Expert Opin Investig Drugs* **21**(12): 1751–1754.
60. Moody TW, Pert CB, Gazdar AF, *et al.* (1981) High levels of intracellular bombesin characterize human small-cell lung carcinoma. *Science* **214**: 1246–1248.
61. Korman LY, Carney DN, Citron ML, Moody TW. (1986) Secretin/VIP stimulated secretion of bombesin-like peptides from human small cell lung cancer. *Cancer Res* **46**: 1214–1218.
62. Cuttitta F, Carney DN, Mulshine J, *et al.* (1985) Bombesin-like peptides can function as autocrine growth factors in human small-cell lung cancer cells. *Nature* **316**(6031): 823–826.
63. Kelley MJ, Linnoila RI, Avis I, *et al.* (1997) Antitumor activity of monoclonal antibody directed against gastrin-releasing peptide in patients with small cell lung cancer. *Chest* **112**(1): 256–261.
64. Jensen RT, Moody TW. (2013) Bombesin peptides. In: Kastin A (ed.), *Handbook of Biologically Active Peptides*. Elsevier, Amsterdam, pp. 506–511.
65. Battey JF, Way JM, Corjay MH, *et al.* (1991) Molecular cloning of the bombesin/gastrin-releasing peptide receptor from Swiss 3T3 cells. *Proc Natl Acad Sci USA* **88**: 395–399.
66. Mahmoud S, Staley J, Taylor J, *et al.* (1991)(Psi^{13,14}) Bombesin analogues inhibit the growth of small cell lung cancer *in vitro* and *in vivo*. *Cancer Res* **51**: 1798–1802.
67. Giaccone G, Battey J, Gazdar AF, *et al.* (1992) Neuromedin B is present in lung cancer cell lines. *Cancer Res* **52**: 2732–2736s.
68. Wada E, Way J, Shapira H, *et al.* (1991) cDNA cloning, characterization and brain region-specific expression of a neuromedin-B preferring bombesin receptor. *Neuron* **6**: 421–430.
69. Moody TW, Staley J, Zia F, *et al.* (1992) Neuromedin B binds with high affinity, elevates cytosolic calcium and stimulates the growth of small-cell lung cancer cell lines. *J Pharm Exp Ther* **263**: 311–317.
70. Reubi JC, Wenger S, Schumuckli-Maurer J, *et al.* (2002) Bombesin receptor subtypes in human cancers: Detection with the universal radoligand (125)I-[D-TYR(6), beta-ALA(11), PHE(13), NLE(14)] bombesin(6-14). *Clin Cancer Res* **8**(4): 1139–1146.

71. Fathi Z, Corjay MH, Shapira H, *et al.* (1993) BRS-3: A novel bombesin receptor subtype selectively expressed in testis and lung carcinoma cells. *J Biol Chem* **268**(8): 5979–5984.
72. Moody TW, Sancho V, Di Florio A, *et al.* (2011) Bombesin-receptor subtype-3 agonists stimulate the growth of lung cancer cells and increase EGF receptor tyrosine phosphorylation. *Peptides* **32**(8): 1677–1684.
73. Moody TW, Jensen RT. (2013) VIP/PACAP receptors. In: Kastin A (ed), *Handbook of Biologically Active Peptides.* Elsevier, Amsterdam, pp. 556–561.
74. Casibang M, Purdom S, Zia F, *et al.* (2001) Prostaglandin E_2 increases vascular endothelial cell growth factor mRNAS in lung cancer cells. *Lung Cancer* **31**: 203–212.
75. Hida T, Makheja A, Ben-Av P, *et al.* (1998) Aspirin and indomethacin inhibit prostaglandin E_2 production and the growth of non-small cell lung cancer cells. *Anticancer Res* **18**: 775–782.
76. Moody TW, Switzer C, Santana-Flores W, *et al.* (2010) Dithiolethione modified valproate and diclofenac increase E-cadherin expression and decrease proliferation of non-small cell lung cancer cells. *Lung Cancer* **68**(2): 154–160.
77. Casibang M, Moody TW. (2002) AH6809 antagonizes non-small cell lung cancer prostaglandin receptors. *Lung Cancer* **35**: 33–42.
78. Zhang Q, Thomas SM, Smithgall TE, *et al.* (2004) SRC family kinases mediate epidermal growth factor receptor ligand cleavage, proliferation, and invasion of head and neck cancer cells. *Cancer Res* **64**(17): 6166–6173.
79. Lui VW, Thomas SM, Zhang Q, *et al.* (2003) Mitogenic effects of gastrin-releasing peptide in head and neck squamous cancer cells are mediated by activation of the epidermal growth factor receptor. *Oncogene* **22**(40): 6183–6193.
80. Zhang Q, Bhola NE, Lui VW, *et al.* (2007) Antitumor mechanisms of combined gastrin-releasing peptide receptor and epidermal growth factor receptor targeting in head and neck cancer. *Mol Cancer Ther* **6**(4): 1414–1424.
81. Moody TW, Berna MJ, Mantey S, *et al.* (2010) Inhibition of Neuromedin B mediated transactivation of EGF receptors in lung cancer cells enhances gefitinib sensitivity. *Eur J Pharmacol* **637**: 38–45.

CHAPTER 11

Childhood and Adolescent B-Cell Lymphoma: Bench to Bedside and Back to Bench

Rodney Miles[*], *Paul Galardy*[†], *Lisa G. Giulino-Roth*[‡], *Stanton Goldman*[§] and *Mitchell S. Cairo*[||,¶]

11.1. INTRODUCTION

Mature pediatric B-cell non-Hodgkin lymphoma (B-NHL) represents 60 percent of all childhood and adolescent NHL. Over the past two decades, there has been a significant improvement of our understanding of the mechanism(s) responsible for pediatric mature B-NHL lymphomagenesis. Expression of surface targets and alterations of specific signaling pathways provide a large host of opportunities of translational research in

[*]Department of Pathology, University of Utah, Salt Lake City, Utah, USA
[†]Department of Pediatric Hematology/Oncology, Mayo Clinic, Rochester, Minnesota, USA
[‡]Department of Pediatric Hematology/Oncology, Weill Cornell Medical College, New York, USA
[§]Division of Pediatric Hematology/Oncology, Medical City Children's Hospital, Dallas, Texas, USA
[||]Departments of Pediatrics, Medicine, Pathology, Microbiology and Immunology and Cell Biology and Anatomy, New York Medical College, Valhalla, New York, USA
[¶]Corresponding author: Mitchell S. Cairo, MD, Chief, Pediatric Hematology, Oncology & Stem Cell Transplantation; Director, Children's and Adolescent Cancer and Blood Diseases Center; Medical and Scientific Director, Cellular and Tissue Engineering Clinical Laboratory; Associate Chairman, Department of Pediatrics; Professor of Pediatrics, Medicine, Pathology, Microbiology & Immunology and Cell Biology & Anatomy, Maria Fareri Children's Hospital at Westchester Medical Center; New York Medical College, Munger Pavilion Room 110A, Valhalla, New York, 10595, USA; E-mail: *mitchell_cairo@nymc.edu*; Tel: +1-914-594-3650; Fax: +1-914-594-3803

pediatric mature B-NHL. In the following chapter, we provide evidence of translational observations of this human cancer that have gone from the bedside to the bench and from the bench back to the bedside. While some investigations have been "lost in translation," progress to date suggests that significant paradigm shifts in clinical research in this disease have benefited significantly from translational investigations.

11.2. EPIDEMIOLOGY OF PEDIATRIC MATURE B-NHL

Burkitt lymphoma (BL) can be divided into three clinical subtypes: endemic, sporadic and immunodeficiency associated. The endemic form has a high incidence in equatorial Africa, where it is the most common childhood cancer. The incidence of BL peaks between ages 4 and 7 years with an increased prevalence among males. Nearly all cases of this endemic form are Epstein Barr virus (EBV) seropositive.[1] The sporadic form of BL occurs primarily in children as well and maintains a predilection among males. The incidence in the US is around 0.6 per 100,000 per year among males and 0.2 per 100,000 among females, ages 0 to 30 years. The classical sporadic presentation is associated with an abdominal mass, typically in the ileocecal region; however, lymph node, gonadal and other organ involvement can be present at presentation. Most commonly, the sporadic form is associated with spread to the bone marrow and/or central nervous system (CNS) at diagnosis. In addition, approximately 30 percent of these cases are EBV positive.[1] Immunodeficiency associated BL occurs in patients with primary or secondary immunodeficiency, especially human immunodeficiency virus (HIV)/acquired immunodeficiency syndrome (AIDS).

Overall, BL has a trimodal incidence pattern across age with peaks near ages 10, 40 and 75 years among males. In the past few decades, an increase in the incidence of BL has been described. This has been attributed to the increasing elderly population, secondary malignancy, and HIV-associated lymphoma.

11.3. HISTOPATHOLOGY OF PEDIATRIC MATURE B-NHL

BL is a malignancy of mature B cells of uniform, intermediate size arranged in diffuse sheets. From lower power, one can appreciate the scattered

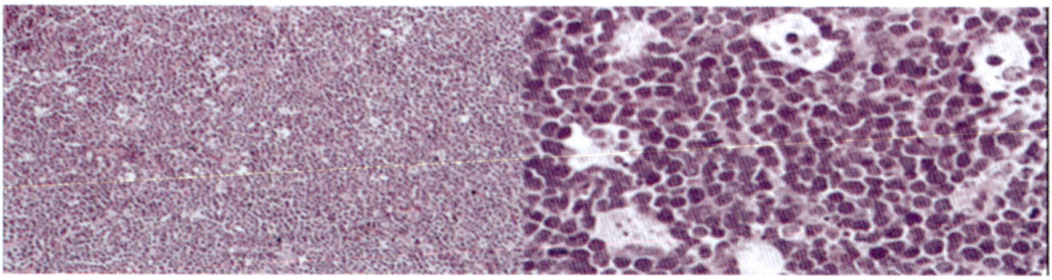

(A) (B)

Fig. 1. Morphology and immunophenotype of BL. (A, B) Hematoxylin & Eosin (H&E); original magnification 200× for A, 1000× for B.

tingible body macrophages that impart the characteristic "starry sky" appearance (Fig. 1A). On higher power examination, the cells demonstrate predominantly round nuclei with finely clumped chromatin and often multiple small, basophilic nucleoli (Fig. 1B). The cytoplasm is scant, basophilic, and demonstrates lipid vacuoles that are best appreciated on touch preparations or aspirate smears. The proliferation rate is extremely high with numerous mitotic figures and apoptotic bodies. The latter, when engulfed by macrophages, represent the "tingible bodies." With the rapid proliferation and tumor growth, areas of necrosis are often present.

Occasional BL cases demonstrate increased nuclear pleomorphism and more prominent nucleoli. Although these have previously been designated atypical BL, gene expression profiling studies[2,3] have demonstrated that they are otherwise similar and thus these cases are now considered part of the morphologic spectrum of BL (see Sec. 11.7).

11.4. DIFFERENTIAL DIAGNOSIS OF PEDIATRIC MATURE B-NHL

The two other entities that are usually considered when making a diagnosis of BL are B lymphoblastic leukemia/lymphoma and diffuse large B-cell lymphoma (DLBCL). Distinction of BL from lymphoblastic leukemia/lymphoma is important, as the treatments differ. Although B lymphoblastic leukemia/lymphoma can morphologically resemble BL with a diffuse proliferation of lymphoid cells and a starry sky background, the former usually demonstrates finer chromatin and less cytoplasm. By immunophenotyping, B lymphoblastic leukemia/lymphoma is usually CD20 negative, TdT positive, and lacks surface light chain expression by flow cytometry with dim to negative CD45 expression. However, rare cases of B lymphoblastic leukemia/lymphoma demonstrate mature features such as surface light chains and CD20 expression. In these cases, cytogenetic analysis including karyotype and fluorescence *in situ* hybridization (FISH) for *MYC* rearrangement may be useful to make a definitive distinction from BL.

In contrast to BL, DLBCL typically shows larger cell size with increased cytoplasm, significantly greater nuclear pleomorphism, and immunophenotypic features such as a lower Ki-67 proliferation index or strong BCL2 staining. However, the distinction becomes more difficult in DLBCL cases that show less pleomorphism and a higher proliferation rate that can approach 100 percent. In these cases, identification of an *MYC*-immunoglobulin translocation would favor BL, while either a *BCL2* or *BCL6* translocation (without an *MYC* translocation) would indicate DLBCL. Some of these cases will be impossible to definitively classify as either BL or DLBCL and thus fall into the new category in the 2008 World Health Organization classification "B-cell lymphoma, unclassifiable, with features intermediate between DLBCL and BL" (indeterminate B-cell lymphoma, IBL).[4] Many of these cases demonstrate a "double hit" with translocations of *MYC* and *BCL2* or, less commonly, *BCL6* in adult patients, but such double-hit lymphomas are distinctly uncommon in children.

11.5. RECURRENT GENETIC ABNORMALITIES IN PEDIATRIC MATURE B-NHL

The primary genetic abnormality in BL is the translocation of *MYC* at 8q24.21 with an immunoglobulin gene locus that brings *MYC* under the control of an immunoglobulin gene enhancer driving high expression. In most cases, *MYC* is partnered with the immunoglobulin heavy chain locus (*IGH@*, 14q32.33), but occasional cases show *MYC* translocations with the light chain genes for kappa (*IGK@*, 2p11.2) and lambda (*IGL@*, 22q11.2). Although the *MYC-IG* translocation is often the only abnormality identified by conventional cytogenetics, additional recurrent secondary chromosomal abnormalities have been recognized with chromosomes 1, 6, 13, 17 and 22 most commonly involved.[5,6] In a large cytogenetic study performed on an international trial in children and adolescents, the main BL-associated chromosomal aberrations were +1q (29 percent), +7q (14 percent) and del(13q) (14 percent).[7] Gain of the long arm of chromosome 1 was due to dup(1q) in 66 percent of cases, while alterations of chromosome 13q were very heterogeneous. The majority (33 of 38) resulted in 13q deletions either isolated or due to various unbalanced translocations without obvious recurrent break points. The most commonly deleted band was 13q34 (82 percent). From a translational perspective from bedside to bench, +7q and del(13q) were independently associated with a significant inferior event-free survival (EFS) [hazard ratio: 2.5 ($p = 0.015$) and 4.0 ($p = 0.0003$), respectively; Fig. 2],[7] which agrees with prior reports suggesting a worse outcome associated with 13q abnormalities.[5,6] Subsequently, Nelson *et al.* utilized FISH to show a worse overall survival in patients with any 13q deletion.[8]

More recently, higher resolution single nucleotide polymorphism (SNP) array assays have been used to characterize copy number variations in BL genomes. Through the use of multiple small probes that target regions distributed across the entire genome, these assays are able to detect

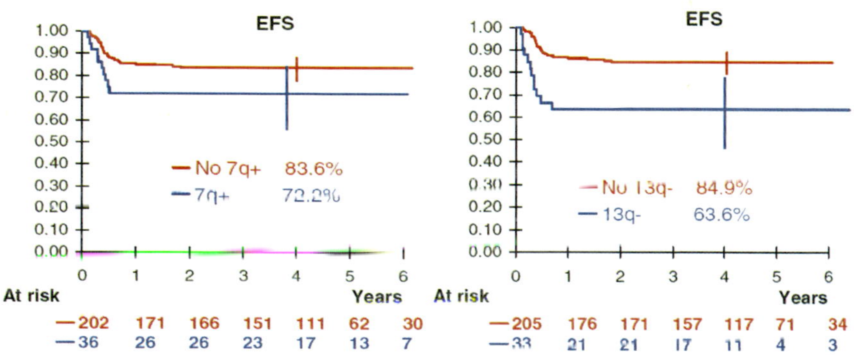

(A) (B)

Fig. 2. The presence of a (A) 7q+ or (B) 13q secondary chromosomal aberration is associated with worse event-free survival in children with B-cell NHL. Reprinted with permission from Ref. 7.

small copy number alterations affecting a few or possibly even a single gene and thus have much higher resolution than conventional cytogenetics. A high-resolution SNP analysis of 39 frozen BL samples found a total of 308 gains and 220 losses,[9] and high resolution gene copy number analysis of formalin-fixed, paraffin embedded pediatric BL samples identified 32 gains and 30 copy number losses with at least one gain or loss in 64 percent of samples.[10] Similar to the conventional cytogenetic findings described earlier, changes on chromosome 1q, 13q and 17p were commonly identified. Scholtysik *et al.* reported gains on 1q localized to minimum common regions (MCRs) at 1q21.1 (26 percent) and 1q31.3 (33 percent).[9] Gain of 13q31 was present in 18 percent, and 17p13.1 showed a copy loss in 18 percent. The results from the study using formalin-fixed samples are very similar, with gain of 1q in 25 percent, gain of 13q in 11 percent, and loss of 17p in 14 percent. Additional recurrent losses identified in both studies included 13q33.1-q34 and Xp22.33.

The recurrent gains on chromosome 13q31 typically include the *MIR-17-92* microRNA cluster, which is oncogenic and accelerates lymphoma development in the mouse E(μ)-*MYC* lymphoma model.[11] *MIR-17-92* inhibits apoptotic pathways downstream of MYC,[12] which suggests a potential pathogenetic role for these microRNAs in BL by suppressing MYC-induced apoptosis and thus shifting the balance towards proliferation. More studies will be required to understand the clinical and pathogenetic significance of this and other recently characterized recurrent copy number changes in BL, which hold potential as prognostic markers and possible therapeutic targets.

The increasing recognition of secondary genetic abnormalities in BL, and especially the association of some of these genetic changes with prognosis, has significant implications for the near future for the translational approach to BL. The fact that BL is not an entirely homogenous disease has already been indicated by the fact that a subset of patients will fail to respond or relapse to conventional therapy while most are cured. The ability to further subdivide BL by recognizing recurrent genetic changes associated with a particularly aggressive subset of the disease will allow more accurate identification of these highest risk patients in future clinical trials. Assays such as FISH for genomic changes associated with poor outcomes can be incorporated into diagnostic work-ups so that high-risk patients can be identified at the time of diagnosis. This would allow these patients to receive alternative, experimental therapies to potentially improve their outcomes without modifying treatment strategies for those patients expected to respond very well to conventional therapies. Finally, recurrent genomic changes reveal aberrant signaling pathways such as microRNA over expression that shed light on the pathogenesis of BL and may represent potential therapeutic targets in the future.

11.6. MINIMAL DISEASE DETECTION TO PREDICT RELAPSE IN PEDIATRIC MATURE B-NHL

Although survival rates are high with current therapies, relapse remains a significant problem and accurate identification of patients at risk for relapse is an active area of investigation. Patients with minimal disease (MD) present after therapy would be predicted to have a higher risk for recurrent disease, so MD detection represents a potential approach to identify high-risk patients. A recent pilot study utilized a polymerase chain reaction (PCR) assay to detect MD based on the *IGH@* variable region gene family (IGHV) usage of the B-cell neoplasm.[13] Diagnostic specimens were all positive when screened by PCR with IGHV primer pools, and then the specific IGHV region involved was identified. The initial specimens included tumor tissue but also blood or bone marrow, which still yielded positive results despite being morphologically negative in most cases. Follow-up specimens were screened with the specific IGHV primer set corresponding to the diagnostic specimen to identify MD. Of the 32 patients with diagnostic specimens available for analysis, MD was detected in seven at the end of induction while 25 were negative. One of these seven patients developed recurrent disease at four months. Of the 25 patients that were MD negative at the end of induction, seven were assayed at the end of therapy; one was positive and developed recurrent disease at 36 months. Although the numbers are small, the findings suggest that MD detection can predict recurrence.

Another approach for MD detection is long distance PCR for t(8;14)(q24;q32), the most common translocation in BL. When performed on bone marrow samples from newly diagnosed pediatric BL patients, the translocation was detected in 26/84 patients (31 percent), which was higher than the rate of morphologic detection (18 percent).[14] Furthermore, a positive result was associated with a lower rate of three-year progression-free survival (68 percent versus 93 percent, $p = 0.03$) and, by multivariate analysis, was the only significant negative prognostic factor in children with high-risk BL. Thus, MD detection can have a role in the prognostic stratification and therapeutic strategy of BL patients, but this will require further investigation in the context of prospective clinical trials for validation.

11.7. BURKITT LYMPHOMA GENOMICS AND TRANSLATIONAL OPPORTUNITIES

The hallmark of BL is the cytogenetic translocation of the MYC proto-oncogene to either the immunoglobulin heavy or light chains. This puts MYC under the regulatory control of the immunoglobulin locus resulting in aberrant MYC expression with effects on cellular growth, proliferation, metabolism and apoptosis. Despite these global cellular changes, MYC translocation alone is insufficient for the development of BL.[15] BL tumors are known to harbor additional cytogenetic and molecular alterations that likely contribute to malignant transformation. Pediatric BL cases in particular frequently demonstrate a complex karyotype with multiple abnormalities in addition to the MYC-IgH translocation.[5,6,16,17] Until recently, however, the consequences of these molecular abnormalities were not well characterized. Advances in microarray and sequencing technology have provided significant insight into the molecular biology of BL, allowing for more precise tumor characterization. Importantly, many of the newly identified molecular alterations are potentially targetable by drugs that are currently in use or are in clinical development. This allows for direct translation of genomic information to the development of novel therapy.

Gene expression profiling defined a unique molecular signature for Burkitt lymphoma in two landmark studies by Hummel *et al.* and Dave *et al.*[2,3] The distinction between BL and DLBCL is not always clear based on morphology, immunophenotype and standard molecular diagnostics. As a result, the World Health Organization has designated a category for cases intermediate between BL and DLBCL.[18] Differentiating the two tumors is particularly relevant in adults where patients with DLBCL receive CHOP (cyclophosphamide, hydroxyl doxorubicin, Oncovin®, prednisone)-based chemotherapy regimens and patients with BL receive more intensive treatment, similar to that used in pediatric BL and DLBCL. Both studies defined a molecular BL signature that included up-regulation of MYC target genes and germinal center B-cell genes as well down-regulation of NF-κB-associated genes (Fig. 3). Both studies also identified a subset of cases that had been diagnosed pathologically as DLBCL but molecularly resembled BL. The outcome for patients with molecular BL (mBL) who were treated with less intense DLBCL regimens

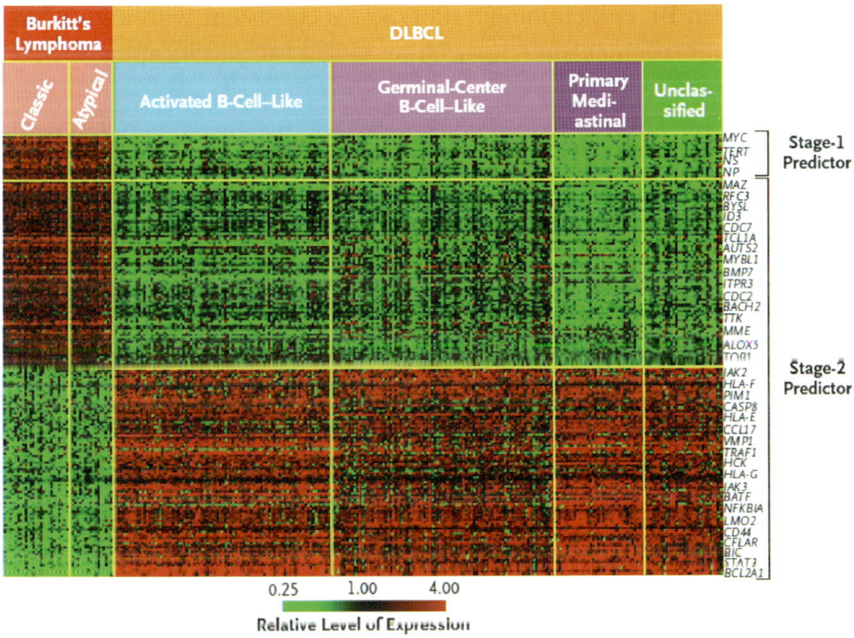

Fig. 3. A molecular classifier of Burkitt lymphoma. The difference in gene expression between Burkitt's lymphoma and diffuse large-B-cell lymphoma (DLBCL) derived from DNA-microarray analysis is shown. The relative levels of gene expression are depicted according to the color scale shown. The genes analyzed in stage 1 of constructing the classifier include c-MYC and its target genes. The 196 genes analyzed in stage 2 include additional genes that distinguish Burkitt's lymphoma from the three subgroups of DLBCL. Only specimens for which the diagnoses based on the pathology review and molecular analysis of gene expression agreed are shown. Reprinted with permission from Ref. 2.

was significantly inferior compared with patients with mBL treated with BL regimens, highlighting the importance of accurate diagnosis and future translational therapeutic strategies.[2]

These initial BL microarray studies were performed on sporadic BL. This work was complemented by a study by Piccaluga *et al.*, who performed gene expression profiling on the sporadic, endemic and HIV-associated forms of BL to evaluate differences among epidemiologic subtypes.[19] Despite relative homogeneity among the sporadic BL, endemic BL and HIV-BL, slight differences were observed, notably in genes relevant in proliferation, cell cycle, transcription, and nucleic acid metabolism. Endemic and HIV-associated BL clustered together, distinct from the sporadic cases and independent of EBV status. This work, indicating molecular differences between BL epidemiologic subtypes, is consistent with known differences in disease incidence, association with EBV, and location of MYC breakpoints.

As the previously described studies did not distinguish between pediatric and adult BL, there have been efforts to understand the molecular distinctions between these clinically different groups. Two studies by Klapper *et al.* and Deffenbacher *et al.* evaluated the gene expression profile of pediatric B-cell non-Hodgkin lymphoma (NHL).[20,21] Both found that, compared with adult cases, the incidence of reclassification of diagnosis based on molecular signature was increased in pediatric tumors. Fifteen to 31 percent of pediatric tumors were reclassified based on molecular signature, compared with 2.7 percent in adult cases. The impact of B-NHL classification on therapy-related decisions, however, is less relevant in pediatrics, where both BL and DLBCL are treated on the same treatment protocols. The importance of this aggressive approach in pediatric DLBCL was confirmed in the Deffenbacher study, where outcome in patients age 15–20 with DLBCL treated with adult CHOP-based regimens was significantly inferior to those treated on pediatric protocols. Differences between pediatric and adult BL based on gene expression signature were also evaluated. The gene signatures of pediatric and adult BL were relatively homogenous, but there were some differentially expressed genes, with pediatric cases being more highly enriched in MYC targets.

While BL tumors are known to frequently harbor alterations in MYC and p53, until recently little was known about additional alterations that may cooperate with MYC to result in tumorigenesis. Advances in sequencing technology have provided an unprecedented opportunity to study the BL genome. Next-generation sequencing allows for high-throughput parallel mass sequencing of tumor specimens, with the potential to identify previously unrecognized oncogenic alterations, as well as targets for novel therapy. As a result, there have been a series of reports utilizing high-throughput sequencing to study BL tumors that have elucidated the catalog of genomic alterations in BL and identified novel mechanisms of tumorigenesis (Table 1).[22–25]

Table 1 Summary of Studies Evaluating BL Using Next-Generation Sequencing

	Schmitz *et al.*[25]	Love *et al.*[23]	Richter *et al.*[24]	Giulino-Roth *et al.*[22]
Sample Source and Size	Primary cases ($n=28$) Cell lines ($n=13$)	Primary cases ($n=51$) Cell lines ($n=8$)	Primary cases ($n=4$)	Primary cases ($n=29$)
BL Subtype in Test Cohort	sBL (eBL, HIV-BL in validation cohort)	sBL	sBL	sBL, eBL, HIV-BL
Age Cohort	Peds + adult	Peds + adult	Peds	Peds
Sequencing Method	RNA-Seq	Whole genome, whole exome	Whole genome, whole exome, RNA-seq	Targeted genomic seq
Primary Findings	ID3/TCF3 alterations in 70% of sBL CCND3 alterations in 38% of sBL, 67% HIV-BL	ID3 mutations in 34% Other frequent alterations: GNA13, RET, PIK3R1, ARId1A, SMARCA4	ID3 mutations in 68% Recurrent alterations in SMARCA4, DDX3x	ARID1A mutations in 17% MCL1 alterations in 22% EBV(−) cases have increased total number of mutations

These studies have utilized whole genome sequencing, whole exome sequencing, transcriptome sequencing, or a combination of these approaches to investigate the BL genome. While there has been heterogeneity in mutations among individual cases as well as differences in findings among the various reports, some common alterations have been found across studies.

One finding documented in almost all studies is recurrent somatic alterations in the inhibitor of DNA binding 3 (ID3). The protein encoded by this gene contains a helix-loop-helix (HLH) motif, which allows it to bind other proteins with HLH domains, resulting in inhibition. Functionally, ID3 is thought to be important in a variety of cellular processes including cell cycle progression and B-cell differentiation. Mutations in ID3 have been identified in 34–68 percent of primary BL tumors.[23–25] Interestingly, these alterations seem to be unique to BL, as they have not been documented in other B-cell lymphomas, including those with MYC translocation. The mutations in ID3 are biallelic in the majority of cases and are associated with a predicted loss of function. Functional studies of ID3 have implicated it as a tumor suppressor. Alterations have also been documented in the ID3 target, TCF3. In contrast to ID3 mutations, the alterations in TCF3 are monoallelic and may be activating. Mutations in either ID3 or TCF3 are predicted to result in TCF3 up-regulation. In a cohort described by Schmitz *et al.*, mutations in ID3 or TCF3 were found in 70 percent of sporadic BL.[25]

In the report by Schmitz *et al.*, extensive functional studies were performed to evaluate the consequences of alterations in ID3 and TCF3. Gene expression profiling identified TCF3 target genes, which included genes crucial for germinal center (GC) B-cell function as well as genes relevant in cell cycle progression. Importantly, they also identified up-regulation of the immunoglobulin heavy and light chains, components of B-cell receptor (BCR) in TCF3 altered cells. They found BL cells to be dependent on TCF3 due to its role in BCR signaling through the AKT/PI3 kinase (PI3K) pathway[25] (Fig. 4). The importance of PI3K in BL was confirmed in an independent study led by Klaus Rajewsky, where genetically modified mice were engineered expressing dysregulated MYC and constitutively active PI3K restricted to GC B cells.[26] These mice developed tumors that not only resembled BL by histology and immunophenotype, but also developed

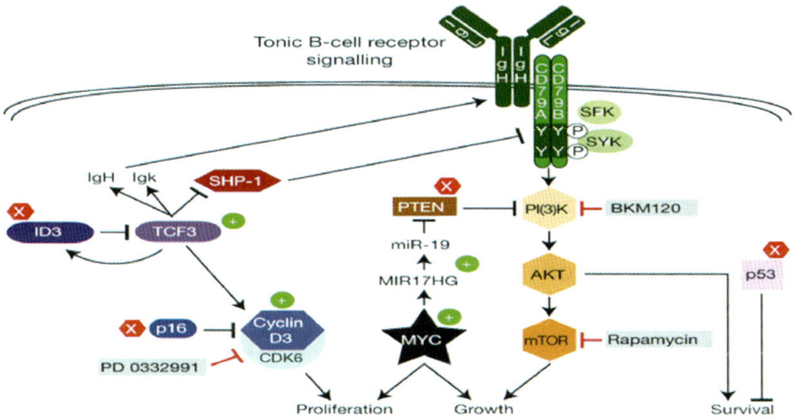

Fig. 4. Schematic of recurrent oncogenic pathways in Burkitt's lymphoma. Gain-of-function and loss-of-function aberrations are indicated by "+" signs and by "×" signs, respectively. Gray boxes indicate drugs that block these deregulated pathways. Reprinted by permission from Ref. 25.

secondary alterations known to be present in BL. These findings implicating the dependence of BL cells on PI3K signaling have direct translational implications. Inhibitors of the PI3K pathway are currently in development and may represent novel treatment approaches for the significant portion of BL patients with PI3K pathway alterations.

In addition to alterations in ID3/TCF3, next-generation sequencing has identified other novel alterations that may contribute to tumorigenesis. Alterations in chromatin remodeling genes were described in multiple cohorts. Mutations in the SWI/SNF family of genes, including ARID1A and SMARCA4, were present in 17–43 percent of samples.[22–25] ARID1A mutations were truncating and resulted in decreased protein expression, implicating this as a tumor suppressor gene. These alterations may also translate to novel therapies. Chromatin modifications are potentially reversible through a variety of agents in development. Mutations in CCND3 were identified in 38 percent of cases in one cohort (Schmitz *et al.*), but the incidence was lower in other cohorts. Differences among epidemiologic subtypes of BL have also been observed. For example, ID3/TCF3 mutations were found in 70 percent of sporadic cases and 67 percent of HIV-associated cases, but only 40 percent of endemic cases.[25] The presence of EBV, an oncogenic herpesvirus, in endemic BL samples may explain the decrease in rate of mutations. BL tumors associated with EBV have a significant decrease in the total number of alterations as compared to EBV negative tumors.[22] This points to the role of EBV as a transforming virus in endemic BL.

While extensive work has been conducted to evaluate the BL genome, further studies are needed to better understand the translational and clinical relevance of alterations. The prognostic significance of the identified mutations remains unknown. This information may aid in risk stratification and therapeutic decisions. Larger studies will also help to elucidate differences in pathogenesis between epidemiologic subtypes of BL as well as differences between pediatric and adult cases. Perhaps most importantly, this work has the potential to identify molecular lesions that could be targeted by novel therapeutics. As the cost and time required for sequencing continues to decline, it is conceivable that this translational technology could be used on each patient at the time of diagnosis to tailor therapy to the specific alterations identified in the tumor genome.

11.8. MOLECULAR SIGNALING PATHWAYS OF THERAPEUTIC INTEREST IN BURKITT LYMPHOMA

11.8.1. MYC

The frequency of the t(8;14) in BL and the strong association of the MYC expression signature in molecular BL makes MYC perhaps the most attractive translational target in BL pathophysiology. It also poses the greatest challenge, as its activity as a transcription factor makes it difficult to target pharmacologically. Underscoring the potential for efficacy of MYC directed therapy, a mouse model was recently used to simulate MYC inhibition using a doxycycline-inducible MYC transgene.[27] In this system, the requirement for MYC was demonstrated in ras-induced lung tumors, with removal of doxycycline leading to rapid regression of established tumors. While this model does not directly address the requirement for ongoing MYC expression in BL, these data combined with results using RNAi in BL cells *in vitro* strongly argue that targeting MYC would be a viable approach. Because of this, a number of direct and indirect strategies have been devised to interfere with MYC function, including therapeutic RNAi, small molecule inhibitors, and promoting the ubiquitin-mediated degradation of MYC. More direct evidence comes from the recent discovery of novel small molecules that inhibit the BET bromodomain proteins that modulate the transcriptional activity of MYC.[28] Potent anti-proliferative effects were seen in mouse models of MYC-dependent multiple myeloma[28] and in xenografts of acute lymphoblastic leukemia.[29] While these efforts have not yet produced a viable clinical product to target BL or other MYC-dependent malignancies, the exciting potential for this holy grail of lymphoma translational therapeutics continues to drive studies in this area.

11.8.2. PI3K-mTOR-Akt

The Akt pro-survival factor is activated on two residues by the activity of two related but distinct pathways.[30] Surface receptor signaling, including signals from the BCR and others, activates phosphoinositol signaling from PI3K that in turn activates PDK1 to phosphorylate Akt on T308 (Fig. 5). The large serine/threonine kinase mTOR, when complexed with

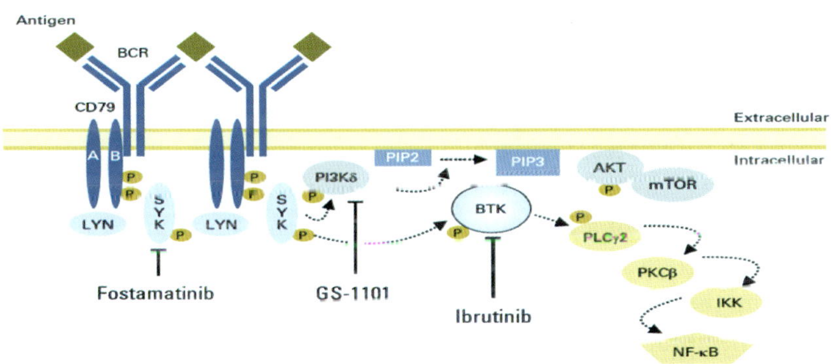

Fig. 5. Antigen-dependent signaling through the B-cell receptor. The most relevant signaling intermediates are shown along with recently developed small molecule inhibitors that are under translational investigation in aggressive NHL. Reprinted with permission from Ref. 47.

rictor to form mTOR complex 2 (mTORC2), catalyzes the phosphorylation of Akt on S473.[31] There is extensive cross-talk between these pathways and phosphorylation of both residues is required for efficient Akt activation. PI3K activity is antagonized by the phosphatase PTEN[32] whereas phosphorylation of Akt by mTOR is counterbalanced by the phosphatase PHLPP.[33] Many cases of mature B-cell lymphoma show signs of increased activity of PI3K as evidenced by heightened phosphorylation of Akt,[34,35] and PTEN loss or reduced expression has been observed in some BL cell lines.[36,37] Further evidence of the importance of this pathway in BL stems from very recent findings in which combined over-activity of MYC and PI3K was found to produce lymphomas in mice with striking similarity to human BL[26] (see Sec. 11.9 for details). Small molecule inhibitors of PI3K induce rapid cell death of BL cell lines *in vitro*.[38,39] There is currently much more available data regarding the efficacy of inhibitory activity of PI3K, mTOR and dual PI3K/mTOR inhibitors in follicular, mantle cell and DLBCL due to its increased prevalence.[40–42] Further work is required to determine if these inhibitors have a translational role in the therapy of BL. Possible roles may include their use as salvage agents, but with more experience one might envision a role in upfront therapy as a means of reducing doses of more toxic chemotherapeutics such as anthracyclines and alkylators.

11.8.3. Bruton's Tyrosine Kinase

Bruton's tyrosine kinase (BTK) is an essential cytoplasmic kinase that participates in B-cell receptor signaling and is mutated in X-linked agammaglobulinema.[43] In this disorder, B cells fail to mature to exit the bone marrow, resulting in a dramatic deficit in peripheral mature B cells.[44–46] Signaling through surface receptors — most notably the B-cell receptor — results in the activation of PI3K and the recruitment of BTK to the plasma membrane through its plekstrin homology (PH) domain, leading to its activation. BTK activity ultimately activates the ras/raf/erk pathway and thereby affects gene transcription. BTK is the target of the small molecule inhibitor ibrutinib, the first-in-class drug targeting this pathway.[47] In recently presented data from a phase 2 trial, ibrutinib monotherapy showed promising activity in patients with refractory DLBCL, including 2/25 patients with the ABC subtype who enjoyed a complete response.[48] Encouraging responses have also been reported for mantle cell[49] and follicular lymphoma,[50] suggesting a broad role for this novel agent. While there are no data regarding this agent and BL, the strong biological importance that is emerging regarding signaling downstream of the BCR suggests this agent may have important translational utility in the disease.

11.9. MOUSE MODELS OF PEDIATRIC MATURE B-NHL

Because of the prominent role of MYC in the pathogenesis of BL, the mouse models for this disease strongly depend on dysregulated expression of this transcription factor. Nearly 30 years ago, the now famous Eμ-MYC transgenic model was developed.[51] This model involved a transgenic approach in which the MYCcDNA was placed downstream of the immunoglobulin heavy chain enhancer (Eμ). This strategy proved highly lymphomagenic, with 100 percent of mice developing fatal lymphoma within the first few months of life.[51,52] While this model provides conclusive evidence of the oncogenic nature of the t(8;14) translocation in BL, the phenotype of the lymphoma that develops in these animals is not an exact phenocopy of human BL, with most murine tumors having more of an immature B-cell signature. The anatomic pattern of disease in these mice is also distinct from that seen in humans, with most mice developing splenic and thymic masses.[52] A subsequent model employed a knock-in approach, placing the human c-MYC into the lambda light chain enhancer region (μ-MYC) in order to more accurately mimic the MYC activation signature seen in human endemic BL.[53] These animals developed B-cell lymphoma with a slightly extended latency (100 percent by eight months) characterized by aggressively infiltrating lymphoma with a striking starry sky appearance. The malignant cells also carried surface markers that closely resemble those seen in BL. Another effort to more closely model the genetic configuration of the immunoglobulin locus involved a knock-in of the mouse c-MYCcDNA in a head-to-head arrangement with the Eμ region (iMYC$^{E\mu}$).[54] Animals carrying this allele develop B-cell lymphomas with a much longer latency and reduced penetrance compared with the prior models, but the lymphomas arise from more mature B cells, with the majority developing lymphoblastic lymphomas followed by DLBCL and plasmacytomas. A more recent model combines the Eμ-MYC transgene with that of a de-ubiquitinase UCH-L1 — a gene whose over expression is part of the gene signature for BL as defined by gene expression profiling.[55] While this model was not thoroughly characterized, there was a notable change in the disease anatomy with frequent abdominal masses as is seen in patients. The UCH-L1 transgene alone also leads to spontaneous B-cell lymphomagenesis, with most cases resembling DLBCL and plasmacytomas. Mechanistically, UCH-L1 was found to be a novel regulator of mTOR activity towards Akt.[56] More work is needed to determine how similar these tumors are to their human counterparts.

Recently, a major breakthrough in modeling human BL in the mouse was accomplished by recognizing the prominent association of increased PI3K signaling in human BL. The model includes combining a MYC transgene with constitutively active PI3K.[26] Both transgenes were introduced into the Rosa26 locus in an inactive form in which the promoter is separated from the transgenes by a "STOP" cassette that is flanked by loxP sites. Transgene activation occurred only in cells undergoing the germinal center reaction by crossing these mice with those expressing the Cre recombinase in early GC B cells by driving it from the Cγ1 promoter. Mice reconstituted with bone marrow from the MYC/PI3K animals developed tumors with 100 percent penetrance. Strikingly, there was a strong tendency of tumors to originate in the Peyer's patches. By immunophenotyping and gene expression profiling, these tumors are very similar to human BL and were clearly distinguished from tumors that arose in the IμHABCL6 model of DLBCL.[26,57] The insights from this model, together with the recent discovery of mutations in TCF3 and ID3 that result in increased PI3K signaling, suggest that the PI3K-Akt-mTOR axis may be particularly important in future therapeutic strategies for BL, and promise a bounty of translational research opportunity for years to come.

11.10. OPPORTUNITIES FOR TRANSLATIONAL THERAPY UTILIZING SURFACE TARGETS IN PEDIATRIC MATURE B-NHL

Surface makers on lymphoma cells represent desirable targets for tumor-directed therapy. Cellular clusters of differentiation (CD) can be exploited through the use of monoclonal antibodies (mAbs). Monoclonal antibody production is the result of pioneering work by Kohler and Milstein, which led to the discovery of hybridoma technology in 1975.[58] While the initial mAbs were used as laboratory reagents, the translational application of this technology was later developed as mAbs were produced with therapeutic intent. In 1997, rituximab, a chimeric mAb to CD20, was the first mAb licensed for the treatment of cancer. Since that time there has been significant focus on the development and refinement of mAbs directed at various cellular surface markers.

11.10.1. Monoclonal Antibody Structure

The original antibodies were composed entirely of mouse protein, which resulted in the development of human anti-mouse antibodies, preventing repeated use. Since then, chimeric, humanized, and now human antibodies have been designed with reduction or elimination of the murine component (Fig. 6). Guidelines exist for the nomenclature of mAbs, which are based on the animal from which the mAb was produced (Table 2). The suffix–mab is used for all mAbs with preceding identifiers to specify the mAb source (o = mouse, xi = chimeric, zu = humanized, u = human).

11.10.2. Mechanism of Action

While the mechanism of action of mAbs is not entirely understood, proposed mechanisms include antibody-dependent cellular cytotoxicity (ADCC), complement-dependent cytotoxicity (CDC), apoptosis and inhibition of cell growth (Fig. 7).[59] Next-generation mAbs have been developed that are conjugated to a radioactive or toxic molecule. This increases cell killing through radio- or chemotherapy delivery directly to the cell of interest.

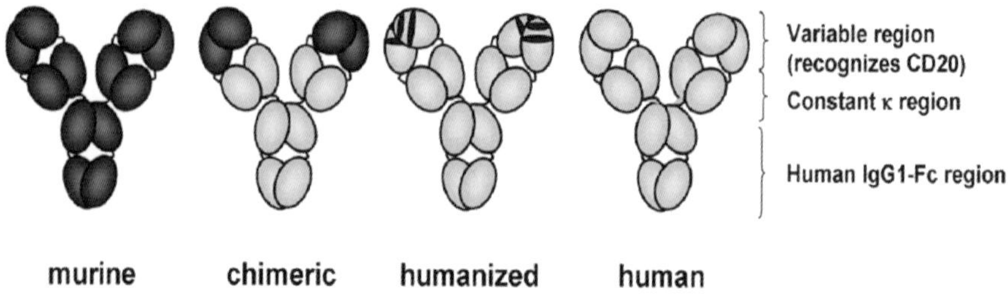

Fig. 6. Development of monoclonal antibodies recognizing CD20. Murine anti-CD20 MoAbsare generated by immunization of mice with $CD20^+$ cells. In chimeric antibodies, the 30 percent that is of murine origin is the variable region that recognizes the CD20 antigen. The variable regions are cloned into a chimeric antibody expression vector, resulting in an antibody that contains the constant κ region and the IgG1-Fc region of human origin. For humanized antibodies, also with cloning techniques, the variable region is modified to be more human. Humanized antibodies contain complementary-determining regions of murine origin, which recognize the CD20 antigen. Only 10 percent of the antibody is of murine origin. Human anti-CD20 MoAbs are derived from human immunoglobulin transgenic mice. The latter antibodies are likely to be non-immunogenic in humans. Reprinted with permission from Ref. 96.

Table 2 Monoclonal-Antibody Nomenclature

Identifier	Ab Source
-emab	Hamster
-imab	Primate
-amab	Rat
-omab	Mouse
-ximab	Chimeric
-zumab	Humanized
-umab	Human

11.10.3. The Ideal Surface Target

When identifying a surface marker for targeted therapy, various criteria should be considered. The ideal target would be preferentially expressed on malignant cells to minimize toxicity. The marker should not circulate in the plasma or be shed or internalized by the cell of interest to increase efficacy.

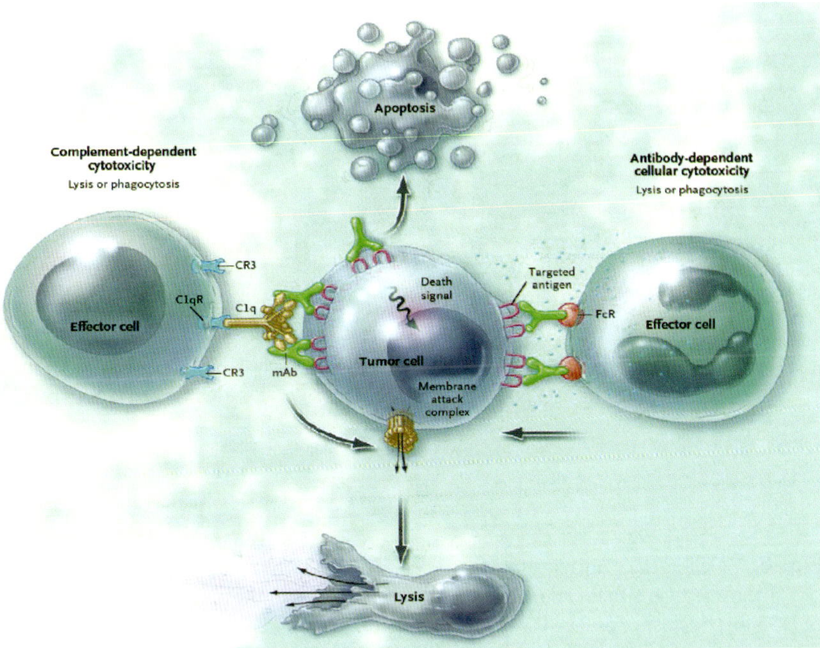

Fig. 7. Potential mechanisms of action of monoclonal antibodies. Monoclonal antibodies have several potential mechanisms of action, including antibody-dependent cellular cytotoxicity, which involves recruitment of effector cells, mediated by Fcγ receptors, complement-dependent cytoxicity, and induction of apoptosis. FcR, Fcγ receptor; mAb, monoclonal antibody. Reprinted with permission from Ref. 97.

The surface target should be necessary for a critical biologic function or survival of the tumor cell. Lastly, the target should not be frequently mutated or modulated, as this could result in resistance. In B-NHL, CD20 meets many but not all of these criteria: CD20 plays a pivotal role in B-cell activation and differentiation; it is not shed or internalized; and it is highly expressed on B-NHL tumors.[60] CD20, however, is expressed on normal B cells but not on plasma cells, which may explain the low risk of severe infections despite marked B-cell depletion. In addition to CD20, many other B-cell surface markers have been identified as possible therapeutic targets (Fig. 8).

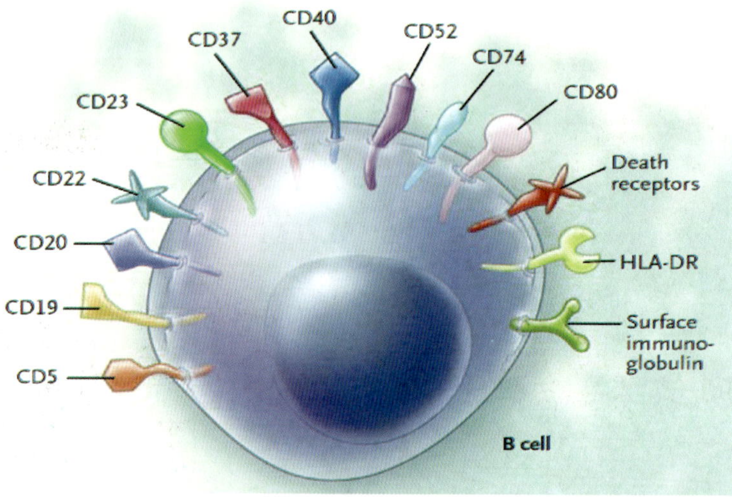

Fig. 8. Cell-surface antigens on the B cell. The B cell has a large number of associated cell-surface antigens that can be exploited for monoclonal-antibody therapy. The presence of CD5 on the surface of B cells varies according to histological type. CD, cluster of differentiation; HLA-DR, human leucocyte antigen-DR. Reprinted with permission from Ref. 97.

11.11. OVERVIEW OF IMMUNOTHERAPY IN PEDIATRIC MATURE B-NHL

BL cells express the B-cell antigens CD19, CD20 (Fig. 9A), and CD22 along with monotypic surface light chains. Consistent with their germinal center origin, the cells express CD10 (Fig. 9B) and BCL6 (Fig. 9C). Nearly all cells (typically more than 99 percent) will express the proliferation antigen Ki-67 (Fig. 9D), which is recognized by the antibody MIB-1. BCL2 is typically negative in the B cells (Fig. 9E), but positivity will be noted in scattered background CD3 positive T cells, which are relatively sparse (Fig. 9F). Although BCL2 may be weakly positive in occasional cases, strong positivity is not typical and should raise consideration of an indeterminate lymphoma (see discussion in Sec. 11.4).

In addition to their diagnostic utility, the epitopes expressed by BL cells also represent potential translational opportunities serving as immunotherapeutic targets with specific antibodies or antibody-drug

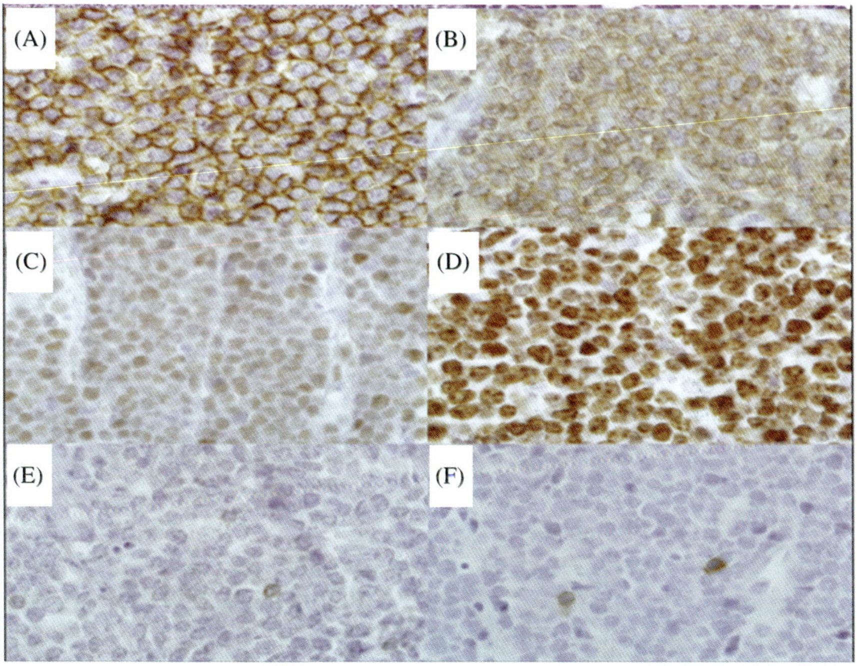

Fig. 9. Morphology and immunophenotype of BL. (A) CD20, (B) CD10, (C) BCL6, (D) MIB-1/Ki-67, (E) BCL2, and (F) CD3. Original magnification 1000× for all.

conjugates (see below). Targeting CD20 with rituximab, a chimeric human/murine monoclonal antibody, has become a mainstay of B-cell lymphoma therapy in adult patients.[61] Obinutuzumab is a newer anti-CD20 monoclonal antibody that appears to have greater potency than rituximab and is currently being directly compared to rituximab in phase III clinical trials in adults with B-cell lymphoma.[62] CD19 can be targeted by blinatumomab, which is a bi-specific T-cell engager (BiTE) that links CD3 and CD19 to target cytotoxic T cells to CD19 positive tumor cells.[63] CD22 on B cells can be targeted by epratuzumab, a humanized monoclonal antibody, as well as two drugs that link a cytotoxic molecule to an anti-CD22 antibody to specifically recognize B cells. Moxetumomab pasudotox works by linking *Pseudomonas* endotoxin to an anti-CD22 monoclonal antibody, which leads to cell death when the toxin is internalized after antigen binding.[64] Inotuzumab ozogamicin links a derivative of calicheamicin, a DNA-binding antibiotic, to an antibody directed against CD22.[65] Epitopes on tumor cells can also be targeted by generating chimeric antigen receptor (CAR) T cells that have been genetically altered to express a protein conjugate that includes the CD3 zeta chain, T-cell co-stimulatory receptor signaling domain(s), and a portion of the antibody (e.g., CD19 or CD20) that provides target specificity.[66] Binding to the target epitope on the tumor cell leads to activation of the modified T cells and cytotoxic death of the target cell.

11.11.1. Unconjugated Antibodies

11.11.1.1. *CD20*

Rituximab: Rituximab is a chimeric anti-CD20 mAb. While initially licensed for use in relapsed/refractory follicular lymphoma, the addition of rituximab to upfront standard chemotherapy has been demonstrated to improve survival in follicular lymphoma,[67,68] mantle cell lymphoma,[69] and DLBCL.[61,70] Data on the use of rituximab in pediatric NHL are limited compared to those in adults. A study of rituximab combined with ICE (ifosfamide, carboplatin, etoposide) in children with relapsed/refractory B-NHL demonstrated the safety of rituximab in combination with chemotherapy and reported an ORR of 60 percent.[71] There have been two cooperative group trials investigating the use of rituximab in the upfront treatment of pediatric B-NHL. The German Berlin–Frankfurt–Munster (BFM) group conducted a window study where rituximab was given prior to conventional chemotherapy with an analysis of response at day 5. Responses were seen in 41.4 percent of patients.[72] A pilot study conducted by the Children's Oncology Group (COG), ANHL01P1, investigated the addition of rituximab to the standard FAB/LMB96 (French–American–British/Lymphome Malins de Burkitt 96) chemotherapy backbone. This primary objective was to assess toxicity with the addition of rituximab. Rituximab was well tolerated,[73] and pharmacokinetic studies demonstrated a sustained peak and prolonged clearance with a half-life of 29 days, similar to that seen in adults.[74] While this study was not powered to evaluate efficacy, the three-year EFS in this group was 95 percent, the highest reported to date in this subset of patients.[73] An international randomized trial has been initiated to evaluate the addition of rituximab to FAB-based therapy in children with mature B-NHL. This study should provide the definitive evidence to evaluate the efficacy of rituximab in pediatric B-NHL.

Other CD20 mAbs: Despite encouraging results with rituximab, resistance has been observed.[75] Newer anti-CD20 mAbs are currently in development with the aim of increasing efficacy and evading proposed mechanisms of resistance. These next-generation anti-CD20 mAbs include: ofatumumab, a fully human mAb with increased CDC[76,77]; obinutuzumab, a humanized mAb with increased FcγRIII binding and increased ADCC[78]; veltuzumab, a humanized mAb with more stable binding[79]; and AME-133, a humanized mAb with increased FcγRIII binding as well as increased ADCC and NK cell activation.[80] Many of these have been investigated in phase I and phase II trials in adults with lymphoma. Ofatumumab has been FDA-approved for use in refractory CLL.

11.11.2. Other mAb Targets

Additional surface markers present on malignant B cells have been targeted by mAbs. Epratuzumab is a humanized mAb directed at CD22 that has shown efficacy for the treatment of aggressive B-NHL in adults.[81,82] Antibodies targeting CD40 are also in development. Dacetuzumab, SGN-40, is reported to have efficacy in early studies in adults with chronic lymphocytic leukemia and NHL.[83] Lucatumumab, also an anti-CD40 mAb, is currently in phase I trials. Antibodies targeting HLA-DR have also been designed. Apolizumab, a humanized anti-HLA-DR, was investigated in B-cell malignancies but found to have limiting toxicities.[84] Milatuzumab, also an anti-HLA-DR mAb, is being investigated in multiple myeloma. These agents have not yet been evaluated in pediatric B-NHL.

11.11.3. Immunoconjugates

11.11.3.1. *Radio immunoconjugates*

Radio immunotherapy refers to the use of an mAb that has been conjugated to a radioisotope, resulting in the targeted delivery of radiation. Two radiolabeled anti-CD20 mAbs, 90-Y-ibritumomab and 131-I-tositumomab, have been FDA approved for relapsed/refractory follicular lymphoma.

90-Y-ibritumomab has been investigated in a phase I trial in pediatric patients with B-NHL[85] where no dose-limiting toxicities were observed. In a phase I/II study of this agent in adults with refractory NHL, responses were seen in 62 percent of patients.[86]

11.11.3.2. *Immunotoxins*

Conjugating an mAb to a chemotherapeutic or toxin has been shown to have great efficacy in the case of brentuximab vedotin, an anti-CD30 antibody drug that has produced impressive responses in relapsed/refractory classical Hodgkin lymphoma and anaplastic large cell lymphoma.[87] Antibody-drug conjugates are also being developed for application in B-cell malignancies. Inotuzumab ozogamicin is a humanized anti-CD22 antibody conjugated to the cytotoxic antibiotic calecheamicin. This agent has been investigated in phase I trials in adults with B-ALL and NHL.[88,89] CAT-3888 is an anti-CD22 mAb fused to a fragment of *Pseudomonas aeruginosa* exotoxin. This agent has had promising results in a phase I study in pediatric patients with B-ALL and NHL.[90]

11.11.4. Targeted Novel Approaches to Pediatric Mature B-NHL

With the success of mAbs in cancer therapeutics, there have been efforts to develop innovative mechanisms to target surface markers on tumor cells. Two particularly promising approaches are the development of bi-specific antibodies and the generation of chimeric antigen receptors. Bi-specific antibodies, composed from two separate mAbs, are engineered to bind both a surface target and an immune effector cell. An example is blinatumomab, a mAb with dual specificity for CD3 and CD19. This agent is currently in phase I trials for pediatric patients with B-cell malignancies. Another novel approach is the adoptive transfer of genetically modified T cells with a CAR. These engineered T cells are programmed to target tumor-specific antigens resulting in tumor cell death through T-cell effector functions. CARs directed at CD19 are currently being evaluated in pediatric and adult patients with B-cell malignancies. This approach demonstrates the true utilization of translational science, where cells are collected from the patient, brought to the laboratory for genetic modification, and then reintroduced into the patient with the intent to eradicate disease.

In summary, mAbs have been utilized in B-NHL and proven to be safe and, in many cases, effective. The success of mAbs may represent a translational opportunity to replace current chemotherapy agents. This could result in substantial improvement in the short- and long-term toxicity associated with conventional chemotherapy.

11.12. CLINICAL AND TRANSLATIONAL THERAPY IN PEDIATRIC MATURE B-NHL

The two major histological subtypes of childhood and adolescent B-cell lymphoma include BL/Burkitt leukemia (approximately 60 percent) and DLBCL (approximately 35 percent). Both subtypes are germinal center-derived malignancies with near 100 percent surface expression of the CD20 antigen. Through application of multiagent cytotoxic chemotherapy including fractionated alkylating agents, anthracyclines and high doses of antimetabolite therapy (methotrexate and cytarabine) in a short pulsatile fashion and prophylaxis of the CNS compartment with direct installation of intrathecal chemotherapy, the cure rate of childhood and adolescent B-cell lymphoma approximates 90 percent in most developed countries. An aspect to the improvement of cure in this disease has been the advancement in supportive care including blood product support, treatment of tumor lysis syndrome, and infectious and nutritional support required for patients undergoing this rigorous treatment. For example, we have previously shown that uric acid nephropathy and resultant kidney dysfunction can be greatly reduced with the use of a recombinant urate oxidase enzyme, which oxidizes uric acid into allantoin.[91] Nevertheless, in patients with advanced disease receiving appropriate chemotherapy, the toxic death rate is approximately 5 percent.[92,93] In addition, certain subsets of patients are at higher risk of treatment failure (and eventual disease-related mortality), including advanced disease stages, combined bone marrow and CNS involvement, and elevated presentation of lactic dehydrogenase (LDH), which reflects disease burden and tumor proliferation.[94]

11.12.1. Reduction of Chemotherapy Unsuccessful in Advanced Pediatric Mature B-NHL

Recent efforts to reduce toxicity in pediatric and adolescent B-cell lymphoma included phase III randomized studies by major cooperative pediatric groups. It is known that infusional high doses of methotrexate are an essential therapy component in this disease. Methotrexate works by depriving cancer cells of folic acid thus shutting down DNA synthesis. Normal proliferative tissues including mucosal surfaces are also sensitive to methotrexate. Besides pain and malnourishment associated with mucositis, there is also a great enhancement in risk of bacterial transmigration over disrupted mucosal surfaces and risk of septicemia and death. For this reason, the BFM attempted to reduce the infusion duration of methotrexate in a randomized controlled fashion. Reduction in methotrexate infusion time was shown to reduce toxicity in all patient risk groups. However, while the failure-free survival (FFS) was not significantly different in patients receiving reduced infusion time of methotrexate with intermediate risk disease, those with the most advanced stages (risk groups 3 and 4) had a significant detriment in FFS. Patients in risk groups 3 and 4 randomized to four-hour methotrexate infusion had a 77 ± 5 percent FFS versus 93 ± 3 percent in those patients receiving the standard 24-hour infusion in the same risk group.[93] The FAB group studied a randomized reduction of doses of cytotoxic agents during consolidation (cytarabine and etoposide) as well as concomitant elimination of three final maintenance cycles in patients with advanced FAB Group C disease (leukemia and/or CNS disease). A non-random component in the therapy was the elimination of CNS irradiation in patients with CNS involvement by additional intrathecal administration and additional course of high-dose methotrexate. The probability of four-year EFS after randomization was 90 ± 3 percent versus 80 ± 4 percent in patients receiving standard versus reduced chemotherapy, respectively. While CNS irradiation could be successfully eliminated without detriment from previous trials, standard intensity FAB therapy (not reduced) was found to be superior.[92] Thus, both studies illustrate that for advanced stage patients, efforts to reduce toxicity in the future while maintaining high cure rates can only come from novel approaches incorporating (or substituting) non-cytotoxic therapies.

11.13. TRANSLATING CD20 EXPRESSION IN PEDIATRIC MATURE B-NHL INTO A THERAPEUTIC STRATEGY

Rituximab has been definitely shown in adult B-cell lymphoma to improve EFS either alone (in low grade follicular) or in combination with standard chemotherapy (in adult DLBCL). In pediatric B-cell lymphoma, it is unknown whether rituximab improves EFS and cure at this point in time. As a first step towards establishing tolerability and activity of rituximab, the BFM conducted a phase II window trial of rituximab prior to multiagent chemotherapy. One standard dose of rituximab was administered and a response by radiographic criteria was measured in short intervals at five days. Of 136 patients enrolled, 49 patients were not evaluable for various reasons. Of the 87 evaluable patients, there was a 41 percent response rate at day 5. Notably, 13 of 16 evaluable patients with Burkitt leukemia were responders. Toxicity encountered in the trial was as expected with infusion reactions and elevated transaminases encountered. This study demonstrated that rituximab is active and tolerable as a single agent in pediatric B-NHL.[72]

Similar to adult aggressive histology, it is more likely that rituximab will be utilized in combination with traditional cytotoxic chemotherapy (i.e., chemoimunotherapy) in pediatric B-cell lymphoma and leukemia. The COG recently published the results of the first pilot incorporating rituximab into the "best" chemotherapy arms of the previous intermediate (FAB B) and high-risk (FAB C) trials. Because of the hypothesized higher tumor burden/rapid disease proliferation, rituximab was administered in a dose-dense fashion during induction with two doses administered in each induction cycle (day −2 and day 0) and one dose in each consolidation cycle (day 0). Eighty-five evaluable patients (45 group B, 40 group C) received rituximab. The intermediate risk patients had no treatment-related (or rituximab-related) toxic deaths with acceptable toxicity profile and did not meet stopping rules for unacceptable mucositis.

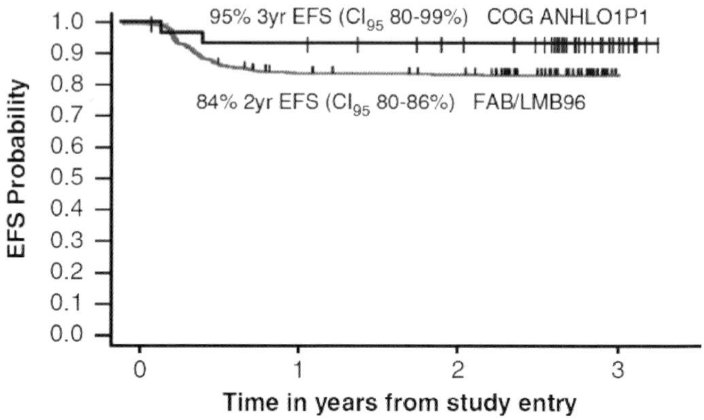

Fig. 10. Probability of EFS of all eligible intermediate-risk patients. Product-limit estimate of probability of EFS in all stage III/IV pilot patients on study compared to all stage III/IV patients treated on FAB/LMB 96 without rituximab. Reprinted with permission from Ref. 73.

The intermediate-risk patients were restricted to only advanced stages (III/IV) of diseases and demonstrated a 95 percent ($95\%_{CI}$ $80 - 99\%$) three-year EFS, which is the best reported to date. A comparison to the previous intermediate stage III/IV FAB group B trial with identical chemotherapy (without rituximab) is shown in Fig. 10.[73] Similarly, we have found acceptable toxicity in patients with high-risk disease with chemoimmunotherapy with remarkably high EFS (93 percent) in patients with CNS disease.[95]

11.14. SUMMARY

Forty years ago, the cure for advanced pediatric mature B-NHL was less than 20 percent with the use of 2.5 years of chemotherapy and radiation therapy. Today, the cure rate in this same group of patients is greater than 90 percent. This remarkable change in outcome is in large part secondary to the observations made at the bedside that were taken to the bench and now back to the bedside. New translational technologies in genomics, immunology and cell biology will further facilitate new translational opportunities for more targeted therapies in the future treatment of mature pediatric B-NHL, which will increase cure rates and decrease acute morbidities and long-term toxicities.

ACKNOWLEDGMENTS

The authors would like to thank Erin Morris, RN, for her expert editorial assistance in the preparation of this chapter. This work was supported in part by the Pediatric Cancer Research Foundation and the Children's Cancer Fund.

REFERENCES

1. Dong HY. (2010) Agressive B-cell lymphomas: Diffuse large B-cell lymphoma and Burkitt lymphoma. In: Jones D(ed). *Neoplastic Hematopathology: Contemporary Hematology* Humana Press, New York, pp. 303–322.
2. Dave SS, Fu K, Wright GW, *et al.* (2006) Molecular diagnosis of Burkitt's lymphoma. *N Engl J Med* **354**: 2431–2342.
3. Hummel M, Bentink S, Berger H, *et al.* (2006) A biologic definition of Burkitt's lymphoma from transcriptional and genomic profiling. *N Engl J Med* **354**: 2419–2430.
4. Swerdlow SH, Campo E, Harris NL, *et al.*eds. (2008) *WHO Classification of Tumours of Haematopoietic and Lymphoid Tissues.* 4th ed. IARC Press, Lyon.
5. Lones MA, Sanger WG, Le Beau MM, *et al.* (2004) Chromosome abnormalities may correlate with prognosis in Burkitt/Burkitt-like lymphomas of children and adolescents: A report from Children's Cancer Group Study CCG-E08. *J Pediatr Hematol Oncol* **26**: 169–178.
6. Onciu M, Schlette E, Zhou Y, *et al.* (2006) Secondary chromosomal abnormalities predict outcome in pediatric and adult high-stage Burkitt lymphoma. *Cancer* **107**: 1084–1092.
7. Poirel HA, Cairo MS, Heerema NA, *et al.* (2009) Specific cytogenetic abnormalities are associated with a significantly inferior outcome in children and adolescents with mature B-cell non-Hodgkin's lymphoma: Results of the FAB/LMB 96 international study. *Leukemia* **23**: 323–331.
8. Nelson M, Perkins SL, Dave BJ, *et al.* (2009) An increased frequency of 13q deletions detected by fluorescence *in situ* hybridization and its impact on

survival in children and adolescents with Burkitt lymphoma: Results from the Children's Oncology Group study CCG-5961. *Br J Haematol* **148**: 600–610.

9. Scholtysik R, Kreuz M, Klapper W, *et al.* (2010) Detection of genomic aberrations in molecularly defined Burkitt's lymphoma by array-based, high resolution, single nucleotide polymorphism analysis. *Haematologica* **95**: 2047–2055.
10. Schiffman JD, Lorimer PD, Rodic V, *et al.* (2011) Genome wide copy number analysis of paediatric Burkitt lymphoma using formalin-fixed tissues reveals a subset with gain of chromosome 13q and corresponding miRNA over expression. *Br J Haematol* **155**: 477–486.
11. He L, Thomson JM, Hemann MT, *et al.* (2005) A microRNA polycistron as a potential human oncogene. *Nature* **435**: 828–833.
12. Hammond SM. (2006) MicroRNAs as oncogenes. *Curr Opin Genet Dev* **16**: 4–9.
13. Shiramizu B, Goldman S, Kusao I, *et al.* (2011) Minimal disease assessment in the treatment of children and adolescents with intermediate-risk (Stage III/IV) B-cell non-Hodgkin lymphoma: A children's oncology group report. *Br J Haematol* **153**: 758–763.
14. Mussolin L, Pillon M, d'Amore ES, *et al.* (2011) Minimal disseminated disease in high-risk Burkitt's lymphoma identifies patients with different prognosis. *J Clin Oncol* **29**: 1779–1784.
15. Janz S, Potter M, Rabkin CS. (2003) Lymphoma- and leukemia-associated chromosomal translocations in healthy individuals. *Genes Chromosomes Cancer* **36**: 211–223.
16. Lai JL, Fenaux P, Zandecki M, *et al.* (1989) Cytogenetic studies in 30 patients with Burkitt's lymphoma or L3 acute lymphoblastic leukemia with special reference to additional chromosome abnormalities. *Ann Genet* **32**: 26–32.
17. Nelson M, Perkins SL, Dave BJ, *et al.* (2010) An increased frequency of 13q deletions detected by fluorescence *in situ* hybridization and its impact on survival in children and adolescents with Burkitt lymphoma: Results from the Children's Oncology Group study CCG-5961. *Br J Haematol* **148**: 600–610.
18. Swerdlow SH, Campo E, Harris NL, *et al.* eds. (2008) *Book WHO Classification of Tumours of Haematopoietic and Lymphoid Tissues* 4th ed. IARC Press, Lyon, France.
19. Piccaluga PP, De Falco G, Kustagi M, *et al.* (2011) Gene expression analysis uncovers similarity and differences among Burkitt lymphoma subtypes. *Blood* **117**: 3596–3608.
20. Deffenbacher KE, Iqbal J, Sanger W, *et al.* (2012) Molecular distinctions between pediatric and adult mature B-cell non-Hodgkin lymphomas identified through genomic profiling. *Blood* **119**: 3757–3766.

21. Klapper W, Szczepanowski M, Burkhardt B, *et al.* (2008) Molecular profiling of pediatric mature B-cell lymphoma treated in population-based prospective clinical trials. *Blood* **112**: 1374–1381.
22. Giulino-Roth L, Wang K, Macdonald TY, *et al.* (2012) Targeted genomic sequencing of pediatric Burkitt lymphoma identifies recurrent alterations in antiapoptotic and chromatin-remodeling genes. *Blood* **120**: 5181–5184.
23. Love C, Sun Z, Jima D, *et al.* (2012) The genetic landscape of mutations in Burkitt lymphoma. *Nat Genet* **44**: 1321–1325.
24. Richter J, Schlesner M, Hoffmann S, *et al.* (2012) Recurrent mutation of the ID3 gene in Burkitt lymphoma identified by integrated genome, exome and transcriptome sequencing. *Nat Genet* **44**: 1316–1320.
25. Schmitz R, Young RM, Ceribelli M, *et al.* (2012) Burkitt lymphoma pathogenesis and therapeutic targets from structural and functional genomics. *Nature* **490**: 116–120.
26. Sander S, Calado DP, Srinivasan L, *et al.* (2012) Synergy between PI3K signaling and MYC in Burkitt lymphomagenesis. *Cancer Cell* **22**: 167–179.
27. Soucek L, Whitfield J, Martins CP, *et al.* (2008) Modelling Myc inhibition as a cancer therapy. *Nature* **455**: 679–683.
28. Delmore JE, Issa GC, Lemieux ME, *et al.* (2011) BET bromodomain inhibition as a therapeutic strategy to target c-Myc. *Cell* **146**: 904–917.
29. Ott CJ, Kopp N, Bird L, *et al.* (2012) BET bromodomain inhibition targets both c-Myc and IL7R in high-risk acute lymphoblastic leukemia. *Blood* **120**: 2843–2852.
30. Hers I, Vincent EE, Tavare JM. (2011) Akt signalling in health and disease. *Cell Signal* **23**: 1515–1527.
31. Laplante M, Sabatini DM. (2012) mTOR signaling in growth control and disease. *Cell* **149**: 274–293.
32. Maehama T, Dixon JE. (1998) The tumor suppressor, PTEN/MMAC1, dephosphorylates the lipid second messenger, phosphatidylinositol 3,4,5-trisphosphate. *J Biol Chem* **273**: 13375–13378.
33. Gao T, Furnari F, Newton AC. (2005) PHLPP: A phosphatase that directly dephosphorylates Akt, promotes apoptosis, and suppresses tumor growth. *Mol Cell* **18**: 13–24.
34. Spender LC, Inman GJ. (2012) Phosphoinositide 3-kinase/AKT/mTORC1/2 signaling determines sensitivity of Burkitt's lymphoma cells to BH3 mimetics. *Mol Cancer Res* **10**: 347–359.
35. Uddin S, Hussain AR, Siraj AK, *et al.* (2006) Role of phosphatidylinositol 3'-kinase/AKT pathway in diffuse large B-cell lymphoma survival. *Blood* **108**: 4178–4186.

36. Gronbaek K, Zeuthen J, Guldberg P, *et al.* (1998) Alterations of the MMAC1/PTEN gene in lymphoid malignancies. *Blood* **91:** 4388–4390.
37. Sakai A, Thieblemont C, Wellmann A, *et al.* (1998) PTEN gene alterations in lymphoid neoplasms. *Blood* **92:** 3410–3415.
38. Brennan P, Mehl AM, Jones M, Rowe M. (2002) Phosphatidylinositol 3-kinase is essential for the proliferation of lymphoblastoid cells. *Oncogene* **21:** 1263–1271.
39. Curnock AP, Knox KA. (1998) LY294002-mediated inhibition of phosphatidylinositol 3-kinase activity triggers growth inhibition and apoptosis in CD40-triggered Ramos–Burkitt lymphoma B cells. *Cell Immunol* **187:** 77–87.
40. Zang C, Eucker J, Liu H, *et al.* (2012) Concurrent inhibition of PI3-Kinase and mTOR induces cell death in diffuse large B-cell lymphomas, a mechanism involving down regulation of Mcl-1. *Cancer Lett*, in press. DOI: 10.1016/j.canlet.2012.11.013. [Epub ahead of print].
41. Kim A, Park S, Lee JE, *et al.* (2012) The dual PI3K and mTOR inhibitor NVP-BEZ235 exhibits anti-proliferative activity and overcomes bortezomib resistance in mantle cell lymphoma cells. *Leuk Res* **36:** 912–920.
42. Bhatt AP, Bhende PM, Sin SH, *et al.* (2010) Dual inhibition of PI3K and mTOR inhibits autocrine and paracrine proliferative loops in PI3K/Akt/mTOR-addicted lymphomas. *Blood* **115:** 4455–4463.
43. Hussain A, Yu L, Faryal R, *et al.* (2011) TEC family kinases in health and disease — Loss-of-function of BTK and ITK and the gain-of-function fusions ITK-SYK and BTK-SYK. *Febs J* **278:** 2001–2010.
44. Bruton OC. (1952) Agammaglobulinemia. *Pediatrics* **9:** 722–728.
45. Tsukada S, Saffran DC, Rawlings DJ, *et al.* (1993) Deficient expression of a B-cell cytoplasmic tyrosine kinase in human X-linked agammaglobulinemia. *Cell* **72:** 279–290.
46. Vetrie D, Vorechovsky I, Sideras P, *et al.* (1993) The gene involved in X-linked agammaglobulinaemia is a member of the src family of protein-tyrosine kinases. *Nature* **361:** 226–233.
47. Wiestner A. (2013) Targeting B-cell receptor signaling for anticancer therapy: The Bruton's tyrosine kinase inhibitor ibrutinib induces impressive responses in B-cell malignancies. *J Clin Oncol* **31:** 128–130.
48. Wilson WH, Gerecitano JF, Goy A, *et al.* (2012) The Bruton's tyrosine kinase (BTK) inhibitor, ibrutinib (PCI-32765), has preferential activity in the ABC subtype of relapsed/refractory de novo diffuse large B-cell lymphoma (DLBCL): Interim results of a multicenter, open-label, phase 2 study. *Blood* (*ASH Annual Meeting Abstract*) **120.**

49. Advani RH, Buggy JJ, Sharman JP, *et al.* (2013) Bruton tyrosine kinase inhibitor ibrutinib (PCI-32765) has significant activity in patients with relapsed/refractory B-cell malignancies. *J Clin Oncol* **31**: 88–94.
50. Fowler NH, Advani RH, Sharman J, *et al.* (2012) The Bruton's tyrosine kinase inhibitor ibrutinib (PCI-32765) is active and tolerated in relapsed follicular lymphoma. *Blood* (*ASH Annual Meeting Abstract*) **120**: 156.
51. Adams JM, Harris AW, Pinkert CA, *et al.* (1985) The c-Myc oncogene driven by immunoglobulin enhancers induces lymphoid malignancy in transgenic mice. *Nature* **318**: 533–538.
52. Harris AW, Pinkert CA, Crawford M, *et al.* (1988) The E mu-myc transgenic mouse. A model for high-incidence spontaneous lymphoma and leukemia of early B cells. *J Exp Med* **167**: 353–371.
53. Kovalchuk AL, Qi CF, Torrey TA, *et al.* (2000) Burkitt lymphoma in the mouse. *J Exp Med* **192**: 1183–1190.
54. Park SS, Kim JS, Tessarollo L, *et al.* (2005) Insertion of c-Myc into Igh induces B-cell and plasma-cell neoplasms in mice. *Cancer Res* **65**: 1306–1315.
55. Hussain S, Foreman O, Perkins SL, *et al.* (2010) The de-ubiquitinase UCH-L1 is an oncogene that drives the development of lymphoma *in vivo* by deregulating PHLPP1 and Akt signaling. *Leukemia* **24**: 1641–1655.
56. Hussain S, Feldman AL, Das C, *et al.* (2013) The ubiquitin hydrolase UCH-L1 destabilizes mTOR complex 1 by antagonizing DDB1-CUL4 mediated ubiquitination of raptor. *Mol Cell Biol* **33**: 1188–1197.
57. Cattoretti G, Pasqualucci L, Ballon G, *et al.* (2005) Deregulated BCL6 expression recapitulates the pathogenesis of human diffuse large B-cell lymphomas in mice. *Cancer Cell* **7**: 445–455.
58. Kohler G, Milstein C. (1975) Continuous cultures of fused cells secreting antibody of predefined specificity. *Nature* **256**: 495–497.
59. Maloney DG, Smith B, Rose A. (2002) Rituximab: Mechanism of action and resistance. *Semin Oncol* **29**: 2–9.
60. Stashenko P, Nadler LM, Hardy R, Schlossman SF. (1980) Characterization of a human B lymphocyte-specific antigen. *J Immunol* **125**: 1678–1685.
61. Coiffier B, Lepage E, Briere J, *et al.* (2002) CHOP chemotherapy plus rituximab compared with CHOP alone in elderly patients with diffuse large-B-cell lymphoma. *N Engl J Med* **346**: 235–242.
62. Owen C, Stewart DA. (2012) Obinutuzumab for the treatment of lymphoproliferative disorders. *Expert Opin Biol Ther* **12**: 343–351.
63. Nagorsen D, Bargou R, Ruttinger D, *et al.* (2009) Immunotherapy of lymphoma and leukemia with T-cell engaging BiTE antibody blinatumomab. *Leuk Lymphoma* **50**: 886–891.

64. Kreitman RJ, Pastan I. (2011) Antibody fusion proteins: Anti-CD22 recombinant immunotoxin moxetumomab pasudotox. *Clin Cancer Res* **17**: 6398–6405.
65. Ricart AD. (2011) Antibody-drug conjugates of calicheamicin derivative: Gemtuzumab ozogamicin and inotuzumab ozogamicin. *Clin Cancer Res* **17**: 6417–6427.
66. Park JH, Brentjens RJ. (2010) Adoptive immunotherapy for B-cell malignancies with autologous chimeric antigen receptor modified tumor targeted T cells. *Discov Med* **9**: 277–288.
67. Hiddemann W, Kneba M, Dreyling M, *et al.* (2005) Frontline therapy with rituximab added to the combination of cyclophosphamide, doxorubicin, vincristine, and prednisone (CHOP) significantly improves the outcome for patients with advanced-stage follicular lymphoma compared with therapy with CHOP alone: Results of a prospective randomized study of the German Low-Grade Lymphoma Study Group. *Blood* **106**: 3725–3732.
68. Herold M, Haas A, Srock S, *et al.* (2007) Rituximab added to first-line mitoxantrone, chlorambucil, and prednisolone chemotherapy followed by interferon maintenance prolongs survival in patients with advanced follicular lymphoma: An East German Study Group Hematology and Oncology Study. *J Clin Oncol* **25**: 1986–1992.
69. Lenz G, Dreyling M, Hoster E, *et al.* (2005) Immunochemotherapy with rituximab and cyclophosphamide, doxorubicin, vincristine, and prednisone significantly improves response and time to treatment failure, but not long-term outcome in patients with previously untreated mantle cell lymphoma: Results of a prospective randomized trial of the German Low Grade Lymphoma Study Group (GLSG). *J Clin Oncol* **23**: 1984–1992.
70. Pfreundschuh M, Trumper L, Osterborg A, *et al.* (2006) CHOP-like chemotherapy plus rituximab versus CHOP-like chemotherapy alone in young patients with good-prognosis diffuse large-B-cell lymphoma: A randomised controlled trial by the MabThera International Trial (MInT) Group. *Lancet Oncol* **7**: 379–391.
71. Griffin TC, Weitzman S, Weinstein H, *et al.* (2009) A study of rituximab and ifosfamide, carboplatin, and etoposide chemotherapy in children with recurrent/refractory B-cell (CD20+) non-Hodgkin lymphoma and mature B-cell acute lymphoblastic leukemia: A report from the Children's Oncology Group. *Pediatr Blood Cancer* **52**: 177–181.
72. Meinhardt A, Burkhardt B, Zimmermann M, *et al.* (2010) Phase II window study on rituximab in newly diagnosed pediatric mature B-cell non-Hodgkin's lymphoma and Burkitt leukemia. *J Clin Oncol* **28**: 3115–3121.

73. Goldman S, Smith L, Anderson JR, *et al.* (2013) Rituximab and FAB/LMB 96 chemotherapy in children with Stage III/IV B-cell non-Hodgkin lymphoma: A Children's Oncology Group report. *Leukemia* **27**: 1174–1177.
74. Barth MJ, Goldman S, Zhi J, *et al.* (2011) Safety and pharmacokinetics (PK) of rituximab (R) in combination with chemotherapy in children and adolescents (C + A) with stage III/IV mature B-NHL: A Children's Oncology Group Report. *AnnOncol* **22**: iv112–iv114.
75. Kennedy GA, Tey SK, Cobcroft R, *et al.* (2002) Incidence and nature of CD20-negative relapses following rituximab therapy in aggressive B-cell non-Hodgkin's lymphoma: A retrospective review. *Br J Haematol* **119**: 412–416.
76. Barth MJ, Hernandez-Ilizaliturri FJ, Mavis C, *et al.* (2012) Ofatumumab demonstrates activity against rituximab-sensitive and -resistant cell lines, lymphoma xenografts and primary tumour cells from patients with B-cell lymphoma. *Br J Haematol* **156**: 490–498.
77. Pawluczkowycz AW, Beurskens FJ, Beum PV, *et al.* (2009) Binding of submaximal C1q promotes complement-dependent cytotoxicity (CDC) of B cells opsonized with anti-CD20 mAbs ofatumumab (OFA) or rituximab (RTX): Considerably higher levels of CDC are induced by OFA than by RTX. *J Immunol* **183**: 749–758.
78. Mossner E, Brunker P, Moser S, *et al.* (2010) Increasing the efficacy of CD20 antibody therapy through the engineering of a new type II anti-CD20 antibody with enhanced direct and immune effector cell-mediated B-cell cytotoxicity. *Blood* **115**: 4393–4402.
79. Goldenberg DM, Rossi EA, Stein R, *et al.* (2009) Properties and structure-function relationships of veltuzumab (hA20), a humanized anti-CD20 monoclonal antibody. *Blood* **113**: 1062–1070.
80. Bowles JA, Wang SY, Link BK, *et al.* (2006) Anti-CD20 monoclonal antibody with enhanced affinity for CD16 activates NK cells at lower concentrations and more effectively than rituximab. *Blood* **108**: 2648–2654.
81. Leonard JP, Coleman M, Ketas J, *et al.* (2005) Combination antibody therapy with epratuzumab and rituximab in relapsed or refractory non-Hodgkin's lymphoma. *J Clin Oncol* **23**: 5044–5051.
82. Micallef IN, Maurer MJ, Wiseman GA, *et al.* (2011) Epratuzumab with rituximab, cyclophosphamide, doxorubicin, vincristine, and prednisone chemotherapy in patients with previously untreated diffuse large B-cell lymphoma. *Blood* **118**: 4053–4061.
83. Advani R, Forero-Torres A, Furman RR, *et al.* (2009) Phase I study of the humanized anti-CD40 monoclonal antibody dacetuzumab in refractory or recurrent non-Hodgkin's lymphoma. *J Clin Oncol* **27**: 4371–4377.

84. Lin TS, Stock W, Xu H, *et al.* (2009) A phase I/II dose escalation study of apolizumab (Hu1D10) using a stepped-up dosing schedule in patients with chronic lymphocytic leukemia and acute leukemia. *Leuk Lymphoma* **50**: 1958–1963.
85. Cooney-Qualter E, Krailo M, Angiolillo A, *et al.* (2007) A phase I study of 90yttrium-ibritumomab-tiuxetan in children and adolescents with relapsed/refractory CD20-positive non-Hodgkin's lymphoma: A Children's Oncology Group study. *Clin Cancer Res* **13**: 5652s–5660s.
86. Morschhauser F, Kraeber-Bodere F, Wegener WA, *et al.* (2010) High rates of durable responses with anti-CD22 fractionated radioimmunotherapy: Results of a multicenter, phase I/II study in non-Hodgkin's lymphoma. *J Clin Oncol* **28**: 3709–3716.
87. de Claro RA, McGinn K, Kwitkowski V, *et al.* (2012) U.S. Food and Drug Administration approval summary: Brentuximab vedotin for the treatment of relapsed Hodgkin lymphoma or relapsed systemic anaplastic large-cell lymphoma. *Clin Cancer Res* **18**: 5845–5849.
88. Ogura M, Hatake K, Ando K, *et al.* (2012) Phase I study of anti-CD22 immunoconjugate inotuzumab ozogamicin plus rituximab in relapsed/refractory B-cell non-Hodgkin lymphoma. *Cancer Sci* **103**: 933–938.
89. Kantarjian H, Thomas D, Jorgensen J, *et al.* (2012) Inotuzumab ozogamicin, an anti-CD22-calecheamicin conjugate, for refractory and relapsed acute lymphocytic leukaemia: A phase 2 study. *Lancet Oncol* **13**: 403–411.
90. Wayne AS, Kreitman RJ, Findley HW, *et al.* (2010) Anti-CD22 immunotoxin RFB4(dsFv)-PE38 (BL22) for CD22-positive hematologic malignancies of childhood: Preclinical studies and phase I clinical trial. *Clin Cancer Res* **16**: 1894–1903.
91. Goldman SC, Holcenberg JS, Finklestein JZ, *et al.* (2001) A randomized comparison between rasburicase and allopurinol in children with lymphoma or leukemia at high risk for tumor lysis. *Blood* **97**: 2998–3003.
92. Cairo MS, Gerrard M, Sposto R, *et al.* (2007) Results of a randomized international study of high-risk central nervous system B non-Hodgkin lymphoma and B acute lymphoblastic leukemia in children and adolescents. *Blood* **109**: 2736–2743.
93. Woessmann W, Seidemann K, Mann G, *et al.* (2005) The impact of the methotrexate administration schedule and dose in the treatment of children and adolescents with B-cell neoplasms: A report of the BFM Group Study NHL-BFM95. *Blood* **105**: 948–958.
94. Cairo MS, Sposto R, Gerrard M, *et al.* (2012) Advanced stage, increased lactate dehydrogenase, and primary site, but not adolescent age (>/= 15 years), are

associated with an increased risk of treatment failure in children and adolescents with mature B-cell non-Hodgkin's lymphoma: Results of the FAB LMB 96 study. *J Clin Oncol* **30**: 387–393.
95. Goldman S, Galardy PJ, Smith L, *et al.* (2011) The efficacy of rasburicase and rituximab combined with FAB chemotherapy in children and adolescents with newly diagnosed stage III/IV BM+ and CNS + mature B-NHL: A Children's Oncology Group Report. *Blood* (*ASH Annual Meeting Abstract*) **118**: 2702.
96. van Meerten T, Hagenbeek A. (2010) CD20-targeted therapy: The next generation of antibodies. *Semin Hematol* **47**: 199–210.
97. Cheson BD, Leonard JP. (2008) Monoclonal antibody therapy for B-cell non-Hodgkin's lymphoma. *N Engl J Med* **359**: 613–626.

CHAPTER 12

Developmental of Translational Sciences Based on Lung Cancer

Eva Szabo

12.1. INTRODUCTION

Despite tremendous recent advances in the understanding of the biology of cancers arising from multiple different target organ sites, the cure for metastatic cancer remains elusive. The development of invasive epithelial cancer is a lengthy process that requires multiple changes to the target tissue, its microenvironment, and the host's immune function, as conceptualized by Hanahan and Weinberg.[1] Abundant data from preclinical studies and from well-designed phase III clinical trials indicate that cancer prevention is a feasible approach to decrease the morbidity and mortality from invasive cancer.[2,3] Since the goal of cancer prevention is to forestall the occurrence of future adverse health events but not impact on current health, it is heavily based on translational research both to identify molecular targets for intervention and to recognize agent efficacy in clinical trials. The purpose of this chapter is to review the principles of chemo preventive drug development, with an emphasis on how translational research informs cancer prevention clinical trials.

Lung and Upper Aerodigestive Cancer Research Group, Division of Cancer Prevention, National Cancer Institute, National Institutes of Health, Bethesda, Maryland, USA

Full address: Eva Szabo, MD, Lung and Upper Aerodigestive Cancer Research Group, Division of Cancer Prevention, National Cancer Institute, National Institutes of Health, 9609 Medical Center Drive, Rm 5E-102, MSC 9781, Bethesda, MD20892, USA; E-mail: *szaboe@mail.nih.gov*; Tel: +1-240-276-7011; Fax:+1-240-276-7848

12.2. CANCER PREVENTIVE AGENT IDENTIFICATION

The identification of appropriate targets for intervention is an iterative process that begins with laboratory insights regarding the pathogenesis of cancers arising at specific target organ sites. Necessary early studies include the demonstration of the presence of the putative target during early phases of carcinogenesis, such as in tissues from individuals with cancer as well as individuals at risk for cancer as the result of environmental exposures (e.g., tobacco for lung cancer), the presence of premalignant lesions (e.g., colorectal adenomas for colon cancer), or due to cancer genetic syndromes (e.g., BRCA1 or 2 for breast or ovarian cancer). Preclinical testing of interventions requires the use of animal systems that model the development of cancer, such as carcinogen exposure-based animal models (e.g., tobacco carcinogens for lung cancer) and transgenic animals harboring genetic mutations implicated in carcinogenesis occurring at specific organ sites [e.g., BRCA1 mutations for breast cancer, APC mutations (Min mice) for colorectal cancer]. Knowledge gleaned from each type of study, either human or animal, should inform the other — for instance, modulation of drug targets *in vitro* and in animal studies should point to markers that should be examined in clinical trials, whereas identification of drug targets only during early or late phases of human carcinogenesis should inform the design of animal studies with regard to the timing of the intervention with respect to carcinogen exposure. In this fashion, data obtained from studying human biospecimens help define the structure of preclinical studies, while conversely, markers modulated by interventions in animal carcinogenesis studies can point to intermediate endpoints that can facilitate early phase human clinical trials.

Selection of appropriate targets for cancer prevention is based on efficacy assessment as well as the potential toxicities resulting from impacting the target. Indications of effectiveness fall into several major categories: knowledge of mechanisms, *in vitro* and animal *in vivo* experimental data, epidemiological case-control and cohort studies, and data from clinical trials, either early phase prevention trials or secondary endpoint analysis from trials performed for other indications (reviewed in Ref. 3). The better the understanding of the process of carcinogenesis and the molecular basis for the evolution of the neoplastic phenotype, the higher is the likelihood of successfully developing interventions to prevent or reverse neoplastic progression.

The efficacy of an agent is dependent on how critical its target is to carcinogenesis, whether the agent can be delivered at the time that its target drives the carcinogenic process, and the potency of the intervention. Different stages of carcinogenesis may be driven by different molecular abnormalities, so it cannot be assumed that a single intervention would be effective at all time points during the evolution of tumor formation. An example of this is the idea of blocking carcinogen metabolism to target DNA damage from tobacco exposure. While this could be highly effective if delivered to current smokers during their entire smoking career, it would not be predicted to be effective in former smokers whose initial DNA damage occurred years prior and who have already accumulated multiple additional genetic defects. A real-world illustration is the use of the tyrosine kinase inhibitor imatinib. This inhibits $p210^{BCR-ABL}$, which causes chronic myelogenous leukemia (CML), and also inhibits c-Kit, which is expressed in small cell lung cancer (SCLC).[4,5] In CML, $p210^{BCR-ABL}$ is necessary and sufficient to cause the disease and imatinib has striking efficacy in the early chronic phase. Chronic CML can be considered a premalignant phase of the leukemic process. However, advanced disease (accelerated phase and blast crisis) is characterized by the accumulation of additional mutations, and imatinib's efficacy is markedly diminished in these disease phases. In SCLC, although c-Kit is frequently expressed, activating c-Kit mutations are not found.[6] Instead, abundant mutations in other genes exist and imatinib is inactive.[7] These two examples point to the importance of identifying processes that are critical to carcinogenesis and targeting them at the appropriate stages of tumor development.

Two additional points need to be underscored. It is becoming increasingly clear that cancers arising within a single target organ may results from different pathogenetic mechanisms involving many different signaling pathways. For instance, breast cancer classification has moved beyond the simple estrogen receptor-positive and estrogen receptor-negative categories, while a variety of molecular alterations, several of which can be specifically targeted for therapy, are known to lead to lung adenocarcinoma.[8,9] This molecular complexity suggests that multiple strategies may well be needed to prevent different types of cancers and thus it becomes critically important to identify the individuals at high risk for specific molecular types of cancer. Second, it is important to remember that phase III cancer prevention trials with tumor incidence endpoints generally test interventions for only a small number of years, so these trials are, by design, testing intervention efficacy on relatively advanced stages of premalignancy. Thus, an intervention that blocks early events in carcinogenesis (e.g., DNA damage) is highly unlikely to prevent cancer in a trial with three to five years of agent administration. In selecting targets for cancer prevention, the ability to perform a clinical trial that is focused on the appropriate cohort, whether by virtue of risk for the specific cancer type or the stage of carcinogenesis, must be taken into account.

12.3. CANCER PREVENTION CLINICAL TRIALS

Important issues in cancer prevention clinical trials include the choice of study cohorts, endpoints to assess efficacy, and actual study design. Although the process of carcinogenesis can be modeled in animal systems, efficacy in human beings can only be accurately assessed in well-designed and well-executed clinical trials. As with all interventions, both the risks and the benefits associated with the preventive interventions need to be weighed to ensure that the balance falls strongly in favor of the intervention. Phase III cancer prevention clinical trials aimed at testing the efficacy of beta carotene for lung cancer prevention showed an increase, rather than decrease, in lung cancer mortality.[10,11] Similarly, the cyclooxygenase-2 inhibitor rofecoxib showed an increase in cardiovascular toxicity in a trial that showed significant decrease in colorectal adenoma recurrence, a result that ultimately led to its withdrawal from the market.[12,13] As a result, there is currently an increased emphasis on early phase cancer prevention trials to better define the intended study cohorts, drug doses, schedules, and safety profiles, and eventual applications of the interventional strategy prior to embarking on large phase III clinical trials.

12.3.1. Cohorts

The choice of study cohort is of particular significance. The goal of prevention trials is to identify a strategy that will prevent the occurrence of cancer, a condition that presumably does not yet exist in the individuals targeted for intervention. In contrast to cancer treatment trials, which focus on easily identifiable populations with cancer, prevention trials need to focus on populations at high risk for cancer who do not yet have cancer and thus do not have easily measurable disease. The reason for this is two-fold. First, a high-risk cohort is needed to decrease the trial size, since the incidence of any given cancer in a non-risk population is actually quite low. Second, toxicities of interventions can only be justified in sufficiently high-risk populations. Whereas chemotherapy with risk of life-threatening toxicities and death can be used in the setting of metastatic cancer where the underlying disease also leads to death, its use cannot be justified in healthy populations that may never develop cancer.

The difficulty lies in identifying such high-risk cohorts. The Gail model has been successfully used to identify high-risk individuals who were found to benefit from tamoxifen for breast cancer prevention, but there is no good algorithm to predict the risk of triple negative breast cancer, a tumor that is not responsive to hormonal interventions.[14,15] Risk prediction models for other cancer types are even less precise. Nevertheless, since all interventions have some side effects, the balance between risk and benefit can be optimized through selection of appropriately high-risk cohort to justify the use of the intended interventions.

12.3.2. Intermediate Endpoints

One of the biggest challenges for cancer preventive agent development is the identification of informative endpoints that demonstrate preliminary efficacy in early phase clinical trials. Cancer incidence is the universally accepted endpoint in phase III clinical trials. However, phase II preliminary efficacy trials need to rely on short-term (intermediate) endpoints that are integrally linked with patient outcomes such as cancer incidence. These endpoints become surrogates for the definitive cancer incidence endpoints and their modulation forms the basis for drug development "go/no-go" decisions. The challenge, then, is to identify measurable markers that meet the criteria for surrogacy. These criteria include: (i) integral involvement in the process of carcinogenesis such that the expression of the marker correlates with the disease course, (ii) differential expression between normal and at-risk epithelium that can be easily and reproducibly measured in specimens that can be obtained in clinical trials, and (iii) modulation by effective interventions and no modulation by ineffective interventions (i.e., minimal spontaneous fluctuation).[16–18] A marker that satisfies these criteria needs validation in prospective clinical trials.[18]

Although no intermediate endpoint marker has been validated to the point that it can replace cancer incidence as an endpoint in clinical trials seeking regulatory approval, translational research has identified many complex molecular mechanisms that help speed early drug development. Aberrantly expressed molecules can potentially serve as biomarkers for risk assessment and for monitoring response to interventions. As an example, recent data indicate that phosphoinositide 3-kinase (PI3K) is frequently mutated in squamous cell carcinomas from the lung or head and neck and that PI3K pathway up-regulation occurs early during lung carcinogenesis.[19–21] In a small phase I chemoprevention trial, intervention with the drug myo-inositol led to regression of bronchial premalignancy and to inhibition of PI3K activation as assessed by gene expression profiling.[21] These results suggest that PI3K activation could be a biomarker of cancer risk in smokers and that it could potentially serve as an endpoint in early phase clinical trials. Further studies, some of which are ongoing, will need to validate these results.

At the current time, histologic precursors to invasive cancer, collectively referred to as intraepithelial neoplasia (IEN), represent the most commonly used intermediate endpoints in phase II cancer prevention trials.[22] Other indices of malignancy, such as increased proliferation, oncogene expression, or panels of markers (such as the gene expression profiles indicative of PI3K activation that are discussed above) can also provide evidence that a drug intervention is affecting its target and interfering with progressive carcinogenesis. As mentioned previously, none of these endpoints is validated and thus none can serve as surrogates for cancer incidence in attempts to obtain regulatory approval for cancer prevention indications. However, strong modulation of such endpoints could provide sufficient evidence of preliminary efficacy to justify subsequent phase III trials. The development of these alternatives to IEN is a perfect example of how clinical trials are critically dependent on translational research. The use of high throughput technologies that can interrogate multiple different markers in a small number of subjects treated with an intervention potentially offers a faster and more efficient way to evaluate drug mechanisms of action and to provide evidence of efficacy than the traditional larger phase IIb prevention trials with IEN as an endpoint.

12.3.3. Early Phase Clinical Trial Designs

A number of early phase clinical trial designs exist to account for differences in target organ tissue accessibility and biology. They range from multi-month interventions aimed at regressing IEN or preventing the re-emergence of an ablated IEN to short-term interventions in a presurgical setting whereby a pharmacodynamic effect or agent accumulation in the target organ is assessed.[23] The common theme among most of these studies is the need for tissue acquisition to assess the primary endpoint in the epithelium of interest, in contrast to radiologic assessments for primary endpoint definition that form the backbone of cancer treatment trials. Longer treatment is believed to be necessary for the tissue remodeling that leads to regression of premalignant lesions, while proliferation, gene or protein expression, or pharmacodynamic endpoints should be able to be modulated within days to a small number of weeks. Consequently, the amount of information learned from these different trial designs varies widely. As an example, prevention of viral infection with human papillomavirus (HPV), which is known to be necessary for cervical carcinogenesis, along with a demonstration of prevention of cervical premalignancy (but not cervical cancer), was sufficient to obtain regulatory approval for the HPV vaccine and an indication for cervical cancer prevention.[24] On the other hand, demonstration that a tyrosine kinase inhibitor accumulates in prostate tissue, for instance, and that the phosphorylation of downstream targets is inhibited only shows drug activity in the target organ. If the signaling pathways that are impacted are irrelevant to carcinogenesis in that target organ, progress has not been made. However, if the signaling pathways are critical to carcinogenesis at that target organ and yet the drug does not get into the organ to adequately inhibit its targets, then this hypothetical study would have demonstrated the need for an alternative drug, formulation or delivery mechanism and would have prevented the investment of valuable resources in a larger, more definitive trial.

Table 1 Early Phase Clinical Trial Designs

Trial Type	Cohort	Duration	Comments
Prevention trial with IEN endpoint	High-risk subjects with IEN	6–12 months	Pre-screening for IEN is necessary
Prevention trial with molecular endpoint(s)	High-risk subjects, no IEN needed	3–6 months	Less pre-screening necessary; less informative
Advanced cancer trial with nested "prevention endpoint"	Cancer patients, +/− IEN	6+ weeks (endpoint assessment time needs to be pre-specified)	Potentially high dropout rate due to progression; agent must be appropriate for prevention; additional ("non-standard of care") tissue acquisition required
Adjuvant trial with nested "prevention endpoint"	Curatively treated cancer patients, +/− IEN	6+ months (endpoint assessment time needs to be pre-specified)	Agent must be appropriate for prevention; additional ("non-standard of care") tissue acquisition
Presurgical trial	Cancer patients prior to definitive surgery	2–6 weeks	Limited duration of treatment, primarily biomarker modulation; tissue acquisition part of "standard of care"

IEN: Intraepithelial neoplasia.

The various prevention trial types are described in Table 1. The most informative design focuses on high-risk populations harboring cancer precursors, which can be studied for progression to cancer, or if removed, for recurrence. A similar trial design with a molecular primary endpoint is potentially less informative, unless the molecular endpoint is known to be causally involved in carcinogenesis at the stage that is being studied. In the modern era of targeted therapies that are less toxic, alternative trial designs include the assessment of "prevention-relevant" endpoints such as premalignant lesions during the course of treatment and adjuvant trials. The main disadvantage of assessing "prevention-relevant" endpoints during treatment of active cancer is the large dropout rates for disease progression. Finally, the main disadvantage of presurgical treatment is the potentially short duration of treatment.

12.4. CONCLUSIONS

Progress in cancer prevention is directly dependent on progress in understanding the biology and heterogeneity of the carcinogenic process occurring at multiple target organs. Translational research lies at the heart of cancer prevention trials, spanning from the identification of relevant targets for intervention to the identification of informative endpoints, cohort selection, and assessment of endpoints during the course of clinical trials. Although intervention in the early phases of carcinogenesis, prior to the development of multiple molecular abnormalities, could potentially be more effective than treatment of late-stage, widely disseminated disease, cancer prevention has proven to be more challenging than previously anticipated. Nevertheless, with an ever-increasing armamentarium of molecular techniques to probe the biology of carcinogenesis, incremental progress in clearly defined, homogeneous high-risk subgroups stands to be made.

REFERENCES

1. Hanahan D, Weinberg RA. (2011) Hallmarks of cancer: The next generation. *Cell* **144**: 646–674.
2. Szabo E. (2008) First do no harm: When is it appropriate to plan a cancer prevention clinical trial? *Nat Clin Pract Oncol* **5**: 348–356.
3. Szabo E. (2006) Selecting targets for cancer prevention: Where do we go from here? *Nat Rev Cancer* **6**: 867–874.
4. Cohen MH, Johnson JR, Pazdur R. (2005) U.S. Food and Drug Administration drug approval summary: Conversion of imatinib mesylate (STI571; Gleevec) tablets from accelerated approval to full approval. *Clin Cancer Res* **11**: 12–19.
5. Blanke CD, Corless CL. (2005) State-of-the art therapy for gastrointestinal stromal tumors. *Cancer Invest* **23**: 274–280.
6. Dy GK, Miller AA, Mandrekar SJ, *et al.* (2005) A phase II trial of imatinib (STI571) in patients with c-kit expressing relapsed small-cell lung cancer: A CALGB and NCCTG study. *Ann Oncol* **16**: 1811–1816.

7. Burger H, den Bakker MA, Stoter G, *et al.* (2003) Lack of *c-kit* exon 11 activating mutations in c-KIT/CD117-positive SCLC tumour specimens. *Eur J Cancer* **39**: 793–799.
8. Peppercorn J, Perou CM, Carey LA. (2008) Molecular subtypes in breast cancer evaluation and management: Divide and conquer. *Cancer Invest* **26**: 1–10.
9. Ding L, Getz G, Wheeler DA, Mardis ER, *et al.* (2008) Somatic mutations affect key pathways in lung adenocarcinoma. *Nature* **455**: 1069–1075.
10. The ATBC Study Group. (1994) The effect of vitamin E and beta carotene on the incidence of lung cancer and other cancers in male smokers. The Alpha-Tocopherol Beta Carotene Cancer Prevention Study Group. *N Eng J Med* **330**: 1029–1035.
11. Omenn GS, Goodman GE, Thornquist MD, *et al.* (1996) Effects of a combination of beta carotene and vitamin A on lung cancer and cardiovascular disease. *N Eng J Med* **334**: 1150–1155.
12. Bresalier RS, Sandler RS, Quan H, *et al.* (2005) Cardiovascular events associated with rofecoxib in a colorectal adenoma chemoprevention trial. *N Eng J Med* **352**: 1092–1102.
13. Baron J, Sandler RS, Bresalier RS, *et al.* (2006) A randomized trial of rofecoxib for the chemoprevention of colorectal cancer. *Gastroenterology* **131**: 1674–1682.
14. Gail MH, Brinton LA, Byar DP, *et al.* (1989) Projecting individualized probabilities of developing breast cancer for white females who are being examined annually. *J Natl Cancer Inst* **81**: 1879–1886.
15. Fisher B, Costantino JP, Wickerham DL, *et al.* (1998) Tamoxifen for prevention of breast cancer: Report of the National Surgical Adjuvant Breast and Bowel Project P-1 Study. *J Natl Cancer Inst* **190**: 1371–1388.
16. Lippman SM, Lee JS, Lotan R, *et al.* (1990) Biomarkers as intermediate end points in chemoprevention trials. *J Natl Cancer Inst* **82**: 555–560.
17. Szabo E. (2010) Assessing efficacy in early-phase cancer prevention trials: The case of the Ki-67 proliferation index in lung cancer prevention. *Cancer Prev Res* **3**: 128–131.
18. Schatzkin A, Gail M. (2002) The promise and peril of surrogate end points in cancer research. *Nat Rev Cancer* **2**: 1–9.
19. Spoerke JM, O'Brien C, Huw L, *et al.* (2012) Phosphoinositide 3-kinase (PI3K) pathway alterations are associated with histologic subtypes and are predictive of sensitivity to PI3K inhibitors in lung cancer preclinical models. *Clin Cancer Res* **18**: 6771–6783.
20. Stransky N, Egloff AM, Tward AD, *et al.* (2011) The mutational landscape of head and neck squamous cell carcinoma. *Science* **333**: 1157–1160.

21. Gustafson AM, Soldi R, Anderlind C, *et al.* (2010) Airway PI3K pathway activation is an early and reversible event in lung cancer development. *Science Trans Med* **2**: 26ra25.
22. O'Shaughnessy JA, Kelloff GJ, Gordon GB, *et al.* (2002) Treatment and prevention of intraepithelial neoplasia: An important target for accelerated new agent development. *Clin Cancer* **8**: 314–346.
23. Szabo E. (2010) Phase II cancer prevention clinical trials. *Sem Oncol* **37**: 359–366.
24. Garland SM, Hernandez-Avila M, Wheeler CM, *et al.* (2007) Quadrivalent vaccine against human papillomavirus to prevent anogenital disease. *N Eng J Med* **356**: 1928–1943.

V. Translational Science in Infectious Diseases

CHAPTER 13

Translational Research in Molecular Diagnostics of Infectious Disease

*Mark Manak** and *Jiuping Ji*[†,‡]

13.1. INTRODUCTION

The application of molecular techniques to the diagnostics of infectious disease has provided important advantages for highly sensitive direct detection of infectious agents in biological fluids and tissues. The greater sensitivity and ability to quantify and directly detect the infectious agent provide additional diagnostic value to molecular techniques that are not achievable with existing antibody, antigen or culture tests, allowing for earlier detection of acute infection, monitoring progress of infection and response to therapies, and differentiation between active and prior or well-established infections. The additional application of sequence analysis provides critical information on prediction of disease severity, evaluation of drug susceptibility and to guide epidemiological and transmission studies. However, the application of nucleic acid methods to routine use in a clinical laboratory is subject to various unique challenges with regard to susceptibility to contamination, high complexity of reagents and methodologies,

*Department of Diagnostics and Monitoring, US Military HIV Research Program (MHRP), HJF, Walter Reed Army Institute of Research, Silver Spring, Maryland, USA.

†National Clinical Target Validation Laboratory, Frederick National Laboratory for Cancer Research, Frederick, Maryland, USA.

‡Corresponding author: Jiuping Ji, PhD, Laboratory Head, National Clinical Target Validation Laboratory, Frederick National Laboratory for Cancer Research, Frederick, MD, USA; E-mail: *jijiupi@mail.nih.gov*; Tel: +1-301-443-2094; Fax: +1-301-443-4679.

and elaborate data analysis requiring sophisticated programming capability to provide a useful clinical interpretation of the data. The goal of translational research is to advance basic research and new technology toward clinical utility.

Techniques developed for quantitative detection of blood-borne pathogens such as human immunodeficiency virus (HIV), hepatitis B and C (HBV/HCV) utilize complex methodologies for sample processing, extraction, amplification and detection to ensure high sensitivity and broad dynamic range of viral load in plasma for use in monitoring progression of disease and effectiveness of therapy. The high complexity of these assays requires sophisticated technologies, instrumentation and often highly specialized training, all of which need to be carefully monitored to ensure accurate results. Furthermore, these assays are faced with the problem of a high degree of variability and continuous evolution of sequence complexity, particularly in the case of HIV testing. Novel approaches to molecular detection of respiratory viruses in nasal secretions allow for earlier and direct detection of infection, but efforts are complicated by the large number of possible agents that can cause respiratory disease. Recent advances in applications of multiplex formats, such as Luminex technology, allow simultaneous detection of multiple infectious agents in the same sample, but are faced with the issue of how to accurately detect and differentiate between many different viruses at the same time. Diagnosis of sexually transmitted bacterial or parasitic agents, such as chlamydia or gonorrhea, have additional challenges in sample preparation and differentiation of pathogenic organisms collected in cervical swabs or urine. Detection of human papilloma virus (HPV) as a risk factor for cervical cancer has the additional challenge of differentiation between carcinogenic and non-carcinogenic subtypes. Molecular testing of infectious agents continues to be hampered by limitations in specimen processing, adequate sample size, and identification of rare strains, or drug-resistant mutations. This chapter will review some of these challenges and the approaches laboratories have taken to implement and validate molecular assays for infectious agents for routine use in clinical diagnosis. The chapter will also briefly address new developments in nucleic acid diagnosis, including the trend toward more multiplexing and therefore greater complexity, applications of digital PCR for more accurate quantitation, and approaches to identify sequence variability for drug resistance or typing of organisms.

13.2. ADVANTAGES OF MOLECULAR TECHNIQUES

The application of molecular techniques to clinical diagnosis has revolutionized the field of infectious disease diagnostics in the clinical laboratory, and molecular methods are rapidly becoming standard laboratory testing tools for fast, accurate and sensitive detection of infectious disease agents. A major advantage of nucleic acid methods over immunoassays is their high sensitivity and specificity in direct identification of the infectious agent compared to conventional culture-based or antigen detection methods, allowing detection even if the organisms are nonviable or nonculturable. Since nucleic acid signals can be amplified to a very large extent, molecular assays can be used to detect extremely low levels of the infecting organisms, such as HIV, and permit diagnosis at very early stages of acute infection, well before the body has a chance to mount an immune response. Amplification of nucleic acids can be precisely controlled, allowing for accurate determination of the levels of infectious agent present in a sample. An accurate assessment of the quantity (rather than merely presence) of virus is particularity important in immunosuppressed patients, such as after a transplant or due to immunosuppressive disease, to alert the physician if a normally quiescent virus becomes reactivated, which can lead to dire consequences. Virus quantitation is also important in monitoring HCV, HBV and HIV levels in patients undergoing antiretroviral therapy to monitor the effectiveness of the treatment and allow for an appropriate change in drug regimen when viral load rises to dangerously high levels. Furthermore, these techniques can detect very specific genetic markers to provide highly selective pathogen typing information, including resolution of specific variants or subtypes, differentiation between pathogenic and non-pathogenic organisms, and identification of mutations that render specific drug resistance.

As more FDA-approved/cleared *in vitro* diagnostic (IVD) devices are becoming available, laboratories need to select the assay that best meets their needs and validate its usage prior to implementation. In addition, as instrumentation and reagents are increasingly becoming available for simplified research applications for sample prep, nucleic acid amplification and detection in standardized formats, sensitive detection reagents, and automated platforms have allowed many hospitals and clinical laboratories to develop or modify their own laboratory-developed molecular assays. Such laboratory-developed assays must be validated in strict accordance with Clinical Laboratory Improvement Act (CLIA) requirements before they can be used in clinical applications to identify new pathogens.[1] Interpretation of the molecular detection of many viral pathogens must validate the use of the clinical specimen to be tested, the quantity of organisms present, the need for quantitative versus qualitative detection, stage of infection, and relevance to disease.

Rapid advances in the field of molecular diagnostics such as automated instrumentation for rapid specimen processing, amplification and detection, coupled with the use of novel chemistries and very sensitive fluorescent probes, have led to the development of highly reliable automated nucleic acid amplification systems for very sensitive detection of pathogens with rapid turn-around time and increasingly greater cost effectiveness.[2] The development of real-time polymerase chain reaction (PCR), with very sensitive hybridization probes and signal detection software packages, allow accurate, rapid and extremely sensitive quantitation of viral load to help guide patient therapy. Closed-tube amplification methods such as real-time PCR have successfully addressed previous concerns of false positive results due to sample carryover, while advances in nucleic acid extraction methods have made possible the application of this technology to detection of infectious agents in various sample types, including plasma, cerebrospinal fluid, nasal secretions, urine and saliva, and various tissue types. Newer sequencing chemistries or melting curve analysis of the amplification products coupled with rapid computer-based phylogenetic analysis software, easily accessible Internet sequence databases, and advanced informatics software have facilitated rapid virus typing, including guidance of appropriate drug therapy particularly for viruses that mutate at high frequency. Such advances have allowed what was originally a very complex technology available only to highly skilled technicians to be brought to routine, cost-effective applications in the clinical laboratory.

13.3. MOLECULAR DIAGNOSTICS OF INFECTIOUS DISEASE

Major applications of infectious disease molecular diagnostics include tests for blood-borne infections such as HIV, HBV and HCV, and for sexually transmitted infections such as *Chlamydia trachomatis* and *Neisseria gonorrhoeae* (CT/NG) and HPV.[3] Sexually transmitted infections are often asymptomatic among females and if left untreated may produce severe long-term effects. As opposed to testing of serum or plasma, diagnosis of these infections requires testing of mucosal cells or tissues, which are collected as swabs of the cervix, urethra, rectum or throat. In some cases, urine specimens can also be used. Detection of CT/NG is normally performed by multiplex nucleic acid tests, which differentiate between the two organisms. Detection of HPV via cervical swabs is an important tool for controlling cervical cancer, which is fully preventable if detected and treated early.[4] The US Food and Drug Administration (FDA) has approved the combination of cervical cytology and HPV DNA testing for primary screening for women aged 30 years and older. Another significant application of nucleic acid testing is the detection of viral pathogens producing respiratory tract infections, which is particularly valuable in the rapid identification of potential outbreaks especially in pediatric patients as well as for patient management allowing for the appropriate use of antibiotic and antiviral drugs.

New directions in applications of molecular diagnostic tests for other infectious disease indications include those for West Nile Virus, *Clostridium difficile* (C-diff), methicillin-resistant *Staphylococcus aureus* (MRSA), respiratory syncytial virus, influenza, pneumonia, *Trichomonas vaginalis*, genital mycoplasma, herpes simplex virus, norovirus, rotavirus, tuberculosis, and meningitis. Of particular interest is the diagnosis of nosocomial infections, or hospital-acquired infections (HAIs), where rapid detection and typing to determine drug susceptibility are finding high value in early detection and intervention.

13.4. CRITICAL ROLE OF TRANSLATIONAL RESEARCH

The goal of translational research is to facilitate the implementation of advances in basic research and development in useful clinical applications. The translation of new scientific discoveries into practical applications requires close interaction between researchers, test kit manufacturers, regulatory agencies, and clinicians in the field. Accurate and informative feedback from the clinician/laboratory technician is critical to a successful implementation strategy. Effective, reiterative communication between researcher, developer, user and regulator is required to ensure rigorous implementation of new technology and stimulate continual progress and innovation. Translational research is a powerful process that continues to drive clinical innovation and stimulate new technological discoveries, bringing to fruition effective and efficient applications of new technological advancements to clinical practice and improved patient care. This chapter will discuss several key considerations in translational research in molecular diagnosis of infectious disease. It will illustrate concepts of clinical validation to meet regulatory requirements, adaptations to various sample types, complications of increased multiplexing for simultaneous detection of multiple analytes, and challenges of utilizing the power of sequence identification to elucidate subtype diversity in infectious agents, variations in pathogenicity, and identification of mutations leading to resistance to antimicrobial drugs.

13.5. BLOOD-BORNE INFECTIONS — MEETING CLIA REQUIREMENTS

Qualitative nucleic acid assays provide a powerful tool for identifying early acute infection and for screening blood products for the presence of infectious agent even before antibody levels develop.[5] HIV antibody tests are not effective in identifying infection within the first four weeks post virus exposure and well after that time. Detectable levels of viral nucleic acids develop very early in infection and provide more useful indicators of early HIV infection than the antibody tests currently used, which may remain negative for weeks or months after initial infection.[6–8] Qualitative assays for sensitive detection of HIV nucleic acids are manufactured by Roche Molecular Systems, Chiron and Gen-Probe and are used in blood screening to ensure the safety of the blood supply, and as supplementary tests in diagnosis.

Quantitative detection of viruses in blood such as HIV, HBV and HCV is used for evaluating progression of infection and monitoring for efficacy of antiviral therapeutics.[9,10] Commercially available assays for quantitative detection of HIV nucleic acids in plasma include the Roche AmpliPrep/COBAS TaqMan v2.0, the Abbott m200, and the Siemens bDNA v3.0 assays, and the bioMérieux NucliSENS nucleic acid sequence-based amplification (NASBA). As additional versions of these assays and assays from other manufacturers are being developed, laboratories will need to evaluate and validate their usage in their operations before they can be implemented for clinical use. The extensive diversity and rapid evolution of HIV pose serious challenges for maintaining reliable serologic and nucleic acid tests (NAT) for blood screening, epidemiological surveillance, diagnosis and clinical management of infected persons.[11] Different test manufacturers target different HIV genes in their nucleic acid tests for screening and quantitative HIV RNA determinations, with varying degrees of success in correctly identifying or quantifying emerging isolates.[12]

Design and implementation of nucleic acid assays used in diagnostics must follow strict design, development and validation guidelines to ensure their proper performance. Guidelines for verification of diagnostic assays are provided by the Clinical and Laboratory Standards Institute (CLSI) and the FDA and include those for both qualitative and quantitative assays.[13,14] The required quality assurance guidelines are detailed in national standards for which compliance is mandated to achieve legislated accreditation. Kit manufacturers must control all steps in the manufacture of kit components, instrumentation and software associated with the test, which goes through a thorough review by the FDA in the US[15] or the European Commission (EC)[16] in Europe prior to release.

In addition, prior to implementation, each laboratory is required to conduct careful performance evaluation before a diagnostic assay can be used for clinical applications. These requirements cover a broad range of issues ranging from specimen processing, kit and instrumentation validation, training of technicians, participation in proficiency programs and quality assurance guidelines. A verification/validation program must be instituted and the validation analyses documented to meet acceptable criteria prior to approval of reporting of test results for patient management. Once a test is implemented, the ongoing performance must be carefully monitored, and problems documented, to ensure the quality of results is maintained. Verifying the performance specification of FDA-cleared or

Table 1 Quality Assurance Parameters that Must be Controlled and Evaluated to Ensure Proper Performance of Nucleic Acid Tests

Verification	Monitoring
Accuracy	Collection, transport and storage
Robustness	Sample suitability
Precision	Negative and weak positive controls
Reproducability	Calibrators (high, medium and low)
Limit of Detection	Laboratory design, air and work flow
Limit of Quantitation	Method validation
Linear Range	Equipment performance
Sensitivity	Staff competency
Specificity	Record keeping
Diagnostic relevance	Proficiency Testing

-approved tests is required by CLIA regulations prior to implementing patient testing. Before introducing new nucleic acid tests, the laboratory must conduct studies to provide evidence of assay accuracy, precision and reportable range. Well-characterized plasma samples are essential for obtaining reliable data to support assay performance verifications. Validation bodies such as the CLIA agencies in each state or the College of American Pathologists (CAP) can provide proficiency testing panels and certification services to verify that the performance of nucleic acid tests meets regulatory requirements. A summary of some of the considerations that must be met is provided in Table 1.

Examples of verification tests conducted in the laboratory for the introduction of the Roche Amplicor HIV, HBV and HCV quantitative nucleic acid tests prior to implementation of a commercial nucleic acid assay are discussed in the following sections. Panels of well-characterized clinical samples and controls obtained from commercial sources or from previously tested materials in the laboratory were used for this verification process.

13.5.1. Accuracy

Verification of accuracy of a new quantitative HIV RNA assay (Roche TaqMan® v2.0) was accomplished by comparing results of tests on reference

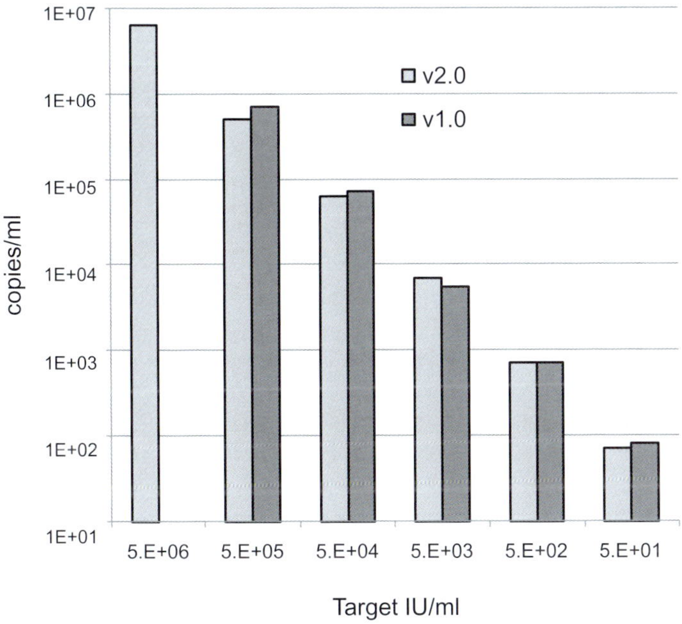

Fig. 1. Evaluation of assay accuracy. A series of controls at different levels of virus quantitation were run on both the new assay and a previously validated predecessor assay to demonstrate performance equivalence.

materials against the results of a previously validated method. The quantitative equivalence of the new method relative to an established method on positive sample material over a range of concentrations was demonstrated by running a series of different level Accurun controls (Sera-Care Life Sciences) on both the new assay (Roche TaqMan v2.0) and the predecessor assay (Roche TaqMan v1.0). As shown in Fig. 1, the performance of the new assay corresponds closely to that of the previously validated assay with coefficient of variation greater than 95 percent. The new assay was also shown to extend the linear range from 50 to above 5,000,000 copies of HIV-1 RNA.

13.5.2. Precision

The precision of the new Roche HIV TaqMan (v2.0) assay was demonstrated by running replicate samples of low and medium viral load control

Table 2 Precision Evaluation of the Roche HIV TaqMan v2.0 Assay

	Mean	SD	%CV	CI	−95% CI	+95% CI
	538	134	24.9%	107	431	645
	873	265	30.4%	212	661	1,086
Series 200	722	309	42.8%	248	475	970
	600	129	21.5%	103	497	704
	703	154	21.9%	123	580	827
Avg	688	198	28.8%	159	529	846
	32,183	7,531	23.4%	6,026	26,157	38,210
	39,950	5,976	15.0%	4,782	35,168	44,732
Series 400	42,500	10,007	23.5%	8,007	34,493	50,507
	37,183	7,037	18.9%	5,631	31,553	42,814
	37,567	5,337	14.2%	4,270	33,296	41,837
Avg	37,877	7,178	19.0%	5,743	32,133	43,620

Replicate aliquots of a low and medium copy number control sample (Accurun 315 Series 200 and Series 400) were run in nine replicate determinations over five different runs and using three different technicians. The means were found to fall within the acceptable range 95 percent confidence interval set for the assay.

samples in multiple runs (three runs) by multiple test operators (three technicians). The assay performed with the present 95 percent confidence interval and was accepted as meeting the precision and reproducibility requirements for use in clinical samples (Table 2).

13.5.3. Linearity

The linear dynamic range of the assay of the Roche HBV TaqMan assay was evaluated in triplicate on a series of serially diluted samples ranging from 33 to 100,000,000 copies per milliliter. The samples at 100,000,000 copies/ml were off the scale on the assay, and thus out of the linear range (Table 3). Similarly, two of three replicate samples at 33 copies were not detected in this assay and were also deemed out of linear range. The remaining samples from 100–10,000,000 copies fell into a linear relationship to expected levels with greater than 0.95 coefficient of correlation, thus establishing the acceptable linear range for this assay.

Table 3 Evaluation of Linear Dynamic Range of the Roche HBV TaqMan Assay

	Roche TaqMan v1.0 Result						Avg/
	Run 1	Run 2	Run 3	Avg	Std Dev	%CV	Target
	> 1.10E + 8	> 1.10E + 8	> 1.10E + 8				
1.00E + 08	> 1.10E + 8	> 1.10E + 8	> 1.10E + 8	Out of Linear Range			
	> 1.10E + 8	> 1.10E + 8	> 1.10E + 8				
	1.34E + 07	2.44E + 07	2.09E + 07				
1.00E + 07	2.63E + 07	1.09E + 08	2.62E + 07	3.78E + 07	3.21E + 07	85%	378%
	2.24E + 07	7.49E + 07	2.28E + 07				
	6.08E + 05	9.27E + 05	1.06E + 06				
1.00E + 06	1.40E + 06	9.93E + 05	1.21E + 06	1.11E + 06	2.89E + 05	26%	111%
	1.61E + 06	9.74E + 05	1.17E + 06				
	1.21E + 04	1.27E + 04	1.46E + 04				
1.00E + 04	2.29E + 04	1.27E + 04	1.54E + 04	1.58E + 04	3.56E + 03	22%	158%
	1.98E + 04	1.60E + 04	1.64E + 04				
	1.51E + 03	1.70E + 03	1.58E + 03				
1.00E + 03	2.10E + 03	1.42E + 03	1.65E + 03	1.72E + 03	2.44E + 02	14%	172%
	2.13E + 03	1.68E + 03	1.67E + 03				
	1.43E + 02	1.11E + 02	1.62E + 02				
1.00E + 02	1.61E + 02	1.22E + 02	1.18E + 02	1.39E + 02	1.87E + 01	13%	139%
	1.46E + 02	1.39E + 02	1.53E + 02				
	5.32E + 01	< 2.90E + 1	4.17E + 01				
3.33E + 01	< 2.90E + 1	3.32E + 01	3.08E + 01	3.73E + 01	7.98E + 00	21%	112%
	3.14E + 01	3.72E + 01	3.33E + 01				

Three replicates of each of a series of serially diluted samples ranging from 33 to 100,000,000 copies/ml were run and the results analyzed. The samples between 100–10,000,000 copies gave on-scale quantitative results with a greater than 0.95 coefficient of correlation, thus establishing the acceptable linear range for this assay.

13.5.4. Subtype Specificity

The subtype specificity of the Roche TaqMan v2.0 assay was evaluated on a series of characterized HIV positive plasma samples from the US (subtype B) and South Africa (subtype C).[17] The quantitation obtained from the Roche TaqMan v2.0 assay was compared to that of the Abbott m2000, as well as the Roche Amplicor v1.5.[18–20] There was excellent agreement between all three assays when the US subtype B samples were evaluated, with a correspondence of greater than or equal to 0.95 coefficient of correlation (Fig. 2). The correspondence was less tight on the subtype C virus isolates, averaging around 0.85. When comparing just the Abbott m2000 and the

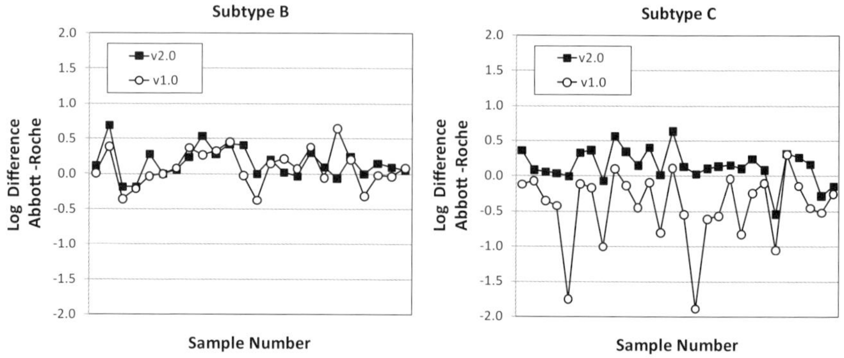

Fig. 2. Evaluation of subtype specificity of HIV Viral load assays. The ratio of the quantitative results of the Roche v1.0 and v2.0 to Abbott m2000 assays was evaluated on a series of clinical plasma samples from HIV infected individuals in the US (all Subtype B) and South Africa (all Subtype C). The Roche v1.0 showed similar results to the Abbott assay on subtype B samples, but underquantitated many of the Subtype C samples. The Roche v2.0 showed similar results to the Abbott on both Subtype B and C samples.

Roche v2.0, which were specifically designed to improve subtype specificity, all samples were within 0.5 log of one another and were deemed to be sufficiently similar to give reliable quantitation of subtype B and C viruses.

13.6. SEXUALLY TRANSMITTED INFECTIONS

Chlamydia trachomatis (CT) and *Neisseria gonorrhoeae* (NG) are the causative agents of the two most common sexually transmitted diseases worldwide, and are the leading causes of pelvic inflammatory disease (PID) and infertility. Whereas NG infection causes symptoms in most men, and approximately 50 percent of women, CT infections are generally asymptomatic in both men and women.[21] The high incidence rates of these infections and their associated morbidity have led public health authorities to recommend screening for CT and NG in all sexually active women at increased risk of infection and intensive behavioral counseling to reduce the risk of infection.[22] Rapid identification of infection is key to initiation of effective treatment and preventing further spread of infection.

Nucleic acid amplification tests (NAATs) are the most sensitive method for diagnosing chlamydia and gonorrhea. A vaginal swab, which can also be self-collected, is the specimen of choice for screening of CT/NG in women, although urine collection is also effective in either women or men, and allowed sensitive and specific detection of CT and NG in the Gen-Probe Aptima assays.[23] First-catch urine specimens and SurePath L-Pap test samples collected with a SurePath cervical broom or ThinPrep cytobrush were equally appropriate specimens for molecular testing.[24] Three FDA-cleared qualitative screening assays for CT and NG dominate the US market: Gen-Probe Aptima Combo 2 (Aptima), Roche Cobas Amplicor CT/NG (Amplicor), and Becton Dickinson ProbeTec ET CT and NG Amplified DNA (ProbeTec).

13.6.1. Evaluation of CT/NG Molecular Assay Performance

Since CT/NG molecular assays are qualitative assays designed for sensitive detection of the infectious agent in swab or urine samples, we wanted to evaluate the relative sensitivity of the various assays for these organisms and ensure adequate stability of infectious agent in the various collection formats. The concentration at the positive cutoff for Aptima, Amplicor and ProbeTec CT/NG assays was determined by testing multiple replicates of a dilution series of cultured CT Elementary Bodies (CT EB) and NG cells. A laboratory-developed TaqMan PCR assay for CT and NG was then used to confirm differing CT and NG analyte content and initiate validation of the three new independent, low positive CT/NG controls for the three qualitative platforms.[25]

The results of testing serial dilutions of the cultured organisms with all three assays are shown in Table 4. Although the sensitivities of the assays varied significantly, all assays reproducibly detected 2,500 copies (cells) or more of the respective organism, with some assays reaching an extremely high sensitivity of 5–10 copies of the infectious agent in a sample. The relative sensitivities at 50 percent and 95 percent confidence intervals were calculated and are shown in Table 5.

The CT/NG assays claim to be suitable for testing either urine or swab samples. The clinical performance of the Roche COBAS Amplicor 4800

Table 4 Comparative Analytical Sensitivities of Three Commercial Assays for CT/NG

	Chlamydia trachomatis % Positive				*Neisseria gonorrhoea* % Positive		
EB/mL	Gen-Probe Aptima	Roche COBAS	BD ProbeTec	Cells/mL	Gen-Probe Aptima	Roche COBAS	BD ProbeTec
0.1	0%	0%	0%	0.1	0%	33%	0%
1	0%	0%	0%	1	0%	67%	0%
5	0%	0%	0%	5	0%	100%	17%
10	100%	17%	8%	10	0%	100%	50%
25	100%	33%		25	0%	100%	67%
50	100%	67%	17%	50	0%	100%	100%
125	100%	100%	33%	125	25%	100%	100%
250	100%	100%		250	50%	100%	100%
625	100%	100%	50%	625	100%	100%	100%
1250	100%	100%	89%	1250	100%	100%	100%
2500	100%	100%	100%	2500	100%	100%	100%
5000	100%	100%	100%	5000	100%	100%	100%

The lowest theoretical concentrations yielding 100 percent positive results for CT and NG using Aptima, Amplicor and ProbeTec were determined. The difference in concentrations for CT and NG equals or exceeds 10-fold. Aptima is most sensitive for CT, but least sensitive for NG. ProbeTec is least sensitive for CT and Amplicor most sensitive for NG.

Table 5 Sensitivity of Three Commercial Assays for CT and NG at 50 percent and 95 percent Confidence Intervals

	Chlamydia trachomatis		*Neisseria gonorrhoeae*	
Assay	50% CI	95% CI	50% CI	95% CI
Gen-Probe Aptima	3	10	250	625
Roche Amplicor	38	75	1	3
BD ProbeTec	625	2500	10	50

CT/NG test to detect CT/NG in both urine and swab was evaluated in 210 sexually active women.[26] As summarized in Table 6, the performance of these tests on urine samples demonstrated similar sensitivity and specificity to those of cervical and urethral swab samples. Thus, the CT/NG assays have

Table 6 Performance of c4800 System for Detection of CT/NG in Swab and Urine Specimens

	C4800Swabs				
Specimen Type	Test Result	Pos	Neg	Sensitivity	Specificity
Chlamydia trachomatis	Pos	28	0	96.6%	100%
Urine (N = 210)	Neg	1	179		
Neisseria gonorrhoeae	Pos	16	0	100%	100%
Urine (N = 210)	Neg	0	192		

an extremely high sensitivity for both organisms and work equally well on swab and urine samples.

13.7. HUMAN PAPILLOMA VIRUS TESTING

Another commonly tested sexually transmitted disease is HPV. The presence of certain types (most commonly 16 and 18) of HPV in the female genital tract is a risk factor for cervical cancer.[27,28] Although HPV cannot be cultured, the virus can be readily detected by molecular assays, and tests for HPV DNA have been widely used in clinical labs. Most clinical laboratories perform the test using swab or brush samples immersed in a transport medium. Since this is a qualitative assay on virus infected cells, we wanted to determine the sensitivity of the assay. Serial dilutions of cultured SiHa cells, which contain 1–2 copies of integrated HPV 16 genome, were prepared in PreservCyt and tested using the Hybrid Capture 2 (HC2) HPV DNA (Digene Corporation).[29] The results of the PreservCyt dilutions are shown in Fig. 3. The HC2 assay was capable of detecting as few as 1,000 HPV infected cells.

The subtype specificity of the HC2 assay was evaluated in various diluents. Full length HPV genomes corresponding to the most common high-cancer-risk types of HPV (type 16, 18, 31 and 11) were generated synthetically and used to transfect human epithelial cells. Transfected cells containing approximately 5,000 genomes were mixed with 500,000 uninfected cells and diluted in PreservCyt or SurePath diluent to resemble an actual clinical specimen representing each of the respective genomes. The samples were tested in the HC2 assays and the results are shown in Table 7.

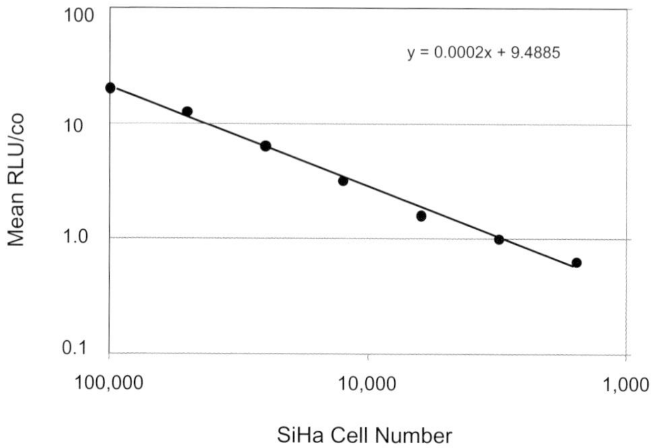

Fig. 3. Sensitivity of Digene HC2 assay for detection of HPV infected cells. Serial dilutions of SiHa cells, which contain 1–2 copies of the HPV genome were diluted in PreservCyt and tested via the HC2 assay. The RLU/CO signal generated was proportional to the number of cells present and was capable of detecting fewer than 1,000 copies of the virus per sample.

Table 7 The Digene HC2 Assay was Capable of Detecting All Major HPV High-risk Subtypes in Either SurePath or PreservCyt Diluent

HPV Subtype	Diluent	N	Mean RLU/co	Std Deviation	%CV
HPV 16	PreservCyt	8	21.4	1.33	6.2%
	SurePath	8	15.2	1.28	8.4%
HPV 18	PreservCyt	8	28.8	2.42	8.4%
HPV 31	SurePath	3	32.3	3.31	10.2%
HPV 11	PreservCyt	8	11.6	1.06	9.2%
	SurePath	8	20.5	2.35	11.4%

The assay successfully detected each of the major high-risk subtypes, and the results from the two diluents were equivalent.

Additional studies were conducted to determine the stability of the virus in cells when preserved in either SurePath or PreservCyt diluent.[30] Replicate samples were generated and subjected to different temperature or freeze–thaw stress conditions. As shown in Figs. 4 and 5, the samples retained positive reactivity throughout the 65-day accelerated stability

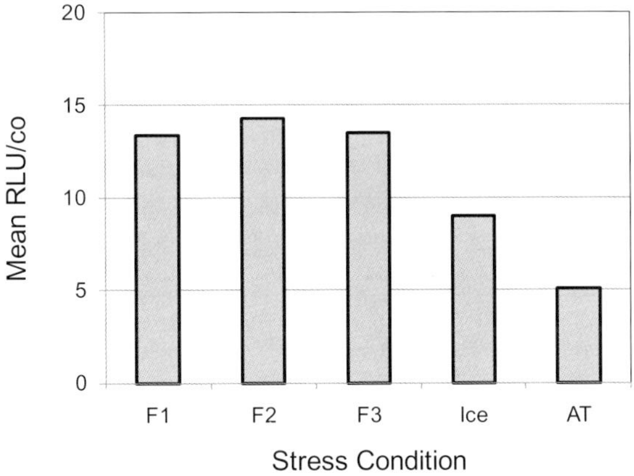

Fig. 4. Stability study by repeated freeze–thaw and shipping. The Digene HC2 assay results showed HPV positive responses for all the samples with similar RLU/CO ratios observed within each set, suggesting the control will be stable during shipping with or without ice packs and remain stable for at least three freeze–thaw cycles. F1, F2 and F3 indicate one, two and three freeze–thaw treatments, respectively. Ice indicates shipping with ice packs and AT indicates shipping at ambient temperature.

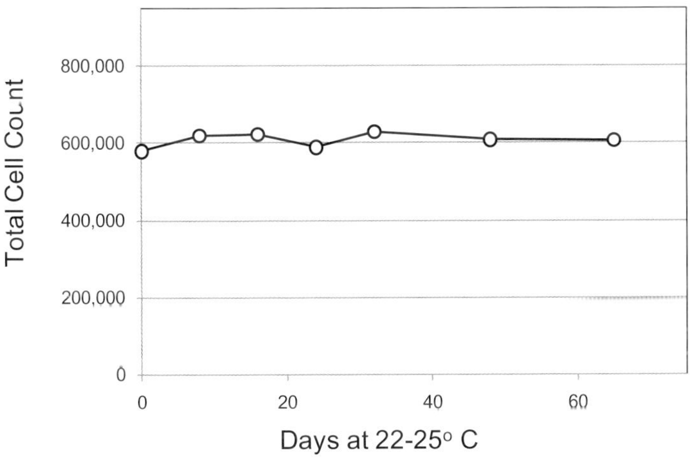

Fig. 5. Stability study at 22–25°C. Digene HC2 assay results showed that all test samples diluted in PreservCyt maintained HPV positive responses with similar HPV DNA signals, suggesting the virus is stable at room temperature for up to two months.

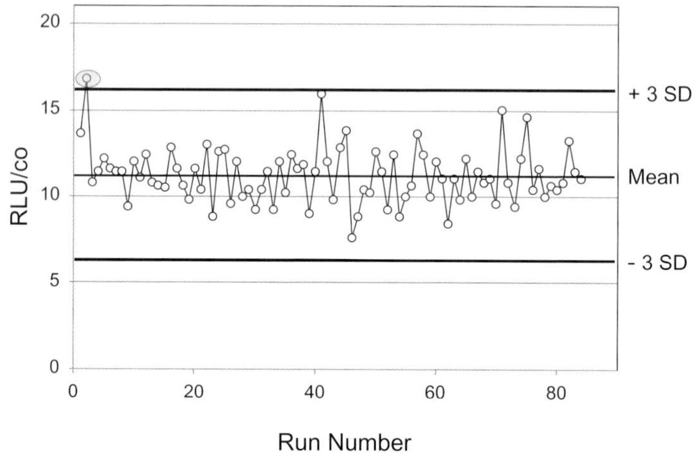

Fig. 6. Levey–Jennings chart of intra-assay performance of the Digene HC2 test on multiple aliquots of the HPV DNA control over 85 different runs. RLU/CO stays within the required limit of three standard deviation limit in all but one run (Run #2), and centers around the mean value with no observable drift in either direction.

study with RLU/CO remaining within a half log of original signal intensity. In addition, all cells remained intact during the 65-day testing period. Freeze–thaw had no effect, with no change in RLU/CO for 1, 2 or 3 freeze–thaw cycles.

The reproducibility of the HC2 assay was also evaluated by running the same control specimens repeatedly over 85 separate runs as a run control. The intra-assay performance of the control was very consistent over this time period with RLU/CO staying within three standard deviations of the mean over the entire study (Fig. 6).

13.8. MOLECULAR DIAGNOSIS VIRAL RESPIRATORY INFECTIONS

Acute respiratory tract infections (ARTIs) are a significant cause of global human morbidity and mortality, particularly in infants, the elderly and immunocompromised patients.[31,32] The most common infections are due to influenza virus and respiratory syncytial virus (RSV), which account for an estimated 325,000 hospitalizations in the US annually.[33] Parainfluenza virus (PIV), human metapneumovirus (hMPV) and adenoviruses (ADV) can cause respiratory disease that is clinically indistinguishable from illness caused by influenza and RSV. Respiratory infections often present with common symptoms such as headache, sore throat, cough, runny nose, chills and coryza, making it difficult to differentiate between infections of viral, bacterial or fungal origins. The rapid, sensitive and specific identification of causative agent(s) of respiratory tract infections is important for proper patient care management, allowing for appropriate decisions for initiation or discontinuation of antivirals and antibiotics, admittance for hospitalization, and taking appropriate infection control measures to reduce nosocomial transmission within healthcare facilities. Rapid respiratory virus diagnosis can lead to significant reduction of total healthcare costs and may include up to a 50 percent reduction in hospital days, a 30 percent reduction in antibiotic use, and a 20 percent reduction in unnecessary diagnostic tests and procedures.[34,35] Moreover, while approximately 75–80 percent of respiratory tract diseases are of viral origin, approximately 55 percent of the 41 million antibiotic prescriptions in the US each year are prescribed for causes unlikely to have a bacterial etiology.[36–38] Several therapies are currently available for the treatment of viral respiratory infections, including influenza A, influenza B, cytomegalovirus pneumonia, and varicella-zoster virus pneumonia, and new drugs continue to be developed.

ARTIs can be caused by bacteria and fungi, but viral infections are most common. Common viral agents of acute respiratory infections may include influenza virus, PIV, ADV, picornavirus (PIC, including rhinovirus and enterovirus), RSV, hMPV, and human coronavirus (HCoV).[39]

The principal methods of diagnosis of respiratory virus infections include virus culture, serology, immunofluorescence/antigen detection, and nucleic acid/PCR-based tests. Traditional culture methods for diagnosis of respiratory virus, although highly sensitive, are often unable to provide results in a timely manner to meaningfully impact patient management. Clinicians have been moving toward more rapid tests such as direct fluorescent antibody (DFA) testing (30–60 min) and rapid cell culture (24–48 hr).[40] These tests work reasonably well on pediatric samples, since children have much higher titers of virus and for longer time periods than adults, but are less useful for testing the elderly or patients with chronic obstructive pulmonary disease.[41,42] Rapid antigen direct tests

(RADTs) — frequently used because of their low cost, ease of use and short time to results — have highly variable sensitivities (10–75 percent) and specificities (50–100 percent) depending on the viral target, age of the patient, sample collection, and duration of symptoms prior to testing.[43] The low sensitivity and specificity of culture and serological assays lead to frequent misdiagnosis of true infections.

Nucleic acid tests (NATs) can be used to detect pathogens that are not easily cultured (e.g., hMPV, bocavirus and parainfluenza virus 4) or are too dangerous to culture (e.g., severe acute respiratory syndrome coronavirus, SARS). Nucleic acid tests are significantly more sensitive than the other available methods, and results can be obtained much faster than with culture.[44] Appropriate specimens for molecular testing of respiratory infection include sputa and nasal swabs, nasopharyngeal swabs, nasopharyngeal aspirates, throat swabs, and bronchoalveolar lavages. NATs provide fast, accurate and sensitive detection of respiratory viruses in clinical specimens and have led to improved understanding of the epidemiology of new emerging viruses such as the pandemic H1N1 influenza virus of 2009, and conventional viruses such as the common cold viruses, including rhinovirus and coronavirus.[45] An important advantage of nucleic acid testing is the ability for multiplexing to allow rapid simultaneous detection of many viruses. A variety of molecular assays are now available to detect viral respiratory tract infection, and new assays continue to be added.[46] These assays utilize nasal and throat swab samples from adult or pediatric patients for detection of the most common respiratory infections, including influenza A and B, RSV, PIV 1–4, ADV, HCoV and hMPV, and can provide highly sensitive and specific results within a few hours.[40,47]

Many manufacturers now provide FDA-cleared assays for diagnosis of respiratory virus infections, particularly for detection of influenza A and B.[48,49] The assays available from the CDC, Focus Technologies, Gen-Probe, Idaho Technologies, Quidel and Qiagen/Artus are high complexity assays requiring highly trained technicians and can be completed in about four hours. Cepheid and IQuum have developed fully self-contained, moderate complexity assays that can be run on a single sample at a time with results in 20–60 minutes. The Cepheid GeneXpert and GeneSTAT incorporate all the steps in the test process in a single test cartridge and have random-access sample-in, result-out reporting to enable laboratories of all sizes to perform rapid, accurate and sensitive molecular diagnostic testing.[50]

An important advantage of molecular assays is their ability to amplify, detect and differentiate between multiple targets simultaneously, and several FDA-cleared multiplex assays are now available for simultaneous detection of multiple respiratory viruses in the same sample.[51] These assays utilize a variety of different amplification and detection platforms to allow automated or semi-automated application of nucleic acid testing, including consolidation of multiple processing steps on a single test platform for streamlined operation in standard clinical use. Table 8 provides a list of FDA-cleared multiplex tests capable of detecting various respiratory viruses in a single assay.

The first widely used multiplex platform for molecular detection of respiratory viruses, the Luminex xTAG Respiratory Virus Panel (Luminex Molecular Diagnostics), can test many samples at a time in a centralized laboratory and can test for 12 viruses or subtypes in a single sample. Nasopharyngeal swab samples collected from persons symptomatic for a respiratory virus infection are used to detect adenovirus, influenza A (A/H1 and A/H3), influenza B, PIV-1, PIV-2, PIV-3, hMPV, rhinovirus, RSV A, and RSV B.[49] The xTAG RVP takes approximately 8–10 hours to complete, depending on the number of samples to be tested. Viral nucleic acids are extracted from clinical samples using the QIAamp MiniElute (Qiagen), easyMAG (bioMérieux) or miniMAG (bioMérieux) extraction platforms, and multiple primers and probes are used to amplify specific target sequences for each virus. The amplicons are labeled with a fluorescent probe and hybridized to color-coded beads to differentiate which target was amplified. Two lasers read each bead; the first identifies the virus-specific color-coded bead, and the second detects the associated fluorescence above a background threshold. Results can be obtained within 8–10 hours and provide excellent sensitivity and specificity for the designated targets.[52] A major advantage of the xTAG RVP assay is the broad spectrum of viruses that can be detected by a single test. However, it does have some limitations, such as decreased sensitivity for certain virus strains, time to final results, number of required steps, technical hands-on time, and a potential for amplicon contamination.

Table 8 FDA-Approved or -Cleared Tests for Multiplex Detection of Respiratory Pathogens

Test name	Manufacturer	Gene Target
Prodesse ProFlu1	Gen-Probe	Influenza A, B, Respiratory Syncitial Virus
xTAG Respiratory Virus Panel (RVP)	Luminex Molecular Diagnostics, Inc.	Influenza A, B, Human Metapneumovirus, Respiratory Syncitial Virus A, B, parainfluenza-1,2, and 3 virus, adenovirus, rhinovirus
x-TAG Respiratory Viral Panel Fast (RVP FAST)	Luminex Molecular Diagnostics, Inc.	Influenza A, B, Human Metapneumovirus, Respiratory Syncitial Virus, adenovirus, rhinovirus
Verigene RespiratoryVirus Nucleic Acid Test	Nanosphere, Inc.	Influenza A, B, Respiratory Syncitial Virus A, B
Verigene RespiratoryVirus Plus Nucleic Acid Test (RV+)	Nanosphere, Inc.	Influenza A, B, Respiratory Syncitial Virus A, B
Simplexa Flu A/B and Respiratory Syncitial Virus	Focus Diagnositcs 3M	Influenza A, B, Respiratory Syncitial Virus
FilmArray Resporatory Panel	Idaho Technologies	Influenza A, B, Human Metapneumovirus, Respiratory Syncitial Virus, PIV-1, 2, 3 and 4, adenovirus, rhinovirus/enterovirus, Coronavirus HKU1, NL63

The Gen-Probe/Prodesse assays reduce the number of steps and handling required, with overall time to results of 4.5–5.5 hours. Automated nucleic acid extraction can be performed on the MagNA Pure LC Instrument (Roche Diagnostics Corp) or the NucliSENS easyMAG system and the Automated Magnetic Extraction Reagents (bio-Mérieux) followed by amplification on the TaqMan SMART Cycler. Multiple SmartCycler instruments can be run simultaneously, giving run size flexibility, and the closed system configuration minimizes risk of amplicon contamination. This assay allows the clinician to mix and match the panel of viruses for testing, allowing greater flexibility. However, a disadvantage is that at most three targets plus an internal control can be run in a single reaction, such that a comprehensive viral diagnostic panel requires multiple amplifications, which add to the time and cost.

The automated Verigene Respiratory Virus Nucleic Acid Test (VRNATsp) (Nanosphere) is a moderately complex test that can be used to detect influenza A and B, and RSV A and B. The Verigene System consists of two instruments (the fully automated Verigene Processor and the Verigene Reader) and single-use test cartridges, which require minimum technical hands-on time, with sample-to-result turnaround time of about 3.5 hours. For this assay, gold nanoparticles containing a high density of sequence-specific oligonucleotides are hybridized to the target and captured on magnetic microparticles (MMPs). Target specific amplicons are captured on a solid substrate (microarray) and labeled with silver-coated gold nanoparticle probes. A light-scattering technique is used to generate a measurable signal, which is detected by the Verigene Reader.

The FilmArray system has the highest multiplexity, with 15 viruses or subtypes, and has a fast turnaround time. This assay handles one sample at a time and may be appropriate for Point of Care testing.

Another important advantage of multiplex testing is the ability to detect dual or multiple infections, which can occur in anywhere from 3 to 20 percent of patients.[52] These tests also allow monitoring of the epidemiologic patterns of respiratory disease and identification of new or re-emerging pathogens. The correct identification of respiratory viruses is also valuable for the evaluation of the efficacy of vaccines. As new antiviral therapeutic agents are being developed, accurate diagnostic tools to identify each virus are needed to guide the rapid implementation of appropriate antiviral therapy and for use in clinical trials to validate the performance of the antiviral therapies as new therapeutic agents.[53] Nucleic acid tests are rapidly fulfilling that need.

Despite the many successes of current molecular assays for respiratory viruses, many challenges remain. The current FDA-approved/-cleared NAATs are useful for detection of the most common viruses, but they miss the atypical pneumonia pathogens. As new viruses or strains emerge, these may not be picked up by existing assays. Laboratories must decide whether to go for a limited number of targets (generally up to three), which provides flexibility and entails lower cost, or more highly multiplex tests (10 or more organisms), which provide more information but are more costly and typically require more technical steps and additional time to result reporting. The selection of the most appropriate panels to run should take into consideration the age of the patient, clinical status, underlying disease, state of immune competence, and the suspected virus(es).

The very high sensitivity of qualitative NAATs has led to concerns that they cannot distinguish between live and dead organisms and therefore, depending on the time for nucleic acid clearance, can continue to give positive signals even after the infection has cleared. In cases with multiple viral infections, determining the relevance of each virus present in the sample is difficult, because any residual virus detected may have been from a previous infection and may not be contributing to the current illness. The very high sensitivity of nucleic acid tests has also raised concerns about possible over-interpretation of positive nucleic acid tests in children. Some studies have shown positive nucleic acid tests for a virus in as much as 41 percent of children without any respiratory symptoms.[54]

Several guidelines for testing of respiratory viruses have been issued and should be considered in implementations of any new respiratory assay.[55] For optimum utility in patient management, tests should be available within a day of sample collection, and preferably within several hours if at all possible. Thus, batching of samples may not be practical for many hospitals, and platforms that allow random access, single sample testing may be beneficial for such applications. Decisions need to be made as to whether it would it be beneficial to select specific panels for targeted risk conditions, such as special risk factors, unusual or severe symptoms, seasonal variations, or possibilities of outbreaks. Complex panels can add to cost, decrease sensitivity, and complicate validations.

Many respiratory viruses demonstrate seasonal variations in prevalence, such that RSV is generally detected from November through March, influenza virus between December and April, and hMPV between December and May in the US. However, with global travel, many "seasonal" viruses are now detected throughout the year, and failure to test off-season can result in missing an important outbreak, such as the 2009 influenza A virus H1N1 pandemic in the US, which began in April 2009 and continued throughout the summer months.

Despite the very high sensitivities and specificities of FDA-cleared molecular assays, interpretations of results need to be taken in the context of the patient's symptoms, risk factors, and potential outbreaks in the community. False negative results can occur due to improper or poor clinical specimen collection, from poor handling of a specimen after collection and before testing, or if the specimen is collected when the patient is no longer shedding detectable virus. Some molecular assays may not specifically identify all currently circulating influenza A virus subtypes. Depending on the test, a negative result for one influenza A virus subtype may not preclude infection with another influenza A virus subtype.

Conversely, a positive result indicates detection of viral RNA, but does not necessarily mean viable virus is present or that the patient is contagious. An influenza positive result can occur in patients who recently received intranasal administration of live attenuated influenza vaccine (LAIV) and it may be possible to detect LAIV strains up to seven days after vaccination.

13.9. SEQUENCE-BASED MOLECULAR DIAGNOSTICS

New molecular assays based on actual genetic sequence analysis are increasingly being used in clinical laboratory applications. Examples of uses for gene sequencing analysis range from prenatal diagnosis to early cancer detection, prognosis, treatment selection and monitoring treatment responses. Sequence based genetic tests are also used to identify patients' genomic variants that affect drug metabolism, drug disposition, and off-site drug targets, which is beyond the scope of this review.[56] Various instruments can perform gene sequencing, though the interpretation of the results can be complex, especially in view of new resistance genes and additional mutations continuously being discovered.

An important application in sequence based diagnostics is HIV drug resistance testing.[58–61] HIV exists in infected individuals as a complex mixture of quasispecies in which many different subpopulations of drug-resistant variants persist in latently infected cells.[62,63] Some of the resistant species are not infectious and require co-infection with a helper virus for proliferation. Other resistant subsets remain dormant in infected tissues and are undetectable in blood, but can be activated after drug treatments.

Phenotypic assays can detect resistant species but are very complex, time consuming and expensive to use. Another difficulty is mutations that cause resistance to more than one drug, or mutations that infer resistance but have not yet been adequately described. Currently, existing assays do not detect resistance to integrase inhibitors or other newly available drugs. This review will focus on the current status of HIV drug resistance testing and the future directions of next-generation sequencing technology in virology diagnosis and monitoring. Clinical laboratories are constantly being challenged for developing, validating and implementing new assays to support HIV patient care.

13.9.1. HIV Drug Resistance Testing for Patient Care

The use of drug resistance testing has become an integral part of HIV clinical care. HIV infection is no longer viewed as a fatal illness, but as a manageable chronic condition in which viral resistance must be closely monitored during the course of treatment. The first clinical description of HIV resistance to antiviral drugs was reported more than 20 years ago. Accumulation of mutations within the reverse transcriptase gene in patients taking zidovudine resulted in a marked increase in drug resistance.[57] As new drugs are developed, new strains of viruses resistant to these drugs are also appearing.[60–63] To date, 36 antiviral products have been approved by the FDA for the treatment of HIV infection. These include 13 nucleoside analog reverse transcriptase inhibitors (NRTIs), six non-nucleoside reverse transcriptase inhibitors (NNRTIs), 11 protease inhibitors (PIs), one fusion inhibitor, one integrase inhibitor and one CCR5 co-receptor antagonist, plus three multiclass combination products. Nearly 50 percent of patients undergoing antiretroviral therapy are infected with virus resistant to one or more antiretroviral drugs. Even in treatment-naive patients, resistance prevalence is between 14 and 23 percent.

The molecular basis of HIV drug resistance is the inherent high mutation rate of HIV associated with the infidelity of HIV reverse transcriptase, which leads to rapid evolution of diverse quasispecies in viral populations even prior to the introduction of antiviral treatment.[64–68] A high viral load during the course of treatment is the consequence of incomplete suppression of viral replication with selected resistant strains or the introduction of a new mutation in the HIV genome, leading to the development of new drug resistant strains. Sequence based information of drug resistance and quantitation provides valuable data to allow clinicians to select and adjust effective antiviral regimens such as specific drug combinations, appropriate drug dosage and duration for effective management of HIV infections.

13.9.2. Selection of Laboratory Tests for Drug Resistance

Drug resistance testing can be classified into phenotypic and genotypic assays. Phenotypic resistance assays are based on the quantitative assessment of viral replication in cell cultures under the selective pressure of increasing concentrations of specific antiretroviral drugs. The testing procedure begins with extraction of HIV RNA from the patient's plasma followed by reverse transcription and amplification of targets by PCR, such as reverse transcriptase (RT) and protease (PR) fragments. The amplified DNA of interest, as well as normal controls, is then inserted into an RT/PR deficient vector. The replication of both recombinant forms in cell culture is measured under different concentrations of antiretroviral drugs.[68–70] Phenotypic assays are not widely used due to their high cost, great complexity and long turnaround time. The clinical utility of phenotypic assays in guiding therapy has also been questioned due to its limited sensitivity and specificity.[71–73]

Genotypic assays for drug resistance are based on identification of sequence mutations associated with resistance to specific antiviral drugs.[74,75] The sequencing-based genotypic assays start with HIV RNA extraction from the patient's plasma, followed by reverse transcription and PCR amplification of RT, PR or other selected target of the viral genome. The amplified fragments are then sequenced by the Sanger sequencing procedure and compared to the wild-type reference sequence via software tools to identify the mutations associated with drug resistance. Two FDA-approved tests for HIV drug resistance are TruGene from Siemens and ViroSeq from Abbott. Several commercial testing services use these FDA-cleared assays or alternative "research use only" HIV drug resistance assays such as VircoType, GeneSeq and GenoSure. "Home-brew" methods are also sometimes used in CLIA laboratories for patient diagnostics following appropriate assay validations.

Home-brew assays are popular due to their relatively low cost and their specific adaptability to the selected subtypes or local populations studied. However, such assays can only be implemented after adequate validation, including evaluating the assay's performance with various HIV-1 drug resistant isolates, subtype panels and circulating recombinant forms, as well as the use of sequence calling software and databases. Laboratory testing quality is dependent on many factors including manufacture source of assay kit or key reagents; specimen collection, handling, storage and processing; sequencing platform; automated versus manual laboratory operations; heterozygosity of sequences; viral subtypes; sequence calling software and databases; and level of experience of technicians and laboratory directors undertaking the analysis and data reporting.[76,77] Depending on the laboratory's expertise and access to bioinformatics support, various sequence alignment software is used to generate resistance reports, including commercial software such as Siemens' OpenGene and home-brew databases and programs.[78,79] Some laboratories rely on the available software and HIV databases from government or university sites, such as Los Alamos National Laboratory (*www.hiv.lanl.gov*), Stanford University (*http://hivdb.stanford.edu*) and the Max Planck Institute (*www.geno2pheno.org*). Only those mutations that have been clinically proven to cause drug resistance can be reported for diagnostic use. Mutations that have not been previously described and validated must be reported as reference information for research use only. Rigorous quality control programs for validation and monitoring performance in testing laboratories must be implemented and maintained to control false positive or negative rates. Internal and external controls and testing calibrators must be used in each run to control for specimen processing, sequencing and reporting. Laboratories must adhere to regular proficiency testing using known mutant strains, and database and software should be checked and updated routinely. A strict QA/QC program must be implemented and documented to ensure that all laboratory processes, sequencing, interpretation and resistance reporting meet the highest quality standards and are in compliance with CLIA or CAP regulations.

13.10. NEXT-GENERATION SEQUENCING FOR VIRAL DIAGNOSTICS AND FUTURE DIRECTIONS

Recent advances in nucleic acid sequencing technologies, chemistry, electronics, engineering and bioinformatics, referred to as next-generation sequencing (NGS), have driven a true revolution and opened new perspectives for viral diagnostic applications with significant increase in speed and throughput of generated sequencing data. NGS has provided promising new solutions for rapid, accurate, low-cost genotyping and drug resistance assays.[80–84]

The primary drawback in conventional sequencing tests is the limited testing sensitivity for detecting minor sequence variants and relevant mutations. In the case of TruGene or ViroSeq, a nucleotide mixture in any specific genome position can be detected only when the minor nucleotide is present in over 20 percent of the total virus population. The existing genotyping assays were designed for mutations involving RT or PR, but do not cover mutations involving the envelope, integrase or any of the regions outside of the targeted mutations in RT and PR. Current NGS technology is capable of sequencing a single genome copy and identifying minor nucleotide changes, even if it is present in less than one per cent of the population, overcoming many of the previous limitations with drug resistance genotyping assays. The improved sensitivity with minimal viral load (~1,000 copies/ml) will allow testing earlier in the drug escape timeline. Furthermore, identification of any mutation across the entire HIV genome is now achievable. NGS makes possible the investigation of previously inaccessible aspects of viral dynamics, such as studying the contribution of various viral reservoirs in the development of replicating infectious viruses, co-receptor usage in minority viral populations from different cell lineages, alterations in the virus that result in drug resistance, and the re-emergence of hidden genomes after ceasing drug treatment.[85–87]

The first next-generation high-throughput sequencing technology, the 454 FLX pyrosequencing platforms, now part of Roche, became available in 2005.[89–90] Many platforms are commercially available, including the Genome Analyzers from Illumina, SOLiD and Ion Torrent PGM from Life Technologies. Both Helicos and Pacific Biosciences released systems for genome sequencing without PCR amplification.[80–84,90–92] Although

Table 9 Next-Generation Sequencing Platforms for Potential Diagnostic Applications

Commercial Availability	Company (Platform)	Sequencing Technology/ Throughput/Running Time
In Market	Roche Diagnostics (454)	Pyrosequencing of template-laden beads prepared by emulsion PCR/0.7 Gb/1 day
	Life Technologies (SOLid)	Ligation for sequencing on beads on glass slide after emulsion PCR/30 Gb/1 week
	Illumina (HiSeq and MiSeq)	Sequencing by synthesis after Bridge PC R amplification and glass slide hybridization with fluorescently labeled reversible terminators/600 Gb/1 week for HiSeq; 1.5 Gb/1 day for MiSeq
	Life Technologies (Ion Torrent)	Semiconductor sensor arrays detect protons released by nucleotide addition with Emulsion PCR amplification/1 Gb/1 day
	Pacific Biosciences	Uses 'zero-mode wave guides' to optically detect real-time nucleotide addition/35 Gb/1 day
	Qiagen (MAX-Seq from IBS)	Sequencing by synthesis with fluorescently labeled reversible terminators/66 Gb/3 days
	Helicos Biosciences	Reversible terminators for sequencing through flow-cell hybridization without any amplification/35 Gb/1 day
Under Development	GenapSys	Electronic detection of thermal/pH changes accompanying nucleotide addition
	Genia	Pairing biological nanopores with semiconductor detection, Fluorescent tag-free for over 5 kb read
	GnuBio	Microfluidic system analyzes DNA nanodroplets with fluorescent primers
	LaserGen	Sequencing by synthesis with fluorescently labeled reversible terminators
	NABSys	Single-molecule analysis revealing genomic location of sequencing probes
	NobleGen Biosciences	Optical detection of 'expanded' DNA templates passing through synthetic pores
	Oxford Nanopore Technologies	Detects changes in current as DNA strands pass through protein nanopores
	Stratos Genomics	Optical sequencing of fluorescently labeled, synthetically expanded templates

sequencing chemistries and detection engineering are dramatically different, all NGS systems use one of two general approaches to assemble individual sequence reads into longer contiguous genomic sequences, the reference-based approach and the de novo assembly approach. The reference-based assembly approach involves mapping each read to a reference genome sequence, similar to conventional methods. The de novo assembly approach compares parallel sequence reads to each other and then overlaps sequences to build longer contiguous sequences.[93] In general sequence assembly, bioinformatics analysis and data reporting for resistant mutations are much more time-consuming than sample handling and sequencing themselves. As summarized in Table 9, this field is rapidly expanding, with novel and improved systems being continuously developed.

Selection of NGS platform is dependent not only underlying chemistries for sequencing, various label tags and sensors for signal detection, sample processing and running time, sequence length and maximum throughput, but also on project needs, genome complexity, laboratory expertise and available resources.[81–85] In general, NGS platforms with longer read lengths and capacity to test multiple samples in one reaction is more attractive for clinical applications. Challenges remain on how to adapt new technologies to viral diagnostics and drug resistance testing, particularly with the analysis and storage of the large amounts of data generated in comparison to conventional genotyping assays. The same principles for clinical laboratory validation as with conventional assays are applicable to NGS assays. As the technology advances, costs decrease and clinical applications become available, we should see smaller, faster and smarter NGS systems entering routine diagnostics laboratories, which in the future will lead not only to better drug regimen treatments for HIV infected patients, but to new understanding of the interaction between virus and host and to identification of new drug targets for individualized patient care.

13.11. CONCLUSION

The application of nucleic acid technology to viral diagnosis offers greater sensitivity, earlier detection, faster turnaround times, more accurate quantitation for staging of infection, and better targeted therapy than had previously been possible with serological or culture-based methods. New molecular targets continue to be discovered as advances in technological and analytical tools open up new opportunities for viral diagnostics. Molecular assays are increasingly being applied to a broader range of biological fluids and tissues, such as nasal secretions, bronchial samples, urine, saliva, buccal swabs, cerebrospinal fluid, whole blood or blood cells, cervical swabs and other mucosal tissues, to allow for better targeted detection of infectious disease at its source. New classes of nucleic acids, such as microRNAs, are being discovered that are highly specific as regulators, with strong potential as biomarkers for fine resolution of both the status of the pathogen and host's response to infection. Improvements in closed-tube amplification methods, greater automation, flexibility in selection of targets, fine discrimination of sequence complexity, high-density microarrays, and massively parallel sequencing will open up increasingly sophisticated applications in specialized testing laboratories and at point of care.

The goal of translational research is to facilitate the implementation of advanced basic research and advance new technologies toward clinical utility. A continuous dialogue between researcher, test developer, regulator and clinician is needed to help refine test specifications and for evaluation and validation of new technologies, studies to support FDA clearance (510 k), implementation in the laboratory and interpretation of results for better patient management. A well-planned and executed translational research activity is critical for ensuring continued advancement of molecular techniques to address the evolving needs of diagnostics and lead to more effective patient care. These advancements in viral molecular diagnostics will provide laboratories and clinicians with information that can be used to personalize the management and treatment of patients, leading to better outcomes, minimizing the impact and side effects of unnecessary treatment, and improving quality of life.

REFERENCES

1. Liotta LA, Petricoin EF, 3rd. (2012) Regulatory approval pathways for molecular diagnostic technology. *Methods Mol Biol* **823**: 409–420.

2. Ratcliff R, Chang G, Kok T, Sloots T. (2007) Molecular diagnosis of medical viruses, *Curr Issues Mol Biol* **9**: 87–102.
3. Witonsky J. (2011) Infectious disease molecular diagnostics: Market review and opportunities. *Gen Eng News* **31**: 20.
4. Li N, Franceschi S, Howell-Jones R, *et al.* (2011) Human papillomavirus type distribution in 30,848 invasive cervical cancers worldwide: Variation by geographical region, histological type and year of publication. *Int J Cancer* **128**: 927–935.
5. Busch MP, Satten GA. (1997) Time course of viremia and antibody seroconversion following human immunodeficiency virus exposure. *Am J Med* **102**: 117–124.
6. Garrett P, Crush-Stanton S, Pickering T, *et al.* (2007) Seroconversion panels: Tools to study evolving infection. *Third European Congress of Virology.* Nürnberg, Germany, 1–5 September.
7. Fiebig EW, Wright DJ, Rawal BD, *et al.* (2003) Dynamics of HIV viremia and antibody seroconversion in plasma donors: Implications for diagnosis and staging of primary HIV infection. *AIDS* **17**: 1871–1879.
8. Peel S, Manak M, Eller L, *et al.* (2012) Evaluation of the Gen-Probe Aptima HIV-1 RNA qualitative assay as a diagnostic tool for identification of acute HIV infection. *19th Conference on Retroviruses and Opportunistic Infections.* Seattle, Washington, USA, March 5–8.
9. Mellors JW, Munoz AM, Giorgi JV. (1997) Plasma viral load and CD4+ lymphocytes as prognostic markers of HIV-1 infection. *Ann Intern Med* **126**: 946–954.
10. Maraschner IC, Collier AC, Coombs RW, *et al.* (1998) Use of changes in plasma levels of human immunodeficiency virus type 1 RNA to assess the clinical benefit of antiretroviral therapy. *J Infect Dis* **177**: 40–47.
11. Buonaguro L, Tornesello M, Buonaguro F. (2007) Human immunodeficiency virus type 1 subtype distribution in the worldwide epidemic: Pathogenetic and therapeutic implications. *J Virol* **81**: 10209–10219.
12. Mendoza C, Soriano V. (2009) Update on HIV viral-load assays: New tech nologies and teasing in resource-limited settings. *Future Virol* **4**(5): 423–430.
13. EP15-A2 and EP12-A2, *www.clsi.org*
14. User Verification of Performance for Precision and Trueness: Approved Guideline, 2nd ed (EP15-A2) and User Protocol for Evaluation of Qualitative Test Performance: Approved Guideline, 2nd ed (EP12-A2), *www.clsi.org*.
15. FDA Guidance to Industry, http://www.fda.gov/downloads/biologicsblood%20vaccines/guidancecomplianceregulatoryinformation/guidances/blood/ucm210270.pdfFDA Guidance to Industry: Nucleic Acid testing for Human

Immunodeficiency Virus Type 1 (HIV-1) and Hepatitis C Virus (HCV): Testing, Product Disposition and Donor Deferral and Reentry.
16. IVD Directive 98/79/EC European Commission.
17. Manak M, Sina S, Anekella B, *et al.* (2012) Pilot studies for development of an HIV subtype panel for surveillance of global diversity. *AIDS Hum Retro Res* **28**: 594–607.
18. De Bel A, Marissens D, Debaisieux L, *et al.* (2010) Correction of underquantification of human immunodeficiency virus type 1 load with the second version of the Roche Cobas AmpliPrep/Cobas TaqMan assays. *J Clin Microbiol* **48**: 1337–1342.
19. Abbott Molecular Inc. (2007) Abbott Real-Time HIV-1. Package Insert.
20. Elbeik T, Charlebois E, Nassos P, *et al.* (2000) Quantitative and cost comparison of ultrasensitive human immunodeficiency virus type 1 RNA viral load assays: Bayer bDNA Quantiplex versions 3.0 and 2.0 and Roche PCR Amplicor Monitor version 1.5. *J Clin Microbiol* **38**: 1113–1120.
21. Mayor MT, Roett MA, Uduhiri KA. (2012) Diagnosis and management of gonococcal infections. *Am Fam Physician* **86**(10): 931–938.
22. Workowski KA, Berman S. (2010). Sexually transmitted diseases treatment guidelines, 2010. *MMWR Recomm Rep* **59**(RR12): 1–110.
23. Chernesky M, Jang D, Smieja M, *et al.* (2009) Validation of the APTIMA Combo 2 assay for the detection of *Chlamydia trachomatis* and *Neisseria gonorrhoeae* in SurePath liquid-based pap test samples taken with different collection devices. *Sex Transm Dis* **36**: 581–583.
24. Schachter J, Chernesky MA, Willis DE, *et al.* (2005) Vaginal swabs are the specimens of choice when screening for *Chlamydia trachomatis* and *Neisseria gonorrhoeae*: Results from a multicenter evaluation of the APTIMA assays for both infections. *Sex Transm Dis* **32**: 725–728.
25. Manak M. (2008) Standardization of *Chlamydia trachomatis* and *Neisseria gonorrhoeae* nucleic acid testing. *SoGAT Clinical Diagnostic Meeting NIBSC.* South Mimms, UK, June 25.
26. Parra-Sánchez M, Palomares JC, Bernal S, *et al.* (2012) Evaluation of the cobas 4800 CT/NG test for detecting *Chlamydia trachomatis* and *Neisseria gonorrhoeae* DNA in urogenital swabs and urine specimens. *Diagn Microbiol Infect Dis* **74**: 338–342.
27. Castle PE, Sadorra M, Lau T, *et al.* (2009) Evaluation of a prototype real-time PCR assay for carcinogenic human papillomavirus (HPV) detection and simultaneous HPV genotype 16 (HPV 16) and HPV 18 genotyping. *J Clin Microbiol* **47**: 3344–3347.

28. Heideman DA, Hesselink AT, Berkhof J, *et al.* (2011) Clinical validation of the cobas 4800 HPV test for cervical screening purposes. *J Clin Microbiol* **49**: 3983–3985.
29. Lathey J, Sharma H, Nguyen L, *et al.* (2006) Development of a cellular HPV control for DNA testing of cervical specimens collected in Tripath's SurePath medium. *22nd Clinical Virology Symposium.* Clearwater Beach, Florida, USA, April 30–May 3.
30. Anekella B, Dryga S, Moskowitz K, *et al.* (2007) Stability of integrated HPV 16 DNA in Various Sample Collection Media. *AMP Annual Meeting.* Los Angeles, California, USA.
31. Klig J, N Shah. (2005) Office pediatrics: Current issues in lower respiratory infections in children. *Curr Opin Pediatr* **17**: 111–118.
32. Christensen K, Holman R, Steiner C, *et al.* (2009) Infectious disease hospitalizations in the United States. *Clin Infect Dis* **49**: 1025–1035.
33. Huijskens E, Biesmans R, Buiting A, *et al.* (2012) Diagnostic value of respiratory virus detection in symptomatic children using real-time PCR. *Virology J* **9**: 276.
34. Hendrickson KJ. (2005) Cost-effective use of rapid diagnostic techniques in the treatment and prevention of viral respiratory infections. *Pediatr Ann* **34**: 24–31.
35. Leonardi GP, Leib H, Birkhead GS, *et al.* (1994) Comparison of rapid detection methods for influenza A virus and their value in health care-management of institutionalized geriatric patients. *J Clin Microbiol* **32**: 70–74.
36. Gonzales R, Malone DC, Maselli JH, Sande MA. (2001) Excessive antibiotic use for acute respiratory infections in the United States. *Clin Infect Dis* **33**: 757–762.
37. Paterson DL. (2006) The role of antimicrobial management programs in optimizing antibiotic prescribing within hospitals. *Clin Infect Dis* **42**: S90–S95.
38. McGeer A, Green KA, Plevneshi A, *et al.* (2007) Toronto Invasive Bacterial Diseases Network. Antiviral therapy and outcomes of influenza requiring hospitalization in Ontario, Canada. *Clin Infect Dis* **45**: 1568–1575.
39. Mahony JB. (2010) Nucleic acid amplification-based diagnosis of respiratory virus infections. *Expert Rev Anti Infect Ther* **8**: 1273–1292.
40. Leland D, Ginocchio CC. (2007) Role of cell culture for virus detection in the age of technology. *Clin Microbiol Rev* **20**: 49–78.
41. Hall CB, Douglas RG Jr, Geiman JM. (1975) Quantitative shedding patterns of respiratory syncytial virus in infants. *J Infect Dis* **132**(2): 151–156.

42. Englund JA, Piedra PA, Jewell A, *et al.* (1996) Rapid diagnosis of respiratory syncytial virus infections in immunocompromised adults. *J Clin Microbiol* **34**: 1649–1653.
43. Casiano-Colon AE, Hulbert BB, Mayer TK, *et al.* (2003) Lack of sensitivity of rapid antigen tests for the diagnosis of respiratory syncytial virus infection in adults. *J Clin Virol* **28**: 169–174.
44. Beck ET, Henrickson KJ. (2010) Molecular diagnosis of respiratory viruses. *Future Microbiol* **5**: 901–916.
45. Morens DM, Folkers GK, Fauci AS. (2008) Emerging infections: A perpetual challenge. *Lancet Infect Dis* **8**: 710–719.
46. Infectious Diseases Society of America. (2011) An unmet medical need: Rapid molecular diagnostics tests for respiratory tract infections. *Clin Infect Dis* **52**(Suppl 4): S384–S395.
47. Yu X, Lu R, Wang Z, *et al.* (2011) Etiology and clinical characterization of respiratory virus infections in adult patients attending an emergency department in Beijing. *PLoS ONE* **7**(2): e32174.
48. Liao RS, Tomalty LL, Majury A, Zoutman DE. (2009) Comparison of viral isolation and multiplex real-time reverse transcription-PCR for confirmation of respiratory syncytial virus and influenza virus detection by antigen immunoassays. *J Clin Microbiol* **47**: 527–532.
49. Ginocchio CC. (2011) Strengths and weaknesses of FDA-approved/cleared diagnostic devices for the molecular detection of respiratory pathogens. *Clin Infect Dis*: **52**(Suppl 4): S312–S325.
50. Ulrich MP, Christensen DR, Coyne SR, *et al.* (2006) Evaluation of the Cepheid GeneXpert® system for detecting *Bacillus anthracis*. *J Appl Microbiol* **100**: 1011–1016.
51. Check W. (2012) For respiratory virus detection, a golden age. *CAP Today* April.
52. Mahony J, Chong S, Merante F, *et al.* (2007) Development of a respiratory virus panel test for detection of twenty human respiratory viruses by use of multiplex PCR and a fluid microbead-based assay. *J Clin Microbiol* **45**: 2965–2970.
53. Poehling KA, Edwards KM, Weinberg GA, *et al.* (2006) The unrecognized burden of influenza in young children. *N Engl J Med* **355**: 31–40.
54. Advani S, Segupta A, Forman M, *et al.* (2012) Detecting respiratory virus in asymptomatic children. *Pediatr Infect Dis J* **31**: 1221.
55. Ginocchio C, McAdam A. (2011) Current best practices for respiratory virus testing. *J Clin Microbiol* **49**(Suppl 9): S44–S48.

56. Morse GD, Maartens G, Maponga CC, Ma Q. (2012) Global HIV/AIDS clinical and translational pharmacology. *AIDS Res Treat* **2012**: 973627.
57. Larder BA, Darby G, Richman DD. (1989) HIV with reduced sensitivity to zidovudine (AZT) isolated during prolonged therapy. *Science* **243**: 1731–1734.
58. WHO. (2012) WHO HIV drug resistance report 2012. The World Health Organization, Geneva, Switzerland. http://aps.who.int/iris/bitstream/10665/75183/1/978924105.
59. FDA. (2012) Antiretroviral drugs used in the treatment of HIV infection. The U.S. Food and Drug Administration, Rockville, Maryland, USA. *www.fda.gov/ForConsumers/ByAudience/ForPatientAdvocates/HIVandAIDSActivities/ucm11891.*
60. Gallant JE. (2006) Antiretroviral drug resistance and resistance testing. *Top HIV Med* **13**: 138-42.
61. Gürtler L. (2012) HIV and drug resistance — Interpretation and therapeutic progress. *Intervirology* **55**: 77–78.
62. Mansky LM. (1998) Retrovirus mutation rates and their role in genetic variation. *J Gen Virol* **79**: 1337–1345.
63. Johnson JA, Li JF, Wei X, *et al.* (2008) Minority HIV-1 drug resistance mutations are present in antiretroviral treatment-naïve populations and associate with reduced treatment efficacy. *PLoS Med* **5**(7): e158.
64. Preston BD, Poiesz BJ, LA Loeb LA. (1988) Fidelity of HIV-1 reverse transcriptase. *Science* **242**: 1168–1171.
65. Ji J, Loeb LA. (1992) Fidelity of HIV-1 reverse transcriptase copying RNA in vitro. *Biochem* **31**. 954–958.
66. Ji J, Loeb LA. (1994) Fidelity of HIV-1 reverse transcriptase copying a hypervariable region of the HIV-1 env gene. *Virology* **199**: 323–330.
67. Napravnik S, Edwards D, Stewart P, *et al.* (2005) HIV-1 drug resistance evolution among patients on potent combination antiretroviral therapy with detectable viremia. *J Acquit Immune Defic Syndr* **40**: 34–40.
68. Eberle J, Gürtler L. (2012) HIV types, groups, subtypes and recombinant forms: Errors in replication, selection pressure and quasispecies. *Intervirology* **55**: 79–83.
69. Hertogs K, de Bethune MP, Miller V, *et al.* (1998). A rapid method for simultaneous detection of phenotypic resistance to inhibitors of protease and reverse transcriptase in recombinant human immunodeficiency virus type 1 isolates from patients treated with antiretroviral drugs. *Antimicrob Agents Chemother* **42**: 269–276.

70. Petropoulos CJ, Parkin NT, Limoli KL, *et al.* (2000) A novel phenotypic drug susceptibility assay for human immunodeficiency virus type 1. *Antimicrob Agents Chemother* **44**: 920–928.
71. Shafer RW. (2002) Genotypic testing for human immunodeficiency virus type 1 drug resistance. *Clin Microbiol Rev* **15**: 247–277.
72. Richman DD. (2004) Benefits and limitations of testing for resistance to HIV drugs. *J Antimicrob Chemother* **53**: 555–557.
73. Panidou ET, Trikalinos TA, Ioannidis JP. (2004) Limited benefit of antiretroviral resistance testing in treatment-experienced patients: A meta-analysis. *AIDS* **18**: 2153–2161.
74. Dunn DT, Green H, Loveday C, *et al.* (2005) Evaluation of resistance assays (ERA) trial investigators. A randomized controlled trial of the value of phenotypic testing in addition to genotypic testing for HIV drug resistance: Evaluation of resistance assays (ERA) trial investigators. *J Acquit Immune Defic Syndr* **38**: 553–559.
75. Stürmer M, Reinheimer C. (2012) Description of two commercially available assays for genotyping of HIV-1. *Intervirology* **55**: 134–137.
76. Zhou Z, Wagar N, DeVos JR, *et al.* (2011) Optimization of a low cost and broadly sensitive genotyping assay for HIV-1 drug resistance surveillance and monitoring in resource-limited settings. *PLoS ONE* **6**(11): e28184.
77. Ji H, Massé N, Tyler S, *et al.* (2010) HIV drug resistance surveillance using pooled pyrosequencing. *PLoS ONE* **5**(2): e9263.
78. Jagodzinski LL, Cooley JD, Weber M, *et al.* (2003) Performance characteristics of human immunodeficiency virus type 1 (HIV-1) genotyping systems in sequence-based analysis of subtypes other than HIV-1 subtype B. *J Clin Microbiol* **41**: 998–1003.
79. Eshleman SH, Crutcher G, Petrauskene O, *et al.* (2005) Sensitivity and specificity of the ViroSeq human immunodeficiency virus type 1 (HIV-1) genotyping system for detection of HIV-1 drug resistance mutations by use of an ABI PRISM 3100 genetic analyzer. *J Clin Microbiol* **43**: 813–817.
80. Liu L, Li Y, Li S, *et al.* (2012) Comparison of next-generation sequencing systems. *J Biomed Biotechnol* **2012**: 251364.
81. Rozera G, Abbate I, Bruselles A, *et al.* (2009) Massively parallel pyrosequencing highlights minority variants in the HIV-1 env quasispecies deriving from lymphomonocyte sub-populations. *Retrovirology* **6**: 15.
82. Capobianchi MR, Giombini E, Rozera G. (2012) Next-generation sequencing technology in clinical virology. *Clin Microbiol Infect* **19**: 15–22.
83. Barzon L, Lavezzo E, Militello V, *et al.* (2011) Applications of next-generation sequencing technologies to diagnostic virology. *Int J Mol Sci* **12**: 7861–7884.

84. Radford AD, Chapman D, Dixon L, *et al.* (2012) Application of next-generation sequencing technologies in virology. *J Gen Virol* **93**: 1853–1868.
85. Simen BB, Simons JF, Hullsiek KH, *et al.* (2009) Low-abundance drug-resistant viral variants in chronically HIV-infected, antiretroviral treatment-naive patients significantly impact treatment outcomes. *J Infect Dis* **199**: 693–701.
86. Wang C, Mitsuya Y, Gharizadeh B, *et al.* (2007) Characterization of mutation spectra with ultra-deep pyrosequencing: Application to HIV-1 drug resistance. *Genome Res* **17**: 1195–1201.
87. Hoffmann C, Minkah N, Leipzig J, *et al.* (2007) DNA bar coding and pyrosequencing to identify rare HIV drug resistance mutations. *Nucleic Acids Res* **35**: e91.
88. Green, RE, Krause J, Ptak SE, *et al.* (2006): Analysis of one million base pairs of Neanderthal DNA. *Nature* **444**: 330–336.
89. Margulies M, Egholm M, Altman WE, *et al.* (2005) Genome sequencing in microfabricated high-density picolitre reactors. *Nature* **437**: 376–380.
90. Andersson AF, Lindberg M, Jakobsson H, *et al.* (2008) Comparative analysis of human gut microbiota by barcoded pyrosequencing. *PLoS ONE* **3**: e2836.
91. Pushkarev D, Neff NF, Quake SR. (2009) Single-molecule sequencing of an individual human genome. *Nat Biotechnol* **27**: 847–850.
92. Rothberg JM, Hinz W, Rearick TM, *et al.* (2011) An integrated semiconductor device enabling non-optical genome sequencing. *Nature* **475**: 348–352.
93. Ng PC, Kirkness EF. (2010) Whole genome sequencing. *Methods Mol Biol* **628**: 215–226.

VI. Translation Research in Endocrinology and Nutrition

CHAPTER 14

Science to Clinical Practice: Lost Opportunities in Obesity

Marian L. Neuhouser

14.1. INTRODUCTION

Translational science and translational medicine have emerged as important approaches for both cancer prevention and cancer treatment.[1,2] Sometimes known as the "bench to bedside" concept, the idea behind translational science is that discoveries made in the laboratory setting should easily translate into clinical trials in humans followed by evidenced-based recommendations and policies for clinical care of patients and widespread dissemination and adoption of new treatment paradigms in the community setting.[1] Ideally, the new approaches become the standard of care to improve patient treatments and outcomes for cancer, cardiovascular disease, diabetes and other diseases. The translational approach operates on a continuum and requires coordinated scientific contributions across multiple disciplines and medical specialties. The theoretical framework for translational research has been described in detail elsewhere.[2–4]

Cancer Prevention Program, Division of Public Health Sciences, Fred Hutchinson Cancer Research Center, Seattle, Washington, USA.
Corresponding address. Marian L. Neuhouser, PhD, RD, Full Member, Cancer Prevention Program, Division of Public Health Sciences, Fred Hutchinson Cancer Research Center, 1100 Fairview Avenue North, M4-B402, Seattle, WA98109-1024, USA; Tel: +1-206-667-4797; Fax: +1-206-667-7850; E-mail: *mneuhous@fhcrc.org*.

The translational science approach is well supported at the US National Institutes of Health (NIH) through the Clinical and Translational Science Awards (CTSA) and the National Cancer Institute's Translational Research Program, which administers the organ-site specific Specialized Programs of Research Excellence (SPOREs).[5] The SPOREs are explicitly charged with rapid discovery of tumor etiology linked with development of promising treatments in the clinical setting. In addition, other federally sponsored programs such as the Transdisciplinary Research on Energetics and Cancer (TREC), Transdisciplinary Tobacco Use Research Centers (TTURC) and Centers for Population Health and Health Disparities (CPHHD) are multi-center team science initiatives whose overarching goals are to merge the knowledge and skills of multiple scientific disciplines into new research paradigms intended to accelerate discovery and applications to clinical practice.[6,7] Many of these transdisciplinary initiatives have embraced a "cells to society" or translational approach to understanding the complex interplay between various risk factors (i.e., tobacco, obesity) and cancer risk and treatment.

Despite the strong support for translational science, "bench to bedside" progress has been slower than initially hoped and many aspects of the translational approach have been unrealized and unfulfilled. The focus of this chapter is to examine the extent to which treatment for obesity has been "lost in translation" with respect to cancer treatment and outcomes.

14.2. OBESITY AND CANCER RISK

Obesity continues to be a major public health problem in the US. The most recent results from the nation's major health surveillance survey, the National Health and Nutrition Examination Survey (NHANES), reported that the age-adjusted prevalence of obesity ($BMI \geq 30.0\ kg/m^2$) was 35.7 percent among all adults while that for overweight plus obesity ($BMI \geq 25.0\ kg/m^2$) was 68.8 percent.[8,9] The obesity prevalence estimates for the years 2009–2010 did not differ from the years 2003–2008, suggesting that little progress has been made in reducing this critical problem.[8,9] The public health ramifications of the obesity epidemic and its relationship to cancer are widespread. Obesity increases risk of several common cancers including cancers of the colon, endometrium, esophagus, pancreas, kidney, gall bladder, liver and postmenopausal breast.[10–13] In addition to these organ sites, obesity increases risk of several hematologic cancers including multiple myeloma, leukemia and lymphoma.[11] The gravity of the obesity–cancer relationship was noted in the 2012 Annual Report to the Nation.[14] This comprehensive report from the American Cancer Society, the Centers for Disease Control and Prevention, the National Cancer Institute, and the North American Association of Central Cancer Registries highlighted the extent to which obesity and lack of physical activity are associated with increased cancer risk. For example, the authors reported that compared to individuals with a normal BMI ($< 25.0\,kg/m^2$), the relative risk of cancer for those who were overweight (BMI 25.0–29.9 kg/m^2) ranged from 1.13 for postmenopausal breast, colorectal and pancreas to 1.6 for esophagus and endometrium. Compared to normal BMI, being obese increased risk further; the relative risks for cancer of the kidney, colon, pancreas and post-menopausal breast were 1.6, 1.4, 1.3 and 1.3, respectively, while the relative risks for endometrial and esophageal cancers more than doubled.[14] In addition to tremendous pain and suffering by patients and their families, the medical treatment for these cancers and the large number of lost workdays represents an enormous burden on the healthcare system and the economy in general. New scientific approaches are urgently needed to reverse these obesity cancer trends.

14.3. OBESITY AND CANCER SURVIVAL

In addition to these well known associations of obesity with cancer risk, increasing evidence suggests that obesity is associated with poor cancer prognosis. In 2003, Calle *et al.* published the landmark report demonstrating the strong link between obesity and cancer-related mortality.[15] In the ensuing years, evidence continued to accumulate showing that cancer patients who are overweight or obese have substantially poorer prognosis and outcomes compared to patients who are normal weight when diagnosed.[16–21] In 2011, the Institute of Medicine (IOM) sponsored the workshop "The Role of Obesity in Cancer Survival and Recurrence," where the overall goals were to examine the biological mechanisms linking obesity with cancer outcomes, to discuss potential human intervention trials and to begin conversations about clinical care and relevant policy recommendations. In essence, the workshop content embraced a translational "bench to bedside" approach. A workshop report and a workshop summary are published.[22,23] Briefly, the report acknowledged that numerous biological pathways are disrupted in obesity and each of these pathways could independently or jointly in a synergistic manner provide the obesity–cancer link. Obesity is well known to disrupt insulin sensitivity and related pathways, such as the insulin-like growth factor (IGF) pathway.[24] Downstream targets of the IGF pathway include activation of the PI3K/Akt and mTOR pathways as well as MAPK pathways. Together these systems up-regulate cell division and fuel mitogenesis.[24] Other biological systems that are disrupted by obesity included sex steroid hormones, various adipokines (e.g., leptin and adiponectin) and inflammatory cytokines (e.g., C-reactive protein, IL-6, TNF-α, IL-1β).[25–27] Each of these systems was discussed in detail by the IOM report[22] and others,[16,23,27] and intense research continues to better understand the etiology of obesity and cancer risk and cancer survivorship.[28] In essence, while there are still gaps in the scientific evidence for these mechanisms, much progress has been made particularly with respect to the "bench" aspects of the obesity–cancer relationship as well as translating the bench discoveries to preclinical models.

14.4. OBESITY TREATMENT AS PART OF THE CANCER PATIENT TREATMENT PLAN: LOST IN TRANSLATION

Given the strong and compelling data that link obesity to poor cancer outcomes (and likely to increased treatment costs and complications with other obesity-related competing health risks), it is rather surprising that obesity treatment is not part of standard clinical care plans for cancer patients. *Obesity treatment for cancer patients has been lost in translation.* In contrast, obesity treatment is a major component of treatment plans for cardiovascular disease and diabetes (and their associated phenotypes such as hypertension and hyperlipidemia). For example, patients who have had a myocardial infarction or various surgical procedures, such as coronary artery bypass graft (CABG), cardiac catheterization or other common procedures, typically will complete a program of cardiac rehabilitation where the overall goal is to reduce risk of recurrence of the particular cardiac event as well as improve overall health and quality of life. Cardiac rehab teams include a range of healthcare providers with broad skill sets designed to provide a comprehensive care plan for improved patient health. One of the critical features of a cardiac rehab program is the recommendation of weight management services for patients who are overweight or obese at the time of the initial cardiac event.[29,30] Nearly 20 years ago, in 1994, the American Heart Association issued a statement on recommendations for cardiac rehabilitation that included recommendations for lifestyle modifications including nutrition, physical activity and weight management.[30] While the use of cardiac rehab services is lower than hoped for eligible patients, the model remains an important one for other chronic diseases for which lifestyle modifications, including weight management/obesity treatment, influence disease outcome. Such recommendations and standards of care do not exist for cancer patients and this represents an important gap in translational medicine.

14.5. HOW DID OBESITY BECOME LOST IN TRANSLATION FOR CANCER TREATMENT?

The US has more than 12 million cancer survivors.[31,32] During active treatment, patients receive care from multiple healthcare providers, which might include the following: surgeon, medical oncologist, radiation oncologist, infusion nurses, physical therapist, psychologist/therapist, dietitian, occupational therapist and medical social worker. When the primary cancer treatments are concluded, patients return to their primary care providers as cancer survivors. Unfortunately, cancer treatments are intense and debilitating, and treatments often leave patients with new medical problems that were previously not present. For example, many patients will have new chemotherapy-induced neuropathies, memory loss, renal and cardiac problems, and weight gain. The recognition of these cancer-treatment related medical issues along with specific proposals for follow-up plans was described in the 2007 joint IOM and National Research Council report "From Cancer Patient to Cancer Survivor: Lost in Translation" and subsequently in an IOM workshop and summary report entitled "Implementing Cancer Survivorship Care Planning."[33] More recently, Wolin *et al.* provided an excellent report that defines and frames a successful plan to disseminate and implement effective cancer survivorship programs.[34] The authors provided a useful six-step plan for implementing and evaluating a specific program for cancer survivors. The example provided in the report is for a smoking cessation program for cancer survivors, but the paradigm is intended to be broadly applicable and could be easily applied to a program of weight loss/weight management for cancer survivors.

Despite these challenges, some progress has been made in the area of post-treatment care for cancer patients, which may include weight management and modification of other lifestyle behaviors. For example, in addition to the recent IOM reports,[33] the American Cancer Society (ACS) recently published an updated "Nutrition and Physical Activity Guidelines for Cancer Survivors."[34] One of the key recommendations in the report was that cancer survivors should achieve and maintain a healthy weight by following a healthy diet and engaging in physical activity. The most successful approach to achieving this may be through structured programs. Weight loss and maintenance of a healthy weight is complex and not at all easy for most people. It is likely to be a significantly greater challenge for cancer survivors, so adequate support and structure is essential for success.

14.6. RECOMMENDATIONS FOR FUTURE RESEARCH, POLICY AND CLINICAL CARE

- Research is needed on particular obesity-related biological pathways affected by cancer and cancer treatment.
- Research is needed on the late effects of cancer treatment, particularly with respect to the effects of chemotherapy on body composition and energy balance.
- Survivorship care plans are needed for all cancer survivors. Comprehensive "cancer rehabilitation" plans should be offered to all cancer patients, in much the same way that cardiac rehabilitation is provided for cardiac patients. These plans need to include programs and referrals for weight management.

- Resources need to be provided to cover these survivorship care plans, either through private insurance coverage or the Centers for Medicare and Medicaid Services.
- Research is needed to identify the most appropriate weight loss approaches for cancer patients. Many patients may have extended symptoms upon completion of treatment including altered taste and olfactory sensations, bowel changes, neuropathies, difficulties with chewing and swallowing, fatigue and psychosocial/body image issues. These symptoms can make it very difficult to be motivated to begin and adhere to a weight loss regimen.
- Research is needed to identify whether diet quality, independent of caloric intake, plays an important role in the energy balance–cancer survivorship equation. Initial studies in this area are promising (George *et al.*, Meyerhardt),[35,36] but more studies are needed in order to provide evidenced-based recommendations.
- While many cancer patients are highly motivated to make dietary and weight changes following a diagnosis (Patterson, Neuhouser),[37,38] others are so overwhelmed with the diagnosis and treatment that initiating and maintaining a weight loss program would be a significant challenge.
- Research is needed to document whether or not tailored cancer survivor care plans that might include weight management strategies are effective in terms of patient reported outcomes as well as recurrence and mortality. These types of data are needed before comprehensive policy and clinical practice guidelines can become the standard of care.

14.7. SUMMARY

Translational medicine requires coordinated scientific contributions across multiple disciplines and medical specialties, and this may be particularly true for the treatment of obesity in cancer patients. Because cancer patients are already cared for by a wide range of specialists and care givers, it could be conveyable to integrate weight management into existing patient care plans. While much convincing and credible data exist with regard to "discovery" or the etiology of the relationship between obesity and cancer survivorship, less data exist with respect to specific human interventions that can be incorporated into policy and clinical care guidelines. This should be the focus of research going forward so that obesity and cancer survivorship is no longer lost in translation.

REFERENCES

1. Lenfant C. (2003) Clinical research to clinical practice — Lost in translation? *New Engl J Med* **349**(9): 868–874.
2. Khoury MJ, Gwinn M, Ioannidis JP. (2010) The emergence of translational epidemiology: From scientific discovery to population health impact. *Am J Epidemiol* **172**(5): 517–524.
3. Hiatt RA. (2008) Epidemiology: Key to translational, team, and transdisciplinary science. *Ann Epidemiol* **18**(11): 859–861.
4. Elena JW, Travis LB, Simon NI, *et al.* (2013) Leveraging epidemiology and clinical studies of cancer outcomes: Recommendations and opportunities for translational research. *J Natl Cancer Inst* **105**: 85–94.
5. Woolf SH. (2008) The meaning of translational research and why it matters. *J Am Med Assoc* **299**(2): 211–213.
6. Patterson RE, Colditz GA, Hu FB, *et al.* (2013) The 2011–2016 Transdisciplinary Research on Energetics and Cancer (TREC) Initiative: Rationale and design. *Cancer Causes Control* **349**(9): 868–874.
7. Parry C, Kent EE, Mariotto AB, *et al.* (2011) Cancer survivors: A booming population. *Cancer Epidemiol Biomarkers Prev* **20**(10): 1996–2005.
8. Ogden CL, Carroll MD, Curtin LR, *et al.* (2006) Prevalence of overweight and obesity in the United States, 1999–2004. *J Am Med Assoc* **295**(13): 1549–1555.
9. Flegal KM, Carroll MD, Ogden CL, Curtin LR. (2010) Prevalence and trends in obesity among US adults, 1999–2008. *J Am Med Assoc* **303**(3): 235–241.
10. Basen-Engquist K, Chang M. (2011) Obesity and cancer risk: Recent review and evidence. *Curr Oncol Rep* **13**: 71–76.
11. World Cancer Research Fund/AICR. (2007) *Food, Nutrition, Physical Activity, and the Prevention of Cancer: A Global Perspective.* AICR, Washington, DC.
12. Neuhouser M, Perrigue M. (2012) The role of energy balance for cancer prevention. *Curr Nutr Rep* **12**: 8–15.
13. Renehan AG, Soerjomataram I, Tyson M, *et al.* (2010) Incident cancer burden attributable to excess body mass index in 30 European countries. *Int J Cancer* **126**(3): 692–702.
14. Eheman C, Henley SJ, Ballard-Barbash R, *et al.* (2012) Annual report to the nation on the status of cancer, 1975–2008, featuring cancers associated with excess weight and lack of sufficient physical activity. *Cancer* **118**(9): 2388–2366.

15. Calle R, Rodriguez C, Walker-Thurmond K, Thun M. (2003) Overweight, obesity, and mortality from cancer in a prospectively studied cohort of U.S. adults. *New Engl J Med* **348**: 1625–1638.
16. Demark-Wahnefried W, Platz EA, Ligibel JA, *et al.* (2012) The role of obesity in cancer survival and recurrence. *Cancer Epidemiol Biomarkers Prev* **21**(8): 1244–1259.
17. Rock CL, Demark-Wahnefried W. (2002) Nutrition and survival after the diagnosis of breast cancer: A review of the evidence. *J Clin Oncol* **20**(15): 3302–3316.
18. Ewertz M, Jensen MB, Gunnarsdóttir KÁ, *et al.* (2011) Effect of obesity on prognosis after early-stage breast cancer. *J Clin Oncol* **29**(1): 25–31.
19. Bessonova L, Marshall SF, Ziogas A, *et al.* (2011) The association of body mass index with mortality in the California Teachers Study. *Int J Cancer* **129**(10): 2492–2501.
20. Sinicrope FA, Foster NR, Sargent DJ, *et al.* (2010) Obesity is an independent prognostic variable in colon cancer survivors. *Clin Cancer Res* **16**(6): 1884–1893.
21. Sinicrope FA, Dannenberg AJ. (2010) Obesity and breast cancer prognosis: Weight of the evidence. *J Clin Oncol* **29**(1): 4–7.
22. National Cancer Policy Forum, Board on Health Care Services, Institute of Medicine, Patlak M, Nass SJ (Rapporteurs). (2012) *The Role of Obesity in Cancer Survival and Recurrence: Workshop Summary.* The National Academies Press, Washington, DC.
23. Hursting SD, Digiovanni J, Dannenberg AJ, *et al.* (2012) Obesity, energy balance, and cancer: New opportunities for prevention. *Cancer Prev Res* **5**(11): 1260–1272.
24. Pollak M. (2008) Insulin and Insulin-like growth factor signalling in neoplasia. *Nat Rev Cancer* **8**(12): 915–928.
25. Shoelson SE, Herrero L, Naaz A. (2007) Obesity, inflammation, and insulin resistance. *Gastroenterology* **132**(6): 2169–2180.
26. Kahn BB, Flier JS. (2000) Obesity and insulin resistance. *J Clin Invest* **106**(4): 473–481.
27. Hursting SD, Berger NA. (2010) Energy balance, host-related factors, and cancer progression. *J Clin Oncol* **28**(26): 4058–4064.
28. Harrop JP, Dean JA, Paskett ED. (2011) Cancer survivorship research: A review of the literature and summary of current NCI-designated cancer center projects. *Cancer Epidemiol Biomarkers Prev* **20**(10): 2042–2047.
29. Ades PA, Savage PD, Harvey-Berino J. (2010) The treatment of obesity in cardiac rehabilitation. *J Cardiopulm Rehab Prev* **30**(5): 289–298.

30. Leon AS, Franklin BA, Costa F, *et al.* (2005) Cardiac rehabilitation and secondary prevention of coronary heart disease. *Circulation* **111**: 369–376.
31. Siegel R, Naishadham D, Jemal A. (2013) Cancer statistics, 2013. *CA Cancer J Clin* **63**: 11–30.
32. Institute of Medicine, Ganz PA, Hewitt M (Rapporteurs). (2007) *Implementing Cancer Survivorship Care Planning*. The National Academies Press, Washington, DC.
33. Wolin KY, Colditz GA, Proctor EK. (2011) Maximizing benefits for effective cancer survivorship programming: Defining a dissemination and implementation plan. *Oncologist* **16**(8): 1189–1196.
34. Rock CL, Doyle C, Demark-Wahnefried W, *et al.* (2012) Nutrition and physical activity guidelines for cancer survivors. *CA Cancer J Clin* **62**: 243–274.
35. George SM, Irwin ML, Smith AW, *et al.* (2011) Postdiagnosis diet quality, the combination of diet quality and recreational physical activity, and prognosis after early-stage breast cancer. *Cancer Causes & Control* **22**(4): 589–598.
36. Meyerhardt JA, Sato K, Niedzwiecki, D, *et al.* (2012) Dietary glycemic load and cancer recurrence and survival in patients with stage III colon cancer: findings from CALGB 89803. *J Nat Cancer Inst* **104**: 1702–1711.
37. Patterson RE, Neuhouser ML, Hedderson MM, *et al.* (2003) Changes in diet, physical activity, and supplement use among adults diagnosed with cancer. *J Am Diet Assoc* **103**: 323–328.
38. Kuiper JG, Phipps AI, Neuhouser ML, *et al.* (2012) Recreational physical activity, body mass index, and survival in women with colorectal cancer. *Cancer Causes & Control* **23**(12): 1939–1948. PMCID: PMC3499635.

CHAPTER 15

Translational Research in Obesity and Type 2 Diabetes

*Michal Ciborowski**, *Edyta Adamska**, *Maria Górska**
*and Adam Kretowski**,†

15.1. INTRODUCTION

Obesity is the most common chronic metabolic disorder in the industrialized world. The prevalence of obesity has been increasing dramatically over the past 30 years and the disorder has become a global pandemic with devastating consequences for health. The most serious clinical problems linked to obesity include increased risk for type 2 diabetes (T2DM), hypertension, hyperlipidemia, atherosclerosis, cardiovascular events, stroke, and various forms of cancer, as well as neurodegenerative diseases and mental disorders.[1–4] Multiple factors (Fig. 1) are considered as potential risk factors for the future development of diabetes and T2DM. As a result, the condition is contributing significantly to the global burden of morbidity and mortality.[5–13] Moreover, the increase in the prevalence of obesity is likely to continue to be a serious health problem in the coming decades.[14,15]

The role of adipose tissue in the development of T2DM has not been fully elucidated. Generally, type 2 diabetes is a result of loss of

*Department of Endocrinology, Diabetology and Internal Medicine, Centre for Clinical Research, Medical University of Bialystok, Bialystok, Poland.
†Corresponding author: Adam Kretowski, Department of Endocrinology, Diabetology and Internal Medicine, Centre for Clinical Research, Medical University of Bialystok, ul. M. Sklodowskiej-Curie 24A, 15-276 Bialystok, Poland; E-mail: *adamkretowski@wp.pl*.

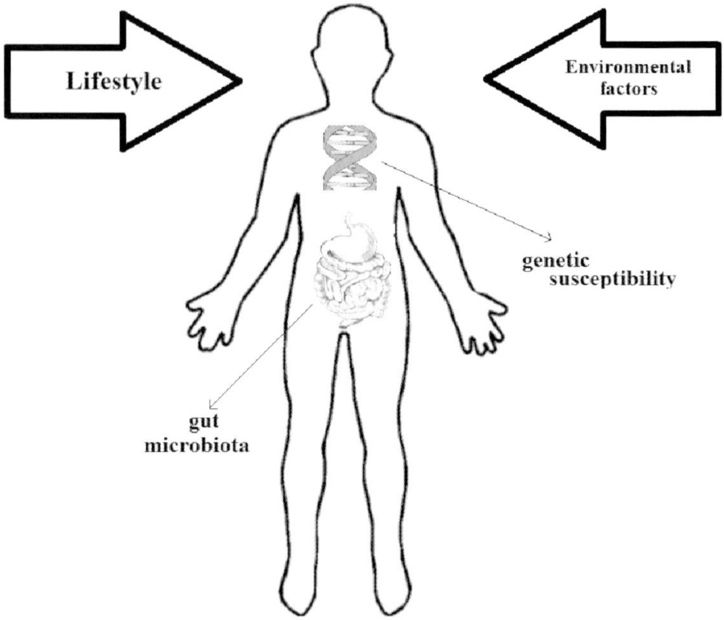

Fig. 1. Factors that contribute to the presence of obesity and type 2 diabetes. The occurrence of obesity and T2DM is dependent on multiple factors, including genetics,[1] composition of gut microbiota,[4] lifestyle,[2] and environmental factors.[3] Known lifestyle factors include diet, alcohol consumption, and physical activity,[2] while environmental factors include polychlorinated biphenyls, pesticides, phenols, phthalates, heavy metals, allergens, and others.[3]

insulin sensitivity and/or impaired insulin secretion, but the mechanisms of obesity-driven insulin resistance are complex and are still being widely investigated.[16–18] Obesity is characterized by excess adipose tissue that results from positive energy balance, whereby energy intake exceeds energy expenditure over a prolonged period of time. However, the increasing prevalence of obesity cannot be explained solely by nutritional habits or by the reduction of energy expenditure through decreased daily physical activity. Mechanisms that regulate energy homeostasis have aroused great interest in the scientific community. Energy homeostasis is partly regulated by signals through the adipose–brain and gut–brain axes. It has been widely noted that energy balance is controlled by the hypothalamus, which is a crucial region for integrating signals from peripheral and central pathways, and plays a major role in appetite regulation. There are many hypothalamic nuclei and neuronal circuits involved in energy homeostasis and interaction with the brainstem and higher cortical centers. The major roles are played by the lateral hypothalamic area (LHA), ventromedial hypothalamic nucleus (VMN), and the arcuate nucleus (ARC). Within the ARC, there are two neuronal populations that influence energy balance and inhibit or stimulate food intake. Neurons that co-express pro-opiomelanocortin (POMC) and cocaine- and amphetamine-regulated transcript (CART) suppress food intake, whereas neurons co-expressing neuropeptide Y (NPY) and agouti-related peptide (AgRP) stimulate feeding. ARC communicates with the paraventricular nucleus (PVN) as well as with other hypothalamic nuclei, including the dorsomedial nucleus (DMN), LHA and VMN. POMC neurons produce α-melanocyte-stimulating hormone (α-MSH), which suppresses food intake by binding melanocortin-4 receptors (MC4R) in the PVN.[19]

POMC/CART and NPY/AgRP neurons are influenced by peripheral metabolic and endocrine signals of such nutrients as glucose, fatty acids and amino acids, as well as by peripheral hormones and many other factors which are released from the gastrointestinal tract and adipose tissue.[20] Gut hormones and signals from adipose tissue can act peripherally and modulate digestion and absorption of nutrients in the intestines, but they also play the role of neurotransmitters to control food intake within the central nervous system. In general, peripheral signals may have direct or indirect (through the autonomous nervous system) effects. They act in two different ways, through afferent vagal fibers to the caudal brainstem, but also directly to the hypothalamus. Upon activation of one of the two mentioned neuronal populations, there are anorexigenic (suppressant) or orexigenic (stimulant) effects. Signals that show anorexigenic effects include peptide YY (PYY), insulin, leptin, pancreatic polypeptide (PP), cholecystokinin (CCK), glucagon-like-peptide-1 (GLP-1), oxyntomodulin (OXM), and amylin. A gastric hormone, ghrelin, which has been consistently associated with increasing appetite and initiation of food intake, is regarded as the main and probably the only known orexigenic hormone.[19] Gut hormones and adipokines act as mediators of feeding behavior, but they also modulate energy expenditure and there is increasing evidence that beneficial effects of bariatric surgery, the most effective treatment modality for obesity, is mediated by surgically induced alterations in circulating gut hormones. Metabolic operations modulate a number of gut hormones that constitute the gut–brain axis and lead to durable weight loss and mitigation of obesity-promoted comorbidities. However, it seems that the metabolic benefits of bariatric surgery, particularly resolution of T2DM, occur independently of weight loss.[21–23] It is also worth noting that different nutrients can modulate levels of factors that regulate energy homeostasis. By contact with multiple sites in the gastrointestinal tract, nutrients may alter peptide and neural signaling. The relationship between postprandial hormone changes induced by meals with different macronutrient content has been widely investigated, but its role in gut hormone release and consequently in appetite regulation remains unclear.[24–26] In addition, recent studies have focused on gut microbiota as an environmental factor that may play an important role in conditions such as obesity, metabolic syndrome and diabetes.[4] It has been suggested that gut microbiota modulates energy yield from diet, regulates peripheral metabolism and thereby influences body weight. There are some relationships between composition of intestinal microbiota and energy extracted from diet as well as synthesis of gut hormones involved in energy homeostasis and the mechanisms that regulate fat storage.[27]

The clinical and translational research goal is the transmission of knowledge between basic and clinical research so that findings in one arena rapidly inform and stimulate research in others. New understanding of disease mechanisms gained in the laboratory should stimulate the development of new methods for diagnosis, therapy and prevention, and their first tests in humans.[28] At the same time, novel observations and problems established at the bedside should be explained and solved by basic laboratory research. The goals of translational research may also be fulfilled by performing studies on animal disease models and subsequently validating the obtained findings on human populations. This allows much smaller human studies to be conducted to confirm results from the more homogeneous populations presented by animal models. The strategy of combined animal and human profiling may complement other more traditional approaches.[29] In most cases, animal studies are performed on genetically modified or diet-induced obese and T2DM rodent models. In comparison to human studies, the use of animal models to study obesity and T2DM has significant advantages when one is investigating potential pathogenic mechanisms and identifying diagnostic/prognostic biomarkers. Diet-induced obesity models are more similar to the development of human obesity compared to genetic models, and better reflect the progression of insulin resistance and the related appearance of diabetes. In animal models, insulin resistance and the resulting development of T2DM can be evoked by high-fat diet (HFD)[30,31] or high-fructose diet.[32] The advantages of genetic T2DM models over diet-induced models include the animals' short generation time, their heritable traits and the lower costs involved. On the other hand, the progressive development of diabetes over a prolonged period of time is lacking in these animals. The two most popular obesity/T2DM models are the db/db model and the obese Zucker (fa/fa) model. Both are characterized by an autosomal recessive defect in the leptin receptor gene that results in obesity and subsequent insulin resistance.[33]

15.2. GENOME-WIDE ASSOCIATION STUDIES (GWAS)

It is well known that obesity and diabetes have a large genetic component. Not everyone exposed to an obesogenic environment become obese, and not all obese people will suffer from diabetes and other complications indicative of a significant genetic heritage. Mutations of genes may cause monogenic forms of obesity, a consequence of single loss-of-function mutations in genes involved in regulation of body weight. However, monogenic forms of obesity seem to be very rare. The first studies looking for genetic factors that predispose to common obesity were based on candidate genes. In these studies, the focus is on genes that are implicated in the pathways controlling food intake and on genes with a suspected role in the metabolism. With the advent of genome-wide association studies (GWAS), the pace of gene discovery has dramatically increased. In fact, GWAS is the most commonly used approach to identify loci associated with particular phenotypes. Across the whole genome, hundreds of thousands of single nucleotide polymorphisms (SNPs) have been tested for their possible association with traits of interest, and at the subsequent stage, SNPs that show the strongest association with particular phenotypes are taken forward into the follow-up phase of the study. So far, at least 50 loci have been identified as associated with obesity, body weight, body fat content, and body fat distribution. The most common significant polymorphic variations associated with obesity were found in or near the FTO and MC4R genes. A strong association with obesity was also confirmed for loci of genetic variants in or near the BDNF, INSIG, GAD2, ENPP1, TMEM18, GNPDA2, SH2B1, MTCH2, KCTD15, NEGR1, ETV5, SEC16B, TFAP2B and NRXN3 genes.[1,34–36] In addition, it is not clear if mutations in genes associated with obesity have any effect on diabetes. It was suggested that some SNPs in the FTO gene may show a strong association with T2DM. However, the link between SNPs in the FTO gene and diabetes could not be maintained when analyses were adjusted for BMI. This indicates that the FTO locus affects T2DM on a pathway through its effect on adiposity.[1]

Common traits such as body weight and body composition, as well as metabolic profiles are the result of genetic and environmental effects that may act in an additive but also in an interactive manner. To examine the effects of this interaction, a very large sample size is required[37] and the problem is further compounded by the difficulty in obtaining accurate measures of lifestyle factors such as diet[38] and physical activity.[39] Variants of genes are linked to phenotypic variation in energy expenditure and food intake, but genetic susceptibility can be attenuated by lifestyle. Some interactions between the FTO gene and diet and physical activity have been observed, which suggests that the FTO gene may be sensitive to lifestyle in general. The results show that the effect of FTO gene variants on BMI was less pronounced in individuals with a low energy intake and with a healthier diet than in individuals with less healthy dietary habits.[40,41] Furthermore, mechanisms that control appetite, food intake, and energy expenditure may be regulated by polymorphic variation in genes. There are mutations in genes encoding known factors regulating energy homeostasis that result in obesity. The FTO locus is associated with increased appetite, reduced satiety as well as with increased energy intake.[42–44] Another important mutation that has been known to lead to extreme and early-onset obesity is located in the MC4R gene. GWAS have also identified some common variants in the locus near MC4R showing an association with obesity in the general population. Moreover, additional loci have been identified near genes that have been shown to carry monogenic mutations resulting in extreme obesity — POMC, SH2B1 and BDNF.[1,45,46]

In conclusion, SNPs may alter the function and expression of genes and play a causal role in different patterns of adiposity. The physiological roles of most of the loci associated with obesity risk are still poorly understood. The identification of new loci is only the starting point of a new series of investigations aimed at increasing our knowledge and understanding of the biological pathways involved in adiposity. Although, several studies show strong evidence of association for each of the investigated loci, they may explain only a fraction of the total variation in body weight. Using genetic risk alleles to assess genetic susceptibility scores is not accurate and has limited value in predicting obesity. Even including many loci in genetic scores to improve the accuracy of the predictions does not seem to be a good approach to discriminate between non-obese and obese individuals and is insufficient to have any clinical application.[47] By identifying obesity susceptibility loci, scientists aim to elucidate its etiology and the mechanisms by which it might influence specific phenotypes, which may provide new insights into body weight regulation. However, continued efforts, using a range of approaches, to detect high-risk populations and improve their cardiometabolic health are eagerly awaited.

15.3. METABOLOMICS

It is beyond doubt that between lean and obese as well as between diabetic and non-diabetic individuals, there are quantitative and qualitative differences in metabolic profiles. Obesity is associated with substantial changes in the function of mechanisms controlling energy homeostasis and metabolic composition, but the pathophysiological processes that influence this bidirectional relationship have not been fully elucidated. The term *metabolomics* is defined as the systematic study of the unique chemical fingerprints that specific cellular processes leave behind.[48] It is the study of the variation of small-molecule metabolites in cells, tissues and organs by measuring the global metabolite profiles. The term *metabonomics* was introduced by Nicholson *et al.*, who defined it as "the quantitative measurement of multiparametric metabolic responses of multicellular systems to pathophysiological stimuli or genetic signaling."[49] *Metabolomics* and *metabonomics* are used synonymously, but the latter is related more to the study of perturbations in metabolism caused by environmental factors (including diet and toxins), disease processes, and the involvement of extra-genomic influences such as gut microflora.[50] Generally, metabol(n)omics approaches involve the use of analytical chemistry techniques to profile as wide a range of metabolites as possible, in a quantitative or semi-quantitative manner, in conjunction with pattern recognition approaches and bioinformatics, to detect and identify metabolites (biomarkers) of specific physiological responses. In the following, we focus on studies that fulfill the above criteria and are devoted to the study of T2DM and obesity.

The analytical methods most commonly used in this type of study are nuclear magnetic resonance (NMR) and mass spectrometry (MS). MS is mainly used in combination with such separation techniques as gas chromatography (GC), liquid chromatography (LC), and capillary electrophoresis (CE). However, any single analytical platform is not able to detect all metabolites. As such, all techniques are complementary to one another, and analysis of a sample via multiple platforms enables a wider range of metabolite detection.[51] Two main approaches are used in metabolomics studies: metabolic profiling and metabolic fingerprinting. Metabolic profiling provides the identification and approximate quantification of groups of metabolites associated to specific pathways[52] or types of metabolites.[53] Metabolic fingerprinting looks at a complete profile, or fingerprint, as a unique pattern characterizing metabolism in particular case. With this approach, several metabolites are detected in one analysis and their intensities are compared between case and control groups. Therefore, it may open new, not previously hypothesized, findings. Typically, MS technology is utilized to obtain those fingerprints, which are then analyzed and compared using multivariate statistics and bioinformatics tools to identify signals (features) responsible for samples separation.[54] Discriminating features are identified based on accurate mass, isotopic pattern distribution, characteristics of MS/MS fragments or analysis of the analytical standard (if possible). Metabolomics studies are typically performed on such biological fluids as serum, urine, saliva and cerebrospinal fluid,[55] but studies on cell cultures,[56] tissue extracts[57] or secretomes[58] are also performed.

Metabolomics is a powerful tool in translational research, a bidirectional process that often begins with the generation of scientific questions based on clinical observations and subsequently involves the application of basic scientific discoveries to patient care and the community at large.

Metabolomics includes the potential discovery of new biomarkers, which can be useful in prognosis, early detection and diagnosis of diseases, and provides novel approaches for therapy. It can also increase knowledge of disease progression and can be used for the determination of treatment efficacy.[59–61] Application of the rapidly growing field of metabolomics has provided new insights into the relationship between obesity and development of T2DM. Studies have been performed in humans as well as in animal models. Validation in human populations of the results obtained with the use of animal models is an important part of translational research. There are several examples of discoveries in the area of obesity, insulin resistance, and T2DM, where studies were performed in animal models and results were later confirmed in humans. A more controlled genetic background as well as controlled environmental and experimental conditions are two of the advantages of using animal models in metabolomics studies, making it feasible to narrow down the number of candidate metabolites to become meaningful therapeutic targets or useful biomarkers. The most important pathways disturbed in obesity and T2DM that were detected by metabolomics technology are highlighted below.

The presence of diabetes evokes disturbances in glucose metabolism, a fact that was known long before the arrival of metabolomics approaches. Figure 2 presents the metabolic pathways that are disturbed by high blood glucose levels. Glucose is catabolized via glycolysis to pyruvate, which under aerobic conditions is converted into acetyl coenzyme A (AcCoA), the entry point into the tricarboxylic acid (TCA) cycle. Under anaerobic conditions, pyruvate is converted to lactate by the enzyme lactate dehydrogenase. As expected, concentrations of lactate in urine, blood or liver tissue were found to be elevated in obese mice induced by HFD, or in obese Zucker rats lacking the leptin receptor, compared to lean controls.[62] The findings of generally higher lactate levels in obese Zucker rats are consistent with higher blood lactate levels in obese humans measured by conventional methods,[63] and by metabolomics technology.[64]

The other group of metabolites that differentiate diabetics from controls are lipids. Fatty acids (FA), FA derivatives, and cholesterol are blood lipids, derived from food intake or adipose tissue and liver. Elevation of free FAs (FFAs) in serum and liver, especially the proportion of saturated fatty acids, has been found to be positively associated with the development

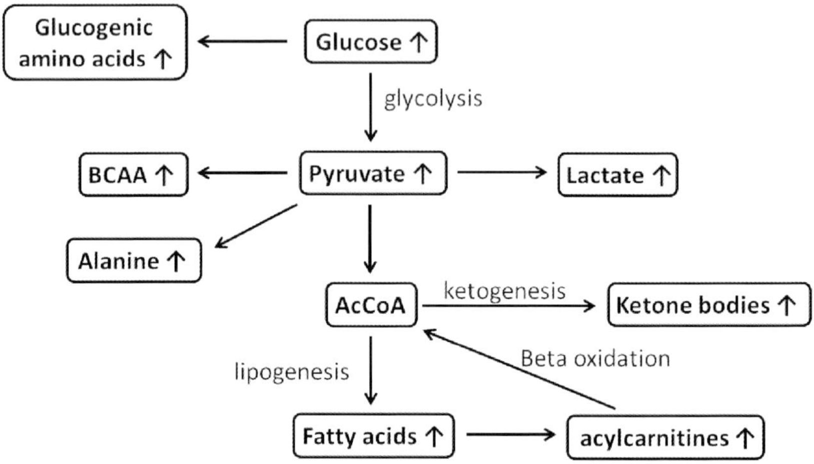

Fig. 2. Metabolic pathways disturbed by high blood glucose level. Glucose is catabolized via glycolysis to pyruvate, so high glucose level leads to an increase in pyruvate. Under aerobic conditions, pyruvate is converted to acetyl coenzyme A (AcCoA), and to lactate under anaerobic conditions. Both were observed to increase in obese/T2DM animals and humans.[62–64] A consequence of high glucose level is also an elevation of glucogenic amino acids (e.g., isoleucine, methionine, glycine, serine, alanine, tyrosine, arginine, phenylalanine, and glutamate). As pyruvate is used to construct such amino acids as alanine and BCAA, the consequence of increased amounts of pyruvate is an elevation of these amino acids. Given than AcCoA is essential in fatty acid metabolism, an increase in fatty acids is observed in obese/T2DM subjects in comparison to controls. A profusion of FFAs can promote fatty acid β-oxidation, which takes place in the mitochondria. Fatty acids can be transported into the mitochondria only after esterification with carnitine. Thus, increased levels of acylcarnitines are observed in obese/T2DM subjects.[75] Additionally, high fatty acid levels lead to a higher β-oxidation rate, an increase in AcCoA, and consequently to the induction of ketogenesis. Thus, elevated levels of ketone bodies are observed in T2DM subjects.[71]

of obesity, diabetes[65] and other diseases.[66,67] In agreement with this, elevation of FFAs in serum and liver of obese animals has been observed by metabolomics analysis,[68,69] and similar results were observed in blood of T2DM patients.[70–72] The profusion of FFAs can promote fatty acid β-oxidation, which takes place in the mitochondria. However, fatty acids can be transported into the mitochondria only after esterification with carnitine. Thus, higher plasma FFAs in obesity may require more carnitine for efficient β-oxidation, and increased levels of acylcarnitines. Consequently, higher levels of acylcarnitines have been observed in diabetic rodents,[73,74] and also in obese and T2DM subjects.[75] Additionally, high fatty acid levels lead to a higher oxidation rate, an increase in AcCoA, and consequently to the induction of ketogenesis. Thus, diabetic animals typically exhibit higher levels of ketone bodies, e.g., β-hydroxybutyrate, acetoacetate or acetone, in comparison to controls.[76,77] Higher levels of ketone bodies were also observed in T2DM subjects.[71] The consequence of increased blood glucose level is an increase in leucine, isoleucine and valine (branched chain amino acids, BCAAs), and alanine.[78] BCAAs, as well as other amino acids like methionine, glycine, serine, alanine, tyrosine, lysine, arginine, phenylalanine, and glutamate, have been shown to display significant obesity-related variations. BCAAs play an important role in the development of diabetes, as they improve glucose metabolism and oxidation, and regulate leptin secretion from fat and food intake.[62] The contribution of BCAAs to obesity-related comorbidities such as insulin resistance and glucose intolerance have been shown by the use of metabolic profiling of obese versus lean humans, which found elevated BCAA levels in serum of obese patients.[63] On the other hand, the opposite results were obtained in two metabolomics studies performed on HFD-fed obese mice, in which depletion of serum levels of BCAAs was reported.[30,79] In another study, higher serum concentrations of citrate when compared to controls were detected by NMR-[30] or GC-MS-based[69] metabolomics in HFD-fed obese animals with insulin resistance. Conversely, a decrease of urinary citrate excretion has also been reported in obese animals with insulin resistance,[69] and lower urinary citrate excretion was reported to be associated with a higher level of insulin resistance in humans.[80] Intriguingly, in another study, higher levels of citrate were observed in urine of T2DM patients.[64] Additional research is required to establish whether there is a difference in urinary citrate level between insulin resistance and T2DM patients. In summary, the application of metabolomics in the study of obesity, and the consequent development of insulin resistance and T2DM in animals and humans, has demonstrated the alteration of several metabolic pathways in those conditions. However, most of the metabolic variations in obesity and T2DM detected using metabolomics approaches (e.g., fatty acids, amino acids, ketone bodies, lactate, and carnitines) were already known.

Interestingly, novel metabolites involved in glucose metabolism were discovered in a study on the changes in plasma metabolic profiles in relation to glucose ingestion, as reported by Shaham *et al.* This study demonstrated changes in the levels of three bile acids (glycocholic acid, glycochenodeoxycholic acid, and taurochenodeoxycholic acid) following the oral glucose tolerance test (OGTT). The levels of these bile acids were found to increase within the first 30 min following glucose ingestion and remained stable thereafter,[81] observations that were later confirmed by other groups.[82,83] The changes in bile acid levels observed in these studies could be connected to the fact that taurine improves insulin sensitivity. Taurine is an important metabolite in bile acid metabolism, and it was found that a taurine-supplemented diet tended to decrease total fat weight in the abdominal cavity and improved insulin sensitivity in a rat model of T2DM.[62] Unfortunately, the effects obtained in animal models have not been observed in humans. Daily supplementation with taurine for eight weeks had no effect on insulin secretion or sensitivity, or on blood lipid levels, suggesting that dietary taurine supplementation cannot prevent the development of T2DM in humans.[84] However, in another study, therapy with bile acid sequestrants led to the expected reductions in the levels of plasma glucose, HbA1c, total cholesterol, and low-density lipoprotein cholesterol as well as improvements in glycemic control in T2DM patients.[85,86] Besides bile acids, several other metabolites were also found to be altered during the OGTT in healthy subjects. An increase in lysophosphatidylcholine and decreases in amino acids, acylcarnitines, and fatty acids were reported. Based on the research applying metabolomics approach to study response to glucose challenge in humans, it can be summarized that various pathways involved in insulin action (i.e., lipolysis, ketogenesis, proteolysis and glucose metabolism) are altered during the OGTT.[81,83,87] The consequences of these results for clinical practice still need to be established.

15.4. PERSPECTIVES FOR METABOLOMICS

Although metabolomics studies comparing the biological fluids of T2DM patients with those of controls have not extended current knowledge about the relationship between obesity and T2DM significantly, metabolomics technology has an undeniable potential to discover novel connections between T2DM and obesity or to measure the efficacy of treatment. One of the areas in which metabolomics has a future, and in which the field has already been used,[88,89] is the investigation of a potential link between gut microbiota, obesity, and the subsequent development of T2DM. The first definite evidence for the role of gut microbiota in the regulation of host energy homeostasis and adiposity came from a group of experiments by Gordon and colleagues, who noticed that germ-free mice had 40 percent less total body fat than control mice, even if their caloric intake was 29 percent higher. Furthermore, colonization of the guts of germ-free mice with a cecum-derived, distal microbial community produced a 57 percent increase in total body fat, a more than two-fold increase in hepatic triglycerides, and a dramatic increase in insulin resistance without affecting chow consumption or energy expenditure.[90] It has been demonstrated, in both mice and humans, that obesity is associated with lower microbial diversity and decreased levels of Bacteroidetes,[89] and also that consumption of a high fat diet results in a decrease of total gut bacterial levels and an increase in Gram-negative bacteria.[91]

The notion that gut microbiota are key players in the onset and development of obesity and diabetes is becoming more widely accepted. As type 2 diabetes is strongly associated with obesity, it is hypothesized that these two conditions could be linked by an underlying physiological process including the disordered regulation of gut bacterial profiles.[91] Based on metabolomics studies, alterations in several intestinal microflora-associated metabolites have been detected in obesity and T2DM. Insulin-deprived T2DM patients exhibited elevated levels of hippurate, dimethylamine or trimethylamine-N-oxide.[64,88] Studies involving genetic and HFD-induced obese/T2DM animal models found alterations in the plasma lipids and in the concentrations of urinary metabolites such as phenylacetate, hydroxyphenylacetylglycine, hydroxyindoleacetic acid, hippurate and dimethylamine.[91] The contribution of microbiota to the development of obesity and diabetes in animal models and humans is evident, but further investigations in this area are needed. Understanding the mechanisms of microbial involvement in these conditions could help in the development of novel therapies for obesity and T2DM.

The importance of gut microbiota in obesity/T2DM can also be supported by the previously mentioned effects of bariatric surgery.[21–23] The idea of bariatric surgery is to enforce dietary compliance either by reducing (e.g., gastric banding and vertical gastroplasty) or eliminating (e.g., Roux-en-Y or biliopancreatic diversion) the presence of food in the proximal small intestine. After such procedures, glycemic control improves rapidly (usually within the first few days), followed by significant weight loss (which takes months).[92] Several hypotheses have been postulated to explain the improved insulin sensitivity post-surgery, including the altered secretion of gut hormones, modifications in intestinal gluconeogenesis, and changes in intramyocellular lipid content.[93] Metabolomics approaches could extend our knowledge about the changes encouraged by bariatric surgery. Thus far, just two studies have applied this novel technology to explain these metabolic changes. One was devoted to tracking general metabolic changes in the serum of patients who underwent surgery, and only five patients were type 2 diabetics.[93] In the other study, the urine of patients before surgery and one month post-surgery was analyzed using NMR fingerprinting, which showed, among other things, changes in such metabolites as hippuric acid, 3-hydroxybutyrate, 2-hydroxyisobutyrate, and trigonelline.[94] More research is necessary to explain the mechanisms behind the treatment of T2DM by bariatric surgery.

Metabolomics also has the potential to be used in progressive studies. Metabolomics has recently been used to search for prognostic biomarkers of diabetes in children and adults. In a study by Orešič and colleagues,[95] reduced serum levels of succinic acid and phosphatidylcholine (PC) at birth, as well as the development of reduced levels of triglycerides and antioxidant ether phospholipids and increased levels of proinflammatory lysoPCs during childhood, were found to be prognostic markers of type 1 diabetes in children. In another study, more than 2,000 normoglycemic individuals were recruited between 1991 and 1995, and followed for 12 years. In this time, about 8 percent of them developed diabetes, and metabolic profiling was performed on the samples collected during the time of recruitment. Five branched-chain and aromatic amino acids (isoleucine, leucine, valine, tyrosine and phenylalanine) had highly significant associations with future diabetes. Additionally, a combination of three amino acids predicted future diabetes with a more than five-fold higher risk for individuals in the top quartile.[96] This type of progressive study could be performed to track obese individuals who go on to develop T2DM.

15.5. GWAS WITH METABOLIC TRAITS (mGWAS)

During the last decade, at least 27 (confirmed and potential) diabetes susceptibility genes[97] and at least 50 loci associated with obesity, body weight, body fat content and body fat distribution have been identified.[1,34–36] Despite such genes and gene–gene interactions being significant type 2 diabetes risk factors, they do not allow a substantially better disease prediction than clinical risk factors alone (e.g., BMI, age, gender, family history of diabetes, fasting glucose level, blood pressure, and plasma triglycerides), nor do they explain the heritability of type 2 diabetes.[97] Hence, alternative approaches, such as correlation analyses of SNPs with standard lab oratory parameters (fasting glucose, cholesterol, insulin resistance, and triglyceride), or global metabolite measurements (e.g., metabolic fingerprinting or metabolic/lipid profiling) may further increase our knowledge about the relationship between obesity and T2DM. Through the integration of genomics, metabolomics and complex disease data, novel pathways involved in the development of these diseases could be revealed. Initial experiments combining metabolomics with GWAS (mGWAS) have been reported recently.[98,99] For instance, it was found that SNP rs1260326 in *GCKR* lowers fasting glucose and triglyceride levels and reduces the risk of type 2 diabetes,[100] and this locus was also found to be associated with different ratios of phosphatidylcholines.[99] Moreover, the polymorphism rs10830963 in the melatonin-receptor gene *MTNR1B* was found to be associated with fasting glucose,[101] and the same SNP has been associated with tryptophan to phenylalanine ratios.[99] Finally, other studies have established an association of SNP rs964184 in the apolipoprotein cluster APOA1-APOC3-APOA4-APOA5 with blood triglyceride levels[102] and phosphatidylcholines.[99]

15.6. CONCLUSIONS

Many years of research are required to better understand the mechanisms and interactions between genes, gut hormones, diet and other environmental factors, as well as to unravel the underlying physiological pathways in the pathogenesis of emerging lifestyle conditions like obesity and T2DM. The introduction of associated genes, SNPs and metabolic pathways into standard prophylactic tests is a matter for the future. For the moment, determination of genetic polymorphisms is too expensive to implement in global populations. Metabolites assumed as potential biomarkers of the disease require validation in much wider populations and the development of accurate, validated laboratory procedures for their determination. However, translation of those discoveries to the mainstream of healthcare might contribute to more targeted preventive strategies and more effective treatment of obesity and associated comorbidities. An understanding of the basis of heterogeneity of each individual provides an opportunity for personalizing prevention and treatment strategies according to the clinical and molecular characteristics of a particular patient. There is evidence-based support for the benefits of a personalized approach to care in patients with certain monogenic forms of diabetes.[103] The combination of metabolomics as a phenotyping tool with GWAS seems to be a promising direction for subclassification of people with obesity and T2DM. This could provide new insights into the genetic mechanisms of disease that are required for personalized medicine. Establishing strategies for individualized diet and/or treatment decisions for people with obesity and/or T2DM is a challenging emerging field for translational research.

REFERENCES

1. Day FR, Loos RJ. (2011) Developments in obesity genetics in the era of genome-wide association studies. *J Nutrigenet Nutrigenom* **4**: 222–238.
2. Patel CJ, Bhattacharya J, Butte AJ. (2010) An environment-wide association study (EWAS) on type 2 diabetes mellitus. *PLoS ONE* **5**: e10746.
3. Villegas R, Delahanty R, Gao YT, *et al.* (2012) Joint effect of genetic and lifestyle risk factors on type 2 diabetes risk among chinese men and women. *PLoS ONE* **7**: e49464.
4. Diamant M, Blaak EE, de Vos WM. (2011) Do nutrient–gut–microbiota interactions play a role in human obesity, insulin resistance and type 2 diabetes? *Obes Rev* **12**: 272–281.
5. Caballero B. (2007) The global epidemic of obesity: An overview. *Epidemiol Rev* **29**: 1–5.
6. Yusuf S, Hawken S, Ounpuu S, *et al.* (2005) Obesity and the risk of myocardial infarction in 27,000 participants from 52 countries: A case-control study. *Lancet* **366**: 1640–1649.

7. Mokdad AH, Ford ES, Bowman BA, *et al.* (2003) Prevalence of obesity, diabetes, and obesity-related health risk factors, 2001. *J Am Med Assoc* **289**: 76–79.
8. Dixon JB. (2010) The effect of obesity on health outcomes. *Mol Cell Endocrinol* **316**: 104–108.
9. Welborn TA, Dhaliwal SS, Bennett SA. (2003) Waist-hip ratio is the dominant risk factor predicting cardiovascular death in Australia. *Med J Aust* **179**: P580–585.
10. Renehan AG, Tyson M, Egger M, *et al.* (2008) Body-mass index and incidence of cancer: A systematic review and meta-analysis of prospective observational studies. *Lancet* **371**: 569–578.
11. Hu G, Jousilahti P, Nissinen A, *et al.* (2006) Body mass index and the risk of Parkinson disease. *Neurology* **67**: 1955–1959.
12. Whitmer RA, Gunderson EP, Quesenberry CP, *et al.* (2007) Body mass index in midlife and risk of Alzheimer disease and vascular dementia. *Curr Alzheimer Res* **4**: 103–109.
13. Scott KM, Bruffaerts R, Simon GE, *et al.* (2008) Obesity and mental disorders in the general population: Results from the world mental health surveys. *Int J Obes (Lond)* **32**: 192–200.
14. Jeffery RW, Sherwood NE. (2008) Is the obesity epidemic exaggerated? No. *Br Med J* **336**: 245.
15. Abelson P, Kennedy D. (2004) The obesity epidemic. *Science* **304**: 1413.
16. Belkina AC, Denis GV. (2010) Obesity genes and insulin resistance. *Curr Opin Endocrinol Diabetes Obes* **17**: 472–477.
17. Stubbs RS, Wickremesekera SK. (2002) Insulin resistance in the severely obese and links with metabolic co-morbidities. *Obes Surg* **12**: 343–348.
18. Succurro E, Marini MA, Frontoni S, *et al.* (2008) Insulin secretion in metabolically obese, but normal weight, and in metabolically healthy but obese individuals. *Obesity (Silver Spring)* **16**: 1881–1886.
19. Suzuki K, Simpson KA, Minnion JS, *et al.* (2010) The role of gut hormones and the hypothalamus in appetite regulation. *Endocr J* **57**: 359–372.
20. Belgardt BF, Okamura T, Bruning JC. (2009) Hormone and glucose signalling in POMC and AgRP neurons. *J Physiol* **587**: 5305–5314.
21. Ashrafian H, le Roux CW. (2009) Metabolic surgery and gut hormones — A review of bariatric entero-humoral modulation. *Physiol Behav* **97**: 620–631.
22. Karra E, Yousseif A, Batterham RL. (2010) Mechanisms facilitating weight loss and resolution of type 2 diabetes following bariatric surgery. *Trends Endocrinol Metab* **21**: 337–344.

23. Laferrère B. (2011) Do we really know why diabetes remits after gastric bypass surgery? *Endocrine* **40**: 162–167.
24. Brennan IM, Luscombe-Marsh ND, Seimon RV, *et al.* (2012) Effects of fat, protein, and carbohydrate and protein load on appetite, plasma cholecystokinin, peptide YY, and ghrelin, and energy intake in lean and obese men. *Am J Physiol Gastrointest Liver Physiol* **303**: G129–G140.
25. Misra M, Tsai PM, Mendes N, *et al.* (2009) Increased carbohydrate induced ghrelin secretion in obese vs. normal-weight adolescent girls. *Obesity* **17**: 1689–1695.
26. Maffeis C, Surano MG, Cordioli S, *et al.* (2010) A high-fat vs. a moderate-fat meal in obese boys: Nutrient balance, appetite, and gastrointestinal hormone changes. *Obesity* (*Silver Spring*) **18**: 449–455.
27. Vrieze A, Holleman F, Zoetendal EG, *et al.* (2010) The environment within: How gut microbiota may influence metabolism and body composition. *Diabetologia* **53**: 606–613.
28. Lauer MS, Skarlatos S. (2010) Translational research for cardiovascular diseases at the National Heart, Lung, and Blood Institute: Moving from bench to bedside and from bedside to community. *Circulation* **121**: 929–933.
29. Griffin JL, Vidal-Puig A. (2008) Current challenges in metabolomics for diabetes research: A vital functional genomic tool or just a ploy for gaining funding? *Physiol Genomics* **34**: 1–5.
30. Shearer J, Duggan G, Weljie A, *et al.* (2008) Metabolomic profiling of dietary-induced insulin resistance in the high fat-fed C57BL/6J mouse. *Diabetes Obes Metab* **10**: 950–958.
31. Kim H-J, Kim JH, Noh S, *et al.* (2010) Metabolomic analysis of livers and serum from high-fat diet induced obese mice. *J Proteome Res* **10**: 722–731.
32. Lin S, Yang Z, Liu H, *et al.* (2011) Beyond glucose: Metabolic shifts in responses to the effects of the oral glucose tolerance test and the high-fructose diet in rats. *Mol Biosyst* 7: 1537–1548.
33. Friedrich N. (2012) Metabolomics in diabetes research. *J Endocrinol* **215**: 29–42.
34. Herbert A, Gerry NP, McQueen MB, *et al.* (2006) A common genetic variant is associated with adult and childhood obesity. *Science* **312**: 279–283.
35. Meyre D, Bouatia-Naji N, Tounian A, *et al.* (2005) Variants of ENPP1 are associated with childhood and adult obesity and increase the risk of glucose intolerance and type 2 diabetes. *Nat Genet* **37**: 863–867.
36. Frayling TM, Timpson NJ, Weedon MN, *et al.* (2007) A common variant in the FTO gene is associated with body mass index and predisposes to childhood and adult obesity. *Science* **316**: 889–894.

37. Wong MY, Day NE, Luan JA, *et al.* (2003) The detection of gene–environment interaction for continuous traits: Should we deal with measurement error by bigger studies or better measurement? *Int J Epidemiol* **32**: 51–57.
38. Westerterp KR, Goris AH. (2002) Validity of the assessment of dietary intake: Problems of misreporting. *Curr Opin Clin Nutr Metab Care* **5**: 489–493.
39. Warren JM, Ekelund U, Besson H, *et al.* (2010) Assessment of physical activity — A review of methodologies with reference to epidemiological research: A report of the exercise physiology section of the European Association of Cardiovascular Prevention and Rehabilitation. *Eur J Cardiovasc Prev Rehab* **17**: 127–139.
40. Ahmad T, Lee IM, Paré G, *et al.* (2011) Lifestyle interaction with fat mass and obesity-associated (FTO) genotype and risk of obesity in apparently healthy U.S. women. *Diabetes Care* **34**: 675–680.
41. Sonestedt E, Roos C, Gullberg B, *et al.* (2009) Fat and carbohydrate intake modify the association between genetic variation in the FTO genotype and obesity. *Am J Clin Nutr* **90**: 1418–1425.
42. Cecil JE, Tavendale R, Watt P, *et al.* (2008) An obesity-associated FTO gene variant and increased energy intake in children. *N Engl J Med* **359**: 2558–2566.
43. Wardle J, Carnell S, Haworth CM, *et al.* (2008) Obesity associated genetic variation in FTO is associated with diminished satiety. *J Clin Endocrinol Metab* **93**: 3640–3643.
44. Speakman JR, Rance KA, Johnstone AM. (2008) Polymorphisms of the FTO gene are associated with variation in energy intake, but not energy expenditure. *Obesity (Silver Spring)* **16**: 1961–1965.
45. Baker M. (2010) Epigenome: Mapping in motion. *Nat Meth* **7**: 181–186.
46. Birney E. (2011) Chromatin and heritability: How epigenetic studies can complement genetic approaches. *Trends Genet* **27**: 172–176.
47. Speliotes EK, Willer CJ, Berndt SI, *et al.* (2010) Association analyses of 249,796 individuals reveal 18 new loci associated with body mass index. *Nat Genet* **42**: 937–948.
48. Fiehn O. (2002) Metabolomics — The link between genotypes and phenotypes. *Plant Mol Biol* **48**: 155–171.
49. Nicholson JK, Lindon JC, Holmes E. (1999) "Metabonomics": Understanding the metabolic responses of living systems to pathophysiological stimuli via multivariate statistical analysis of biological NMR spectroscopic data. *Xenobiotica* **29**: 1181–1189.
50. Robertson DG. (2005) Metabonomics in toxicology: A review. *Toxicol Sci* **85**: 809–822.

51. Kusano M, Fukushima A, Redestig H, Saito K. (2011) Metabolomic approaches toward understanding nitrogen metabolism in plants. *J Exp Bot* **62**: 1439–1453.
52. Cheng S, Rhee EP, Larson MG, *et al.* (2012) Metabolite profiling identifies pathways associated with metabolic risk in humans. *Circulation* **125**: 2222–2231.
53. Waszczuk-Jankowska M, Markuszewski MJ, Markuszewski M, Kaliszan R. (2012) Comparison of RP-HPLC columns used for determination of nucleoside metabolic patterns in urine of cancer patients. *Bioanalysis* **4**: 1185–1194.
54. Shulaev V. (2006) Metabolomics technology and bioinformatics. *Brief Bioinform* **7**: 128–139.
55. Lu X, Zhao X, Bai C, *et al.* (2008) LC-MS-based metabonomics analysis. *J Chromatogr B Analyt Technol Biomed Life Sci* **866**: 64–76.
56. Khoo SH, Al-Rubeai M. (2007) Metabolomics as a complementary tool in cell culture. *Biotechnol Appl Biochem* **47**: 71–84.
57. Wu H, Southam AD, Hines A, Viant MR. (2008) High-throughput tissue extraction protocol for NMR- and MS-based metabolomics. *Anal Biochem* **372**: 204–212.
58. Ciborowski M, Martin-Ventura JL, Meilhac O, *et al.* (2011) Metabolites secreted by human atherothrombotic aneurysms revealed through a metabolomic approach. *J Proteome Res* **10**: 1374–1382.
59. Serkova NJ, Standiford TJ, Stringer KA. (2011) The emerging field of quantitative blood metabolomics for biomarker discovery in critical illnesses. *Am J Respir Crit Care Med* **184**: 647–655.
60. Spratlin JL, Serkova NJ, Eckhardt SG. (2009) Clinical applications of metabolomics in oncology: A review. *Clin Cancer Res* **15**: 431–440.
61. Mayr M. (2008) Metabolomics: Ready for the prime time? *Circ Cardiovasc Genet* **1**: 58–65.
62. Xie B, Waters MJ, Schirra HJ. (2012) Investigating potential mechanisms of obesity by metabolomics. *J Biomed Biotechnol* **2012**: 805683.
63. Newgard CB, An J, Bain JR, *et al.* (2009) A branched-chain amino acid-related metabolic signature that differentiates obese and lean humans and contributes to insulin resistance. *Cell Metab* **9**: 311–326.
64. Messana I, Forni F, Ferrari F, *et al.* (1998) Proton nuclear magnetic resonance spectral profiles of urine in type II diabetic patients. *Clin Chem* **44**: 1529–1534.
65. Laaksonen DE, Lakka TA, Lakka HM, *et al.* (2002) Serum fatty acid composition predicts development of impaired fasting glycaemia and diabetes in middle-aged men. *Diabet Med* **19**: 456–464.

66. Ohrvall M, Berglund L, Salminen I, *et al.* (1996) The serum cholesterol ester fatty acid composition but not the serum concentration of alpha tocopherol predicts the development of myocardial infarction in 50-year-old men: 19 years follow-up. *Atherosclerosis* **127**: 65–71.
67. Green R, Kwok S, Durrington PN. (2002) Preventing cardiovascular disease in hypertension: Effects of lowering blood pressure and cholesterol. *Q J Med* **95**: 821–826.
68. Serkova NJ, Jackman M, Brown JL, *et al.* (2006) Metabolic profiling of livers and blood from obese Zucker rats. *J Hepatol* **44**: 956–962.
69. Li H, Xie Z, Lin J, *et al.* (2008) Transcriptomic and metabonomic profiling of obesity-prone and obesity-resistant rats under high fat diet. *J Proteome Res* **7**: 4775–4783.
70. Yi L, Yuan D, Che Z, *et al.* (2008) Plasma fatty acid metabolic profile coupled with uncorrelated linear discriminant analysis to diagnose and biomarker screening of type 2 diabetes and type 2 diabetic coronary heart diseases. *Metabolomics* **4**: 30–38.
71. Suhre K, Meisinger C, Döring A, *et al.* (2010) Metabolic footprint of diabetes: A multiplatform metabolomics study in an epidemiological setting. *PLoS ONE* **5**: e13953.
72. Li X, Xu Z, Lu X, *et al.* (2009) Comprehensive two-dimensional gas chromatography/time-of-flight mass spectrometry for metabonomics: Biomarker discovery for diabetes mellitus. *Analytica Chimica Acta* **633**: 257–262.
73. Connor SC, Hansen MK, Corner A, *et al.* (2010) Integration of metabolomics and transcriptomics data to aid biomarker discovery in type 2 diabetes. *Mol Biosyst* **6**: 909–921.
74. Gipson GT, Tatsuoka KS, Ball RJ, *et al.* (2008) Multi-platform investigation of the metabolome in a leptin receptor defective murine model of type 2 diabetes. *Mol Biosyst* **4**: 1015–1023.
75. Mihalik SJ, Goodpaster BH, Kelley DE, *et al.* (2010) Increased levels of plasma acylcarnitines in obesity and type 2 diabetes and identification of a marker of glucolipotoxicity. *Obesity* **18**: 1695–1700.
76. Zhao X, Fritsche J, Wang J, *et al.* (2010) Metabonomic fingerprints of fasting plasma and spot urine reveal human pre-diabetic metabolic traits. *Metabolomics* **6**: 362–374.
77. Salek RM, Maguire ML, Bentley E, *et al.* (2007) A metabolomic comparison of urinary changes in type 2 diabetes in mouse, rat, and human. *Physiol Genomics* **29**: 99–108.

78. Mochida T, Tanaka T, Shiraki Y, *et al.* (2011) Time-dependent changes in the plasma amino acid concentration in diabetes mellitus. *Mol Genet Metab* **103**: 406–409.
79. Duggan GE, Hittel DS, Sensen CW, *et al.* (2011) Metabolomic response to exercise training in lean and diet-induced obese mice. *J Appl Physiol* **110**: 1311–1318.
80. Cupisti A, Meola M, D'Alessandro C, *et al.* (2007) Insulin resistance and low urinary citrate excretion in calcium stone formers. *Biomed Pharmacother* **61**: 86–90.
81. Shaham O, Wei R, Wang TJ, *et al.* (2008) Metabolic profiling of the human response to a glucose challenge reveals distinct axes of insulin sensitivity. *Mol Syst Biol* **4**: 214.
82. Matysik S, Martin J, Bala M, *et al.* (2011) Bile acid signaling after an oral glucose tolerance test. *Chem Phys Lipids* **164**: 525–529.
83. Zhao X, Peter A, Fritsche J, *et al.* (2009) Changes of the plasma metabolome during an oral glucose tolerance test: Is there more than glucose to look at? *Am J Physiol Endocrinol Metab* **296**: E384–E393.
84. Brons C, Spohr C, Storgaard H, *et al.* (2004) Effect of taurine treatment on insulin secretion and action, and on serum lipid levels in overweight men with a genetic predisposition for type II diabetes mellitus. *Eur J Clin Nutr* **58**: 1239–1247.
85. Zieve FJ, Kalin MF, Schwartz SL, *et al.* (2007) Results of the glucose-lowering effect of WelChol study (GLOWS): A randomized, double-blind, placebo-controlled pilot study evaluating the effect of colesevelam hydrochloride on glycemic control in subjects with type 2 diabetes. *Clin Ther* **29**: 74–83.
86. Kondo K, Kadowaki T. (2010) Colestilan monotherapy significantly improves glycaemic control and LDL cholesterol levels in patients with type 2 diabetes: A randomized double-blind placebo-controlled study. *Diabetes Obes Metab* **12**: 246–251.
87. Spégel P, Danielsson AH, Bacos K, *et al.* (2010) Metabolomic analysis of a human oral glucose tolerance test reveals fatty acids as reliable indicators of regulated metabolism. *Metabolomics* **6**: 56–66.
88. Dumas M-E, Barton RH, Toye A, *et al.* (2006) Metabolic profiling reveals a contribution of gut microbiota to fatty liver phenotype in insulin-resistant mice. *Proc Natl Acad Sci USA* **103**: 12511–12516.
89. Velagapudi VR, Hezaveh R, Reigstad CS, *et al.* (2010) The gut microbiota modulates host energy and lipid metabolism in mice. *J Lipid Res* **51**: 1101–1112.

90. Bäckhed F, Ding H, Wang T, *et al.* (2004) The gut microbiota as an environmental factor that regulates fat storage. *Proc Natl Acad Sci USA* **101**: 15718–15723.
91. Holmes E, Li JV, Athanasiou T, *et al.* (2011) Understanding the role of gut microbiome-host metabolic signal disruption in health and disease. *Trends Microbiol* **19**: 349–359.
92. Flatt PR, Day C, Bailey CJ. (2009) Bariatric surgery: To treat diabesity. *Br J Diabetes Vasc Dis* **9**: 103–107.
93. Mutch DM, Fuhrmann JC, Rein D, *et al.* (2009) Metabolite profiling identifies candidate markers reflecting the clinical adaptations associated with Roux-en-Y gastric bypass surgery. *PLoS ONE* **4**: e7905.
94. Friedrich N, Budde K, Wolf T, *et al.* (2012) Short-term changes of the urine metabolome after bariatric surgery. *OMICS* **16**: 612–620.
95. Orešič M, Simell S, Sysi-Aho M, *et al.* (2008) Dysregulation of lipid and amino acid metabolism precedes islet autoimmunity in children who later progress to type 1 diabetes. *J Exp Med* **205**: 2975–2984.
96. Wang TJ, Larson MG, Vasan RS, *et al.* (2011) Metabolite profiles and the risk of developing diabetes. *Nat Med* **17**: 448–453.
97. Staiger H, Machicao F, Fritsche A, Häring HU. (2009) Pathomechanisms of type 2 diabetes genes. *Endocr Rev* **30**: 557–585.
98. Tukiainen T, Kettunen J, Kangas AJ, *et al.* (2012) Detailed metabolic and genetic characterization reveals new associations for 30 known lipid loci. *Hum Mol Genet* **21**: 1444–1455.
99. Illig T, Gieger C, Zhai G, *et al.* (2010) A genome wide perspective of genetic variation in human metabolism. *Nat Genet* **42**: 137–141.
100. Vaxillaire M, Cavalcanti-Proença C, Dechaume A, *et al.* (2008) The common P446L polymorphism in GCKR inversely modulates fasting glucose and triglyceride levels and reduces type 2 diabetes risk in the DESIR prospective general French population. *Diabetes* **57**: 2253–2257.
101. Prokopenko I, Langenberg C, Florez JC, *et al.* (2009) Variants in MTNR1B influence fasting glucose levels. *Nat Genet* **41**: 77–81.
102. Kathiresan S, Melander O, Guiducci C, *et al.* (2008) Six new loci associated with blood low-density lipoprotein cholesterol, high-density lipoprotein cholesterol or triglycerides in humans. *Nat Genet* **40**: 189–197.
103. Malandrino N, Smith RJ. (2011) Personalized medicine in diabetes. *Clin Chem* **57**: 231–240.

CHAPTER 16

Translating Science into Practice: What Are the Needs of People with Obesity and/or Diabetes?

Wieland Kiess[*,†], *Sabine Herget*[*], *Jana Markert*[*], *Andreas Hiemisch*[*], *Stefanie Naumann*[*], *Madlen Neef*[*], *Ruth Gausche*[*], *Mandy Vogel*[*], *Antje Körner*[*] *and Roland Pfaeffle*[*]

16.1. INTRODUCTION

Translating science into clinical practice is not an easy task. Many researchers in biology, biomedicine, psychology, or even the social sciences and humanities are ambitious people with career well-defined goals. As with professionals in any given area, there is a natural tendency among researchers to compete and strive for power and influence. In the worst cases, this can hinder scientific advancement and diminish the benefits for the wider society. The need to apply for funding and resources exerts tremendous pressure on individual researchers: the means to provide for equipment, personnel and consumables have to be secured both within an institution and from outside. Scientists are kept extremely busy by the

[*]Hospital for Children and Adolescents, Department for Women and Child Health, Centre for Pediatric Research, University of Leipzig, Leipzig, Germany.

[†]Corresponding author: Prof. Wieland Kiess, MD, Hospital for Children and Adolescents, Department for Women and Child Health, Centre for Paediatric Research, University of Leipzig, Liebigstr. 20a, D-04103 Leipzig, Germany; Tel: +49-341-972-6000; Fax: +49-341-972-6009; E-mail: *wieland.kiess@medizin.uni-leipzig.de*.

constant requirement to write and review grants, evaluate whether or not milestones have been reached, and ensure deliverables have been delivered and goals have been achieved. Ultimately, that pressure can divert researchers' attention from following up projects, for example, and most importantly, from the task of actively and decisively meeting the needs of patients. Inevitably, this state of affairs influences the choice of topics, areas of interest and even the questions that are being asked: without money, biomedical research cannot be carried out. Researchers very often focus on areas where applications for financial support have been successful and chances are high that additional grants are available. As a consequence, scientists may choose to follow mainstream research: working in an area where everyone else works and researching topics with tools that everyone else is using ("state-of-the-art") enable scientists to form large research groups, increase their social power, and — last but not least — stay in business.

Science has become a business with many stakeholders and interest groups involved. The questions that are being asked are not necessarily the questions that need to be answered in order to improve our quality of life, reduce suffering from illness, or increase the survival of patients. An area where the current research system has been particularly weak is prevention, and this is especially true for obesity and diabetes prevention. Asking fundamental questions is still very important and the very essence of science. Basic questions should always be allowed to be asked without the expectation of an immediate benefit for the patient or society. However, asking questions without asking why one should answer the question in the long run, and what society expects from the answer, is a self-serving enterprise. Today, billions of dollars from public sources are spent on research on the pathogenesis and/or pathophysiology of obesity and type 2 diabetes. In comparison, extremely little is spent on actually preventing diabetes and obesity and their comorbidities. Huge sums have been invested in genetic and biomedical research without real breakthroughs and with very little gain for the general public.[1–3] On the other hand, very conspicuous questions about how society has become obesogenic and why the obesity epidemic has risen and spread so rapidly have not been tackled adequately.[4,5] This chapter puts forward some obvious and therefore provocative hypotheses, with a view to answering the question: What needs to be done in order to develop a real translational research program to combat obesity and type 2 diabetes?

16.2. WHAT IS THE PROBLEM?

In general, researchers make use of common knowledge, available technologies [e.g., Sanger sequencing, matrix-assisted laser desorption/ionization-time of flight (MALDI-TOF) mass spectrometry, protein electrophoresis, positron emission tomography/magnetic resonance imaging (PET/MRI)], and clinical investigations.[6,7] They take advantage of available resources to try to answer old and new questions, and to advance scientific thinking. In most cases, therefore, we follow old routes and easily accessible paths. Table 1 lists the kind of topics relating to questions that are constantly being asked again and again in the area of metabolism.

We live at a time when a wealth of information is available and, most importantly, is readily accessible for many people in most countries around the world, for example through electronic means and open access sources. There is huge diversity and variety of information. On the other hand, importantly, the question of what information may be true and in the widest sense "correct" is not readily answerable. There is a constant need to look for "truth" in any given information — without ever being certain that we will ever know the answer.

In the present era of advertising and media manipulation, questions of correctness and truth have become more important and pressing than ever. For the public, there is a conspicuous lack of quality control of the available information. For instance, the question of whether or not a given diet may help to reduce body weight cannot be answered readily but may be experienced only after a potentially arduous personal trial. Expert opinion versus truth versus evidence is not readily comprehensible from the Internet

Table 1 Some General Research Questions in Obesity and Diabetes Research that are Constantly being Asked But have not been Sufficiently Answered

How does a beta-cell know that it resides in an obese body?
How does beta-cell failure occur?
Which tissue/organ contributes to disease and bodily failure to what extent and how?
How does hyperglycemia contribute/lead to beta-cell failure?
How does atherosclerosis follow from hyperglycemia?
Why do people continue to eat beyond their physiological need?
Why do people eat unhealthy food and do not exercise regularly?
Why do people not adhere to the rules of healthy lifestyle?
Why do people not participate in anti-obesity programs?
Why do many people not take their medications?

Table 2 Examples of the Conditions in the Current Research Environment Provided for Metabolic Research. However, It is Understood that there Is More Money Available in Cancer Research, Cardiology and Hepatology, for example

Modern laboratories and field technologies
Well-educated researchers
International research networks/societies
Common research languages
Focused research programs
Financial support
Societal acceptance of science/research
Modern communication
Data/sample banking

or other electronic or publicly available sources. As a result, society is being fragmented into parties of stakeholders and so-called (self-perceived) experts.

16.3. WHAT ARE WE GOOD AT?

Modern societies have been good at developing new technologies and research tools and for stating dogmas (Table 2). A wealth of information has become widely available and accessible. Well-trained and dedicated staff migrate from around the world to countries with good funding opportunities and well-developed scientific infrastructure: high-quality facilities and technologies as well as excellent ethical standards are available in some areas of the world, though not in all. International networks ensure good communication and global interaction between scientists in widely dispersed geographical locations. Excellent training and education opportunities are available. Thus, many scientists are put in the position of pursuing their own research focus and their own research questions — sometimes in a somewhat self-centered manner (Table 3).

16.4. WHAT ARE WE DOING?

In recent years, researchers in obesity and diabetes research have focused their attention both on rare diseases, such as congenital lipodystrophies[8]

Table 3 Examples of How and Where Research into Metabolic Disorders may Lead to False Results or may be Misleading in General Terms. This List of Threats to True Scientific Advancement is also Applicable to Research Fields Outside Obesity and Diabetes

Wrong focus of research
Outside mainstream research or well within mainstream thinking
Too much or not enough money
Missed opportunities
Too many patients for common diseases
Not enough patients for rare diseases
Not enough/not well-trained scientists
Lack of supervision
Lack of quality management
Lack of ethical consideration
Lack of public control
Lack of interaction with general society
Lack of strategic thinking/planning

Table 4 Topics Investigated or Pursued by Researchers in Metabolic Research Centers Around the World

Rare diseases such as lipodystrophies and congenital diabetes
Common disorders and diseases such as obesity and type 2 diabetes
Molecular mechanisms of disease such as beta-cell function or neuronal control of appetite
Epidemiology (for example, of obesity or diabetes)
Prevention research and clinical trials
Imaging techniques (for example, neuroimaging and single-cell imaging)
Laboratory tests including whole genome sequencing
Documenting, storing and monitoring data
Data analysis (biostatistics)
Writing grants and papers
Administrating large research groups and centers

and forms of congenital diabetes, and on common disorders and diseases, such as obesity and type 2 diabetes (Table 4).

Molecular mechanisms of disease and the epidemiology of common disorders are under investigation. In addition, research into preventive strategies and well-controlled randomized trials to test treatments are under way. Such interventional studies are often based on findings from basic research studies. Imaging techniques, in particular neuroimaging and metabolic imaging such as PET scanning, and refined laboratory tests including high-throughput sequencing, MALDI-TOF and proteomics are helping to generate a wealth of data and knowledge in the area of metabolic health and disease.[9–13]

These are all good examples of true translational research. However, in reality and day-to-day practice, many researchers and highly specialized scientists spend most of their time writing grants and publishing papers in an effort to "stay in business." It can be hypothesized that an enormous amount of time, energy and money is being spent simply on keeping the business of the science running. In some instances, these business aspects are overshadowing any real scientific approaches and displacing the humanitarian and ethical issues,[14–16] threatening to undermine authentic scientific thinking and the scientific endeavor.

16.5. WHAT SHOULD WE DO?

It has become apparent that scientists need to involve themselves more in strategic thinking and analyzing what they are actually doing. In principle, scientists need to ask questions, develop hypotheses and test hypotheses. Issues of patient care, treatment efficacy, and the occurrence of unwanted side effects of therapies are important areas of metabolic research. Very often, treatment endpoints are not defined well enough. Metabolic research should focus on matters that are most likely to help families and society as a whole to live and cope with disorders and disease. There is a need to train and educate physician-scientists. Multidisciplinary approaches need to be employed more often. Researchers with biomedicine and basic science backgrounds (including chemistry, physics and mathematics) need to work together. Researchers in the social and cultural sciences including sociology, psychology, history and geography can help by elucidating, for example, the origins of obesity and the global obesity epidemic. This latter fact is very often neglected in a way that we can no longer afford.

16.6. WHAT DO WE FAIL TO DO?

Modern societies have failed to advance ethical principles and answer fundamental questions (Tables 4 and 5). Many metabolic researchers have the wrong focus. Instead of spending huge amounts of time and money on

Table 5 What should be Done in Day-to-Day Metabolic Research?

Ask questions
Analyze patient care
Define treatment endpoints
Help families and society
Train physician-scientists
Involve interdisciplinary approaches

elucidating the very tiny contributions of individual gene variants on the development of obesity by investigating increasing numbers of affected people, more research should address the social and socioeconomic conditions of these patients. There needs to be a greater focus on questions outside mainstream research: spending a lot of money is sometimes not the best way to answer a research question. Basic science is important, but only with the appropriate translation into patient care and application in a societal context.

16.7. SOLUTIONS TO THE PROBLEM

In order to achieve real translational effects in metabolic research, scientists need to understand the socioeconomic impact and etiology of obesity and diabetes. The wide array of research tools needs to be applied prudently and only to ask clearly defined questions; "fishing expeditions" without hypotheses may not lead to true discoveries. Education and training, both of scientists and the public, is essential. While investors and pharmaceutical companies, for example, are stakeholders and should be partners, they cannot drive improvements in patient care or a better understanding of disease as long as their principal interest is in making money. To reap the benefits from translational medicine, both basic research and interdisciplinary research are vitally important.

16.8. DISCUSSION

Translation of research findings into day-to-day life and in particular into routine clinical practice has not yet been widely realized. The time has come to change the scope of research and scientists' individualized thinking. While the merits of basic metabolic research are clear and important discoveries have been made, critical questions concerning topics related to the health and well-being of the general public have not been asked — or at least have not been answered as yet (Tables 6 and 7).

Table 6 Areas Where True Translational Approaches are Needed in Obesity and Diabetes Research

Organization and aims of inpatient care
Organization and aims of outpatient care
Community healthcare delivery
All aspects of prevention
Clinical relevance, affordability, cost–benefit ratio of diagnostic tools
Behavior science questions
Societal, cultural and socioeconomic impacts
Barriers to participation
Psychology, psychobiology
Nursing
Management
Quality of life
Humanities

Table 7 (a) What Scientists are Particularly Good at, and (b) What Scientists are Occasionally Not Good at

(a)	Asking questions
	Spending money
	Competing with peers
	Adhering to old behavioral patterns
	Paying too little or too much attention to public opinion
	Neglecting the needs of people and society
	Dwelling on the past
(b)	Communicating with one another
	Talking and listening to the public
	Behaving in an altruistic manner
	Considering society
	Thinking globally
	Acting in an interdisciplinary manner
	Focusing on the challenges of the present
	Looking to the future

REFERENCES

1. Scott RA, Lagou V, Welch RP, *et al.* (2012) Large-scale association analyses identify new loci influencing glycemic traits and provide insight into the underlying biological pathways. *Nat Genet* **44**: 991–1005.
2. Horikoshi M, Yaghootkar H, Mook-Kanamori DO, *et al.* (2012) New loci associated with birth weight identify genetic links between intrauterine growth and adult height and metabolism. *Nat Genet* **45**: 76–82.
3. Ichimura A, Hirasawa A, Poulain-Godefroy O, *et al.* (2012) Dysfunction of lipid sensor GPR120 leads to obesity in both mouse and human. *Nature* **483**: 350–354.
4. Zhang M, Guo F, Tu Y, *et al.* (2012) Further increase of obesity prevalence in Chinese children and adolescents — Cross-sectional data of two consecutive samples from the city of Shanghai from 2003 to 2008. *Pediatr Diabetes* **13**: 572–577.
5. Blüher S, Meigen C, Gausche R, *et al.* (2011) Age-specific stabilization in obesity prevalence in German children: A cross-sectional study from 1999 to 2008. *Int J Pediatr Obes* **6**: e199–e206.
6. Sabin MA, Clemens SL, Saffery R, *et al.* (2010) New directions in childhood obesity research: How a comprehensive biorepository will allow better prediction of outcomes. *BMC Med Res Methodol* **10**: 100–107.
7. Quante M, Hesse M, Döhnert M, *et al.* (2012) The LIFE child study: A life course approach to disease and health. *BMC Public Health* **12**: 1021–1029.
8. Jin J, Cao L, Zhao Z, *et al.* (2007) Novel BSCL2 gene mutation E189X in Chinese congenital generalized lipodystrophy child with early onset diabetes mellitus. *Eur J Endocrinol* **157**: 783–787.
9. Landgraf K, Friebe D, Ullrich T, *et al.* (2012) Chemerin as a mediator between obesity and vascular inflammation in children. *J Clin Endocrinol Metab* **97**: E556–E64
10. Bernhard F, Landgraf K, Klöting N, *et al.* (2013) Functional relevance of genes implicated by obesity genome-wide association study signals for human adipocyte biology. *Diabetologia* **56**(2): 311–322.
11. Körner A, Wiegand S, Hungele A, *et al.* (2012) Longitudinal multicenter analysis on the course of glucose metabolism in obese children. *Int J Obes (Lond)*, doi: 10.1038/ijo.2012.163. [Epub ahead of print].
12. Flechtner-Mors M, Thamm M, Wiegand S, *et al.* (APV initiative and the BMBF Competence Network Obesity). (2012) Comorbidities related to BMI category in children and adolescents: German/Austrian/Swiss Obesity Register APV compared to the German KiGGS Study. *Horm Res Paediatr* **77**: 19–26.

13. Melchior C, Schulz A, Windholz J, *et al.* (2012) Clinical and functional relevance of melanocortin-4 receptor variants in obese German children. *Horm Res Paediatr* **78**: 237–246.
14. Alff F, Markert J, Zschaler S, *et al.* (2012) Reasons for (non)participating in a telephone-based intervention program for families with overweight children. *PLoS ONE* **7**: e34580.
15. Wagner IV, Sabin MA, Pfäffle RW, *et al.* (2012) Effects of obesity on human sexual development. *Nat Rev Endocrinol* **31**: 246–254.
16. Bereket A, Kiess W, Lustig RH, *et al.* (2012) Hypothalamic obesity in children. *Obes Rev* **13**: 780–798.

VII. Translation Research and Neuroscience

CHAPTER 17

Translational Neurosciences: From Mathematical Modeling to Clinical Practice

Zofia H. Czosnyka, Wojciech Maksymowicz†,‡ and Marek Czosnyka**

17.1. INTRODUCTION

All technologically dependent areas of clinical medicine have a natural potential to be branded *translational*, a term that is rather vague but unquestionably fashionable nowadays. Translation from the basic sciences — physics, chemistry, biology, and so on — to applied sciences, such as medicine, has a long and fascinating history. Part of this history began 800 years ago when scholar-monks from Oxford left to study basic sciences (not only theology and other applied subjects, such as medicine) and settled in the swamps of East Anglia, out of which grew one of the most prestigious institutions in the world: the University of Cambridge. By comparison, the Brain Physics Laboratory at the Academic Neurosurgical Unit in Cambridge has a comparatively short history of just 20 years, but the experience we wish to relate spans almost our entire professional lives — and is destined to continue well into the future. Our story begins in 1980s at the Warsaw University of Technology and the Warsaw Medical University,

*Neurosurgical Unit, Department of Clinical Neurosciences, University of Cambridge, UK
†Department of Neurosurgery and Stem Cell Research Laboratory, University of Warmia and Mazury, Olsztyn, Poland
‡Corresponding author: Wojciech Maksymowicz, MD, Department of Neurosurgery and Stem Cell Research Laboratory, University of Warmia and Mazury, ul. Warszawska 30, 10-082 Olsztyn, Poland; E-mail: *wmaksymowicz@interia.pl*

and encompasses numerous journeys, diversions, and unexpected changes in scenery.

A brain shielded by a stiff box of bone is difficult to monitor. In the majority of acute brain diseases, monitoring must replace direct neurological assessment, for example if a patient needs to be kept in a pharmacological coma. In turn, the majority of brain-monitoring techniques require the use of invasive probes. To minimize risk/gain ratios in the clinical neurosciences, a series of mathematical models have been formulated to describe the circulation of cerebrospinal fluid (CSF), and global and local cerebral blood flow, with increasing complexity over the past six decades. The role of models is not intuitive, but probably rightly. One can imagine that if not everything in the brain can be monitored directly, some of the monitored variables can be used as input signals to a model, which in turn can generate secondary output data, characterizing the state of the organ in a more descriptive manner.

The simplest CSF model consists of a handful of elements that can be reliably identified during the so-called infusion test and have proven useful in clinical practice for diagnosing patients suffering from hydrocephalus. The addition of more complex phenomena, such as regulation of cerebral blood flow, requires a significant increase in the number of independent model parameters. Therefore, the application of expanded models progressively shifts towards providing a testing ground for ideas based on the literature or clinical/experimental practice. Generalizations prevail over the interpretation of individual measurements. In this way, the more complex models can be used to improve our understanding of dynamical interactions between primary monitored variables (intracranial pressure, cerebral perfusion, cerebral blood flow, etc.) and express them as clinical indices. Some of these indices, such as cerebrospinal compensatory reserve, cerebral autoregulation and cerebrovascular pressure-reactivity, have already gained wider interest in clinical neurosciences.

17.2. MODEL OF CSF CIRCULATION AND ITS USE IN MANAGEMENT OF HYDROCEPHALUS

Popular mathematical models applied to hydrocephalus simulate brain tissue displacement, usually showing deformation of the anatomical structure and distribution of stress-strain in the tissue. Models of CSF circulation describe the hydrodynamics of CSF flow visualized non-invasively with phase-coded or spin-labeling MRI techniques, or the dynamics of intracranial pressure (ICP), which may be measured invasively in clinical practice with a pressure transducer. Models of CSF dynamics have established clinical applications in the diagnosis and management of several diseases, including hydrocephalus, idiopathic intracranial hypertension and syringomyelia.

Many theoretical/modeling studies on CSF dynamics were published before the 1970s.[1–4] However, Professor Anthony Marmarou was one of the first[5,6] who integrated all the various components — CSF production, circulation, absorption and storage — in one elegant theoretical structure expressed as an electrical circuit. He analyzed three basic maneuvers: bolus CSF withdrawal, addition and constant rate infusion. This model has withstood the test of time and, with only a very few "cosmetic" modifications, is still used today. As a result, hydrocephalus and other disorders of CSF circulation are now characterized using parameters from this model, such as resistance to CSF outflow, elasticity, and pressure volume index (PVI).

To give the reader a flavor of the approach, we will look at some of the basic mathematics involved. Under normal conditions, without long-term fluctuations of the cerebral blood volume, production of CSF is balanced by its storage and reabsorption in the sagittal sinus:

$$\text{Production of CSF} = \text{Storage of CSF} + \text{Readsorption of CSF}. \qquad (1)$$

Production of CSF is assumed to be constant, although this may not always be the case. Reabsorption is proportional to the difference between CSF pressure (p) and the pressure in the sagittal sinus (p_{ss}):

$$\text{Reabsorption} = \frac{p - p_{SS}}{R}. \qquad (2)$$

p_{ss} is the sagittal sinus pressure, considered to be a constant parameter determined by central venous pressure. The coefficient R (R_{CSF} is also used) is termed the resistance to CSF reabsorption or outflow [units: mmHg/(ml/min)]. Normal resistance is typically between 5 and 10 mmHg/(ml/min). Elevated resistance to CSF outflow [greater than 13 mmHg/(ml/min)] indicates disturbed CSF circulation.

Storage of CSF is proportional to the cerebrospinal compliance C (units: ml/mmHg) and the rate of change of CSF pressure dp/dt:

$$\text{Storage} = C \cdot \frac{dp}{dt}. \tag{3}$$

The compliance of the cerebrospinal space is inversely proportional to the difference between the CSF pressure p and the reference pressure p_0:

$$C = \frac{1}{E \cdot (p - p_0)}. \tag{4}$$

Some authors suggest that Eq. (4) is valid only above a certain pressure level, called the "optimal pressure."[7] The coefficient E is termed the cerebral elasticity (or elastance coefficient) (units: ml^{-1}). Elevated elasticity (greater than 0.18 ml^{-1}) signifies a poor pressure–volume compensatory reserve.[8] This coefficient has recently been confirmed to be useful in predicting a patient's response to third ventriculostomy.[9] Equation (4) expresses the most important law of the cerebrospinal dynamic compensation: When the CSF pressure increases, the compliance of the brain decreases.

A combination of (1) with (2) and (4) gives the final equation:

$$\frac{1}{E \cdot (p - p_0)} \cdot \frac{dp}{dt} + \frac{p - p_b}{R} = I(t), \tag{5}$$

where $I(t)$ is the rate of external volume addition and p_b is a baseline CSF pressure.

The model described by this equation may be presented in the form of its electric circuit equivalent[6] (Fig. 1). Equation (5) can be solved for various types of external volume additions $I(t)$. The most common in clinical practice are as follows:

(a) A constant infusion of CSF $[I(t) = 0$ for $t < 0$ and $I(t) = I_{\text{inf}}$ for $t > 0]$ (see Fig. 2):

$$P(t) = \frac{\left[I_{\text{inf}} + \frac{p_b - p_0}{R}\right] \cdot [p_b - p_0]}{\frac{p_b - p_0}{R} + I_{\text{inf}} \cdot \left[e^{-E\left[\frac{p_b - p_0}{R} + I_{\text{inf}}\right] \cdot t}\right]} + p_0. \tag{6}$$

The analytical curve (6) can be matched to the real recording of the pressure during the test, which results in an estimation of the unknown parameters: R, E and p_0 (see Fig. 2A).

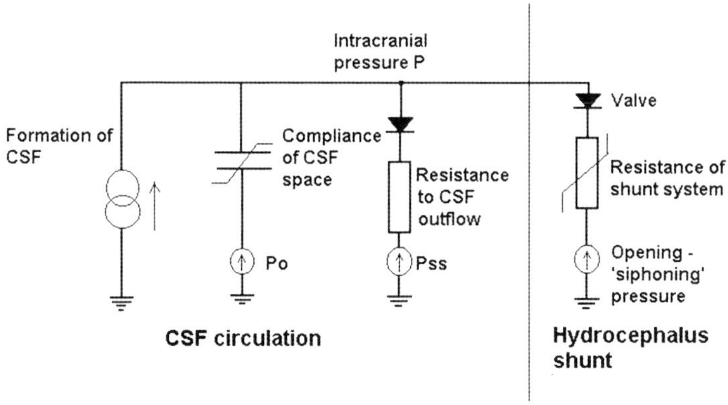

Fig. 1. The electrical model of CSF dynamics according to Marmarou. The current source represents the formation of CSF; the resistor and diode represent unilateral absorption to sagittal sinus (voltage source p_{ss} represents sagittal sinus pressure); the capacitor represents nonlinear compliance of CSF space. The part to the right of the vertical line shows the modification of the model when the hydrocephalus shunt is implanted.

(b) A bolus injection of CSF (volume ΔV):

$$P(t) = \frac{(p_b - p_0) \cdot e^{E[\Delta V + \frac{p_b - p_0}{R} \cdot t]}}{1 + e^{E\Delta V} \cdot \left[e^{E \cdot \frac{p_b - p_0}{R} \cdot t} - 1\right]} + p_0. \tag{7}$$

The bolus injection can be used for calculation of the pressure–volume index (PVI), defined as the volume added externally to produce a ten-fold increase in the pressure[12]:

$$\text{PVI} \stackrel{\text{def}}{=} \frac{\Delta V}{\log_{10}\left(\frac{p_p - p_0}{p_b - p_0}\right)} \quad \text{and} \quad \text{PVI} \cong \frac{1}{0.434 \cdot E}. \tag{8a, 8b}$$

p_p in Eq. (8a) is the peak pressure recorded just after addition of the volume ΔV. PVI is theoretically proportional to the inverse of the brain elastance coefficient E. The pressure–volume compensatory reserve is insufficient when PVI $<$ 13 ml, and a PVI value above 26 ml signifies an "over-compliant" brain. These norms are valid for the PVI calculated as an inverse of E [according to Eq. (8b)] using slow infusion. If the bolus test is used, norms for PVI are higher (the threshold equivalent to 13 ml is around 25 ml[10]).

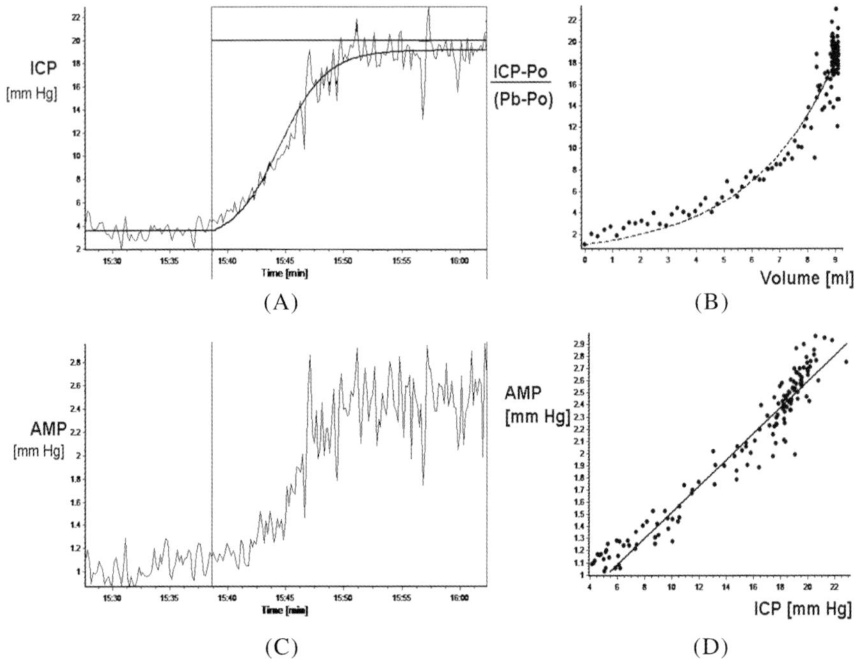

Fig. 2. Methods of identification of the model of CSF circulation during constant rate infusion studies. (A) Recording of CSF pressure (ICP) versus time increasing during infusion with interpolated modeling curve (7). Infusion at a constant rate of 1.5 [ml/min] starts from the vertical line. (B) Recording of pulse amplitude (AMP) during infusion. Rise in AMP is usually well correlated with rise in ICP. (C) Pressure–volume curve. Effective volume increase is plotted on the x-axis (i.e., infusion and production minus reabsorption of CSF). On the y-axis: increase in pressure measured as a gradient of current pressure minus reference pressure p_0, relative to baseline pressure p_b. (D) Linear relationship between pulse amplitude and mean ICP. Intercept of the line with x-axis (ICP) theoretically indicates the reference pressure p_0. Screenshot from the software supporting the constant rate infusion test.

Formula (7) for time $t = 0$ describes the shape of the relationship between the effective volume increase ΔV and the CSF pressure, called the pressure–volume curve (Fig. 2B):

$$p = (p_b - p_0) \cdot e^{E\Delta V} + p_0. \tag{9}$$

Finally, Eq. (7) can be helpful in the theoretical evaluation of the relationship between the pulse wave amplitude of ICP and the mean CSF pressure. If we presume that the rise in blood volume after a heart contraction is equivalent to a rapid bolus addition of CSF fluid at the baseline pressure p_b, the pulse amplitude (AMP) can be expressed as:

$$\mathrm{AMP} = p_p - p_b = (p_b - p_0) \cdot (e^{E\Delta V} - 1). \tag{10}$$

In almost all cases, when CSF pressure is being increased by the addition of an external volume, the pulse amplitude rises[7,8] (see Figs. 2C and 2D). The gradient of the regression line between AMP and p is proportional to the elasticity. Point of intersection, theoretically, marks the reference pressure p_0.

From its initial publication,[5] this model proved to be extremely useful in the diagnosis of hydrocephalus, using bolus, constant-rate or constant-pressure infusion studies. In the following, we summarize the most important clinical applications of the model.

- The servo-controlled constant pressure infusion test[11] is used for assessment of CSF disorders. The aim of the test is to evaluate the resistance to CSF outflow in a repetitive and reliable way.
- Full identification of the model, including elasticity can be made using a computerized constant rate infusion test[12] supported by the dedicated software ICM+ (*www.neurosurg.cam.ac.uk/icmplus*). Increased resistance to CSF outflow can be corrected by shunting or third ventriculostomy (depending on location of obstruction). Increased elasticity can be corrected by third ventriculostomy.[9]
- Use of the constant rate infusion test in many centers contributed to the definition of profiles of ICP and its pulse amplitude in different possible clinical scenarios, including normal pressure hydrocephalus, brain atrophy, acute hydrocephalus and in non-disturbed CSF circulation (see Fig. 3)
- Analysis of the constant rate infusion test in shunted patients can be helpful in shunt assessment *in vivo*. The electrical circuit model proposed by Marmarou is supplemented by a branch-defining nonlinear pressure–flow performance curve of the shunt. Direct knowledge of the curve, as assessed in shunt evaluation laboratories,[13] allows *in vivo* identification of the model and sensitive prediction of whether the shunt is working properly, under- or over-draining.
- The proportional increase in the amplitude of the ICP pulse waveform with mean ICP has been explained by Marmarou[10] as a

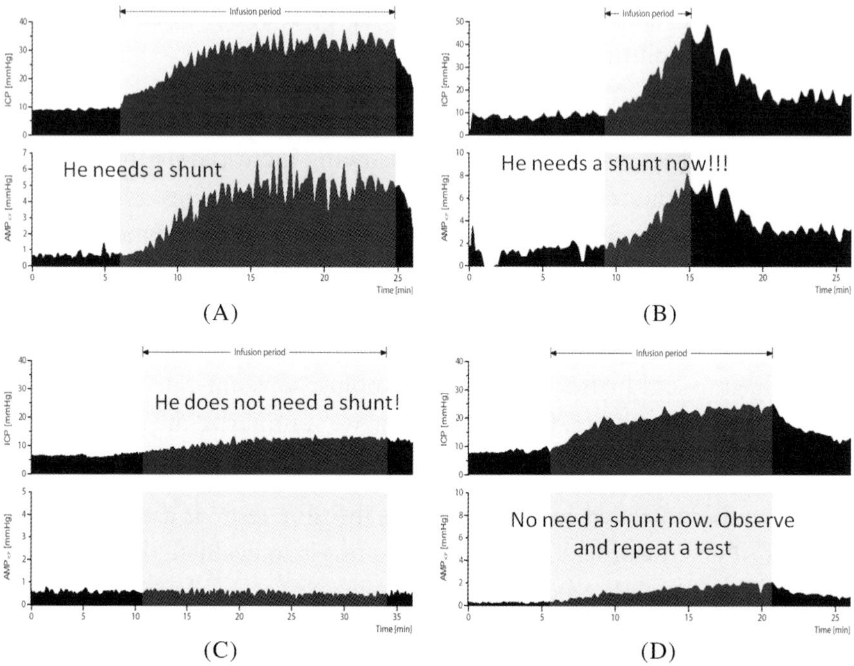

Fig. 3. "Who needs a shunt from CSF dynamics point of view?" Examples of the constant rate infusion test. ICP: mean ICP (10 sec average) and AMP: pulse amplitude of ICP. Horizontal lines above signify the duration of constant rate infusion (either 1 or 1.5 ml/min). (A) Normal pressure hydrocephalus (NPH): although the baseline pressure is normal, the resistance to CSF outflow is increased, there are lots of strong vasogenic waves, and changes in pulse amplitude are fairly well correlated with changes in mean ICP. (B) Acute hydrocephalus post-SAH: the normal baseline pressure was measured, but the resistance to CSF outflow is high. Good response to shunt surgery was expected. (C) Cerebral brain atrophy: the baseline pressure is low and the resistance to CSF outflow is low. No vasogenic waves were recorded and pulse amplitude does not respond. (D) Normal: the baseline pressure, the resistance to CSF outflow and other parameters are normal. If clinical symptoms persist, the infusion study should be repeated in 2–3 months' time.

consequence of the exponential pressure–volume curve. However, further works demonstrated that in a system with a good pressure–volume compensatory reserve, the pressure–volume curve is linear,[7,8] and at higher pressures, the curve becomes exponential. This led to analysis of a moving correlation coefficient (20 sec to 2 min) between mean ICP and AMP. The resulting RAP coefficient indicates the state of compensatory reserve. RAP = 0 suggests good compensatory reserve; RAP = 1, poor compensatory reserve.[14]

- The idea of a vasogenic component of ICP led to modification of Davson's equation[2]:

  $\text{ICP} = R_{CSF} * \text{CSF formation} + P_{SS} + \text{"Arterial Vasogenic Component"}$.

  The "arterial vasogenic component" is an ICP that is derived by detection of pulsatile blood flow in nonlinear elements of the cerebrospinal space (intracranial and arterial bed compliance, resistance of collapsible bridging veins, and autoregulation-controlled main cerebrovascular resistance).

17.3. COMBINED MODEL OF CSF AND CBF DYNAMICS

The previously described model of the mechano-elastic properties of the brain was related to the CSF circulation only and included the non-linear pressure–volume relationship of the intracranial compartment. The advent of modern computing technology has led to attempts to integrate the intracranial CSF circulation with cerebral blood flow.[15–17]

CSF pressure results from the dynamic equilibrium between the volumetric changes in brain tissue, CSF volume, and cerebral blood volume.[4,18] Any malfunction may generate a pressure response affecting the cerebrovascular circulation. Several stabilizing feedback loops are involved, including cerebrovascular autoregulation/reactivity, neurogenic innervation, intraparenchymal water fluxes, and secretion/reabsorption of CSF. The model contains two major flow pathways (Fig. 4). The CBF pathway starts with the arterial blood inflow to the brain through the resistance of a large intracranial artery (R_a) but is unable to simulate phenomena resulting from the complex topography of the basal cerebral arteries included in the circle of Willis. Arterial blood is stored in a high-pressure arterial compliance, C_a. Forward flow through the cerebrovascular resistance vessels (CVR) is controlled by cerebral autoregulation. Capillary and venous blood is stored in a compliance C_v. Finally, venous blood flows out to the sagittal sinus through bridging veins R_b. The CSF pathway consists of CSF formation (I_f), storage in the distensible fluid structures formed by the ventricles and basal cisterns (C_i) and reabsorption through the arachnoid villi (R_{CSF}) to the sagittal sinus.

Using this structure, described with a set of differential equations, three basic phenomena were simulated.

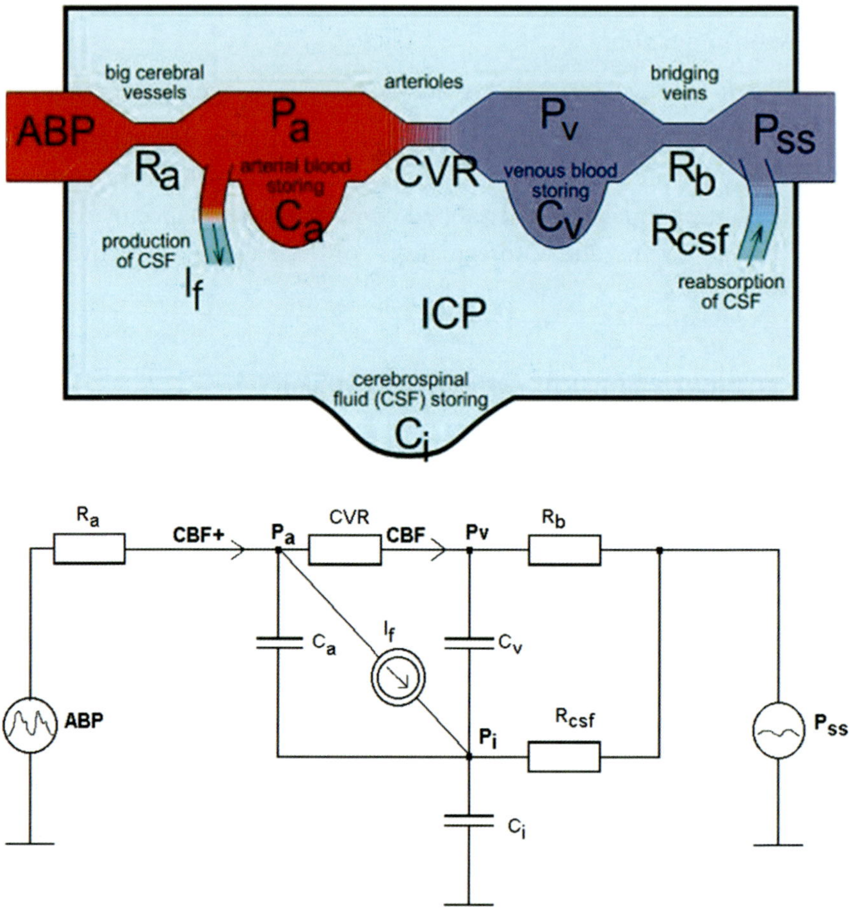

Fig. 4. Hydrodynamic equivalent of the model, comprising pathways of cerebral blood flow and cerebrospinal fluid circulation. A rigid skull is represented by the outer box, with a compensatory reserve C_i associated with the compliant dural sac within the lumbar channel. Bottom: electrical equivalent of the hydrodynamic structure.

17.4. SHORT-TERM HYPOPERFUSION: TRANSIENT HYPEREMIC RESPONSE TEST

A response to compression was simulated by a short-term increase in the resistance of the big cerebral arteries (CVR) from 0.01 to 0.08 mm Hg/(ml/min). Simulation was conducted with intact autoregulation and with autoregulation impaired by equalizing the levels of maximal vasodilatation

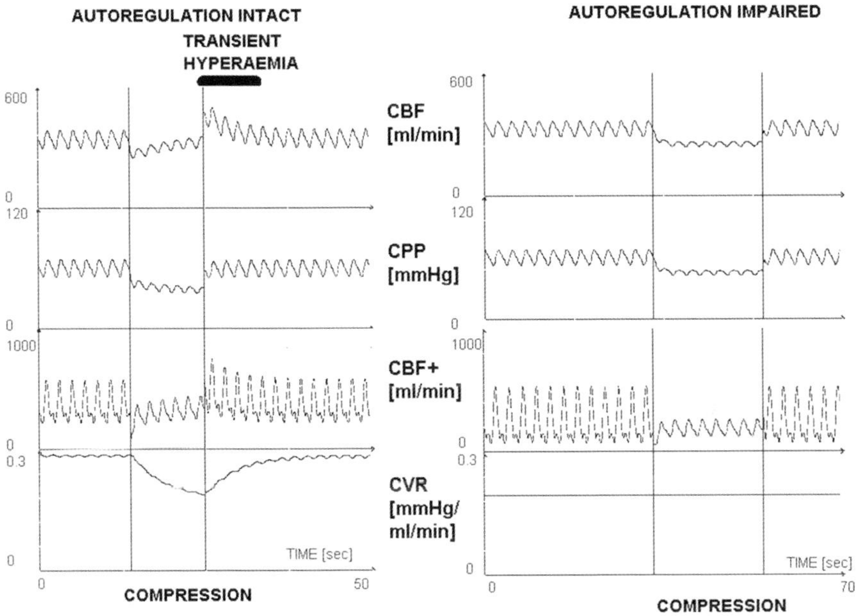

Fig. 5. Dynamic response to a simulated 7-sec compression of the common carotid artery. CBF, flow through small cerebral vessels; CBF+, flow through big cerebral vessels; CVR, the resistance of small cerebral vessels. Compression causes transient hyperemia in auto regulating system (left graph) and a passive recovery of the flow to the baseline in the non-autoregulating system (right graph). Screenshot from the modeling software

and maximal vasoconstriction to the value of 0.2 mm Hg/(ml/min). In both cases, a significant reduction of cerebral perfusion pressure (CPP $= P_a - P_v$) was recorded during compression. In the auto-regulating system, the cerebral vessels dilated, which was demonstrated as a gradual decrease in CVR with a time constant equivalent to the delay of autoregulation. The modeled blood flow through the big cerebral arteries (CBF+) and arterioles (CBF) decreased immediately during the compression, and then started to increase, as the cerebral arterioles dilated (Fig. 5a). After a release of compression, the CPP increased abruptly towards the baseline. As the vessels remained pre-dilated, a transient hyperemia was recorded until CVR returned to the baseline.

When autoregulation was impaired, the reduction in CPP did not induce the vasodilatation (CVR remained constant). After the release of compression, CBF and CBF+ returned passively to the baseline

(Fig. 5b). Hence, post-compression hyperemia is consistent with presumed autoregulation.

17.5. ARTERIAL HYPOTENSION

A gradual decrease in arterial blood pressure was simulated in autoregulating cerebrovascular systems (Fig. 6). The time averaged arteriolar CBF (mCBF) demonstrated good stabilization until mean CPP decreased below the lower limit of autoregulation set at 40 mm Hg. A gradual decrease in CPP towards the lower limit of autoregulation produced a gradual increase in ICP. The systolic flow in the big cerebral arteries (CBF+) increased and diastolic CBF+ decreased, increasing the pulse amplitude of CBF+. The cerebral arterioles dilated, as indicated by a decrease in CVR, until the vessels dilated maximally at the lower limit of autoregulation at the time point A. Below this limit, the mean CBF and ICP started to decrease when ABP decreased further. Coincidentally, with the mean CPP reaching the lower limit of autoregulation, the diastolic CPP started to fall below the critical closing pressure. This was manifested by a momentary pulsatile increase in CVR, initially for a short part of each pulse, and then during most of the pulse cycle. The diastolic CBF+ fell to zero as the arterioles started to close intermittently. Finally, the systolic CBF+ started to fall when the systolic CPP fell below the lower limit of autoregulation.

17.6. INTRACRANIAL HYPERTENSION

An increase in intracranial pressure was modeled as a response to an external infusion of CSF with a stepwise increase in rate, a technique frequently used in the laboratory. In addition to the parameters simulated for systemic hypotension, the compliance of the big cerebral arteries (C_a) was also simulated (Fig. 6).

CPP fell with increasing ICP. The amplitude of the ICP pulsations and the compliance of the big cerebral arteries increased as both the arteriolar resistance and the amplitude of the CPP pulsations decreased. The time averaged CBF+ was constant with the systolic value increasing and the diastolic slightly decreasing. mCBF was maintained constant until the mean

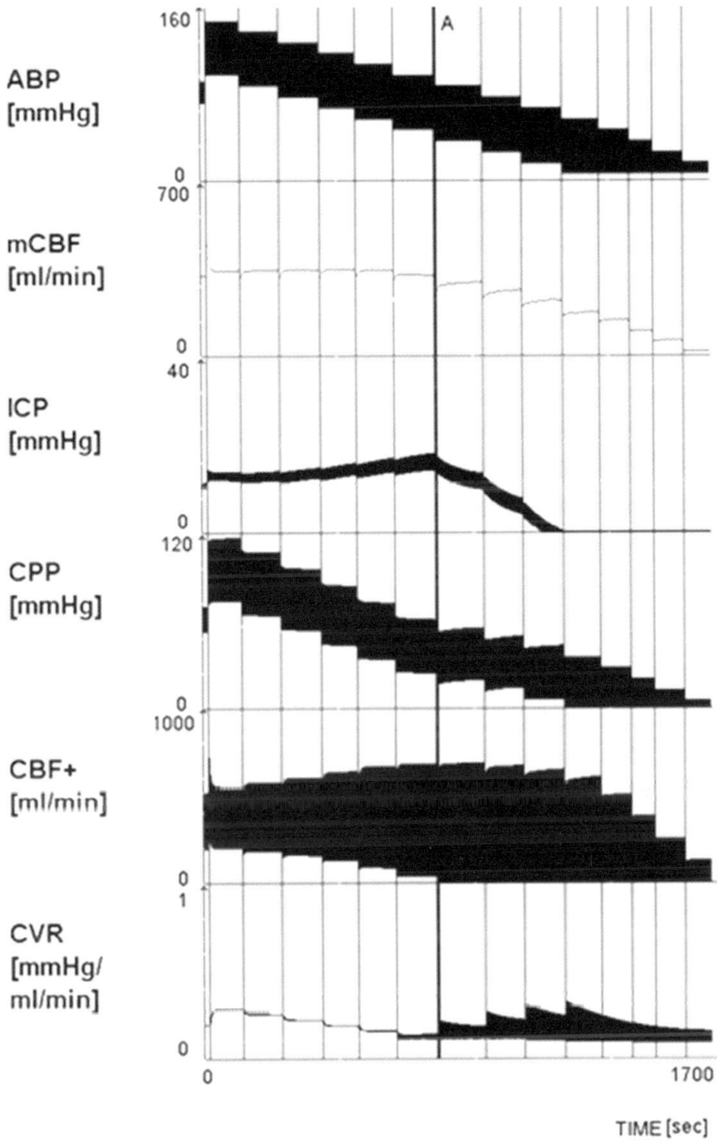

Fig. 6. The effect of stepwise decrease in arterial blood pressure was modeled in autoregulating cerebrovascular systems. Vertical line A shows limit of autoregulation, other lines show moments of step changes in arterial pressure (ABP). mCBF, time averaged cortical blood flow; ICP, intracranial pressure; CPP, cerebral perfusion pressure; CBF+, pulsatile blood flow through big cerebral arteries; CVR, cerebrovascular resistance. Screenshot from the modeling software.

CPP decreased below the lower limit of autoregulation at time point A. Just below the lower limit of autoregulation, the diastolic CPP decreased below the critical closing level. As with simulations for arterial hypotension, CVR started to pulsate, indicating transient arteriolar closure during diastole of the CPP pulse. The diastolic CBF+ decreased to zero. Because the pressure in the big cerebral arteries was greater than in the cerebral arterioles, the compliance C_a was maintained. Beyond point B, CPP became too low to keep the big arteries open. The compliance C_a started to fall, causing a steep decrease in the systolic CBF+. The pulse amplitude of the ICP waveform also started to decrease.

17.7. FROM MODEL TO CLINICAL PRACTICE

Carotid artery compression was introduced as a test of cerebral autoregulation many years ago and was recently revived,[19] although patients at risk of carotid atheroma cannot be examined using this method. Thus, we perform a careful carotid artery Doppler study before the test to exclude patients not suitable for compression.

The presence of transient hyperemia following compression and release of the common carotid artery may be interpreted as evidence of intact autoregulation. The height of the hyperemic overshoot is proportional to the percentage decrease in CVR during compression, and related to the gradient of the static rate of autoregulation. The principal difficulty with the interpretation of this test, which produces "yes-no" results, is that autoregulation is not an "all-or-none" phenomenon. The test is widely used, particularly in patients suffering from subarachnoid hemorrhage (SAH). Recent work[20] with a group of nearly 100 patients after SAH show that early deterioration of autoregulation, before vasospasm is observed, correlates with incidence of delayed ischemia — a common secondary complication after SAH.

The simulation results (see Fig. 7) suggest that the analysis of changes in the systolic and time averaged blood flow velocities, when CPP fluctuates spontaneously, would be useful for detection of breakpoints of autoregulation. A negative correlation between the changes in CPP and systolic flow velocity, with non-significant changes in the time averaged flow velocity, would indicate good autoregulation. A pressure-passive decrease in time

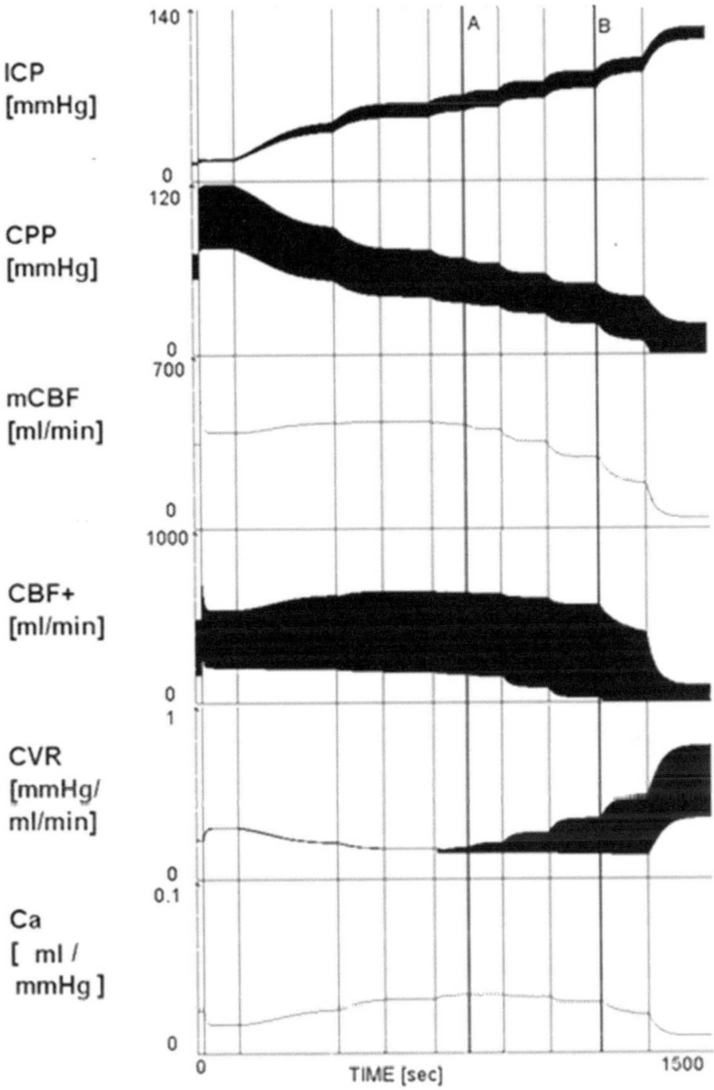

Fig. 7. The effect of stepwise increase in intracranial pressure (ICP) was modeled in auto regulating cerebrovascular systems. Line A shows limit of autoregulation; line B shows critical closing of cerebral arteries. Other vertical lines denote changes in the rate of the simulated external infusion. ICP, intracranial pressure; CPP, cerebral perfusion pressure; mCBF, time averaged cortical blood flow; CBF+, pulsatile blood flow through big cerebral arteries; CVR, cerebrovascular resistance; Ca, compliance of big cerebral arteries. Screenshot from the modeling software.

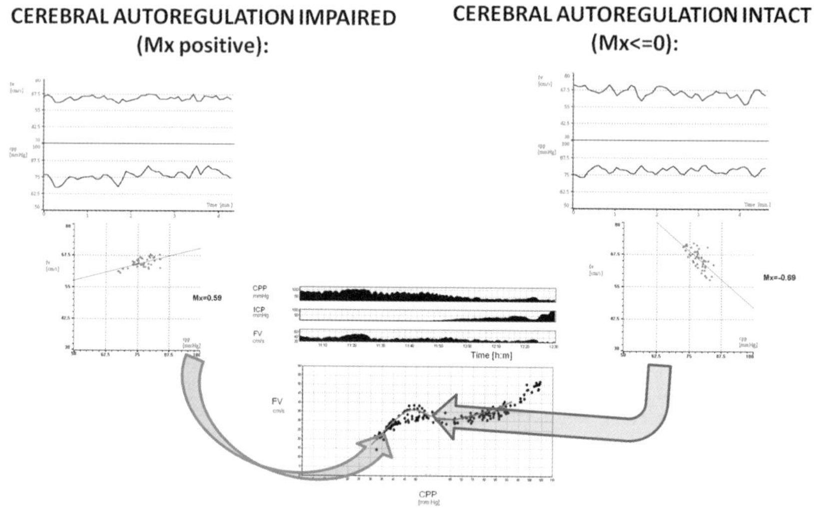

Fig. 8. Calculation of autoregulation index Mx, by correlating slow changes in CPP and mean blood flow velocity. Below and above lower/upper limit of autoregulation seen on Lassen's curve (see middle panel), correlation (and respectively Mx) is positive, while within the autoregulatory limits, it is negative or zero.

averaged and systolic flow velocities, when CPP decreases, signifies impaired autoregulation. An intermediate situation, with time averaged flow velocity falling and systolic remaining constant when CPP is decreasing, marks the state where autoregulation is compromised but still intact. Clinical evaluations made in patients with head injury[21] are compatible with this conclusion. Using computer waveform analysis, such a correlation of fluctuating CPP with changes in the blood flow velocity waveform can be expressed as a time-dependent index of the cerebral autoregulatory reserve, Mx[22] (see Fig. 8). The index is currently used in clinical practice in various group of patients: after traumatic brain injury, carotid artery stenotic disease, and cardiopulmonary bypass surgery.[23] (In these two latter cases, mean blood pressure takes the place of CPP.)

Simulations (Fig. 6) illustrate another clinical observation: Fluctuations in the arterial blood pressure produce inverse changes in ICP when autoregulation is intact. The correlation becomes positive when autoregulation is impaired. Hence, a running correlation coefficient between the time averaged ICP and arterial pressure could be of clinical utility. From early mathematical simulations, pressure-reactivity index (PRx) became

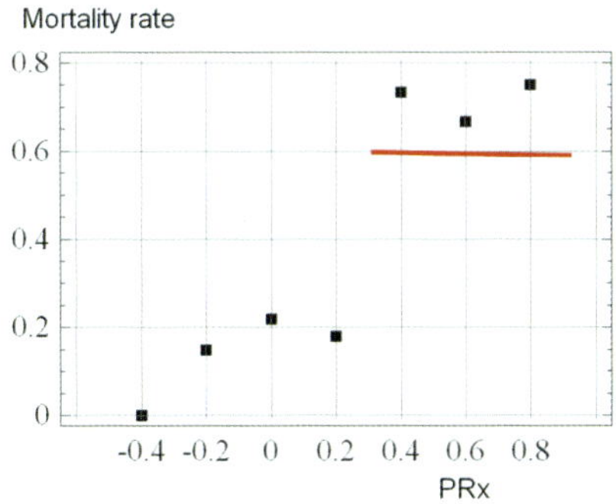

Fig. 9. Pressure reactivity index (PRx) compared with mortality rate in nearly 500 patients after TBI. Increasing PRx from 0.2 to 0.3 (average value for total monitoring time) dramatically increases mortality rate from 20 to 70 percent.

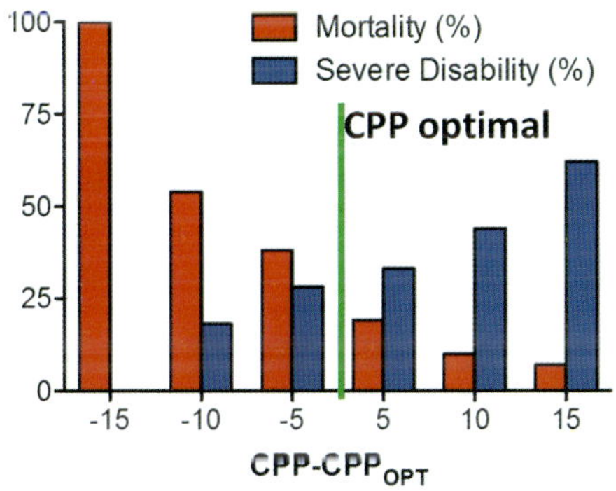

Fig. 10. Distribution of outcomes ($N = 320$ patients[27]) versus averaged difference between median CPP and "optimal CPP." Too-low CPP is associated with greater mortality rate while too-high CPP is associated with greater incidence of severe disability. CPP around "optimal CPP"maximizes favorable outcome.

very popular in continuous monitoring of cerebral autoregulation.[24] It has been validated against several other measures of autoregulation, including the gold standard, PET-CBF static rate of autoregulation.[25] The difference between normal and impaired cerebrovascular reactivity most dramatically implicates mortality rate (see Fig. 9). It proved to be helpful in a new technique for managing patients after severe traumatic brain injury (TBI) at adequate CPP (called "optimal CPP") which preserves cerebral autoregulation.[26,27] Patients with too-low CPP (below "optimal CPP") tend to die more frequently and those treated at too-high CPP (above "optimal CPP") more frequently achieve severe disability outcomes (see Fig. 10).

17.8. WHAT WAS "LOST IN TRANSLATION"?

From our perspective, it is difficult to say what was "lost in translation," as it is not clearly evident. What was lost yesterday, one month, or even several years ago may be found tomorrow. A lot of new techniques (Mx, PRx, "optimal CPP", transient hyperemic response test, CSF infusion test) that were initiated thanks to modeling studies are used in current clinical practice. New techniques are continuously emerging, such as near infrared spectroscopy, thermal dilution monitoring of CBF, microdialysis, etc. They are sending us back to "modeling bench," and new studies, new indices, new software and new hardware solutions are under continuous development. Some of them will come into clinical practice as useful tools; some, without question, will be "lost in translation." This continuous whirlpool of innovation — supported by the fresh ideas and enthusiastic brains of new generations of PhD students at the Brain Physics Lab in Cambridge and the new Stem Cell Research Laboratory, University of Warmia and Mazury in Olsztyn, Poland — leaves us with hope for the future.

REFERENCES

1. Benabid AL. (1970) *Contribution à l'Étude de l'Hypertension Intracranienne Modele Mathematique.* MD Thesis. Grenoble University, France.
2. Davson H, Hollingsworth JR, Segal MD. (1970) The mechanism of drainage of the cerebrospinal fluid. *Brain* **93**: 665–678.
3. Guinane JE. (1972) An equivalent circuit analysis of cerebrospinal fluid hydrodynamics. *Am J Physiol* **223**: 425–430.
4. Lofgren J, Zwetnow NN. (1973) The pressure-volume curve of the cerebrospinal fluid space in dogs. *Acta Neurologica Scand* **49**: 557–574.
5. Marmarou A. (1973) *A Theoretical and Experimental of Cerebrospinal Fluid System.* PhD Thesis, Drexel University, Philadelphia, PA, USA.
6. Marmarou A, Shulman K, Rosende RM. (1978) A non-linear analysis of CSF system and intracranial pressure dynamics. *J Neurosurg* **48**: 332–344.
7. Sliwka S. (1980) *A Clinical System for the Evaluation of Selected Dynamic Properties of the Intracranial System* (in Polish). PhD Thesis, Polish Academy of Sciences, Warsaw, Poland.
8. Avezaat CJJ, Eijndhoven JHM. (1984) Cerebrospinal Fluid Pulse Pressure and Craniospinal Dynamics. Phd Thesis, The Jongbloed en Zoon Publishers, The Hague.

9. Tisell M, Edsbagge M, Stephensen H, *et al.* (2002) Elastance correlates with outcome after endoscopic third ventriculostomy in adults with hydrocephalus caused by primary aqueductal stenosis. *Neurosurgery* **50**: 70–76.
10. Marmarou A, Schulman K, La Morgese J. (1975) Compartmental analysis of compliance and outflow resistance of cerebrospinal fluid system. *J Neurosurg* **43**: 523–534.
11. Eklund A, Lundkvist B, Koskinen LO, Malm J. (2004) Infusion technique can be used to distinguish between dysfunction of a hydrocephalus shunt system and a progressive dementia. *Med Biol Eng Comput* **42**(5): 644–649.
12. Weerakkody RA, Czosnyka M, Schuhmann MU, *et al.* (2011) Clinical assessment of cerebrospinal fluid dynamics inhydrocephalus. Guide to interpretation based on observational study. *Acta Neurol Scand* **124**(2): 85–98.
13. Czosnyka Z, Czosnyka M, Richards HK, *et al.* (1998) Posture-related overdrainage: Comparison of the performance of 10 hydrocephalus shunts *in vitro*. *Neurosurgery* **42**(2): 327–333.
14. Kim DJ, Czosnyka Z, Keong N, *et al.* (2009) Index of cerebrospinal compensatory reserve in hydrocephalus. *Neurosurgery* **64**(3): 494–501.
15. Hoffmann O. (1985) Ein mathematisches Modell zur Simulation und Analyse der intrakraniellen Liquor und Hämodynamik. Habilitationsschrift. Justus-Liebig-Universitat, Giesen, Germany.
16. Sorek S, Bear J. (1986) *Models of Cerebral System Mechanics.* Scientific Report No. 2. Technion Israel Institute of Technology, Haifa, Israel.
17. Ursino M. (1988) A mathematical study of human intracranial hydrodynamics. Part 1 — The cerebrospinal fluid pulse pressure. *Ann Biomed Eng* **16**: 379–401.
18. Pickard JD, Czosnyka M. (1993) Management of raised intracranial presure. *J Neurol Neurosurg Psychiat* **56**: 845–858.
19. Giller CA. (1991) A bedside test for cerebral autoregulation using transcranial Doppler ultrasound. *Acta Neurochir* (*Wien*) **108**: 7–14.
20. Budohoski KP, Czosnyka M, Smielewski P, *et al.* (2012) Impairment of cerebral autoregulation predicts delayed cerebral ischemia after subarachnoid hemorrhage: A prospective observational study. *Stroke* **43**(12): 3230–3237.
21. Czosnyka M, Smielewski P, Piechnik S, *et al.* (2001) Cerebral autoregulation following head injury. *J Neurosurg* **95**(5): 756–763.
22. Czosnyka M, Smielewski P, Kirkpatrick P, *et al.* (1996) Monitoring of cerebral autoregulation in head-injured patients. *Stroke* **27**(10): 1829–1834.
23. Joshi B, Brady K, Lee J, *et al.* (2010) Impaired autoregulation of cerebral blood flow during rewarming from hypothermic cardiopulmonary bypass and its potential association with stroke. *Anesth Analg* **110**(2): 321–328.

24. Czosnyka M, Smielewski P, Kirkpatrick P, *et al.* (1997) Continuous assessment of the cerebral vasomotor reactivity in head injury. *Neurosurgery* **41**(1): 11–17.
25. Steiner LA, Coles JP, Johnston AJ, *et al.* (2003) Assessment of cerebrovascular autoregulation in head-injured patients: A validation study. *Stroke* **34**(10): 2404–2409.
26. Steiner LA, Czosnyka M, Piechnik SK, *et al.* (2002) Continuous monitoring of cerebrovascular pressure reactivity allows determination of optimal cerebral perfusion pressure in patients with traumatic brain injury. *Crit Care Med* **30**(4): 733–738.
27. Aries MJ, Czosnyka M, Budohoski KP, *et al.* (2012) Continuous determination of optimal cerebral perfusion pressure in traumatic brain injury. *Crit Care Med* **40**(8): 2456–2463.

CHAPTER 18

Alzheimer's Disease: Discussing the "Bench-to-Bed" and the "Bed-to-Bench" Pathway Linking Preclinical and Clinical Research

Vito A. Baldassarro[*], *Laura Calzà*[*], *Mercedez Fernández*[*]
L. Giardino[*,†,‡], *A. Giuliani*[†], *L. Lorenzini*[*],
C. Mangano[†] *and S. Sivilia*[†]

Abbreviations; AD, Alzheimer's Disease; APP, amyloid precursor protein; PSEN, presenilin; A ββ-amyloid; KPI, Kunitz protease inhibitor; BACE, β-site APP cleaving enzyme; AICDs, APP intracellular domains; APO, apoliproteins; SAD, sporadic Alzheimer's Disease; FAD, familial Alzheimer's Disease; LTP, long-term potentiation; ChAT, choline acetylesterase; GABA, gamma-aminobutyric acid; NGF, nerve growth factor; NMDA, N-methyl-D-aspartate; VGLUT, vesicular glutamate transporters; PDGF-β, platelet derived growth factor-β.

[*] Interdepartmental Center for Industrial Research (HST-ICIR), University of Bologna, Bologna, Italy.
[†] Department of Veterinary Medical Sciences and Health Science and Technologies, University of Bologna, Bologna, Italy.
[‡] IRET Foundation, Ozzano dell'Emilia, Bologna, Italy.
[§] Corresponding author: Laura Calzà, MD, Health Science and Technologies Interdepartmental Center for Industrial Research (HST-ICIR), University of Bologna, Via Tolara di Sopra 41/E, 40064 Ozzano Emilia, Bologna, Italy; E-mail: laura.calza@unibo.it.
Authors are listed in alphabetic order, and each contributed equally to the article.

18.1. ALZHEIMER'S DISEASE: FROM PATIENT GENOME TO HYPOTHESIS-ORIENTED MODELS

Alzheimer's disease (AD) is a devastating progressive neurodegenerative disease that leads to cognitive deficits and brain atrophy. It is characterized by the presence of extracellular plaques rich in β-amyloid (Aβ aggregates), intraneuronal neurofibrillary tangles rich in hyper phosphorylated tau (NFTs), loss of synapse density, neuroinflammation and neuronal death. As for most neurological disorders, translational research represents a driving strategy for advancement in AD diagnosis and therapy. A multidisciplinary bi-directional path links *in vitro* cell models, animal models and experimental animal science, and neuropathological, genetic and biomarkers studies in human subjects.[1]

While the disease was described at the beginning of the 1900s, the biggest advances have been made over the last few decades thanks to genetic and molecular studies. In particular, genetic studies have provided the first insight into developing hypothesis-oriented models. Based on mutations in three genes observed in a few hundred families around the world, the familial form of the disease has been described: the amyloid precursor protein (APP) gene, presenilin 1 (PSEN1), and presenilin 2 (PSEN2). This early onset (EOAD) or familial (FAD) form of the disease accounts for 4–5 percent of cases. More complex is the genetic background for the late-onset (LOAD) or sporadic (SAD) form of AD, which account for the majority of cases of the disease, and where a risk factor has been associated with the ε4 allele of the APOE gene.[2]

A relevant goal of translational medicine for AD is to develop and characterize animal models that recapitulate all aspects of Alzheimer's disease in humans.[3] A "perfect" animal model of disease should be able to replicate symptoms and lesions but also causes of the disease. Thus, APP and PSEN1/2 human mutations have been used to generate transgenic animals and mutated cells. In this chapter, we will focus on APP-related models. We will illustrate how genetic studies in humans have provided information on creating cell and *in vitro* models; how these models have contributed to disease understanding, diagnosis improvement and therapy development; and how this multidisciplinary effort is now redefining the APP working hypothesis for AD.

18.2. APP METABOLISM AND THE AMYLOID CASCADE HYPOTHESIS

In the rare familial forms of AD, several APP or PSEN1/2 mutations have been described. The APP gene is located on chromosome 21 and contains 18 exons. With alternative splicing, the APP gene may codify three different isoforms of the APP transmembrane protein but the role of these proteins is still poorly understood in normal brain function. APP695 (lacking the gene sequence from exons 7 and 8), APP751 (lacking exon 8) and APP770 isoforms are three isoforms containing the specified number of amino acids. The two larger isoforms are expressed in most tissues and contain the Kunitz protease inhibitor (KPI) region, a 56-amino-acid extracellular domain that is not present in APP695 (predominantly expressed in neurons). Alterations in splicing mechanisms are reported in AD patient brains, leading to an increase in APP isoforms containing the KPI domain and Aβ generation.[4] APP-like protein 1 and 2 (APLP1 and APLP2), two type I integral membrane protein homologs of APP, were also identified. Even if these proteins show conserved domains, Aβ and KPI sequences are unique to APP.

APP can be processed through two mutually exclusive pathways involving a first cleavage within the luminal domain by β- or α-secretase and a subsequent cleavage of the resulting C-terminal fragments by γ-secretase[5] (Fig. 1). Aβ is generated in different cellular compartments (endoplasmatic reticulum, Golgi apparatus and trans-Golgi-network) where APP is synthesized and can be transported in secretory vesicles to the cell surface. Here it can be cleaved by γ-secretase or reinternalized via an endosomal/lysosomal system that can generate Aβ fragments. Only a small fraction of the protein is present at the plasma membrane, where it can then be internalized and delivered to the endosomes. Internalized APP can be recycled to the plasma membrane or degraded in lysosomes.

The α-secretase cleavage takes place within the Aβ domain between amino acids Lys16 and Leu17 precluding the Aβ generation and resulting in the release of a large soluble ectodomain (sAPPα) in the cytosol, and leaves behind the carboxyl terminal fragment (C83) bound to the membrane. ADAMs (a disintegrin and metalloproteinase), type I transmembrane glycoproteins present at the cell surface, are the main α-secretases involved in the nonamyloidogenic APP processing.[6] Some authors have described

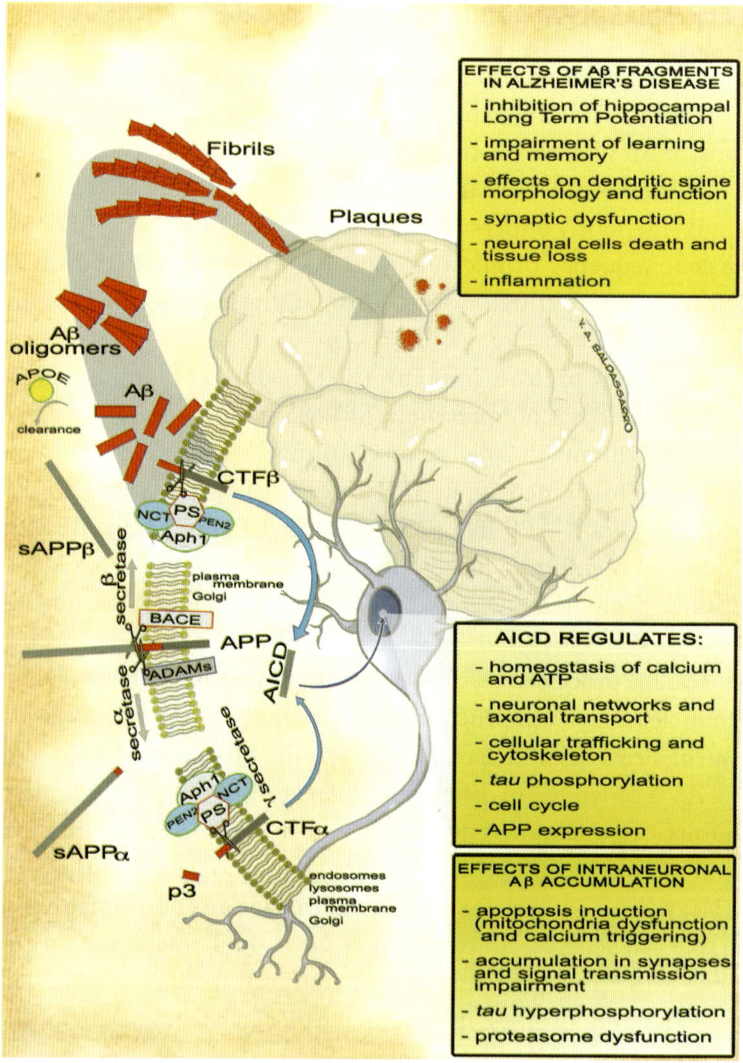

Fig. 1. Figure shows the intracellular processing of the amyloid precursor protein (APP). The first step in Aβ formation is γ-secretase (BACE1 and 2) cleavage. The resulting C-terminus fragment β (CTFβ) is once again cleaved by the γ-secretase complex (NCT, nicastrin; PS, presenilins; PEN2, presenilin enhancer 2; Aph1, anterior pharynx-defective 1) producing Aβ fragments. Amyloid monomers can aggregate in soluble oligomers, protofibrils, fibrils and plaques, leading to neuronal cell damage (bottom panel) and brain injuries (top panel). AICD (APP intracellular domain) fragments of different sizes are produced by the γ-secretase complex cleaving both CTF-β and -α. AICDs migrate into the nucleus acting as transcription factor, thereby regulating the expression of genes involved in different processes (central panel). Other abbreviations: Aβ, β-amyloid; ADAMs, a disintegrin and metalloproteinase; sAPP, soluble amyloid precursor protein.

their neuroprotective and growth factor roles in *in vitro* and *in vivo* models.[7–9]

APP can be also cleaved by β-secretases, resulting in the formation of the soluble APPβ and the membrane-bound C99 containing the β-amyloid domain. The most important proteins showing this β-secretase activity, localized to the late Golgi/trans-Golgi-network, endosomes and cell surface, are called β-site APP-cleaving enzyme 1 and 2 (BACE1 and BACE2). This APP cleavage is the first step in the β-amyloid formation. The sAPPβ has not been particularly well studied and even if it shows a difference of only 17 aminoacids with respect to sAPPα,[10] its role in the cell system seems to be controversial due to evidence of positive effects on neuronal growth and differentiation[11,12] and its involvement in cell death processes.[13]

The short APP C-terminal fragments C83 and C99, resulting from α- and β-cleavage, are substrates for other enzymes involved in the γ-secretase complex. The enzymatic complex consists of four major proteins: presenilin (PS), nicastrin, anterior pharynx-defective-1 (APH1) and presenilin enhancer-2 (PEN2). This complex can cleave C83 and C99, leading to the formation of p3and Aβ fragments, respectively. Both cleavages also yield various APP intracellular domains (AICDs). These fragments are linked to different cellular processes, including regulation of cell-death pathways through Fas-associated protein with death domain (FADD)[14] and p53 factors,[15] modulation of intracellular calcium and ATP,[16] and regulation of neprilysin, one of the main β-amyloid-degrading enzymes.[17]

The γ-secretase complex can cleave APP at multiple sites, producing peptides ranging from 38 to 43 aminoacids. It also mediates ζ- and ε-cleavage generating, respectively, Aβ46 and Aβ49, and various AICDs of different sizes. The majority of Aβ peptides are 40 aminoacids long[18] and their physiological concentration is in the picomolar range. The Aβ40-mediates induction of newly generated neurons in the hippocampus and its involvement in synaptic activity *in vitro* have been described.[19] Aβ42, the most amyloidogenic fragment, accounts for less than 10 percent of secreted Aβ, and its production increases in familial Alzheimer's disease-linked APP mutations, just beyond the C-terminus of the Aβ domain. Mutations in presenilins can also influence the γ-secretase cleavage, increasing the Aβ42/40 ratio. Other cytotoxic fragments can be generated by a caspase-independent cleavage at the APP C-terminus, releasing a short C31 peptide and the Jcasp fragment.[20]

Genes involved in the Aβ clearance processes are also genetic risk factors for AD. Different apolipoproteins (APOE, APOA and APOJ) are involved in Aβ clearance and specific isoforms of the APOE gene are recognized as risk factors for AD.[21]

This network of enzymatic complexes — in addiction to other enzymatic processes mediated by aminopeptidases, glutaminyl cyclase, isomerases and phosphorylation reactions[22] — results in a mixture of Aβ fragments that differ in size, solubility, biological properties and toxicity. Aβ monomers can aggregate in soluble forms of oligomers, protofibrils, fibrils and plaques that are deposited in the intra- and extracellular space.[23] The major pathological hallmark of the disease is the formation of neuritic plaques composed primarily of fibrils of the Aβ39–42 peptides. Aβ42 fragments have the ability to form stable oligomers significantly more toxic than protofibrils and fibrils, probably due to their secondary structures.[24] Although the fundamental role of a pool of soluble Aβ of different sizes has been demonstrated, *in vitro* and *in vivo* experiments show how Aβ42, the most-studied Aβ soluble fragment, can initiate amyloid fibril formation leading to amyloidogenesis through a polymerization mechanism.[25]

These soluble Aβ species seem to be the main causes of the functional deficits in cognitively impaired transgenic mice in which Aβ plaques occupy less than 5 percent of the neuropil. Monomeric, oligomeric and protofibrillary Aβ species are thought to be the main culprits in initiating disease in AD patients, given the lack of correlation between Aβ plaque deposition level and the degree of cognitive impairment.[26]

18.3. HIGHLIGHTS OF THE Aβ CASCADE HYPOTHESIS

18.3.1. Transgenic Animals

Since SAD has an unknown etiology, initial animal models have been based on genetic knowledge associated with FAD. Individuals carrying mutations in autosomal dominant APP, PSEN1 or PSEN2 are characterized by an overproduction of Aβ and a tendency to develop the disease earlier compared with SAD patients. Transgenic mice for investigating APP overproduction develop Aβ brain plaques that are structurally very similar to those in humans. They appear as diffuse plaques consisting mainly of Aβ42, develop a dense Aβ42 core, and then incorporate Aβ40 and other non-Aβ components such as ubiquitin and α-synuclein.[27]

The first transgenic mouse models of AD, dating back to the mid 1990s, are (i) PDAPP, (ii) Tg2576, and (iii) APP23. All three models support the amyloidogenic cascade hypothesis, showing a progressive deposition of Aβ in both diffuse and neuritic plaques, cerebral amyloid angiopathy, astrocytosis, microgliosis, (limited) hippocampal atrophy, synaptic and neurotransmitter alterations, and cognitive and behavioral deficits.[3] The PDAPP mouse model shows an over expression of the gene encoding for the Indiana mutation, APPV717F, under the control of the promoter PDGF-β. In this mouse model, APP expression levels are 10 times higher than endogenous ones, with amyloid plaques appearing around the age of 6–8 months.[28] Gliosis, synaptic deficits and hippocampus atrophy were also observed. The Tg2576 mouse expresses the human APP gene carrying the Swedish mutation (APP695.K670N-M671L) under the control of the hamster prion protein (PrP) promoter. This model shows a rapid increase in levels of Aβ around the age of 6 months, with the development of amyloid plaques at 9–12 months, along with cognitive impairment.[28] The TgAPP23 mouse model expresses the human APP gene carrying the Swedish mutation (APP695.K670N-M671L) but under the control of the promoter Thy1. These mice show Aβ plaques at the age of approximately 6 months. These animals have serious problems with memory and learning that occur progressively from 3 months up to the formation of plaques. More aggressive AD models with double and triple mutations have also been developed. For instance, TgCRND8 mice (carrying the double Swedish and Indiana mutations) show early manifestation of the disease with amyloid deposits visible at the age of 3 months. The TgAPPSweArc model (carrying the triple Swedish, Arctic and Indiana mutations) shows abundant Aβ plaques already at the age of 2 months. In contrast, other animal models expressing the Swedish double mutation, such as the C3-3 mouse, are less aggressive and plaques do not develop before the age of 18 months.[28]

As mentioned, the discovery of the early onset of AD in individuals with mutations in the presenilin (PS) gene led to the development of transgenic models with human PSEN1 and PSEN2 mutations.[3] In these mouse models, although there is an increased Aβ40/Aβ42 ratio, there is no appreciable injury and the behavioral deficits are also very modest.

However, in this model, slowing of axonal transport and hyper phosphorylation of tau have been observed.[28] The important role of PS has been demonstrated thanks to transgenic models with APP/PS double mutation. The co-transfection of human mutated PS1 (M146L or 146V) significantly reduces the timing of plaque formation compared to models with APP single mutation.[28] Crossing Tg2576 mice with mice expressing human PS1 (M146L), amyloid deposits have been observed at 6 months, instead of 9 months in Tg2576 animals. When C3-3 mice were crossed with mice expressing human PS1, the plaques were detected at 9 months, instead of 18 months.

Another interesting model is the "Down" mouse model, in which different parts of human chromosome 21 are replicated in mouse chromosome 16. There are two different models of trisomy 21: (i) the Ts65Dn line, where a large segment of chromosome 16 including the APP gene is triplicated, and (ii) the Ts1Cje line, where the smaller segment not including the APP gene is triplicated. As expected, only in Ts65Dn is it possible to observe increased levels of Aβ (at the age of 6 months). In addition, only in this model have increased levels of APP mRNA and the protein itself been detected in the striatum by the age of 6–8 months and in the hippocampus and parietal cortex by the age of 13–16 months.[28]

The main disadvantage of all the above-mentioned transgenic mice models is the lack of NFT formation, although many of them show an increase in hyper phosphorylated tau.[27] The lack of NFT development has been partially overcome by the development of transgenic mice expressing mutant human tau, and subsequent models derived from the breeding of APP- and these mice. Expression of human tau containing the most common FTDP-17 mutation (P301L) results in motor and behavioral deficits in transgenic mice, with age- and gene dose-dependent development of NFT. This phenotype occurred as early as 6.5 months in hemizygous and 4.5 months in homozygous animals.[29] In humans the P301S mutant causes an earlier onset of clinical signs of frontotemporal dementia than the P301L mutation.[30] For TauP301S, homozygous mice develop severe paralysis at the age of 5–6 months due to degeneration of the brain and spinal cord with loss of neurons. However, mutant tau models have a very severe phenotype, due to cytoskeleton deterioration in different brain and spinal cord regions. Thus, other mice have been generated with regionally specific tau pathology. For example, transgenic tau is expressed only in the hippocampus in TauV337M mouse. These mice increase their spontaneous locomotion in the open field test and higher memory deficits in the elevated plus maze, but no significant impairment in the Morris water maze.[31] A combination of these features has been sought by developing the double mutant tau/APP mouse. In this model, an increase in tau phosphorylation, NFT formation, and neuronal loss has been observed in addition to increased amyloid deposition, thereby supporting the amyloid cascade hypothesis stating that Aβ pathology mediates tau pathology.[32] Subverting expectations, there is no co-localization of Aβ plaques and NFT in AD-relevant brain regions in APP/tau mice. This shortcoming was countered with the development of the triple transgenic (3xTg) mouse. 3xTg mice develop Aβ plaques prior to NFT pathology with a temporal and spatial profile equivalent to AD.[28] These mice express the Swedish APP, PS1 M146V and MAPT P301L mutations, developing plaques at 6 months and tau clusters at 12 months.[33]

18.3.2. Age-dependent Behavioral Impairment

A major contribution from preclinical research to AD patients derives from the study of cognitive performance in AD animal models. In fact, while the initial link between amyloid pathology and cognitive defect was attributed to amyloid plaque deposition and Aβ peptide aggregation, the study of cognitive performance in AD animal models provided extensive evidence that learning and memory defects are present prior to plaque deposition.[34] Accordingly, attention has been redirected toward the pre-aggregation stages of Aβ biology. Extensive work on animal models provided evidence that soluble Aβ fragments are indeed toxic for dendritic spine morphology and function,[35] impairing hippocampal long-term potentiation (LTP) and thus learning and memory.[36] In this section, we briefly present the main behavioral test used for assessing learning and memory, and illustrate the principal studies proving cognitive defects in AD mice in relation to amyloid plaque deposition.

Behavioral neuroscience has developed a great number of tests, tools and tasks able to investigate cognitive performance in a region- and function-specific manner. In particular, behavioral tasks used to examine cognition in animals are divided into either associative or operant learning tasks. Associative learning tasks use environmental cues to condition a specific response. Operant learning tasks induce a particular response to a specific stimulus in order to receive an outcome. Cognitive tasks are further divided into groups depending on the type of memory being tested. Working memory is defined as a short-term memory for an object, stimulus or location that is used within a testing session, but not typically between sessions. Reference memory is typically acquired with repeated training and persists from days to months.[37]

The most often used tasks to determine cognitive changes in mouse models, transgenic or otherwise, are:

1. spatial memory tasks, including the Morris water maze, the radial arm maze, and the radial arm water maze;
2. contextual memory, including fear conditioning and passive-avoidance learning;
3. working memory/novelty/activity, including Y-maze, T-maze, and object recognition.

For translational purposes, video tracking and computerized analysis of animal behavior is highly recommended in order to maintain a record of the row data (video) of individual animals.

The Morris water maze (MWM) is one of the most common behavioral tasks used to determine hippocampal spatial memory deficits.[38] The MWM assesses the ability of a rat or mouse to escape the water by swimming to reach a platform located just below the water's surface. The animal uses a series of spatial cues placed around the pool. The time taken to reach the platform (latency), swimming velocity and distance swam are parameters used to determine learning deficits. At the end of training sessions, a trial is used to define the capability to retain learned information or to develop new strategies.

The radial arm maze (RAM) consists of a series of arms radiating from a central arena. At the end of some arms a reward is positioned (food or water), which is not visible from the central platform. The aim of the test is to have the animal visit each arm only once, in order to obtain the greatest result in the shortest time. In this way, the test stimulates both working memory, a short-term memory (inter-trial), and reference memory, a long-term memory that allows animals to remember the right strategy over a period of days. The major limitation of this test is that food or water deprivation is recommended before testing animal.[39,40]

By employing a radial arm maze inside a circular pool, the radial arm water maze (RAWM) addresses the shortcomings of the two previously described tests (MWM and RAM). Here, the animal must swim to reach the submerged platforms located at the ends of the arms. This more challenging test impels the animal to use the spatial cues and working memory to remember where platforms are located. Several variations of this task, using different numbers of platforms and different platform organizations, have been used to examine spatial memory under different conditions, such as pharmacological treatment,[41,42] across species[43] and genders,[44] and to study different models of AD.[40,45]

Fear conditioning (FC) is a behavioral paradigm in which animals learn to predict aversive events.[46] An aversive stimulus (e.g., an electrical shock) is associated with a particular neutral context (e.g., a cage) or neutral stimulus (e.g., a tone), resulting in the expression of fear responses to a context or stimulus that was originally neutral. Normally, the neutral stimulus is defined as the "conditioned stimulus" (CS) while the aversive stimulus is the "unconditional stimulus" (US). The state of fear (freezing) in rodents is defined as the lack of movement except that required to breathe. FC is a widely used test to measure hippocampal-dependent associative learning. The test is thought to be sensitive to emotion-associated learning and therefore is a useful measure of communication between the amygdala and hippocampal regions.

Passive-avoidance learning (P-AL) is a test in which the animal has to learn to avoid an adverse stimulus. The associated apparatus is composed of two adjacent compartments, one well illuminated and one dark. Although rodents have a natural tendency to take refuge in dark places, if an aversive stimulus is placed in the dark compartment, they have to learn to suppress this tendency and to stay in the well-illuminated compartment. Animals that do not remember the aversive stimulus will cross over earlier than animals that remember it. The parameters used to determine learning deficits are the time taken to cross over to the unsafe compartment (latency) and the percentage of animals from each experimental group that cross the threshold within an allocated time.[47,48]

The Y-maze consists of three arms of the same length (30 to 35 cm) radiating from a central area at 120-degree intervals. This test is based on the innate preference of rodents to explore the different arms of the maze. In the most often used version of this task, the animal is free to explore the maze for five or eight minutes, and the number of arms entered and sequence of entries are recorded. An alternation is defined as an entry into each of the three arms consecutively with no repetitions.

The T-maze test is widely used for cognitive behavioral testing mediated by the medial prefrontal cortex and hippocampus in both mice and rats. The T-maze apparatus is made of a central and two lateral arms (shorter than the central one) positioned at 90 degrees to the central arm, forming a "T" shaped maze. The animal is positioned at the base of the central arm and it chooses one of the two lateral arms. Rodents tend to choose the arm not previously visited, reflecting memory of their first choice.

The object recognition (OR) test is based on the natural tendency of rodents to investigate a novel environment or a novel object instead of a familiar one. The apparatus consists of an open field with dark walls and floor. In a common version of the test, animals are free to explore the empty area to get used to the new environment. After 24 hours, two identical objects located on the back wall are presented to the animal. On the third day, an object is replaced with a new one different in form, color and, sometimes, material. The number of objects or their locations may vary. The time spent exploring the new object with respect to the familiar one is used as a parameter to investigate memory deficits.

Some key contributions from animal behavioral studies to the redefining of the amyloid hypothesis in AD are presented in Fig. 2.

The compromise of spatial working memory tested by MWM begins in Tg2576 mice at the age of 8 months. Stewart *et al.* compared results from different research groups on the behavioral tests performed on Tg2576 mice at different ages, and found that 64 percent of cohorts in the range of 8–11 months of age reported an impairment compared to littermates of the same age.[49] For the Y-maze test, the parameter used to evaluate working memory deficit being spontaneous alternation, animals tested before 8 months of age gave conflicting results. According to some authors, 3-month-old Tg2576 mice showed a performance similar to non-transgenic animals,[50,51] while others described impairment.[52,53]

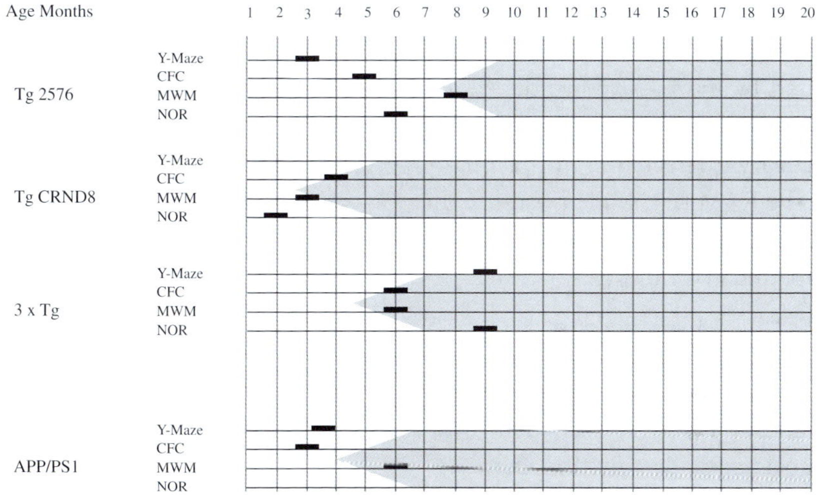

Fig. 2. Relation between the age of plaque formation and memory deficit in the most widely used Alzheimer transgenic mouse models. The horizontal bar refers to the age of the animal. The tip of the arrow indicates the beginning of Aβ aggregation leading to plaque deposition. The marks indicate the earliest age at which the impairment of the corresponding test was described. Abbreviations: CFC, contextual fear conditioning; MWM, Morris water maze; NOR, novel object recognition; PA, passive avoidance; RAWM, radial arm water maze.

With contextual FC, contextual memory is evaluated as time spent freezing in a new context after exposure to an aversive stimulus. At 5 months of age (20 weeks), prior to the deposition of amyloid plaques, a decrease in the freezing time in Tg2576 mice compared to non-Tg littermates has been observed.[54] In the novel object recognition test, using visual working memory to assess the ability of mice to explore a novel object more than a familiar one, Tg2576 mice showed an impairment of performance at the pre-plaque ages of 6 and 7 months.[54,55] TgCRND8 mice have been tested in the reference memory version of MWM. At 10 weeks of age, these mice showed severe deficits in their ability to form a spatial memory.[56] OR memory assessed at pre-plaque age showed a deficit in TgCRND8 mice by 8 weeks,[57] showing impairment in context and cue learning at 5 and 6 months.[58] The first clear sign of cognitive impairment in the 3xTg-AD model is already evident at 4 months after the onset of Aβ deposits as tested with the learning phase of MWM[59] and are confirmed with respect to memory at 6 months of age, with the performance of females being worse than that of males.[60] Context memory is impaired at 6 months of age as tested by the passive avoidance test.[60] Deficits in visual memory (NOR) and working memory (Y-maze) appear at 9 months of age.[60,61] Working memory is affected in pre-plaque 3-month-old APP/PS1 mice as reported by the RAM test, while reference memory is impaired only at 6–8 months, when plaque deposition is already present[62]; contextual memory is already impaired at 3 months.[63]

18.3.3. Synapse and Neurotransmitter Dysfunction

Some of the most relevant data from animal studies have led to the discovery that synaptic dysfunction characterizes the initial phase of AD pathology and is responsible for learning and memory deficits.[64] Soluble assembly states of Aβ peptides can cause cognitive problems by disrupting synaptic function in the absence of significant neurodegeneration, also impairing LTP in AD transgenic mice.[59,65] A strong correlation exists between axonal and synaptic damage and progressive accumulation of Aβ oligomers.[23] Loss of dendritic spines similar to the synapse loss observed in human AD has been reported in several mouse models that develop amyloid and tau pathology.[26] Moreover, recent two-photon microscopy studies showed that spine loss is caused by soluble oligomeric Aβ,[66] secreted by neuron and glial cells but also mobilized by surrounding plaques, which can be formed quite rapidly.[67] In APP transgenic AD mouse models, there are significant alterations in hippocampal synaptic transmission and plasticity at excitatory glutamatergic synapses. These alterations appear sometimes in young animals long before Aβ is deposited in plaques, although compensatory phenomena might occur.[26] However, from 6 months onwards, most AD transgenic mice show significant deficits in basal synaptic transmission, as indicated by LTP experiments and loss/deterioration of dendritic spines.

This synaptic dysfunction is coupled with a complex neurotransmitter rearrangement. Major neurotransmitter systems connected with AD are the cholinergic, monoaminergic and opioid systems, as well as excitatory inhibitory amino acid-like glutamate and gamma-aminobutyric acid (GABA). The neurotransmitter systems described below are strictly interconnected and likely exert contemporaneous effects on AD pathology.

Several studies have indicated a strong involvement of the cholinergic system in AD manifestations, leading to the so-called cholinergic hypothesis of geriatric memory dysfunction.[68] Progressive loss of neurons projecting to the cortex and hippocampus, reduction of choline acetylesterase (ChAT) activity,[69,70] degradation and loss of functionality as well as impairment in acetylcholine receptor signaling have been highlighted as probable causes of the onset of memory deficit.[71] Age-related modifications of the cholinergic system have been extensively investigated in AD mice, with contrasting results.[72] However, most recently, several studies have correlated cholinergic deficit associated to cognitive impairment and the presence of Aβ fragments, which have been shown to negatively regulate acetylcholine (ACh) synthesis and release.[73] Moreover, results obtained from the PC12 cell line *in vitro* have revealed the binding between nicotinic receptor α7nAChR and Aβ42, and this fragment seems to act as a nicotinic receptor antagonist increasing AChE levels and tau phosphorylation.[74] Nerve growth factor (NGF) also plays an important role in modulating cholinergic system functionality.

Other transmitter-identified pathways are altered in AD, including serotonin, noradrenaline, glutamate and opiate. For the purposes of this chapter, we will briefly compare data derived from AD brains and animal models. In the serotoninergic system, a reduction of raphe nuclei neurons, changes in 5-HT levels, and degeneration of serotoninergic fibers in various regions of the human brain have been described.[75] However, to date, the loss of neurons is a controversial aspect of the disease. Discrepancies are observed in different transgenic animals, possibly related to the model used. For example, a loss of serotonergic neurons[76] and fiber degeneration were reported in APPswe/PS1ΔE9 transgenic mice after plaque deposition, which may be due to amyloid-induced neurotoxicity.[77]

The neurodegeneration of the locus coeruleus was reported and linked to the progression of dementia in post-mortem AD brains. In APP23 mice, lesion of the noradrenergic system increased β-amyloid deposition and cognitive deficit.[78] A reduction in locus coeruleus volume associated with a reduction in newborn neurons in the olfactory bulb and olfactory memory deficit before β-amyloid accumulation have also been shown in Tg2576 mice.[79]

The opioid system has also been associated with AD onset, including modulation of opioid peptide and receptor expression. In transgenic hAPP mice, elevated levels of enkephalin, through the activation of the mu-opioid receptor, correlates with behavioral alteration and may contribute to cognitive impairment.[80]

Deserving of a special mention is the link between glutamate and AD pathology. Non-essential amino acid glutamate plays a key role in synaptic plasticity, learning and memory, but its concentration and compartmentalization has to be severely regulated because of its toxicity. Glutamate-mediated transmission is severely altered in AD, although the underlying molecular changes are not clear.[81] Soluble oligomeric Aβ has been shown to interact with glutamatergic receptors of the N-methyl-D-aspartate (NMDA) type and proteins responsible for maintaining glutamate homeostasis such as uptake and release.[82] Moreover, due to its metabolic role and excitotoxicity, glutamate constitutes a molecular link between many different triggers (energy deficiency, oxidative stress, mitochondrial dysfunction, calcium overload, etc.) and neuron death.[83] Indeed, glutamatergic neurons are located in the region of the brain that is vulnerable to the disease in which neuronal loss has been reported during the early phase of disease. Independent studies have shown a reduction of the vesicular glutamate transporter VGLUT1 in the human prefrontal cortex and preferential accumulation of Aβ peptides in synapses positive for VGLUT1/2. The role of Aβ peptides in controlling glutamate metabolism and glutamate-dependent transmission was also demonstrated in different *in vitro* systems. Low levels of Aβ peptides may exert physiological roles in synaptic plasticity, demonstrated by viability experiments on cultured neurons. Conversely, high levels of soluble Aβ depressed synaptic activity in neuronal cells.[81]

The possible implication of inhibitory amino acid GABA in AD pathology has also been evaluated. A PS1/APP transgenic mice model was used to investigate the somatostatin (SOM)-positive/neuropeptide Y (NPY)-positive GABA interneuron population in the hippocampal system. It was found that cortical and hippocampal SOM-containing interneurons are strongly affected in AD brains, where reductions in NPY levels and NPY receptor densities were also reported. A reduction in GABAergic neurons containing SOM/NPY in the hippocampus (stratum oriens of CA1 and CA3 and dentate gyrus), without compromising other neurotransmitter systems, was observed in 6-month-old PS1/APP mice, demonstrating the early degeneration of the SOM/NPY GABAergic population.[84]

18.3.4. In vitro Models for AD

Cellular models are fundamental tools in the study of pathology mechanisms and for the development of drug screening systems. Moreover, they are also key players in the translational process, with respect to the reduction, where possible, in the number of animals used in AD studies. Cell lines and primary cultures are widely used in the study of neurodegenerative disease. Furthermore, new and more efficient techniques are enabling the creation of more complete cellular models for studying specific mechanisms.

One of the most widely used is the SN56 cell line, generated by fusing mouse embryonic septal neurons with N18TG2 neuroblastoma cells, in which cholinergic differentiation is induced by retinoic acid. These differentiated cells display neuronal morphology and express cholinergic markers: they may be used to study diseases with a component of cholinergic dysfunction, like AD, to study APP metabolism and its role in cellular processes. Furthermore, this cell system can be used as a model for APP toxicity studies on cholinergic neurons, to analyze the effect of Aβ on gene[85] and protein[86] expression, and the protective effect of different compounds on APP toxicity mechanisms.[87]

Among the neuron-like cell lines available, human neuroblastoma derived cells are widely used in the AD field. A neuroblast-like sub line called SH-SY5Y was developed from SK-N-SH cells isolated from human neuroblastomas. Their differentiation can be driven by different molecules and growth substrates. The SH-SY5Y cell line is a useful platform for AD study, given the ability of these cells to differentiate into mature neuronal phenotypes expressing neuron-specific markers (β-tubulin, NeuN, Sv2), and for studying the physiological hallmarks of AD. These cells express APP and, when properly differentiated, also tau protein, resembling the quantity and cellular localization of *in vivo* neurons.[88] This model is useful to study how neurotransmitters, growth factors and their receptors are involved in, or affected by, Aβ toxicity mechanisms. These cells have also been transfected to express pathological human APP or tau genes.[89] From SH-SY5Y, it is possible to create transgenic cells expressing the human mutated forms of tau to obtain *in vitro* models of tauopathies.[90,91] It is also possible to create a FAD model developing cell lines expressing the APP gene carrying the Swedish mutation.[92,93]

Primary cell cultures represent another way to perform *in vitro* studies. It is possible to isolate cells from different regions of the brain to obtain pure or mixed cultures of several cell types. Cortical, hippocampal or cerebellar neurons isolated from mice or rats are widely used to perform studies on Aβ and tau pathology mechanisms.[94] Even if primary cultures are a more powerful cellular model compared to cell lines, the disadvantages are the low cell numbers and time-consuming techniques involved. It is also difficult to achieve human primary cultures, from the fetus or post-mortem human subjects,[95] limiting the target exclusively to animal models. A step forward in the development of *in vitro* systems based on primary cell cultures is the isolation of specific cell types from animal models of neurodegenerative disease. It is possible to isolate primary neurons using different transgenic mice models to investigate the effect of the mutated proteins in different conditions,[96] in order to compare sensitivity to toxic stimuli[97] and for drug screening.[62] Adult neural progenitors can be isolated from fetal, newborn or adult mouse brain.[98] These "neurospheres" are used to study the different expression patterns due to transgenic genes. It is also possible to differentiate them and to study their development.

It is widely accepted that microglial cells play an important role in neuronal damage and cognitive loss in AD. Primary microglia derived from mouse or rat brain has high phenotypic similarities to *in vivo* cells.[99] In the study of the mechanisms of AD, these primary cultures were useful in understanding how the neuronal damage, due to the Aβ oligomers, may be emphasized and driven by activating microglial cells. These activated M2 microglia have the ability to phagocytize Aβ fragments. This function is inhibited by cytokines that shift cell type to the pro-inflammatory state M1. Rat BV2 and mouse N9 immortalized cell lines are similar to primary microglia cultures, both in terms of morphology and gene expression, and also for the production of nitric oxide (NO) and cytokines and for Aβ phagocytosis.[99]

The final, most powerful arrow in the *in vitro* models' quiver is the induced pluripotent stem (iPS) system. Since 2006, when Nobel Prize winner Shinya Yamanaka described the technique to obtain embryonic stem-like cells from adult differentiated cells,[100] different uses have been proposed for these cells. In recent years, different protocols have been developed to obtain differentiated neurons from iPS cells derived from neurodegenerative disease patients, including sufferers of Parkinson's disease, amyotrophic lateral sclerosis, spinal muscular atrophy and AD.[101,102] These cells recapitulate the *in vivo* phenotypes, demonstrating their important role in the development of efficient human disease models.[103]

18.3.5. Biomarkers for Clinical Studies

Advances in the diagnosis of AD have been achieved thanks to the growing knowledge of the molecular mechanisms involved in the disease through research performed in animal models. These multidisciplinary translational studies have contributed greatly to the development of new approaches for diagnosis and specific therapies applicable to humans. In this context, translational research should not be considered unidirectional ("bench-to-bed"), as data obtained from clinical studies might pilot/condition basic research ("bed-to-bench"). This is evident in the "biomarkers" field, where data from AD patients are more numerous than from AD animal models. In the context of dementia, the term *biomarker* refers to: (i) cognitive tests, (ii) imaging and (iii) biochemistry of biological fluids. For the purposes of this chapter, we will consider biochemistry of biological fluids only. In particular, cerebrospinal and plasma biomarkers will be considered and discussed from a translational perspective.

Amyloid peptides, in particular Aβ40 and Aβ42, have been proposed for the study of the deposition of amyloid plaques, known to be a very early event in AD that leads to axonal, synaptic and neuronal damage and consequently to synaptic dysfunction. Among the first and most widely studied, these proteins have been found in early AD brains as full-length proteins (Aβ40 and Aβ42) and also as C- or N-terminally truncated forms (AβN-40 and Aβ N-42).[104]

The potential use of plasma biomarkers instead of (or together with) cerebrospinal fluid (CSF) biomarkers has the advantage of being less invasive. However, results for Aβ40 and Aβ42 plasma level proteins have been contradictory. Some studies have described Aβ42 plasma levels as being higher in cases of familial AD, and have suggested that elevated Aβ42 plasma levels together with low Aβ40 levels and a reduced Aβ40/Aβ42 ratio in old subjects might predict the risk of potential dementia (mild cognitive impairment, MCI, or AD) in normal cognitive subjects. Other studies instead found that decreased Aβ42 plasma levels might be an indicator of the change from normal cognitive or MCI subjects to AD subjects.[105] These contrasting results may be differentially explained[105]: (i) The levels of plasma Aβ proteins could be influenced by peripheral and brain APP processing (metabolism and clearance) and this has been found to be different between subjects (high intra- and inter-subject variability). (ii) Standardization of sample taking has not yet been achieved. Oddly enough, changes in Aβ production and clearance are influenced by many physiological factors, such as the circadian cycle sleep/wakefulness, renal function, starving, etc., within the same individual. Moreover, Aβ42 plasma levels are influenced by ongoing therapies. (iii) Methods for quantifying Aβ proteins in plasma have not yet been standardized. The accurate and reproducible measurement of these proteins in biological fluids is very difficult because of the "sticky" nature of Aβ peptides (hydrophobic and heterogeneous). In this context, the Alzheimer's Disease Neuroimaging Initiative (ADNI, *http://adni.loni.ucla.edu*) has attempted to standardize methods across certain participating laboratories. They proposed using a kit from Innogenetics (Ghent, Belgium), INNO-BIA plasma Aβ forms, for the simultaneous quantification of plasmatic Aβ40 and Aβ42 using the Luminex platform (xMAP technology). All the laboratories that participated in this study used kits with the same lot number, and processed the same samples, diluted or not in the described way. From this study, named Round Robin INNO-BIA plasma Aβ forms, important conclusions came out regarding factors that can markedly influence results: patient preparation before sample taking, sample collection, vials used for sample storage, sample storage and handling, and so on.

All the above-described observations have a lot in common with what happens in animals, since Aβ peptides possess the same physicochemical characteristics. High inter- and intra-animal variability has been also observed in studies performed with different animal models for AD.[106,107]

It is well established that neuroinflammation has a key role in AD pathology and progression.[108] Activated microglia have been found in damaged brain areas in which β-amyloid plaques, NFT and damaged neurons coexist. Evidence from human studies shows that activated microglia in AD afflicted subjects release pro-inflammatory cytokines, tumor necrosis factor α (TNF-α) and interleukin-β (IL-β), among others. Epidemiologic studies revealed the lower incidence of dementia in elderly subjects that were regular users of non-steroidal anti-inflammatory drugs (NSAIDs). On the other hand, studies performed in different transgenic mouse models for AD (Tg2576, APP/PS1, APPV717I) have demonstrated the decrease in amyloid plaque burden and neuroinflammation after early and long-term treatment with some NSAIDs such as ibuprofen, curcumin or NCX-2216. Cytokines such as TNF-α and IL-β, and the soluble form of CD40 ligand (sCD40L) have been studied in both human and animal AD models, as potential biomarkers of neuroinflammation. It has been described that microglial activation due to Aβ accumulation is associated with increasing expression of the transmembrane receptor CD40 (a tumor necrosis receptor super-family member) and its ligand (CD40L), as well as with an increase in the circulating levels of soluble forms of CD40 (sCD40) and CD40L (sCD40L).[109] On the other hand, TNF-α has been described to be involved in the pathogenesis of AD.[110] Recently published data from a phase I clinical study describe the modulation of sCD40L level in plasma and CSF after multiple oral administrations of the ibuprofen-like drug, CHF5074, in a dose-dependent way. It has also been found that TNF-α level is decreased in CSF treatment but not in plasma after CHF5074.[111]

CSF amyloid protein quantification as a biomarker is a hallmark of early AD diagnosis and progression. Decreased CSF Aβ42 constitutes one of the first pieces of evidence of AD in normal cognitive subjects. Many studies have demonstrated that Aβ42 levels in CSF are around half lower in AD patients compared with healthy subjects or subjects at early clinical disease stages.[112] Tau and the hyperphosphorylated form of this protein, p-tau, are the principal and more abundant components, respectively, of the NFT present in neuronal cell bodies. More importantly, the combination of Aβ42, total tau and p-tau values, more than each individual marker, constitutes the most useful/important information to best discriminate AD from healthy subjects of the same age with higher sensitivity and specificity, and assess the clinical progression to AD from MCI (Aβ42, tau and p-tau, core CSF AD biomarkers). This is very important in the context of clinical trials.[112,113] On the other hand, Aβ40 levels in CSF can be used as a good indicator of individual global circulating amyloid load.[114] Moreover, CSF Aβ40/Aβ42 ratio is also correlated to clinical dementia rating (CDR).[115] Thus, although CSF Aβ40 level cannot be used as a monitoring biomarker for the evolution of cognitive impairment, it can be used to better characterize the biochemical profile of some neurodegenerative dementias,[116] given that CSF Aβ40 level is the only parameter showing limitations in distinguishing AD from other types of dementia such as vascular dementia, frontotemporal dementia, and Lewy body dementia.[117]

Finally, there is an increasing amount of literature from animal and human studies describing new CSF biomarker candidates, but these results have not been reproduced. Some of these new proteins are the BACE1 protein; neuronal and synaptic proteins as markers for cognitive status and disease prognosis [e.g., visinin-like protein 1 (VSNL1), neurofilaments (NF), synaptotagmin, synaptosomal-associated proteins (SNAP-25)]; inflammatory, signaling and oxidative stress marker proteins (interleukins, TNF-α, IFN-β, TGF-β, etc.).[112]

As in the case of plasma, there are some problems regarding the standardization of methods for the quantification of CSF AD biomarkers (subject conditions at the time of sample taking, fluid storage conditions, technical approaches followed, commercial kits used for quantification, etc.). From the recent literature on biomarkers, it can be concluded that the scientific community is devoting efforts to the standardization of specific methods for the quantification of potential/accepted AD biomarkers. A particular effort is also being made by some manufacturers to validate methods for the single and (much more often used) multi parametric quantification of potential biomarkers of AD, such as Aβ42, tau and p-tau.[118] Round robin studies performed in plasma and CSF, not only by kit manufacturers' research teams but also by different laboratories around the world, are of huge importance for improving and standardizing methods for biomarker studies.

At the same time, the increasing importance of working in accordance with certified good practice (e.g., GLP, GCP and GXP) must be taken into account. Although this is very expensive for laboratories, working at any of these certified levels would lead to standardized methods and to the harmonization of applications in early diagnosis and progression of disease. GLP-level validation of one of the most widely used kits in diagnostics for the quantification of CSF Aβ42 protein, the INNOTEST Aβ42 ELISA (Ghent, Belgium), has been published. This study constitutes a very important contribution to diagnostic methodologies, since crucial technical aspects such as minimum required sample dilution, Aβ42 adsorption vial test, standard curve optimization, among others, have been studied in depth.[119]

Another inconvenient aspect of the quantification of proteins as potential biomarkers of AD is that no validated methods are available for their accurate and reproducible quantification, and/or no methods exist for specific species (animal or human) for use in the required biological fluid (plasma, serum, CSF, cell supernatant, etc.). This is the case for sCD40L quantification in human CSF, for which researchers have dedicated effort and money to properly modify commercially validated methods for specific biological fluids, e.g., plasma, to be used in others, for instance, CSF.[111]

Moreover, studies have been also performed comparing different methodologies for the quantification of specific proteins (e.g., ELISA versus multiparametric platforms)[120] as well as studies proposing new advanced methods [tandem mass spectrometry (TMS), liquid chromatography combined with mass spectrometry (LC–MS), stable isotope labeling kinetics (SILK), etc.] for application in animal and clinical studies.[112]

18.4. CONCLUSIONS

The multidisciplinary translational science in AD has contributed in a fundamental way to the progress in our understanding of AD pathology, thus providing key information for novel diagnostic and therapeutic developments. Starting from human genetic studies, animal and cell models have explored the so-called amyloid cascade hypothesis, proving that cognitive phenotype is not associated to plaques or tangles, but to early synaptic dysfunction, which appear well before the histopathological hallmarks of AD. In the meantime, animal studies have provided indications concerning the early appearance of neuroinflammation, supporting the inclusion of neuroinflammation-related biomarkers in clinical monitoring of the disease and drug efficacy profiles.

With this redefinition of the amyloid cascade hypothesis, as well as data from SAD patients and incoming results from genome-wide association studies, other animal and cell models are under development and will soon be available to support the global alliance to combat this devastating disease.

REFERENCES

1. Honig LS. (2012) Translational research in neurology: Dementia. *Arch Neurol* **69**: 969–977.
2. Mihaescu R, Detmar SB, Cornel MC, *et al.* (2010) Translational research in genomics of Alzheimer's disease: A review of current practice and future perspectives. *J Alzheimers Dis* **20**: 967–980.
3. Van Dam D, De Deyn PP. (2011) Animal models in the drug discovery pipeline for Alzheimer's disease. *Br J Pharmacol* **164**: 1285–1300.
4. Zhang YW, Thompson R, Zhang H, Xu H. (2011) APP processing in Alzheimer's disease. *Mol Brain* **4**: 3.
5. Zhang H, Ma Q, Zhang YW, Xu H. (2012) Proteolytic processing of Alzheimer's beta-amyloid precursor protein. *J Neurochem* **120**(Suppl 1): 9–21.
6. Gough M, Parr-Sturgess C, Parkin E. (2011) Zinc metalloproteinases and amyloid beta-peptide metabolism: The positive side of proteolysis in Alzheimer's disease. *Biochem Res Int* **2011**: 721463.
7. Ma T, Zhao Y, Kwak YD, Yang Z, *et al.* (2009) Statin's excitoprotection is mediated by sAPP and the subsequent attenuation of calpain-induced truncation events, likely via rho-ROCK signaling. *J Neurosci* **29**: 11226–11236.
8. Siemes C, Quast T, Kummer C, *et al.* (2006) Keratinocytes from APP/APLP2-deficient mice are impaired in proliferation, adhesion and migration *in vitro*. *Exp Cell Res* **312**: 1939–1949.
9. Taylor CJ, Ireland DR, Ballagh I, *et al.* (2008) Endogenous secreted amyloid precursor protein-alpha regulates hippocampal NMDA receptor function, long-term potentiation and spatial memory. *Neurobiol Dis* **31**: 250–260.
10. Chasseigneaux S, Allinquant B. (2012) Functions of Abeta, sAPPalpha and sAPPbeta: Similarities and differences. *J Neurochem* **120**(Suppl 1): 99–108.

11. Chasseigneaux S, Dinc L, Rose C, *et al.* (2011) Secreted amyloid precursor protein beta and secreted amyloid precursor protein alpha induce axon outgrowth *in vitro* through Egr1 signaling pathway. *PLoS ONE* **6**: e16301.
12. Freude KK, Penjwini M, Davis JL, *et al.* (2011) Soluble amyloid precursor protein induces rapid neural differentiation of human embryonic stem cells. *J Biol Chem* **286**: 24264–24274.
13. Nikolaev A, McLaughlin T, O'Leary DD, Tessier-Lavigne M. (2009) APP binds DR6 to trigger axon pruning and neuron death via distinct caspases. *Nature* **457**: 981–989.
14. Passer B, Pellegrini L, Russo C, *et al.* (2000) Generation of an apoptotic intracellular peptide by gamma-secretase cleavage of Alzheimer's amyloid beta protein precursor. *J Alzheimers Dis* **2**: 289–301.
15. Ozaki T, Li Y, Kikuchi H, Tomita T, *et al.* (2006) The intracellular domain of the amyloid precursor protein (AICD) enhances the p53-mediated apoptosis. *Biochem Biophys Res Commun* **351**: 57–63.
16. Hamid R, Kilger E, Willem M, *et al.* (2007) Amyloid precursor protein intracellular domain modulates cellular calcium homeostasis and ATP content. *J Neurochem* **102**: 1264–1275.
17. Nalivaeva NN, Beckett C, Belyaev ND, Turner AJ. (2012) Are amyloid-degrading enzymes viable therapeutic targets in Alzheimer's disease? *J Neurochem* **120**(Suppl 1): 167–185.
18. Thinakaran G, Koo EH. (2008) Amyloid precursor protein trafficking, processing, and function. *J Biol Chem* **283**: 29615–29619.
19. Teich AF, Arancio O. (2012) Is the amyloid hypothesis of Alzheimer's disease therapeutically relevant? *Biochem J* **446**: 165–177.
20. Lu DC, Soriano S, Bredesen DE, Koo EH. (2003) Caspase cleavage of the amyloid precursor protein modulates amyloid beta-protein toxicity. *J Neurochem* **87**: 733–741.
21. Kim J, Basak JM, Holtzman DM. (2009) The role of apolipoprotein E in Alzheimer's disease. *Neuron* **63**: 287–303.
22. De Strooper B. (2010) Proteases and proteolysis in Alzheimer disease: A multifactorial view on the disease process. *Physiol Rev* **90**: 465–494.
23. Crews L, Rockenstein E, Masliah E. (2010) APP transgenic modeling of Alzheimer's disease: Mechanisms of neurodegeneration and aberrant neurogenesis. *Brain Struct Funct* **214**: 111–126.
24. Ahmed M, Davis J, Aucoin D, *et al.* (2010) Structural conversion of neurotoxic amyloid-beta(1–42) oligomers to fibrils. *Nat Struct Mol Biol* **17**: 561–567.

25. Benilova I, Karran E, De Strooper B. (2012) The toxic Abeta oligomer and Alzheimer's disease: An emperor in need of clothes. *Nat Neurosci* **15**: 349–357.
26. Spires-Jones T, Knafo S. (2012) Spines, plasticity, and cognition in Alzheimer's model mice. *Neural Plast* **2012**: 319836.
27. LaFerla FM, Green KN. (2012) Animal models of Alzheimer disease. *Cold Spring Harb Perspect Med* **2**.
28. Duyckaerts C, Potier MC, Delatour B. (2008) Alzheimer disease models and human neuropathology: Similarities and differences. *Acta Neuropathol* **115**: 5–38.
29. Lewis J, McGowan E, Rockwood J, *et al.* (2000) Neurofibrillary tangles, amyotrophy and progressive motor disturbance in mice expressing mutant (P301L) tau protein. *Nat Genet* **25**: 402–405.
30. Bugiani O, Murrell JR, Giaccone G, *et al.* (1999) Frontotemporal dementia and corticobasal degeneration in a family with a P301S mutation in tau. *J Neuropathol Exp Neurol* **58**: 667–677.
31. Tanemura K, Murayama M, Akagi T, *et al.* (2002) Neurodegeneration with tau accumulation in a transgenic mouse expressing V337M human tau. *J Neurosci* **22**: 133–141.
32. Ribe EM, Perez M, Puig B, *et al.* (2005) Accelerated amyloid deposition, neurofibrillary degeneration and neuronal loss in double mutant APP/tau transgenic mice. *Neurobiol Dis* **20**: 814–822.
33. Oddo S, Caccamo A, Shepherd JD, *et al.* (2003) Triple-transgenic model of Alzheimer's disease with plaques and tangles: Intracellular Abeta and synaptic dysfunction. *Neuron* **39**: 409–421.
34. D'Alton S, George DR. (2011) Changing perspectives on Alzheimer's disease: Thinking outside the amyloid box. *J Alzheimers Dis* **25**: 571–581.
35. Yu W, Lu B. (2012) Synapses and dendritic spines as pathogenic targets in Alzheimer's disease. *Neural Plast* **2012**: 247150.
36. Mucke L, Selkoe DJ. (2012) Neurotoxicity of amyloid beta-protein: Synaptic and network dysfunction. *Cold Spring Harb Perspect Med* **2**: a006338.
37. Dudchenko PA. (2004) An overview of the tasks used to test working memory in rodents. *Neurosci Biobehav Rev* **28**: 699–709.
38. Morris R. (1984) Developments of a water-maze procedure for studying spatial learning in the rat. *J Neurosci Methods* **11**: 47–60.
39. de Toledo-Morrell L, Morrell F, Fleming S. (1984) Age-dependent deficits in spatial memory are related to impaired hippocampal kindling. *Behav Neurosci* **98**: 902–907.

40. Morgan D, Diamond DM, Gottschall PE, *et al.* (2000) A beta peptide vaccination prevents memory loss in an animal model of Alzheimer's disease. *Nature* **408**: 982–985.
41. Shear DA, Dong J, Haik-Creguer KL, *et al.* (1998) Chronic administration of quinolinic acid in the rat striatum causes spatial learning deficits in a radial arm water maze task. *Exp Neurol* **150**: 305–311.
42. Bimonte HA, Denenberg VH. (1999) Estradiol facilitates performance as working memory load increases. *Psycho neuroendocrinology* **24**: 161–173.
43. Hyde LA, Hoplight BJ, Denenberg VH. (1998) Water version of the radial-arm maze: Learning in three inbred strains of mice. *Brain Res* **785**: 236– 244.
44. Bimonte HA, Hyde LA, Hoplight BJ, Denenberg VH. (2000) In two species, females exhibit superior working memory and inferior reference memory on the water radial-arm maze. *Physiol Behav* **70**: 311–317.
45. Arendash GW, Gordon MN, Diamond DM, *et al.* (2001) Behavioral assessment of Alzheimer's transgenic mice following long-term Abeta vaccination: Task specificity and correlations between Abeta deposition and spatial memory. *DNA Cell Biol* **20**: 737–744.
46. Maren S. (2001) Neurobiology of Pavlovian fear conditioning. *Annu Rev Neurosci* **24**: 897–931.
47. Senechal Y, Kelly PH, Dev KK. (2008) Amyloid precursor protein knockout mice show age-dependent deficits in passive avoidance learning. *Behav Brain Res* **186**: 126–132.
48. McGaugh JL. (1966) Time-dependent processes in memory storage. *Science* **153**: 1351–1358.
49. Stewart S, Cacucci F, Lever C. (2011) Which memory task for my mouse? A systematic review of spatial memory performance in the Tg2576 Alzheimer's mouse model. *J Alzheimers Dis* **26**: 105–126.
50. Hsiao K, Chapman P, Nilsen S, *et al.* (1996) Correlative memory deficits, Abeta elevation, and amyloid plaques in transgenic mice. *Science* **274**: 99–102.
51. King DL, Arendash GW, Crawford F, *et al.* (1999) Progressive and gender-dependent cognitive impairment in the APP(SW) transgenic mouse model for Alzheimer's disease. *Behav Brain Res* **103**: 145–162.
52. Holcomb LA, Gordon MN, Jantzen P, *et al.* (1999) Behavioral changes in transgenic mice expressing both amyloid precursor protein and presenilin-1 mutations: Lack of association with amyloid deposits. *Behav Genet* **29**: 177–185.

53. King DL, Arendash GW. (2002) Behavioral characterization of the Tg2576 transgenic model of Alzheimer's disease through 19 months. *Physiol Behav* **75**: 627–642.
54. Balducci C, Mehdawy B, Mare L, *et al.* (2011) The gamma-secretase modulator CHF5074 restores memory and hippocampal synaptic plasticity in plaque-free Tg2576 mice. *J Alzheimers Dis* **24**: 799–816.
55. Giuliani A, Beggiato S, Baldassarro VA, *et al.* (2012) CHF5074 restores visual memory ability and pre-synaptic cortical acetylcholine release in pre-plaque Tg2576 mice. *J Neurochem* **124**(5): 613–620.
56. Yiu AP, Rashid AJ, Josselyn SA. (2011) Increasing CREB function in the CA1 region of dorsal hippocampus rescues the spatial memory deficits in a mouse model of Alzheimer's disease. *Neuro psychopharmacology* **36**: 2169–2186.
57. Francis BM, Kim J, Barakat ME, *et al.* (2012) Object recognition memory and BDNF expression are reduced in young TgCRND8 mice. *Neurobiol Aging* **33**: 555–563.
58. Greco SJ, Bryan KJ, Sarkar S, *et al.* (2010) Leptin reduces pathology and improves memory in a transgenic mouse model of Alzheimer's disease. *J Alzheimers Dis* **19**: 1155–1167.
59. Oddo S, Caccamo A, Tran L, *et al.* (2006) Temporal profile of amyloid-beta (Abeta) oligomerization in an *in vivo* model of Alzheimer disease. A link between Abeta and tau pathology. *J Biol Chem* **281**: 1599–1604.
60. Clinton LK, Billings LM, Green KN, *et al.* (2007) Age-dependent sexual dimorphism in cognition and stress response in the 3xTg-AD mice. *Neurobiol Dis* **28**: 76–82.
61. Caccamo A, Oddo S, Billings LM, *et al.* (2006) M1 receptors play a central role in modulating AD-like pathology in transgenic mice. *Neuron* **49**: 671–682.
62. Trinchese F, Liu S, Battaglia F, *et al.* (2004) Progressive age-related development of Alzheimer-like pathology in APP/PS1 mice. *Ann Neurol* **55**: 801–814.
63. Gong B, Vitolo OV, Trinchese F, *et al.* (2004) Persistent improvement in synaptic and cognitive functions in an Alzheimer mouse model after rolipram treatment. *J Clin Invest* **114**: 1624–1634.
64. Wang H, Megill A, He K, *et al.* (2012) Consequences of inhibiting amyloid precursor protein processing enzymes on synaptic function and plasticity. *Neural Plast* **2012**: 272–374.
65. Chang L, Bakhos L, Wang Z, *et al.* (2003) Femtomole immunodetection of synthetic and endogenous amyloid-beta oligomers and its application

to Alzheimer's disease drug candidate screening. *J Mol Neurosci* **20**: 305–313.
66. Shankar GM, Bloodgood BL, Townsend M, *et al.* (2007) Natural oligomers of the Alzheimer amyloid-beta protein induce reversible synapse loss by modulating an NMDA-type glutamate receptor-dependent signaling pathway. *J Neurosci* **27**: 2866–2875.
67. Meyer-Luehmann M, Spires-Jones TL, Prada C, *et al.* (2008) Rapid appearance and local toxicity of amyloid-beta plaques in a mouse model of Alzheimer's disease. *Nature* **451**: 720–724.
68. Bartus RT. (2000) On neurodegenerative diseases, models, and treatment strategies: Lessons learned and lessons forgotten a generation following the cholinergic hypothesis. *Exp Neurol* **163**: 495–529.
69. Gsell W, Jungkunz G, Riederer P. (2004) Functional neurochemistry of Alzheimer's disease. *Curr Pharm Des* **10**: 265–293.
70. Nordberg A. (1992) Neuroreceptor changes in Alzheimer disease. *Cerebrovasc Brain Metab Rev* **4**: 303–328.
71. Xu Y, Yan J, Zhou P, *et al.* (2012) Neurotransmitter receptors and cognitive dysfunction in Alzheimer's disease and Parkinson's disease. *Prog Neurobiol* **97**: 1–13.
72. Contestabile A. (2011) The history of the cholinergic hypothesis. *Behav Brain Res* **221**: 334–340.
73. Auld DS, Kornecook TJ, Bastianetto S, Quirion R. (2002) Alzheimer's disease and the basal forebrain cholinergic system: Relations to beta-amyloid peptides, cognition, and treatment strategies. *Prog Neurobiol* **68**: 209–245.
74. Dziewczapolski G, Glogowski CM, Masliah E, Heinemann SF. (2009) Deletion of the alpha 7 nicotinic acetylcholine receptor gene improves cognitive deficits and synaptic pathology in a mouse model of Alzheimer's disease. *J Neurosci* **29**: 8805–8815.
75. Rodriguez JJ, Noristani HN, Verkhratsky A. (2012) The serotonergic system in ageing and Alzheimer's disease. *Prog Neurobiol* **99**: 15–41.
76. Bernedo V, Insua D, Suarez ML, *et al.* (2009) Beta-amyloid cortical deposits are accompanied by the loss of serotonergic neurons in the dog. *J Comp Neurol* **513**: 417–429.
77. Liu Y, Yoo MJ, Savonenko A, *et al.* (2008) Amyloid pathology is associated with progressive monoaminergic neurodegeneration in a transgenic mouse model of Alzheimer's disease. *J Neurosci* **28**: 13805–13814.
78. Hawkes C. (2003) Olfaction in neurodegenerative disorder. *Mov Disord* **18**: 364–372.

79. Guerin D, Sacquet J, Mandairon N, *et al.* (2009) Early locus coeruleus degeneration and olfactory dysfunctions in Tg2576 mice. *Neurobiol Aging* **30**: 272–283.
80. Cai Z, Ratka A. (2012) Opioid system and Alzheimer's disease. *Neuromol Med* **14**: 91–111.
81. Revett TJ, Baker GB, Jhamandas J, Kar S. (2013) Glutamate system, amyloid ss peptides and tau protein: Functional interrelationships and relevance to Alzheimer disease pathology. *J Psychiatry Neurosci* **38**: 6–23.
82. Danysz W, Parsons CG. (2012) Alzheimer's disease, beta-amyloid, glutamate, NMDA receptors and memantine — Searching for the connections. *Br J Pharmacol* **167**: 324–352.
83. Mehta A, Prabhakar M, Kumar P, *et al.* (2012) Excitotoxicity: Bridge to various triggers in neurodegenerative disorders. *Eur J Pharmacol* **698**: 6–18.
84. Ramos B, Baglietto-Vargas D, del Rio JC, *et al.* (2006) Early neuropathology of somatostatin/NPY GABAergic cells in the hippocampus of a PS1xAPP transgenic model of Alzheimer's disease. *Neurobiol Aging* **27**: 1658–1672.
85. Heinitz K, Beck M, Schliebs R, Perez-Polo JR. (2006) Toxicity mediated by soluble oligomers of beta-amyloid(1–42) on cholinergic SN56.B5.G4 cells. *J Neurochem* **98**: 1930–1945.
86. Joerchel S, Raap M, Bigl M, *et al.* (2008) Oligomeric beta-amyloid(1–42) induces the expression of Alzheimer disease-relevant proteins in cholinergic SN56.B5.G4 cells as revealed by proteomic analysis. *Int J Dev Neurosci* **26**: 301–308.
87. Pirondi S, Giuliani A, Del Vecchio G, *et al.* (2010) The galanin receptor 2/3 agonist Gal2–11 protects the SN56 cells against beta-amyloid 25–35 toxicity. *J Neurosci Res* **88**: 1064–1073.
88. Agholme L, Lindstrom T, Kagedal K, *et al.* (2010) An *in vitro* model for neuroscience: Differentiation of SH-SY5Y cells into cells with morphological and biochemical characteristics of mature neurons. *J Alzheimers Dis* **20**: 1069–1082.
89. Sokolova TV, Furaev VV, Rychkova MP, *et al.* (2008) PC12 cells transfected with human mutant gene causing one of Alzheimer's disease forms have a high sensitivity to oxidative stress. *Zh Evol Biokhim Fiziol* **44**: 26–31.
90. Bloom GS, Ren K, Glabe CG. (2005) Cultured cell and transgenic mouse models for tau pathology linked to beta-amyloid. *Biochim Biophys Acta* **1739**: 116–124.
91. Loffler T, Flunkert S, Taub N, *et al.* (2012) Stable mutated tau441 transfected SH-SY5Y cells as screening tool for Alzheimer's disease drug candidates. *J Mol Neurosci* **47**: 192–203.

92. Stoppelkamp S, Bell HS, Palacios-Filardo J, *et al.* (2011) *In vitro* modelling of Alzheimer's disease: Degeneration and cell death induced by viral delivery of amyloid and tau. *Exp Neurol* **229**: 226–237.
93. Cai Z, Li B, Li K, Zhao B. (2012) Down-regulation of amyloid-beta through AMPK activation by inhibitors of GSK-3beta in SH-SY5Y and SH-SY5Y-AbetaPP695 cells. *J Alzheimers Dis* **29**: 89–98.
94. Wang C, Wurtman RJ, Lee RK. (2000) Amyloid precursor protein and membrane phospholipids in primary cortical neurons increase with development, or after exposure to nerve growth factor or Abeta(1–40). *Brain Res* **865**: 157–167.
95. Konishi Y, Lindholm K, Yang LB, *et al.* (2002) Isolation of living neurons from human elderly brains using the immunomagnetic sorting DNA-linker system. *Am J Pathol* **161**: 1567–1576.
96. Burger S, Yafai Y, Bigl M, *et al.* (2010) Effect of VEGF and its receptor antagonist SU-5416, an inhibitor of angiogenesis, on processing of the beta-amyloid precursor protein in primary neuronal cells derived from brain tissue of Tg2576 mice. *Int J Dev Neurosci* **28**: 597–604.
97. Ray S, Howells C, Eaton ED, *et al.* (2011) Tg2576 cortical neurons that express human Ab are susceptible to extracellular Abeta-induced, K+ efflux dependent neurodegeneration. *PLoS ONE* **6**: e19026.
98. Ahmed S. (2009) The culture of neural stem cells. *J Cell Biochem* **106**: 1–6.
99. Stansley B, Post J, Hensley K. (2012) A comparative review of cell culture systems for the study of microglial biology in Alzheimer's disease. *J Neuroinflammation* **9**: 115.
100. Takahashi K, Yamanaka S. (2006) Induction of pluripotent stem cells from mouse embryonic and adult fibroblast cultures by defined factors. *Cell* **126**: 663–676.
101. Park IH, Arora N, Huo H, *et al.* (2008) Disease-specific induced pluripotent stem cells. *Cell* **134**: 877–886.
102. Qiang L, Fujita R, Yamashita T, *et al.* (2011) Directed conversion of Alzheimer's disease patient skin fibroblasts into functional neurons. *Cell* **146**: 359–371.
103. Israel MA, Yuan SH, Bardy C, *et al.* (2012) Probing sporadic and familial Alzheimer's disease using induced pluripotent stem cells. *Nature* **482**: 216–220.
104. Sergeant N, Bombois S, Ghestem A, *et al.* (2003) Truncated beta-amyloid peptide species in pre-clinical Alzheimer's disease as new targets for the vaccination approach. *J Neurochem* **85**: 1581–1591.

105. Jellinger KA, Janetzky B, Attems J, Kienzl E. (2008) Biomarkers for early diagnosis of Alzheimer disease: "ALZheimer ASsociated gene" — A new blood biomarker? *J Cell Mol Med* **12**: 1094–1117.
106. Imbimbo BP, Giardino L, Sivilia S, *et al.* (2010) CHF5074, a novel gamma-secretase modulator, restores hippocampal neurogenesis potential and reverses contextual memory deficit in a transgenic mouse model of Alzheimer's disease. *J Alzheimers Dis* **20**: 159–173.
107. Chakravarthy B, Gaudet C, Menard M, *et al.* (2010) Amyloid-beta peptides stimulate the expression of the p75(NTR) neurotrophin receptor in SHSY5Y human neuroblastoma cells and AD transgenic mice. *J Alzheimers Dis* **19**: 915–925.
108. Weitz TM, Town T. (2012) Microglia in Alzheimer's disease: It's all about context. *Int J Alzheimers Dis* **2012**: 314185.
109. Giunta B, Rezai-Zadeh K, Tan J. (2010) Impact of the CD40-CD40L dyad in Alzheimer's disease. *CNS Neurol Disord Drug Targets* **9**: 149–155.
110. Kelley BJ, Petersen RC. (2007) Alzheimer's disease and mild cognitive impairment. *Neurol Clin* **25**: 577–609.
111. Imbimbo BP, Frigerio E, Breda M, *et al.* (2012) Pharmacokinetics and pharmacodynamics of CHF5074 after short-term administration in healthy subjects. *Alzheimer Dis Assoc Disord.*
112. Blennow K, Zetterberg H, Fagan AM. (2012) Fluid biomarkers in Alzheimer disease. *Cold Spring Harb Perspect Med* **2**: a006221.
113. Holtzman DM. (2011) CSF biomarkers for Alzheimer's disease: Current utility and potential future use. *Neurobiol Aging* **32**(Suppl 1): S4–S9.
114. Wiltfang J, Esselmann H, Bibl M, *et al.* (2007) Amyloid beta peptide ratio 42/40 but not A beta 42 correlates with phospho-Tau in patients with low- and high-CSF A beta 40 load. *J Neurochem* **101**: 1053–1059.
115. Fagan AM, Roe CM, Xiong C, *et al.* (2007) Cerebrospinal fluid tau/beta-amyloid(42) ratio as a prediction of cognitive decline in nondemented older adults. *Arch Neurol* **64**: 343–349.
116. Verbeek MM, Kremer BP, Rikkert MO, *et al.* (2009) Cerebrospinal fluid amyloid beta(40) is decreased in cerebral amyloid angiopathy. *Ann Neurol* **66**: 245–249.
117. Tarawneh R, Holtzman DM. (2010) Biomarkers in translational research of Alzheimer's disease. *Neuropharmacology* **59**: 310–322.
118. Kang JH, Vanderstichele H, Trojanowski JQ, Shaw LM. (2012) Simultaneous analysis of cerebrospinal fluid biomarkers using microsphere-based xMAP multiplex technology for early detection of Alzheimer's disease. *Methods* **56**: 484–493.

119. Cullen VC, Fredenburg RA, Evans C, *et al.* (2012) Development and advanced validation of an optimized method for the quantitation of Abeta42 in human cerebrospinal fluid. *AAPS J* **14**: 510–518.
120. Fagan AM, Shaw LM, Xiong C, *et al.* (2011) Comparison of analytical platforms for cerebrospinal fluid measures of beta-amyloid 1–42, total tau, and p-tau181 for identifying Alzheimer disease amyloid plaque pathology. *Arch Neurol* **68**: 1137–1144.

CHAPTER 19

Neural Stem Cell-based Oncolytic Virotherapy Against Glioblastoma Multiforme: Translational Aspects

Brenda Auffinger, Esther Rincon*, Atique U. Ahmed**
and Maciej S. Lesniak,†*

19.1. INTRODUCTION

Glioblastoma multiforme is the most common and aggressive primary brain tumor in adults. Even with the combination of thorough surgical resection, radiation and chemotherapy, it is still related to high morbidity and short life expectancy (median survival of ~14 months).[1] The presence of highly infiltrative malignant cells that escape conventional therapy is responsible for nearly 100 percent of tumor recurrence. Other factors that contribute to glioblastoma resistance are the incapacity of many chemotherapeutic agents to cross a selective blood-brain barrier (BBB), the inability of agents to reach the tumor site in a concentration high enough to eradicate remaining resistant cells with low toxicity to non-cancerous brain tissues, the presence of multi-drug resistance genes in the residual malignant tissue, and the constant repopulation of the tumor by cancer stem cells.[2]

*The Brain Tumor Center, The University of Chicago, Chicago, Illinois, USA.
†Corresponding author: Maciej S. Lesniak, The Brain Tumor Center, The University of Chicago Pritzker School of Medicine, 5841 South Maryland Ave, M/C 3026, Chicago, IL 60637, USA; Tel: +1-773-834-4757; Fax: +1-773-834-2608; E-mail: *mlesniak@surgery.bsd.uchicago.edu*

In light of these challenges, oncolytic virotherapy has emerged as an exciting alternative for anti-glioma therapy. It entails the use of conditionally replicative adenoviruses (CRAds), which are able to selectively infect and lyse malignant cells, while sparing non-neoplastic tissues.[3] These genetically engineered viruses are able to specifically hijack the tumor cell machinery, actively replicate and release viable viral progeny to neighboring neoplastic cells. As a consequence, oncolytic cytotoxicity is not only limited to the initial target site, but it can spread to adjacent neoplastic tissues that escaped initial infection and enhance viral distribution throughout the targeted tumor bed.[4] Oncolytic viruses also present other important advantages. Their well-known and considerably large backbone allows for the insertion of therapeutic genes, which makes them excellent vectors for targeted anti-tumor gene therapy.[5] Next, by infecting and lysing neoplastic tissues, they induce a major exposure of tumoral antigens, which may lead to a prolonged acquired anti-tumor immunity.[6,7] In addition to being safe and effective for anti-glioma therapy in both humans and animal models, oncolytic viruses are able to demonstrate potent anti-tumor activity either alone or when combined with standard therapies.[8–10] Finally, they have also proven to effectively target both neoplastic cells and cancer stem cells, allowing for a more efficient eradication of resistant malignant populations.[11]

Despite initially encouraging results, oncolytic virotherapy still faces important limitations that need to be overcome in order to allow its broad clinical application. First, pre-existing host antivirus immunity considerably hampers viral spread to neighboring neoplastic tissues. Second, uneven intratumoral virus distribution and inefficient delivery to distant tumor foci are still major challenges.[12,13] A potential strategy that may surpass these obstacles is the use of carrier stem cells as delivery vehicles of oncolytic viruses to targeted neoplastic tissues. Neural stem cells (NSCs) possess unique properties that make them a great candidate to enhance viral delivery and overcome host antivirus immunity. Their migratory properties towards neoplastic tissues allows for an efficient virus transport and targeted delivery. This characteristic is also important for a successful targeting of distant tumor foci and even intratumoral payload distribution. In addition to being permissive to virus replication, their distinctive immunosuppressive quality allows NSCs to shield viruses from host immune surveillance and amplify such selective agents at the targeted tumor site. Lastly, they can be genetically modified with the addition of conditionally cytotoxic genes in order to produce a synergistic tumoricidal effect, thus maximizing the therapeutic potential of oncolytic viruses.[14–16]

In this chapter, we will survey the mechanisms of targeted toxicity exerted by oncolytic viruses, their main benefits and drawbacks, and how the combination of such an approach with carrier neural stem cells would lead this combined anti-glioma therapy closer to clinical practice.

19.2. ANTI-GLIOMA ONCOLYTIC VIROTHERAPY

The oncolytic viruses that are currently employed in anti-glioma therapy are commonly divided according to their reproductive abilities into replication-defective or replication-competent vectors. Replication-defective vectors are important tools in anti-cancer gene therapy since they are able to deliver or modify specific genes in malignant cells. This targeted approach can, for instance, induce the over expression of tumor-suppressor genes, such as p53, in defective brain tumor cells and consequently activate intratumor pro-apoptosis pathways.[17,18] Although highly specific, replication-defective vectors cannot efficiently spread within the neoplastic area and, after intratumoral inoculation, their *in vivo* transgene expression has been reported to be limited to as little as 5 mm from the initial injection site.[18] On the other hand, in addition to a targeted gene therapy, replication-competent viral vectors are capable of offering an enhanced infectivity, replication, transgene expression and oncolysis. They are able to replicate within the initial target site, spread their therapeutic potential to other neighboring tumor areas, and cause a targeted oncolytic virotherapy.

19.2.1. Oncolytic Adenoviruses in Anti-Glioma Therapy

In contrast to other viral vectors, adenoviruses present many appealing features that render them excellent tools for anti-glioma oncolytic virotherapy. They are able to grow in high titers, present a stable structure, have broad tropism and exhibit efficient transduction, and their large backbone allows for the insertion of many therapeutic genes of interest. In addition, adenoviruses present a safe profile for clinical application, since in humans they only cause a mild infection of the upper respiratory tract with no major complications. So far, anti-cancer adenoviral-based gene therapy has been tested in more than 15,000 patients in clinical trials with no mortality or severe adverse reaction due to treatment.[19,20] Adenoviral vectors are also an attractive choice for anti-glioma therapy because they are able to infect either dividing and non-dividing cancer cells, a characteristic that renders them able to target not only malignant glioma cells, but also non-dividing glioma stem cells. Furthermore, upon infection, adenovirus DNA is not integrated into the host cell genome, which precludes unwanted insertional mutagenesis of the host DNA. Taken together, these features have made adenoviruses one of the most commonly used systems in clinical trials for anti-cancer gene therapy and an exciting source for anti-glioma therapy.[21]

19.2.2. Adenoviral Biology

An adenoviral particle is composed of a non-enveloped icosahedral capsid that encloses a double-stranded DNA genome of up to 38 kb.[22] Three major proteins comprise the virus capsid: the hexon protein, the penton base and the fiber knob.[21] Hexon is the most abundant protein in the virus capsid, building the structure of the viral facets. Penton bases are present on each vertex that joins two consecutive facets. They serve as a support for the fiber knob, which plays an important role as a major attachment and recognition point of the adenovirus structure to receptors on the host cell membrane (Fig. 1A). In the majority of host cells, viral recognition is mediated by a Coxsackie-adenovirus receptor (CAR). Upon a highly specific binding of the viral fiber knob to CAR, the viral vector is internalized by the host cell in a clathrin-coated vesicle through a process known as endocytosis.[23,24] This internalization is mediated by a secondary interaction between the arginine-glycine-aspartate (RGD) motif on the viral penton base and cellular alpha(v)beta integrins.[25] In the cytoplasm, the clathrin-coated vesicle is fused with endosomes, the virus is disassembled and the viral genome is transported to the nucleus and genomic transcription starts.[26,27] Early (E1A), immediate early (E1B, E2, E3 and E4), intermediate (IVa2 and IX) and late genes (L1 to L5) compose the adenovirus transcriptional genome region. These genes are placed in independent transcription units that overlap one another and run in a bidirectional manner (Fig. 1A).[21] The viral

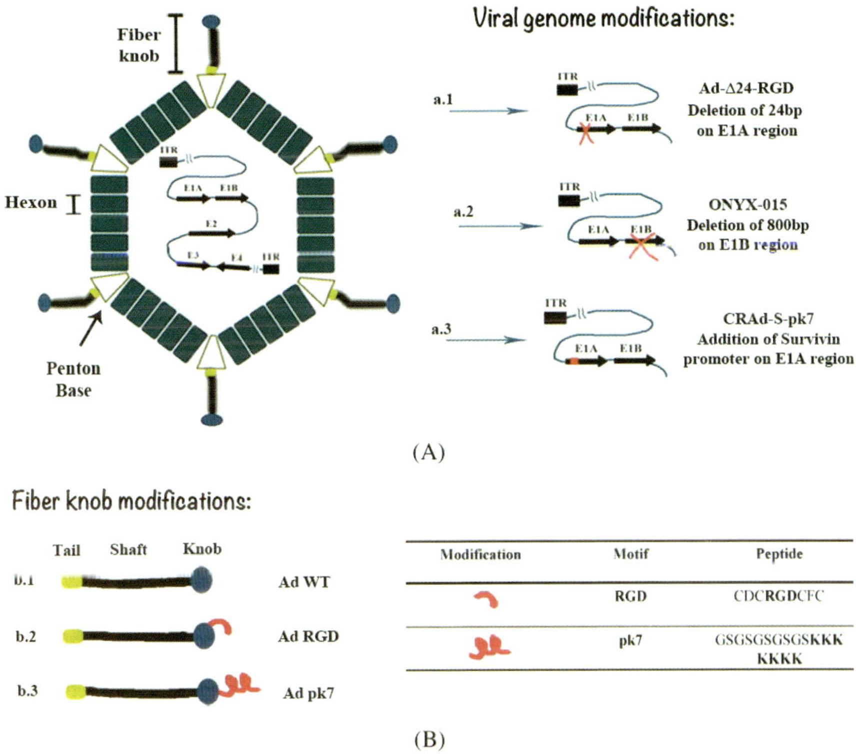

Modification	Motif	Peptide
	RGD	CDCRGDCFC
	pk7	GSGSGSGSGSKKK KKKK

Fig. 1. (A) Schematic representation of adenoviral particle structure, genome organization and related genomic modifications that are required to produce genetically engineered CRAds. (1) depicts the genomic alteration that is found in Ad-Δ24-RGD, which possesses a partial 24-bp E1A deletion, (2) refers to ONYX 015, which presents a full 800-bp E1B deletion, and (3) describes CRAd-S-pk7, which has the survivin promoter on the E1A genomic region. (B) Specific modifications that are performed on the viral fiber knob to enhance virus transduction in the host cell. (1) describes the wild-type (WT) adenoviral fiver knob, (2) depicts the addition of the RGD motif (CDC**RGD**CFC) on the HI loop (a surface-exposed loop) of the fiber knob so as to produce Ad-RGD, and (3) illustrates,in turn, the addition of the pk7 motif (GSGSGSGSGS**KKKKKKK**), which is responsible for creating CRAd-pk7.

genome hijacks the cell machinery and the cell now produces innumerous new viral particles that will lead to an eventual cytolysis. These newly formed viruses are released in the intercellular matrix and vasculature and will infect neighboring cells.

19.2.3. Conditionally Replicative Adenoviruses

Conditionally replicative adenoviruses (CRAds) are naturally selected or genetically engineered adenoviruses that preferentially replicate in and lyse neoplastic cells, sparing the non-neoplastic tissue.[28,29] This selective replication is achieved by genetic modifications on the virus backbone or fiber knob that renders the vector specific for cancer cells. Therefore, each viral reproductive cycle will culminate in selective cancer cell destruction and release of innumerous oncolytic viruses to neighboring cancer cells, leading to a widespread tumoral infection and tumor destruction.[30,31] Three main viral modifications can be performed in order to improve the specificity of transgene expression and viral replication to cancer cells and avoid toxicity in non-malignant tissues. Such modifications include (a) deletion of transcriptional genomic regions that are dispensable for virus replication in cancer cells, (b) insertions on the adenoviral fiber knob so as to facilitate viral transduction in tumor cells, and (c) insertion of tumor specific promoters on the adenoviral genome in order to enhance viral transcriptional targeting.

(a) *Deletion of transcriptional genomic regions.* Viral selectivity and tropism to malignant cells can be enhanced by the deletion of specific transcriptional genomic regions that are not important for adenovirus replication in cancer cells (Fig. 1A). As opposed to normal cells, tumor cells present several deregulations on DNA checkpoints, such as defective p53 and Rb (retinoblastoma) tumor suppressor pathways, which allow these mutant cells to escape from apoptosis. Two important adenoviruses that take advantage of these deficiencies to selectively replicate in tumor cells are: ONYX-015 and Ad-Δ24. ONYX-015 has been engineered to replicate in neoplastic cells with a deficient p53 pathway, which is responsible for inducing apoptosis in mutant cells.[8] As approximately 50 percent of all glioma cells harbor a p53 mutation, it is believed that such an approach would improve the selectivity of CRAds in anti-glioma therapy.[32] In normal cells infected by adenoviruses, the viral E1B genomic region encodes a 55-kDa protein that binds and inactivates pro-apoptotic p53 protein. As a result, the host cell machinery is successfully hijacked and viral replication continues. ONYX-015 is a genetically engineered CRAd that presents an 800-bp deletion in the E1B region. Therefore, it cannot bind to p53 protein in normal cells, preventing viral replication from proceeding. However, this deletion renders the modified virus fully active in p53 defective tumor cells, allowing selective viral replication and tumor cell lysis. *In vivo* results showed that ONYX-015 was able to successfully replicate in human glioma xenografts[32] and that radiation therapy could enhance this effect.[33] Such results led to a phase I clinical trial in patients with recurrent malignant glioma. Although the efficacy was not determined, the virus was well tolerated with no related toxicity.[8]

CRAd-Δ24 is another candidate for selective anti-glioma therapy. It effectively exploits a deficiency in the p16/Rb cell cycle checkpoint pathway that is present in most human cancers. The Rb tumor suppressor exerts a central role in controlling the cell cycle by binding to and consequently inhibiting transcription factors of the E2F family. In normal cells, when pRb is bound to E2F, the complex works as a growth suppressor and prevents the cell cycle from progressing from the G1 (gap 1 phase) to the S (synthesis) phase.[34] During adenoviral infection in cells with a functional Rb pathway, the CR2 (constant region 2) region of viral E1A binds to Rb protein, which consequently renders E2F active, leading to viral DNA synthesis, vector replication and cell lysis (Fig. 2A). Genetically engineered CRAd-Δ24 presents a 24-bp deletion in the CR2 region of viral E1A. Viral E1A is therefore unable to bind to active Rb protein in non-neoplastic cells. As a result, functional Rb binds to transcriptional E2F, rendering it inactive. The process of oncolytic viral replication is then stopped and the normal cell survives (Fig. 2B).[28,35] However, in cancer cells, the partially deleted E1A region is not important for viral replication since these mutant cells already present a deficient Rb protein. In this case, transcriptional E2F is free and active, leading to an activated viral DNA synthesis, adenoviral replication and selective tumor cell lysis,

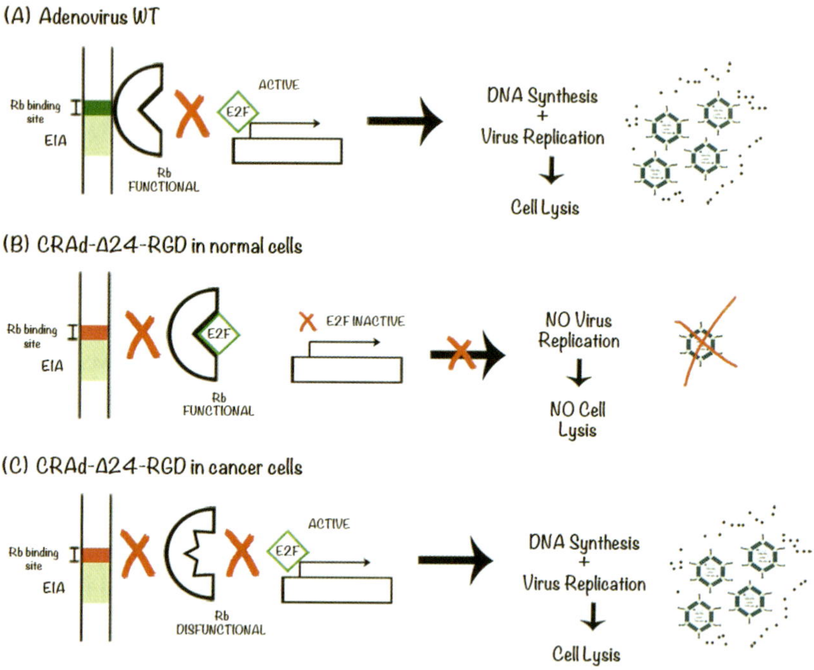

Fig. 2. Synopsis of the mechanism of function of CRAd-Δ24-RGD. (A) In the wild-type (WT) adenovirus, the 24-bp genomic region of E1A binds to and inactivates functional Rb in the host cell, thereby leaving E2F active. This leads to viral replication and lysis of the infected host cell. (B) CRAd-Δ24-RGD is a genetically engineered virus that selectively replicates in neoplastic cells. It possesses a partial 24-bp E1A deletion that renders the virus unable to bind to intracellular Rb. When CRAd-Δ24-RGD infects normal cells, functional Rb links to E2F, rendering it inactive. This process impedes virus replication in the host cell, which survives. (C) Most neoplastic cells present a dysfunctional Rb protein. As disrupted Rb does not link to E2F, rendering it active, CRAd-Δ24-RGD infection leads to viral replication and selective cytolysis of malignant tissues.

thereby sparing non-malignant tissues (Fig. 2C).[28,35] When compared to E1B-deleted CRAd, Ad-Δ24 was more effective in suppressing tumor growth in both intracranial and subcutaneous glioma xenograft models.[36]

(b) *Facilitation of viral transduction in tumor cells.* Enhanced viral transduction and increased targeting of glioma-specific receptors can be achieved by specific modifications on the adenoviral fiber knob, such as the insertion of RGD or pk7 motifs. As previously discussed, in normal cells, adenovirus infection depends on initial recognition of the viral fiber knob by host cell surface CAR receptors, followed by viral internalization through an RGD-alpha(v)beta integrin-mediated interaction. As glioma cells express low levels of CAR and high levels of alpha(v)beta integrins, a CAR-independent viral internalization would significantly enhance tumor-specific viral transduction. Therefore, inserting an RGD motif (ACDC**RGD**CFCG) into the HI loop of the viral fiber knob in order to transform CRAd-Δ24 in CRAd-Δ24-RGD would enable an effective retargeting of initial CAR-mediated internalization to an alpha(v)beta integrin-dependent mechanism, leading to enhanced viral internalization in CAR-deficient malignant cells (Fig. 1B).[37] Preclinical studies showed that CRAd-Δ24-RGD presented higher transduction and induced extended survival in glioma models.[38,39] Additional reports demonstrated that CRAd-Δ24-RGD was able to target both glioma stem cells and non-stem cell populations, leading to a significantly improved survival in glioma-bearing mice.[40] Due to such exciting results, CRAd-Δ24 is now entering two phase I clinical trials recruiting patients with recurrent glioblastoma (NCT00805376, NCT01582516) (Table 1).

Another CAR-independent pathway that has shown to improve adenoviral transduction in CAR-deficient tumor cells comprises the incorporation of a polylysine (pk7) peptide into the C-terminal end of the viral fiber knob domain (Fig. 1B). Thus, instead of binding to CAR, the modified viral fiber knob will bind to heparan sulfate proteoglycans present on the host cell surface.[42] Genetically engineered CRAd-pk7 viruses exhibited potent *in vitro* and *in vivo* anti-tumor activity and significantly increased survival in intracranial glioma xenograft models.[43] Although this therapeutic approach has not yet reached clinical trials, it has shown very promising preclinical results with enhanced tumor-specific viral transduction and important animal survival. Further studies evaluating its toxicity and safety are necessary in order to advance the application of this approach to a future clinical setting.

(c) *Insertion of tumor-specific promoters on the adenoviral genome.* Neoplastic cells commonly over-express tumor-specific promoters such as survivin,[44] human telomerase reverse transcriptase (hTERT)[45]

Table 1 Completed and Ongoing Clinical Trials Using Adenovirotherapy as a Therapeutic Approach Against Malignant Glioma

Virus	Genetic Modification	Study Type	Delivery Method	Status of Trial	Benefit	Toxic Effects	References
Ad-Δ24-RGD	Partial E1A deletion and received RGD motif	Phase I/II	Intracranially by CED	Recruiting patients	—	—	NCT01582516
Ad-Δ24-RGD	Partial E1A deletion and received RGD motif	Phase I	Intratumor/ Resection cavity	Recruiting patients	—	—	NCT00805376
ONYX-015	E1B-800 bp deletion	Phase I	Resection cavity	Completed	No significant differences found	No	Ref. 8
Ad-p53	E1 region replaced with wt p53 gene driven by CMV promoter	Phase I	Intratumor/ Resection cavity	Completed	Transduced cells found only at a short distance from the injection site	No	Ref. 18
Ad-tk/VCV	Thymidine kinase (tk) incorporation	Phase Ib	Resection cavity	Completed	33 percent survival at two years and 25 percent at three years	No	Ref. 41
Ad-tk/VCV	Thymidine kinase (tk) incorporation	Phase II	Resection cavity	Recruiting patients	—	—	NCT00589875

Abbreviations: Ad, adenovirus; E1A, adenovirus early region 1A; RGD, arginyl-glycyl-aspartic acid motif; CED, convectional enhanced delivery; E1B, adenovirus E1B protein; bp, base pairs; p53, protein 53; wt, wild type; CMV, cytomegalovirus; tk, thymidine kinase; VCV, valacyclovir.

or midkine,[46] which render them a more invasive and aggressive phenotype. The specificity of CRAds to neoplastic cells can be enhanced by the insertion of some of these tumor-specific promoters on the adenoviral genome. Such modification would limit viral infection to malignant cells bearing such promoters. Based on this principle, Komata *et al.* engineered a viral vector with a constitutively expressed caspase-6, a pro-apoptotic enzyme, under the influence of the hTERT promoter.[45] hTERT is a well-known regulator of telomerase activity, which is over expressed in approximately 85 percent of all gliomas and remains undetectable in normal brain tissues.[47,48] By adding the sequence "TTAGGG" to the 3' end of the DNA strand, the enzyme telomerase is able to maintain the chromosome integrity, thus avoiding cell death and allowing uncontrollable cell divisions in neoplastic tissues. Komata *et al.* showed that the hTERT-driven viral vector was able to selectively eliminate cancer cells that over expressed such promoters and successfully suppress tumor growth in nude mice bearing subcutaneous glioma xenografts.

Survivin is another well-studied apoptosis-inhibitor promoter whose function is up-regulated in almost 90 percent of malignant glioma samples.[44] It significantly impacts patient survival by playing an important role in oncogenesis and tumor progression.[49,50] By incorporating the survivin promoter into a viral vector, van Houdt *et al.* produced a tumor-specific CRAd that proved highly effective for *in vivo* anti-glioma therapy.[51] Further studies demonstrated that CRAd-S-pk7 was able to efficiently infect and replicate in a large panel of glioma cell lines, with minimal toxicity to non-neoplastic tissues.[52,53] Intratumoral injection of this vector in U87MG glioma xenografts resulted in successful inhibition of tumor growth and significantly increased animal survival (greater than 110 days).[43] Likewise, genetically engineered CRAds expressing the tumor-specific midkine promoter demonstrated enhanced cytolytic effects in midkine-positive glioma xenografts, with no related toxicity in non-neoplastic brain tissues.[54] Although this therapeutic approach has not yet been tested in human patients, it presents exciting preclinical results that are mostly replicable in distinct animal models and among different research groups.

19.3. DELIVERY OF ONCOLYTIC ADENOVIRUSES

In order to achieve clinically relevant therapeutic efficacy, oncolytic viruses must primarily escape the host-related anti-virus immunity, successfully reach the tumor site in a concentration high enough to be able to infect and lyse as many neoplastic cells as possible, spread to nearby tumoral areas, and finally induce a secondary anti-tumor immune response. However, there are a few major obstacles that currently impede oncolytic virotherapy in achieving such clinically significant effects. For instance, limited tissue penetration with uneven intratumoral virus spread, lack of efficient virus delivery to distant tumor foci, and pre-existing host-related antivirus immunity are frequent drawbacks that need to be overcome.

Three main approaches are used to deliver oncolytic viruses to the targeted tumor site: intravenous administration, local delivery with intracranial injection, and convectional enhanced delivery (CED). All three methods have reached clinical trials and have proven to be safe for humans. Tumor targeting through systemic adenoviral delivery has shown to be inefficient due to liver sequestration of intravenously administered viruses and the presence of pre-existing immunity against adenoviral vectors. Local delivery with intracranial injection has proven to present superior efficacy than systemic delivery both in animal models and in clinical trials. In humans, most oncolytic viruses are usually applied during craniotomy over the tumor resection bed (NCT00589875). Despite direct delivery, the transduction efficacy of this method is still modest. This is mainly due to the inability of oncolytic viruses to effectively spread beyond certain physical barriers within the complex tumor micro environment and due to anti-vector immune response. Areas of extracellular matrix constitute an important physical barrier that hampers viral vectors from reaching scattered areas of infiltrative tumor cells. Therefore, pretreatment of the tumor bed with enzymes that is able to disrupt such barriers, such as elastase,[55] trypsin,[56] collagenase[57] or human hyaluronidase,[58] has proven to enhance virus transduction in neoplastic tissues.

CED is a recently developed therapeutic approach that tries to overcome such limited intratumoral virus distribution.[59] It relies on the convective distribution of high concentrations of oncolytic viruses through constant infusion via intracranial catheters. It is able to treat large volumes of targeted neoplastic tissue and has shown to effectively increase viral transduction in glioma xenografts.[60,61] A phase I/II clinical trial using CED to intracranially infuse Ad-Δ24-RGD in solid and infiltrative recurrent malignant glioma tumors is now underway. The main goal of this study is to test the maximum tolerated dose (MTD) of the CRAd-based anti-tumor therapy, as well as the safety of the approach and preliminary signs of therapeutic efficacy (NCT01582516).

Despite having reached clinical trials, all three of the above methods share a common limitation: host-related antivirus immunity. Pre-existing host-related immunity against adenoviral vectors is present in approximately 90 percent of the human population.[62] In particular, pre-existing protection against the most commonly used adenoviruses in anti-cancer therapy (Ad2 and Ad5) occurs, respectively, in around 88 percent and 68 percent of the adult population.[63] This leads to increased titers of viral neutralizing antibodies in human patients after both intravenous and intratumoral injections.[8,18] One possible way to overcome this problem is either the use of other adenoviral serotypes, such as Ad 3, 11, 16 or its variants (Ad5/3), which have shown efficient transduction and replication in glioma cells,[43,64] or the use of cell carriers as vehicles for adenovirus delivery to the targeted tumor site. Amongst other cell carriers, neural and mesenchymal stem cells are especially attractive for this application, because they have proven to be permissive for virus replication, to be able to hide viruses from the host immune surveillance, and to migrate efficiently to the targeted tumor area and deliver their payload in an optimal concentration. An additional important feature is their unique oncotropic property that allows them to target distant tumor foci, decreasing levels of tumor recurrence. As a result of their inherent tumor-tropic and immunosuppressive properties, as well as their ability to integrate into the host brain without disturbing the usual brain function, NSC carriers seem to be more suitable for anti-cancer therapy when compared to other delivery vehicles. In this chapter, we will survey the main characteristics of NSCs as tumor-specific carriers of oncolytic viruses, their synergistic effect in anti-glioma therapy, and the main limitations related to such an approach.

19.4. NSCs AS CARRIERS FOR TARGETED DELIVERY OF THERAPEUTIC AGENTS

Neural stem cells (NSCs) are self-renewing, multipotent populations that have the capability to differentiate into glial and neuronal cell lineages triggered by specific stimuli from the brain microenvironment.[65] These cells have received special attention because of their therapeutic potential for neurological malignancies.[66] Since the beginning of this century, many studies have shown the unique and inherent properties of NSCs and their ability to migrate throughout the brain and target invasive solid tumors, including gliomas. Such properties make these cells exceptional carriers for delivery of therapeutic agents, such as oncolytic adenoviruses.[14–16,67–69] In addition, a significant amount of preclinical data suggests that they have immunosuppressive properties, which allow for the protection of loaded therapeutic agents from host immunosurveillance.[70]

19.4.1. NSCs Used in Anti-Cancer Research

There are several NSC lines currently available for therapeutic research. These cells mainly differ according to their required culture conditions, migratory abilities, methods of immortalization, and capacity to express therapeutic agents.[14,71,72] All of them come from fetal brain tissue and some have been scaled up under GMP-grade conditions and are available for clinical trials.[73] However, as there is no consensus on a common classification, it remains unclear whether cultured NSCs that are being used in research laboratories are identical to resident populations that have been reported *in vivo*. Also, similarly named NSCs may differ among different research groups. In the future, for the translation of NSC-based anti-cancer therapy to the clinic, researchers will have to reach a consensus on a common characterization criterion.

To improve the stability of NSCs in culture, as well as their ability to sustain the expression of therapeutic agents, most NSCs have been immortalized using different genes. Some examples are the addition of human telomerase, SV40 large T antigen, and the c-*myc* oncogene.[74–76] One of the main concerns in the use of these modified cells is their potential for developing secondary malignancies. Therefore, before their wide use in the clinical setting, it is essential to carefully characterize these cells and rule out any possible tumorigenicity.

Another major concern surrounding the clinical use of the currently available NSCs is a possible host-related rejection as a result of HLA mismatches,[77] since these transplanted cells are derived from human donors that are not related to their recipients (allogeneic origin). To overcome this problem, patient immunosuppression may be required before local transplantation of allogeneic NSCs. The use of autologous NSCs (derived from the patient itself) would be a better fit. However, so far, this approach has been beyond our capabilities, since currently available technology does not allow the unlimited expansion of autologous primary cells that are capable of expressing therapeutic agents.[78]

19.4.2. NSCs as Carriers of Oncolytic Adenoviruses in Anti-Glioma Therapy

In contrast to other stem cell carriers, there are some important characteristics that render NSCs a good fit for combination with anti-glioma oncolytic virotherapy. The first is their natural permissiveness for replication of loaded viruses, which turns these carriers into local factories and allows viruses to continue replicating within the cell vehicle for days after transplantation,[79] amplifying the therapeutic payload at the tumor site. The second is their inherent oncotropism, which allows them to migrate efficiently, navigating obstacles such as the interstitial matrix, towards primary or infiltrative neoplastic tissues and effectively deliver their therapeutic payload to distant tumor foci. Last is their intrinsic immunosuppressive property, which renders NSCs natural vehicles that shield the therapeutic payload from the pre-existing host-related immunosurveillance. All of these characteristics make the use of NSC carriers a promising strategy to address traditional limitations of oncolytic virotherapy.

(a) *Permissiveness for viral replication.* A characteristic that confers NSCs the quality of a good carrier is their inherent permissiveness for adenovirus replication. Such permissiveness mainly occurs due to the expression of many Ad-targeted receptors on the surface of carrier NSCs. Common receptors include alpha(v)beta3 and alpha(v)beta5 integrins, adhesion proteins targeted by vectors possessing RGD motifs, CAR, mCD46, syndecan, perlecan and heparan sulfate proteoglycans.[68] In addition to working as cellular vehicles, NSCs allow adequate CRAd genome amplification at the targeted tumor site, which is essential for the success of CRAd-loaded NSC therapy.[68,80] As a result, carrier NSCs may serve as cellular factories that churn out increased numbers of oncolytic viruses to both primary and infiltrative neoplastic areas.

Our laboratory was the first to demonstrate that CRAd-loaded NSCs could be used as an efficient therapy for intracranial gliomas.[68] We have also determined the optimal *ex vivo* conditions to load oncolytic adenoviruses into NSCs for *in vivo* delivery in an orthotopic human malignant glioma model.[79,80] In all of these efforts, it was clear that the delivery of NSCs loaded with CRAds was able to improve the anti-glioma therapeutic efficacy when compared with the administration of CRAd alone.

(b) *Inherent oncotropic properties.* The inefficiency of viral delivery and distribution at tumor sites is one of the main obstacles in anti-cancer virotherapy.[13] However, with the use of oncolytic virus-loaded NSCs, it is possible to overcome this limitation by different routes. One of them is the targeted delivery of oncolytic adenoviruses to both infiltrative areas and distant tumor foci. Several groups have demonstrated that NSCs display inherent tumor-tropic properties that can be exploited for targeted delivery of anti-cancer agents to tumor cells.[14,16,68,79,80] Aboody and colleagues showed the first proof that NSCs could migrate towards intracranial gliomas. Using an immortalized murine NSC line expressing β-galactosidase, the authors were able to localize NSCs within the intracranial tumor following either intracranial or intravenous injections.[14] While the reason NSCs migrate to tumors remains unclear, one hypothesis is that these cells are recruited to the tumor site in order to repair damaged tissues.[69,81]

The exact mechanism responsible for the *in vivo* tumor-tropic properties of NSCs is not well understood. However, available data suggest that gradients of agents such as chemokines and pro-angiogenic growth factors produced in the tumor microenvironment may act as chemoattractants for NSCs.[16] Candidate cytokine/receptor pairs include SDF-1/CXCR4,[82] SCF/c-Kit,[83] MCP-1/CCR2.[84] Brain tumor neovasculogenesis could also be involved in the regulation of this response through local production of chemoattractants such as VEGF.[85] Hypoxia is another important feature of gliomas that could affect the migration of NSCs. In 2008, Zhao *et al.* demonstrated that NSCs would be preferentially distributed in hypoxic areas within intracranial glioma xenografts.[86]

Strikingly, NSCs were able to target not only primary brain tumors, but also invasive tumor cells.[14,15,87,88] The ability to infiltrate tumor bulks and distribute their therapeutic compounds throughout neoplastic tissues have made carrier NSCs capable of mediating a more comprehensive and robust anti-tumor response when compared to other vehicles with less distribution capacity, such as modified liposomes, antibodies or naked oncolytic adenoviruses.[89] All these attractive migratory features have caught researchers' attention, since understanding the mechanism that underlies these properties will be crucial for improving the use of NSCs as carriers of therapeutic payloads for both primary and invasive tumor cells.

(c) *Immune system evasion.* It is well known that most of the genetically engineered CRAds developed so far undeniably trigger a host-related immune response, which is the main thing responsible for preventing an adequate anti-tumor therapeutic effect in the clinical setting.[8,38,90] Loading oncolytic viruses in NSCs can effectively overcome this shortcoming. In addition to behaving as immunosuppressive agents, these carriers are also able to protect loaded viruses from the host immunosurveillance[13,70] (Fig. 3).

The immunosuppressive properties of NSCs have been extensively described in models of experimental autoimmune encephalomyelitis (EAE).[70,91,92] In these models, transplanted NSCs have been shown to reduce brain inflammation and improve clinical outcome. We have recently observed that NSCs loaded with oncolytic viruses express immunosuppressive cytokines such as IL-10. As a result, the delivery of these virus-loaded NSCs into the animal brain significantly reduces vector mediated neuroinflammation.[80] Furthermore, NSCs do not express the major histocompatibility complex (MHC) class II and express low levels of CD80 and CD86 co-stimulatory molecules, which make them particularly resistant to immune-mediated cytolysis.[70]

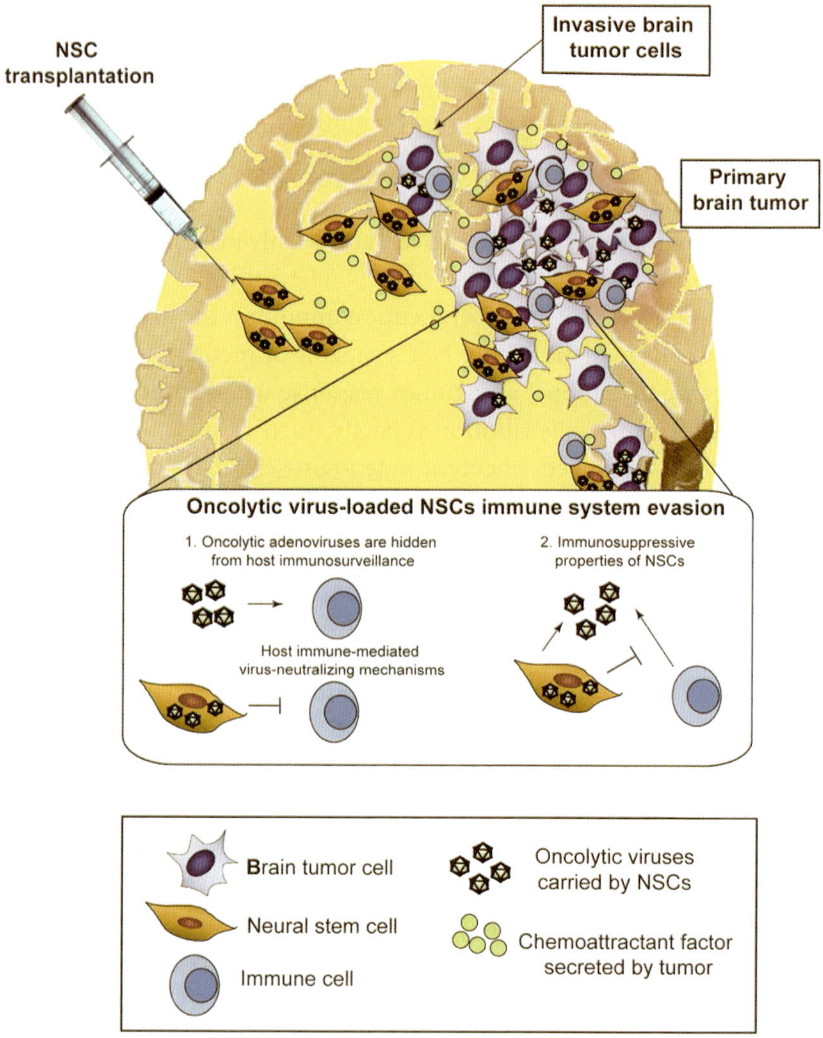

Fig. 3. Simplified overview of oncolytic adenovirus-loaded NSC migration and payload delivery. After transplantation, NSCs are attracted to primary and invasive tumors due to gradients of agents produced in the tumor microenvironment (such as chemokines and pro-angiogenic growth factors). The use of NSCs as carriers of oncolytic adenoviruses allows these viruses not only to be hidden from the host immune-mediated virus-neutralizing mechanism, but also to replicate and multiply inside the NSC carriers. It has also been suggested that NSCs alone play a significant role as immunosuppressants, a characteristic that would be an additional protection for oncolytic adenoviruses against the host immune surveillance. Once inside the tumor, NSCs evenly spread to different neoplastic areas and effectively deliver their payload (oncolytic adenoviruses), leading to the selective extermination of tumor cells.

Altogether, these data suggest that NSCs may serve as ideal carriers for oncolytic adenovirotherapy.

Although there are many questions regarding the possible role of NSCs as immunosuppressants, it is expected that a better understanding and characterization of NSC-mediated immunosuppression will enhance the therapeutic anti-cancer efficacy of oncolytic adenoviruses.

19.5. GENETICALLY ENGINEERED NSCs

Genetically engineered NSCs may work in a synergistic way with oncolytic virotherapy to amplify the anti-glioma therapeutic effect at the targeted tumor site. During the last decade, NSC carriers have been modified using two different approaches for anti-glioma gene therapy. In the first approach, NSCs were genetically engineered to express various therapeutic genes and to carry these products to infiltrative tumor areas. Examples of such genes include pro-drug activating enzymes (cytosine deaminase, HSV1-TK), interleukins (IL-4, IL-12), apoptosis-promoting genes (TRAIL) and metalloproteinases (PEX). These modifications are summarized in Table 2.

The well-established delivery potential of carrier stem cells for gene therapy in intracranial models has prompted researchers to investigate the use of genetically engineered NSCs as delivery vehicles for oncolytic adenoviruses as well. Our laboratory[68,79,80,94] has extensively studied this second approach. Up to now, the majority of studies on NSC-based anti-cancer therapy have used an enzyme pro-drug suicide gene therapy system. Following promising preclinical results, the US FDA recently allowed Aboody and colleagues from City of Hope (California, USA) to conduct the first human phase I study of genetically engineered NSCs carrying a suicide gene for the treatment of patients with recurrent high-grade gliomas. This trial tests an extensively characterized allogeneic NSC line, HB1.F3.CD, which is derived from the fetal telencephalon and has been immortalized with the addition of v-*myc*. This cell line was also genetically modified to express cytosine deaminase (CD), an enzyme that converts the pro-drug 5-fluorocytosine (5-FC) into the active chemotherapeutic 5-fluorouracil (5-FU).[66] All patients receive injections of HB1.F3.CD at the tumor resection bed. Then, 5-FC is orally administered to all patients.

Table 2 Relevant Examples of NSC-Mediated Therapies for Experimental Gliomas

Therapeutic Load	Target	Current Application	Therapeutic Effect	Reference
Cytosine deaminase (CD)	Activation of pro-drug 5-FC into 5-fluorouracil in tumor cells	Preclinical models and phase I clinical trial	Dramatic (~80 percent) reduction in tumor mass post-systemic 5-FC administration	Ref. 14 (NCT01172964)
HSV1-TK	Activation of pro-drug ganciclovir into GCV-triphosphate in tumor cells	Preclinical models	Strong bystander effect + elimination of ~70 percent of glioma cells post-GCV addition	Ref. 93
Oncolytic CRAds	U87MG intracranial glioma xenografts	Preclinical models	Significantly increased CRAd therapeutic delivery and median survival in glioma-bearing mice treated with CRAd-loaded NSCs as opposed to MSCs	Ref. 94
IL-4	Intracranial syngeneic glioma xenografts	Preclinical models	Extended mice survival	Ref. 15
IL-12	GL26 intracranial glioma xenografts	Preclinical models	Extended mice survival, enhanced T-cell infiltration in tumor microsatellites and long-term anti-tumor immunity	Ref. 95
IL-23	GL26 intracranial glioma xenografts	Preclinical models	Induction of anti-tumor immunity	Ref. 96

(*Continued*)

Table 2 (*Continued*)

Therapeutic Load	Target	Current Application	Therapeutic Effect	Reference
TRAIL	U343MG intracranial glioma xenografts	Preclinical models	Dramatic induction of apoptosis and significant inhibition of tumor growth	Ref. 97
PEX	U87MG intracranial glioma xenografts	Preclinical models	90 percent reduction of tumor volume and 44.8 percent decreased angiogenesis	Ref. 98
TSP-1	Gli36-EGFRvIII-FD intracranial glioma xenografts	Preclinical models	Reduced tumor vessel density, inhibition of tumor progression and increased mice survival	Ref. 99

Abbreviations: CD, cytosine deaminase; 5-FC, 5-fluorocytosine; HSV-1 TK, herpes simplex virus 1 thymidine kinase; GCV, ganciclovir; CRAds, conditionally replicative adenoviruses; NSCs, neural stem cells; MSCs, mesenchymal stem cells; IL-4, interleukin-4; IL-12, interleukin-12; IL-23, interleukin-23; TRAIL, tumor necrosis factor-related apoptosis inducing ligand; PEX, hemopexin like protein; TSP-1, trombospondin; EGFRvIII, endothelial growth factor receptor variant III.

The introduction of the CD gene in the tumor should induce the activation of the pro-drug 5-FC into 5-FU, resulting in intratumoral chemotherapy and, consequently, tumor shrinkage (NCT 01172964).

An emerging field in the use of stem cells as carriers of therapeutic agents is the modification of these cells to express intact or single-chain antibodies with anti-tumor effect. Recently, human NSCs have been modified to express breast cancer-specific anti-HER2 antibody. Similarly, our laboratory was able to modify mesenchymal stem cells (MSCs) so as to express a cell surface-bound single-chain antibody targeting glioma associated with EGF receptor variant III.[72,100,101] However, it is important to keep in mind that the introduction of such modifications can induce mutagenesis in stem cell carriers and enhance their ability to form tumors. One possibility to overcome this problem that can be further explored is the combination of oncolytic viruses with these cell carriers. This would not only allow the combination of two potent anti-tumor therapeutic agents using the same carrier, but also create a safeguard against abnormally growing transplanted stem cell carriers by utilizing their own payload (oncolytic viruses) against themselves once their delivery function is complete.

19.6. METHODS TO TRACK NSC FATE

One important aspect of using NSCs as carriers of therapeutic anti-glioma agents is to identify their ultimate fate after *in vivo* transplantation. This would give invaluable information about their spatial distribution, dosing, optimization, efficacy and safety concerns.[66,102,103] Overall, there are two approaches that allow effective tracking of carrier cells. The first is called direct cell labeling, in which cells are marked with certain tags that can be detected with suitable imaging equipment. The second is indirect cell labeling, which typically uses a reporter gene approach.[104] A considerable drawback with this latter approach is that the reporter gene is not suitable for final cells such as those used in clinical trials. There are three main techniques that are currently employed for tracking NSCs in glioma models: bioluminescence imaging (BMI), fluorescence, and magnetic resonance imaging (MRI).

(a) *BMI.* The first experimental evidence of the migratory abilities of luciferase-expressing murine neural progenitor cells toward brain tumors was given in 2003 by Tang *et al.* Utilizing routine BMI, they were able to visualize *in vivo* migration of NSCs and they also demonstrated NSC persistence in brain tumor tissues four weeks after implantation in living mice.[105] BMI is a technique in which a charge-coupled device camera detects light emitted from the substrate of the enzyme luciferase. The luciferase gene may be incorporated into, for example, a lentiviral vector, and this vector in turn codifies for the luciferase indicator protein into the defined stem cell population.[83] In a later study, the same group used NSCs transduced with both luciferase and soluble TRAIL to simultaneously monitor the migration of NSCs and their effects on glioma burdens in real time.[87] In our laboratory, we have used this approach to effectively track the migration of oncolytic adenovirus-loaded NSCs after intracranial implantation in nude mice.[79,94]

(b) *Fluorescence.* The use of fluorescence is another common technique to track NSCs in pre-clinical models. These cell carriers can be either modified to express a fluorescent protein or directly labeled with imaging agents, such as quantum dots (QDs). QDs are semiconductor particles with physical properties that enable labeled cells to emit fluorescent light from 525 to 800 nm. QDs are capable of entering stem cell carriers through passive loading, receptor-mediated endocytosis or transfection.[106] In 2007, Slotkin *et al.* demonstrated that fluorescent semiconductor QDs could be effectively used to label mammalian neural stem and progenitor cells *in vivo.*[107] In addition to QDs, nanoshells are a new class of optically tunable nanoparticles that may provide novel abilities to image NSC migration. They also provide therapeutic photothermal therapy to treat glioma cells.[108] Loo *et al.* engineered immunotargeted nanoshells that are able to scatter light in the near-infrared region, enabling an efficient imaging of the targeted tumor. These nanoshells are also able to absorb selected wavelengths that are harmless to normal tissue, but selectively induce high temperatures within the nanoparticle-loaded tumor. As a consequence, there is a discriminatory extermination of malignant tissue, while sparing the non-neoplastic tissue.[108] This combined imaging and therapeutic modality has great potential in gliomas.

(c) *MRI.* Another powerful imaging technique is the use of MRI for *in vivo* tracking and recovery of NSCs.[109] MRI is an imaging technique in which magnetic fields are used to detect variations in the nuclear spin of molecules. The benefits of MRI include high resolution, no exposure to ionizing radiation, clinical applicability and 3D anatomical imaging capability.[110] The drawbacks include low sensitivity and difficulty in quantifying a labeled cell population.[111] There are different cellular markers that can be used to track cells for MRI, although labeling with nanoparticles is the most commonly used for NSC tracking.[102,112] In 2004, Zhang *et al.* labeled neural progenitor cells with lipophilic dye-coated super paramagnetic particles, which allowed MRI to trace the NSC migration towards intracranial gliomas after injection into the cisterna magna or the rat-tail vein.[88]

One promising cell-tracking approach for monitoring NSCs via MRI involves pre-loading with super paramagnetic iron oxide particles (SPIOs) just prior to administration and subsequently tracking their distribution over time via MRI. Pre-clinical studies in mice have demonstrated the effective use of MRI to track iron-labeled NSCs.[113,114] In addition, the safe use of iron oxide-based MRI contrast agents has been demonstrated in clinical research studies for CNS tumor visualization and diagnostic MRI.

Recently, a very interesting approach has been described for targeted delivery of NSCs to the brain using MRI-guided focused ultrasound (MRIgFUS).[115] This is a novel method for noninvasive delivery of systemically administered stem cells to the brain by opening the blood-brain barrier (BBB) in specific regions. This study[115] used MRI guidance to direct the ultrasound beam, thereby delivering the iron-labeled green fluorescent protein (GFP)-expressing NSCs specifically to the striatum and the hippocampus of the rat brain. This is a promising strategy that could facilitate progression of NSCs towards clinical use, since it could decrease the risks associated with invasive intracranial surgery, which is currently the mainstay technique to deliver such carriers to brain tumors.

19.7. LIMITATIONS OF NSC-BASED ONCOLYTIC VIROTHERAPY

Although the combination of oncolytic adenoviruses loaded in NSCs is capable of surpassing most of the delivery issues of naked oncolytic viruses, there are still some important drawbacks that need to be overcome in order to enable a broad clinical application of such a joint approach. The first obstacle is the decreased lifespan of NSCs after *in vivo* transplantation, which considerably decreases the number of viable carriers that actually reach infiltrative areas around the primary tumor. The second is the current use of cell carriers that possess an allogeneic origin, which increases the chances of host-related rejection due to HLA mismatches. A third limitation is the inaccuracy of the currently available preclinical animal models that are used to study local or distant delivery of NSC-loaded oncolytic viruses. Such models are not truly representative of the complex and heterogeneous nature of human gliomas, and they do not allow a reliable application to humans in terms of the distance that the cell carrier needs to travel in order to effectively reach infiltrative neoplastic areas.

(a) *Decreased lifespan of NSCs after in vivo transplantation.* Stem cell carriers (MSCs and NSCs) loaded with oncolytic viruses have a relatively limited survival time after *in vivo* transplantation.[116,117] The main reason for this is their permissiveness for virus replication, which allows considerable viral amplification at the tumor site. Thaci *et al.* have recently demonstrated that CRAd-S-pk7 oncolytic adenoviruses require approximately five days to reach their maximum intracellular titer and complete their replication cycle in a stem cell carrier.[79] Although most loaded carriers effectively manage to reach the targeted tumor site and deposit their therapeutic payload, there is still a concern about viral release in non-neoplastic areas trafficked by these cells.[79,94,117] Reaching an efficient and reliable regulation of virus replication in cell carriers is very difficult. Therefore, in order to achieve timely virus release at the targeted site, any therapeutic schedule using such a strategy should take into consideration the half-life of their chosen carriers. An approach that tries to overcome this problem is the pre-treatment of loaded cell vehicles with mimosine, an alkaloid that arrests dividing cells in the G1 phase by inhibiting DNA replication. By adopting this strategy, Herrlinger *et al.* stopped the replication of rRp450, a mutant HSV-1, in neural progenitor cells (NPCs), thus allowing increased survival and efficient migration of these cell carriers to neoplastic areas in the mouse brain.[116] This approach opens doors for the generation of additional combinations that would increase the survival of loaded cell carriers until they reach the desired neoplastic area.

(b) *Use of stem cell carriers with an allogeneic origin.* The current use of stem cell carriers possessing an allogeneic origin could be an important drawback for the application of such a strategy in the clinic, since it could lead to host-related rejection due to HLA mismatches. As previously discussed, the cell carriers that are presently used in preclinical studies are derived from unrelated donors. This approach permits unlimited *in vitro* expansion and stocking of both original and modified stem cells in lower passages. However, when transplanted into humans, such loaded carriers could suffer host rejection. Immune rejection of fetal NSCs grafts (allogeneic origin) due to alloimmunisation to donor antigens was observed in a phase II clinical trial with Huntington's disease patients.[118] Although immunosuppressive treatment was able to reverse the rejection reaction, such studies opened a discussion about the use of stem cell carriers from an autologous source, which, in theory, would overcome this problem. However, the technology necessary to efficiently extract, isolate and expand autologous stem cells from the adult patient still faces some important limitations, since it requires invasive procedures that typically obtain a small number of viable cells, which is difficult to expand in culture.[78] Until the technology required for an efficient expansion of stem cells from an autologous origin becomes available, the therapeutic use of well-characterized NSC carriers is still the best option.

(c) *Inaccuracy of the currently available preclinical animal models.* Due to their small size, easy breeding, well-known genome and high homology with humans, mice are the most commonly used mammals to study brain tumor biology and its therapeutic applications. There are two main models that are currently used to study the characteristics of malignant glioma: intracranially injected cells [expanded in culture and derived from mice (syngeneic models) or humans] and spontaneously formed tumors in genetically engineered mice (GEM).[119] The first major drawback of both models is that they are not truly representative of the complex and heterogeneous nature of human gliomas. Although GEM models are mostly successful in modeling glioblastoma tumorigenesis and spread, they still fail to reproduce the multiple genetic alterations present in the human-derived tumor.[120] The second major limitation is that, when studying local or distant delivery of NSC-loaded oncolytic viruses, mice models do not allow a reliable comparison to humans in terms of the distance that the cell carrier needs to travel in order to effectively reach infiltrative neoplastic areas. Therefore, it is still not known whether, in the human brain, NSC carriers would be able to fulfill their main goal, namely to migrate sufficiently so as to deliver their therapeutic payload to distant tumor foci. In pre-clinical models, the dog brain could offer a more reliable reference in terms of migration and distant delivery. But this model still has many drawbacks, such as the high cost of animal maintenance, the challenges associated with long-term breeding, and the difficulty of obtaining identical animals in order to decrease intra-experimental variations.[121] The first clinical trial testing the therapeutic efficacy of carrier NSCs in malignant glioma patients is now underway (NCT01172964). The results of this study may answer many of these questions, opening the way for the optimization of such strategies so that they may be further exploited in other trials.

19.8. CONCLUSION

Pre-clinical studies on NSC-based oncolytic adenovirotherapy have confirmed that this is a promising approach against malignant glioma, since these cell carriers are able to effectively reach the primary tumor site and surrounding infiltrative areas, release their therapeutic payload and significantly improve animal survival. Clinical trials in human patients have demonstrated the safety of oncolytic viruses in anti-cancer therapy. However, the efficient delivery of oncolytic viruses in stem cell carriers requires not only the integration of many different techniques, such as genetic engineering of viral vectors and preparation/modification of cell carriers, but also an appropriate interaction of the therapeutic package with the host microenvironment that will receive it. Therefore, investments should be made in alternatives that enhance migration efficiency and improve survival of therapeutic cell carriers. In addition, other important drawbacks such as the feared host-related allorejection could be avoided through the optimization of technologies that focus on the extraction and *in vitro* expansion of allogeneic NSCs. Another important point that deserves to be highlighted is that, although highly effective against malignant glioma in pre-clinical trials, stem cell-based oncolytic virotherapy alone may not be enough to eradicate such a heterogeneous and complex disease. As a result, in order to be introduced into the clinical practice, this novel and encouraging therapeutic modality should be combined with other currently established strategies, such as chemo- and radiotherapy. The synergistic effect between these approaches should lead to enhanced and efficient clinical application of this new technology.

ACKNOWLEDGMENTS

This work was supported by the National Cancer Institute (R01CA122930, R01CA138587), the National Institutes of Health (R01NS077388), the National Institute of Neurological Disorders and Stroke (U01NS069997), and the American Cancer Society (RSG-07-276-01-MGO).

REFERENCES

1. Stupp R, Mason WP, van den Bent MJ, *et al.* (2005) Radiotherapy plus concomitant and adjuvant temozolomide for glioblastoma. *N Engl J Med* **352**(10): 987–996.
2. Dean M, Fojo T, Bates S. (2005) Tumour stem cells and drug resistance. *Nat Rev Cancer* **5**(4): 275–284.
3. Bischoff JR, Kirn DH, Williams A, *et al.* (1996) An adenovirus mutant that replicates selectively in p53-deficient human tumor cells. *Science* **274**(5286): 373–376.
4. Heise CC, Williams A, Olesch J, Kirn DH. (1999) Efficacy of a replication-competent adenovirus (ONYX-015) following intratumoral injection: Intratumoral spread and distribution effects. *Cancer Gene Ther* **6**(6): 499–504.
5. Martuza RL, Malick A, Markert JM, *et al.* (1991) Experimental therapy of human glioma by means of a genetically engineered virus mutant. *Science* **252**(5007): 854–856.

6. Bluming AZ, Ziegler JL. (1971) Regression of Burkitt's lymphoma in association with measles infection. *Lancet* 2(7715): 105–106.
7. Taqi AM, Abdurrahman MB, Yakubu AM, Fleming AF. (1981) Regression of Hodgkin's disease after measles. *Lancet* 1(8229): 1112.
8. Chiocca EA, Abbed KM, Tatter S, *et al.* (2004) A phase I open-label, dose-escalation, multi-institutional trial of injection with an E1B-Attenuated adenovirus, ONYX-015, into the peritumoral region of recurrent malignant gliomas, in the adjuvant setting. *Mol Ther* **10**(5): 958–966.
9. Markert JM, Liechty PG, Wang W, *et al.* (2009) Phase Ib trial of mutant herpes simplex virus G207 inoculated pre-and post-tumor resection for recurrent GBM. *Mol Ther* **17**(1): 199–207.
10. Papanastassiou V, Rampling R, Fraser M, *et al.* (2002) The potential for efficacy of the modified (ICP 34.5(-)) herpes simplex virus HSV1716 following intratumoural injection into human malignant glioma: A proof of principle study. *Gene Ther* **9**(6): 398–406.
11. Cripe TP, Wang P-Y, Marcato P, *et al.* (2009) Targeting cancer-initiating cells with oncolytic viruses. *Mol Ther* **17**(10): 1677–1682.
12. Parker JN, Bauer DF, Cody JJ, Markert JM. (2009) Oncolytic viral therapy of malignant glioma. *Neurotherapeutics* **6**(3): 558–569.
13. Ferguson SD, Ahmed AU, Thaci B, *et al.* (2010) Crossing the boundaries: Stem cells and gene therapy. *Discov Med* **9**(46): 192–196.
14. Aboody KS, Brown A, Rainov NG, *et al.* (2000) Neural stem cells display extensive tropism for pathology in adult brain. Evidence from intracranial gliomas. *Proc Natl Acad Sci USA* **97**(23): 12846–12851.
15. Benedetti S, Pirola B, Pollo B, *et al.* (2000) Gene therapy of experimental brain tumors using neural progenitor cells. *Nat Med* **6**(4): 447–450.
16. Aboody KS, Najbauer J, Danks MK. (2008) Stem and progenitor cell-mediated tumor selective gene therapy. *Gene Ther* **15**(10): 739–752.
17. Ichikawa T, Chiocca EA. (2001) Comparative analyses of transgene delivery and expression in tumors inoculated with a replication-conditional or -defective viral vector. *Cancer Res* **61**(14): 5336–5339.
18. Lang FF, Bruner JM, Fuller GN, *et al.* (2003) Phase I trial of adenovirus-mediated p53 gene therapy for recurrent glioma: Biological and clinical results. *J Clin Oncol* **21**(13): 2508–2518.
19. Kanerva A, Raki M, Hemminki A. (2007) Gene therapy of gynaecological diseases. *Expert Opin Biol Ther* **7**(9): 1347–1361.
20. Ribacka C, Pesonen S, Hemminki A. (2008) Cancer, stem cells, and oncolytic viruses. *Ann Med* **40**(7): 496–505.

21. McConnell MJ, Imperiale MJ. (2004) Biology of adenovirus and its use as a vector for gene therapy. *Hum Gene Ther* **15**(11): 1022–1033.
22. Russell WC. (2000) Update on adenovirus and its vectors. *J Gen Virol* **81**(Pt 11): 2573–2604.
23. Bergelson JM, Cunningham JA, Droguett G, *et al.* (1997) Isolation of a common receptor for Coxsackie B viruses and adenoviruses 2 and 5. *Science* **275**(5304): 1320–1323.
24. Tomko RP, Xu R, Philipson L. (1997) HCAR and MCAR: The human and mouse cellular receptors for subgroup C adenoviruses and group B coxsackieviruses. *Proc Natl Acad Sci USA* **94**(7): 3352–3356.
25. Wickham TJ, Mathias P, Cheresh DA, Nemerow GR. (1993) Integrins alpha v beta 3 and alpha v beta 5 promote adenovirus internalization but not virus attachment. *Cell* **73**(2): 309–319.
26. Meier O, Boucke K, Hammer SV, *et al.* (2002) Adenovirus triggers macropinocytosis and endosomal leakage together with its clathrin-mediated uptake. *J Cell Biol* **158**(6): 1119–1131.
27. Strunze S, Trotman LC, Boucke K, Greber UF. (2005) Nuclear targeting of adenovirus type 2 requires CRM1-mediated nuclear export. *Mol Biol Cell* **16**(6): 2999–3009.
28. Heise C, Hermiston T, Johnson L, *et al.* (2000) An adenovirus E1A mutant that demonstrates potent and selective systemic anti-tumoral efficacy. *Nat Med* **6**(10): 1134–1139.
29. Jiang H, Conrad C, Fueyo J, *et al.* (2003) Oncolytic adenoviruses for malignant glioma therapy. *Front Biosci* **8**: d577–d588.
30. Alemany R, Balague C, Curiel DT. (2000) Replicative adenoviruses for cancer therapy. *Nat Biotechnol* **18**(7): 723–727.
31. Lin E, Nemunaitis J. (2004) Oncolytic viral therapies. *Cancer Gene Ther* **11**(10): 643–664.
32. Geoerger B, Grill J, Opolon P, *et al.* (2002) Oncolytic activity of the E1B-55 kDa-deleted adenovirus ONYX-015 is independent of cellular p53 status in human malignant glioma xenografts. *Cancer Res* **62**(3): 764–772.
33. Geoerger B, Grill J, Opolon P, *et al.* (2003) Potentiation of radiation therapy by the oncolytic adenovirus dl1520 (ONYX-015) in human malignant glioma xenografts. *Br J Cancer* **89**(3): 577–584.
34. Sherr CJ. (1996) Cancer cell cycles. *Science* **274**(5293): 1672–1677.
35. Fueyo J, Gomez-Manzano C, Alemany R, *et al.* (2000) A mutant oncolytic adenovirus targeting the Rb pathway produces anti-glioma effect *in vivo*. *Oncogene* **19**(1): 2–12.

36. Jiang H, Gomez-Manzano C, Alemany R, *et al.* (2005) Comparative effect of oncolytic adenoviruses with E1A-55 kDa or E1B-55 kDa deletions in malignant gliomas. *Neoplasia* 7(1): 48–56.
37. Fueyo J, Alemany R, Gomez-Manzano C, *et al.* (2003) Preclinical characterization of the anti-glioma activity of a tropism-enhanced adenovirus targeted to the retinoblastoma pathway. *J Natl Cancer Inst* **95**(9): 652–660.
38. Jiang H, Gomez-Manzano C, Lang FF, *et al.* (2009) Oncolytic adenovirus: Preclinical and clinical studies in patients with human malignant gliomas. *Curr Gene Ther* **9**(5): 422–427.
39. Lamfers ML, Grill J, Dirven CM, *et al.* (2002) Potential of the conditionally replicative adenovirus Ad5-Delta24RGD in the treatment of malignant gliomas and its enhanced effect with radiotherapy. *Cancer Res* **62**(20): 5736–5742.
40. Jiang H, Gomez-Manzano C, Aoki H, *et al.* (2007) Examination of the therapeutic potential of Delta-24-RGD in brain tumor stem cells: Role of autophagic cell death. *J Natl Cancer Inst* **99**(18): 1410–1414.
41. Chiocca EA, Aguilar LK, Bell SD, *et al.* (2011) Phase IB study of gene-mediated cytotoxic immunotherapy adjuvant to up-front surgery and intensive timing radiation for malignant glioma. *J Clin Oncol* **29**(27): 3611–3619.
42. Wickham TJ, Tzeng E, Shears LL 2nd, *et al.* (1997) Increased *in vitro* and *in vivo* gene transfer by adenovirus vectors containing chimeric fiber proteins. *J Virol* **71**(11): 8221–8229.
43. Ulasov IV, Zhu ZB, Tyler MA, *et al.* (2007) Survivin-driven and fiber-modified oncolytic adenovirus exhibits potent anti-tumor activity in established intracranial glioma. *Hum Gene Ther* **18**(7): 589–602.
44. Yang L, Cao Z, Li F, *et al.* (2004) Tumor-specific gene expression using the survivin promoter is further increased by hypoxia. *Gene Ther* **11**(15): 1215–1223.
45. Komata T, Kondo Y, Kanzawa T, *et al.* (2001) Treatment of malignant glioma cells with the transfer of constitutively active caspase-6 using the human telomerase catalytic subunit (human telomerase reverse transcriptase) gene promoter. *Cancer Res* **61**(15): 5796–5802.
46. Mishima K, Asai A, Kadomatsu K, *et al.* (1997) Increased expression of midkine during the progression of human astrocytomas. *Neurosci Lett* **233**(1): 29–32.
47. Le S, Zhu JJ, Anthony DC, *et al.* (1998) Telomerase activity in human gliomas. *Neurosurgery* **42**(5): 1120–1124; discussion 1124–1125.
48. Langford LA, Piatyszek MA, Xu R, *et al.* (1995) Telomerase activity in human brain tumours. *Lancet* **346**(8985): 1267–1268.

49. Kajiwara Y, Yamasaki F, Hama S, *et al.* (2003) Expression of survivin in astrocytic tumors: Correlation with malignant grade and prognosis. *Cancer* **97**(4): 1077–1083.
50. Das A, Tan WL, Teo J, Smith DR. (2002) Expression of survivin in primary glioblastomas. *J Cancer Res Clin Oncol* **128**(6): 302–306.
51. Van Houdt WJ, Haviv YS, Lu B, *et al.* (2006) The human survivin promoter: A novel transcriptional targeting strategy for treatment of glioma. *J Neurosurg* **104**(4): 583–592.
52. Zheng S, Ulasov IV, Han Y, *et al.* (2007) Fiber-knob modifications enhance adenoviral tropism and gene transfer in malignant glioma. *J Gene Med* **9**(3): 151–160.
53. Sonabend AM, Ulasov IV, Han Y, *et al.* (2009) Biodistribution of an oncolytic adenovirus after intracranial injection in permissive animals: A comparative study of Syrian hamsters and cotton rats. *Cancer Gene Ther* **16**(4): 362–372.
54. Kohno S, Nakagawa K, Hamada K, *et al.* (2004) Midkine promoter-based conditionally replicative adenovirus for malignant glioma therapy. *Oncol Rep* **12**(1): 73–78.
55. Maillard L, Ziol M, Tahlil O, *et al.* (1998) Pre-treatment with elastase improves the efficiency of percutaneous adenovirus-mediated gene transfer to the arterial media. *Gene Ther* **5**(8): 1023–1030.
56. Kuriyama N, Kuriyama H, Julin CM, *et al.* (2000) Pretreatment with protease is a useful experimental strategy for enhancing adenovirus-mediated cancer gene therapy. *Hum Gene Ther* **11**(16): 2219–2230.
57. McKee TD, Grandi P, Mok W, *et al.* (2006) Degradation of fibrillar collagen in a human melanoma xenograft improves the efficacy of an oncolytic herpes simplex virus vector. *Cancer Res* **66**(5): 2509–2513.
58. Ganesh S, Gonzalez-Edick M, Gibbons D, *et al.* (2008) Intratumoral coadministration of hyaluronidase enzyme and oncolytic adenoviruses enhances virus potency in metastatic tumor models. *Clin Cancer Res* **14**(12): 3933–3941.
59. Bobo RH, Laske DW, Akbasak A, *et al.* (1994) Convection-enhanced delivery of macromolecules in the brain. *Proc Natl Acad Sci USA* **91**(6): 2076–2080.
60. Mardor Y, Rahav O, Zauberman Y, *et al.* (2005) Convection-enhanced drug delivery: Increased efficacy and magnetic resonance image monitoring. *Cancer Res* **65**(15): 6858–6863.
61. Sanftner LM, Sommer JM, Suzuki BM, *et al.* (2005) AAV2-mediated gene delivery to monkey putamen: Evaluation of an infusion device and delivery parameters. *Exp Neurol* **194**(2): 476–483.

62. Pandey A, Singh N, Vemula SV, *et al.* (2012) Impact of preexisting adenovirus vector immunity on immunogenicity and protection conferred with an adenovirus-based H5N1 influenza vaccine. *PLoS ONE* 7(3): p. e33428.
63. Kremer EJ, Boutin S, Chillon M, Danos O. (2000) Canine adenovirus vectors: An alternative for adenovirus-mediated gene transfer. *J Virol* **74**(1): 505–512.
64. Skog J, Edlund K, Widegren B, *et al.* (2004) Efficient internalization into low-passage glioma cell lines using adenoviruses other than type 5: An approach for improvement of gene delivery to brain tumours. *J Gen Virol* **85**(Pt 9): 2627–2638.
65. Gage FH. (2000) Mammalian neural stem cells. *Science* **287**(5457): 1433–1438.
66. Aboody K, Capela A, Niazi N, *et al.* (2011) Translating stem cell studies to the clinic for CNS repair: Current state of the art and the need for a Rosetta stone. *Neuron* **70**(4): 597–613.
67. Tabatabai G, Wick W, Weller M. (2011) Stem cell-mediated gene therapies for malignant gliomas: A promising targeted therapeutic approach? *Discov Med* **11**(61): 529–536.
68. Tyler MA, Ulasov IV, Sonabend AM, *et al.* (2009) Neural stem cells target intracranial glioma to deliver an oncolytic adenovirus *in vivo. Gene Ther* **16**(2): 262–278.
69. Muller FJ, Snyder EY, Loring JF. (2006) Gene therapy: Can neural stem cells deliver? *Nat Rev Neurosci* 7(1): 75–84.
70. Einstein O, Ben-Hur T. (2008) The changing face of neural stem cell therapy in neurologic diseases. *Arch Neurol* **65**(4): 452–456.
71. Cho T, Bae JH, Choi HB, *et al.* (2002) Human neural stem cells: Electrophysiological properties of voltage-gated ion channels. *Neuroreport* **13**(11): 1447–1452.
72. Flax JD, Aurora S, Yang C, *et al.* (1998) Engraftable human neural stem cells respond to developmental cues, replace neurons, and express foreign genes. *Nat Biotechnol* **16**(11): 1033–1039.
73. Hayden EC. (2008) California institute to help stem-cell biotechs. *Nature* 455(7212): 436–437.
74. Truckenmiller ME, Vawter MP, Zhang P, *et al.* (2002) AF5, a CNS cell line immortalized with an N-terminal fragment of SV40 large T: Growth, differentiation, genetic stability, and gene expression. *Exp Neurol* 175(2): 318–337.
75. Xu G, Li X, Bai Y, Bai J, *et al.* (2004) Improving recovery of spinal cord-injured rats by telomerase-driven human neural progenitor cells. *Restor Neurol Neurosci* 22(6): 469–476.

76. Kim S-K, Kim SU, Park H, *et al.* (2006) Human neural stem cells target experimental intracranial medulloblastoma and deliver a therapeutic gene leading to tumor regression. *Clin Cancer Res* **12**(18): 5550–5556.
77. Ubiali F, Nava S, Nessi V, *et al.* (2007) Allorecognition of human neural stem cells by peripheral blood lymphocytes despite low expression of MHC molecules: Role of TGF-beta in modulating proliferation. *Int Immunol* **19**(9): 1063–1074.
78. Mitrecic D, Gajovic S, Pochet R. (2009) Toward the treatments with neural stem cells: Experiences from amyotrophic lateral sclerosis. *Anat Rec* (*Hoboken*) **292**(12): 1962–1967.
79. Thaci B, Ahmed AU, Ulasov IV, *et al.* (2012) Pharmacokinetic study of neural stem cell-based cell carrier for oncolytic virotherapy: Targeted delivery of the therapeutic payload in an orthotopic brain tumor model. *Cancer Gene Ther* **19**(6): 431–442.
80. Ahmed AU, Thaci B, Alexiades NG, *et al.* (2011) Neural stem cell-based cell carriers enhance therapeutic efficacy of an oncolytic adenovirus in an orthotopic mouse model of human glioblastoma. *Mol Ther* **19**(9): 1714–1726.
81. Kim SU, de Vellis J. (2009) Stem cell-based cell therapy in neurological diseases: A review. *J Neurosci Res* **87**(10): 2183–2200.
82. Xu Q, Yuan X, Xu M, *et al.* (2009) Chemokine CXC receptor 4-mediated glioma tumor tracking by bone marrow-derived neural progenitor/stem cells. *Mol Cancer Ther* **8**(9): 2746–2753.
83. Sun L, Lee J, Fine HA. (2004) Neuronally expressed stem cell factor induces neural stem cell migration to areas of brain injury. *J Clin Invest* **113**(9): 1364–1374.
84. Magge SN, Malik SZ, Royo NC, *et al.* (2009) Role of monocyte chemoattractant protein-1 (MCP-1/CCL2) in migration of neural progenitor cells toward glial tumors. *J Neurosci Res* **87**(7): 1547–1555.
85. Schmidt NO, Przylecki W, Yang W, *et al.* (2005) Brain tumor tropism of transplanted human neural stem cells is induced by vascular endothelial growth factor. *Neoplasia* 7(6): 623–629.
86. Zhao D, Najbauer J, Garcia E, *et al.* (2008) Neural stem cell tropism to glioma: Critical role of tumor hypoxia. *Mol Cancer Res* **6**(12): 1819–1829.
87. Shah K, Bureau E, Kim DE, *et al.* (2005) Glioma therapy and real-time imaging of neural precursor cell migration and tumor regression. *Ann Neurol* **57**(1): 34–41.
88. Zhang Z, Jiang Q, Jiang F, *et al.* (2004) *In vivo* magnetic resonance imaging tracks adult neural progenitor cell targeting of brain tumor. *Neuroimage* **23**(1): 281–287.

89. Waehler R, Russell SJ, Curiel DT. (2007) Engineering targeted viral vectors for gene therapy. *Nat Rev Genet* **8**(8): 573–587.
90. Fulci G, Breymann L, Gianni D, *et al.* (2006) Cyclophosphamide enhances glioma virotherapy by inhibiting innate immune responses. *Proc Natl Acad Sci USA* **103**(34): 12873–12878.
91. Pluchino S, Gritti A, Blezer E, *et al.* (2009) Human neural stem cells ameliorate autoimmune encephalomyelitis in non-human primates. *Ann Neurol* **66**(3): 343–354.
92. Pluchino S, Quattrini A, Brambilla E, *et al.* (2003) Injection of adult neurospheres induces recovery in a chronic model of multiple sclerosis. *Nature* **422**(6933): 688–694.
93. Uhl M, Weiler M, Wick W, *et al.* (2005) Migratory neural stem cells for improved thymidine kinase-based gene therapy of malignant gliomas. *Biochem Biophys Res Commun* **328**(1): 125–129.
94. Ahmed AU, Tyler MA, Thaci B, *et al.* (2011) A comparative study of neural and mesenchymal stem cell-based carriers for oncolytic adenovirus in a model of malignant glioma. *Mol Pharm* **8**(5): 1559–1572.
95. Ehtesham M, Kabos P, Kabosova A, *et al.* (2002) The use of interleukin 12-secreting neural stem cells for the treatment of intracranial glioma. *Cancer Res* **62**(20): 5657–5663.
96. Yuan X, Hu J, Belladonna ML, *et al.* (2006) Interleukin-23-expressing bone marrow-derived neural stem-like cells exhibit anti-tumor activity against intracranial glioma. *Cancer Res* **66**(5): 2630–2638.
97. Ehtesham M, Kabos P, Gutierrez MA, *et al.* (2002) Induction of glioblastoma apoptosis using neural stem cell-mediated delivery of tumor necrosis factor-related apoptosis-inducing ligand. *Cancer Res* **62**(24): 7170–7174.
98. Kim SK, Cargioli TG, Machluf M, *et al.* (2005) PEX-producing human neural stem cells inhibit tumor growth in a mouse glioma model. *Clin Cancer Res* **11**(16): 5965–5970.
99. van Eekelen M, Sasportas LS, Kasmieh R, *et al.* (2010) Human stem cells expressing novel TSP-1 variant have anti-angiogenic effect on brain tumors. *Oncogene* **29**(22): 3185–3195.
100. Balyasnikova IV, Ferguson SD, Sengupta S, *et al.* (2010) Mesenchymal stem cells modified with a single-chain antibody against EGFRvIII successfully inhibit the growth of human xenograft malignant glioma. *PLoS ONE* **5**(3): e9750.
101. Balyasnikova IV, Franco-Gou R, Mathis JM, Lesniak MS. (2010) Genetic modification of mesenchymal stem cells to express a single-chain antibody against EGFRvIII on the cell surface. *J Tissue Eng Regen Med* **4**(4): 247–258.

102. Cromer Berman SM, Walczak P, Bulte JW. (2011) Tracking stem cells using magnetic nanoparticles. *Wiley Interdiscip Rev Nanomed Nanobiotechnol* **3**(4): 343–355.
103. Lin D, Najbauer J, Salvaterra PM, *et al.* (2007) Novel method for visualizing and modeling the spatial distribution of neural stem cells within intracranial glioma. *Neuroimage* **37**(Suppl 1): S18–S26.
104. Hong H, Yang Y, Zhang Y, Cai W. (2010) Non-invasive cell tracking in cancer and cancer therapy. *Curr Top Med Chem* **10**(12): 1237–1248.
105. Tang Y, Shah K, Messerli SM, *et al.* (2003) *In vivo* tracking of neural progenitor cell migration to glioblastomas. *Hum Gene Ther* **14**(13): 1247–1254.
106. Rosen AB, Kelly DJ, Schuldt AJ, *et al.* (2007) Finding fluorescent needles in the cardiac haystack: Tracking human mesenchymal stem cells labeled with quantum dots for quantitative *in vivo* three-dimensional fluorescence analysis. *Stem Cells* **25**(8): 2128–2138.
107. Slotkin JR, Chakrabarti L, Dai HN, *et al.* (2007) *In vivo* quantum dot labeling of mammalian stem and progenitor cells. *Dev Dyn* **236**(12): 3393–3401.
108. Loo C, Lowery A, Halas N, *et al.* (2005) Immunotargeted nanoshells for integrated cancer imaging and therapy. *Nano Lett* **5**(4): 709–711.
109. Chang NK, Jeong YY, Park JS, *et al.* (2008) Tracking of neural stem cells in rats with intracerebral hemorrhage by the use of 3T MRI. *Korean J Radiol* **9**(3): 196–204.
110. Kim D, Hong KS, Song J. (2007) The present status of cell tracking methods in animal models using magnetic resonance imaging technology. *Mol Cells* **23**(2): 132–137.
111. Frangioni JV, Hajjar RJ. (2004) *In vivo* tracking of stem cells for clinical trials in cardiovascular disease. *Circulation* **110**(21): 3378–3383.
112. Budde MD, Frank JA. (2009) Magnetic tagging of therapeutic cells for MRI. *J Nucl Med* **50**(2): 171–174.
113. Guzman R, Uchida N, Blisset TM, *et al.* (2007) Long-term monitoring of transplanted human neural stem cells in developmental and pathological contexts with MRI. *Proc Natl Acad Sci USA* **104**(24): 10211–10216.
114. Thu MS, Najbauer J, Kendall SE, *et al.* (2009) Iron labeling and pre-clinical MRI visualization of therapeutic human neural stem cells in a murine glioma model. *PLoS ONE* **4**(9): e7218.
115. Burgess A, Ayala-Grosso CA, Ganguly M, *et al.* (2011) Targeted delivery of neural stem cells to the brain using MRI-guided focused ultrasound to disrupt the blood-brain barrier. *PLoS ONE* **6**(11): e27877.
116. Herrlinger U, Woiciechowski C, Sena-Esteves M, *et al.* (2000) Neural precursor cells for delivery of replication-conditional HSV-1 vectors to intracerebral gliomas. *Mol Ther* **1**(4): 347–357.

117. Sonabend AM, Ulasov IV, Tyler MA, *et al.* (2008) Mesenchymal stem cells effectively deliver an oncolytic adenovirus to intracranial glioma. *Stem Cells* **26**(3): 831–841.
118. Krystkowiak P, Gaura V, Labalette M, *et al.* (2007) Alloimmunisation to donor antigens and immune rejection following foetal neural grafts to the brain in patients with Huntington's disease. *PLoS ONE* **2**(1): e166.
119. Fomchenko EI, Holland EC. (2006) Mouse models of brain tumors and their applications in preclinical trials. *Clin Cancer Res* **12**(18): 5288–5297.
120. Hu X, Holland EC. (2005) Applications of mouse glioma models in preclinical trials. *Mutat Res* **576**(1–2): 54–65.
121. Candolfi M, Curtin JF, Nichols WS, *et al.* (2007) Intracranial glioblastoma models in preclinical neuro-oncology: Neuropathological characterization and tumor progression. *J Neurooncol* **85**(2): 133–148.

VIII. Stem Cells and Translation Research

CHAPTER 20

Challenges in Stem Cells and Translational Research

*Dhruv Kumar**, *Sharmila Shankar*†,‡ *and Rakesh K. Srivastava**,‡

20.1. INTRODUCTION

Stem cell research has been evolving as one of the most interesting research areas providing answers to various unsolved problems related to health. Stem cells are undifferentiated/unspecialized cells that have the ability to renew themselves and generate highly specific cells for specialized functions. The human body contains more than 200 different cell types that are organized into tissues and organs with highly specific functions. The origins of stem cell research have allowed us to understand how tissues are maintained in adult life, rather than how different cell types arise in the embryo. It has long been discussed that the differentiated cells that form structurally and functionally different tissues, such as the skin, blood and intestinal epithelium, have a short lifespan and are unable to renew themselves. This directed the discussion to the notion that such tissues are maintained

*Department of Pharmacology, Toxicology and Therapeutics, and Medicine, The University of Kansas Medical Center, Kansas City, USA.

†Department of Pathology and Laboratory Medicine, The University of Kansas Medical Center, Kansas City, USA.

‡Corresponding authors: Sharmila Shankar, Department of Pathology and Laboratory Medicine, The University of Kansas Medical Center, 3901 Rainbow Boulevard, Kansas City, KS 66160, USA; E-mail: *sshankar@kumc.edu*; Rakesh K. Srivastava, Department of Pharmacology, Toxicology and Therapeutics, and Medicine, The University of Kansas Medical Center, 3901 Rainbow Boulevard, Kansas City, KS 66160, USA; E-mail:*rsrivastava@kumc.edu*.

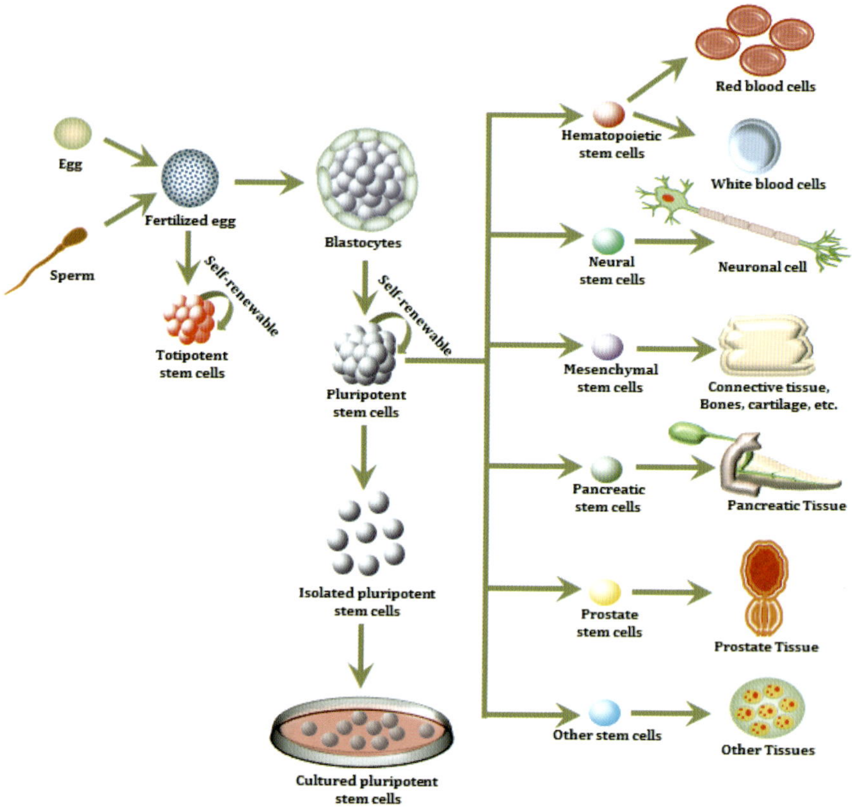

Fig. 1. The origin of stem cells and the generation of different tissues from stem cells. Pluripotent stem cells can form all the cell types of the adult organism. Totipotent stem cells can form the extraembryonic tissues of the embryo.

by cells with extensive renewal capacity and the ability to regenerate, cells that can undergo further differentiation called "stem cells."[1] Such cells generate only the differentiated families that are appropriate for the tissue in which they are present and are thus referred to as multipotent/unipotent stem cells (Fig. 1).

Initially, stem cell research was focused on only three types of tissues: those, such as in the epidermis, with a rapid turnover of differentiated cells; those, such as in the brain, in which there appeared to be no self-renewal; and those, such as in the liver, in which cells divided to give two daughter cells that were functionally equivalent.[2] While it remains true that different adult tissues differ in terms of the proportion of proliferative cells and the nature of the differentiation compartment, in recent years it has become apparent that some tissues that appeared to lack the self-renewal ability do indeed contain stem cells[3] and others contain a previously unrecognized cellular heterogeneity.[4] These cells have received widespread attention in recent years.[5–7]

20.2. STEM CELLS

Stem cells are defined as undifferentiated cells found in the body that have the potential to develop into many different cell types during early life and growth which are structurally and functionally different from one another.

20.2.1. Why Stem Cell Research Is Important

With their remarkable potential to develop into many different cell types in the human body system, stem cells have been steadily gaining ground as a leading area of scientific research into disease. It has been found that stem cells serve as a sort of internal repair system, dividing essentially without limit to replenish other cells. Stem cells divide to form either new stem cells or other cell types with more specialized functions. The following characteristics distinguish stem cells from other cell types: (i) they are unspecialized cells capable of renewing themselves through cell division, sometimes after long periods of inactivity, and (ii) under certain physiologic or experimental conditions, they can be induced to become tissue or organ-specific cells with special functions.

Scientists have mainly worked with two kinds of stem cells from animals and humans: embryonic stem cells and non-embryonic somatic or adult stem cells. Human embryonic stem cells were first isolated in 1998, when stem cells were derived from human embryos and cultured in the laboratory. In 2006, researchers successfully "reprogrammed" some specialized adult cells and those genetically reprogrammed cells assumed a stem cell-like state, a new type of stem cell called induced pluripotent stem cells.

Stem cells are important for living organisms for many reasons. In the three- to five-day-old embryo, called a blastocyst, the inner cells give rise to the entire body of the organism, including all of the many specialized cell types and organs such as the lung, heart, skin, eggs, sperm and other tissues. In some adult tissues, such as bone marrow, muscle and brain, discrete populations of adult stem cells generate replacements for cells that are lost through normal wear and tear, injury or disease. Given their unique regenerative abilities, stem cells provide us a new potential for treating several diseases, such as cancer, diabetes, stroke and heart disease (Fig. 2). Work is already in progress to screen new drugs and to develop model

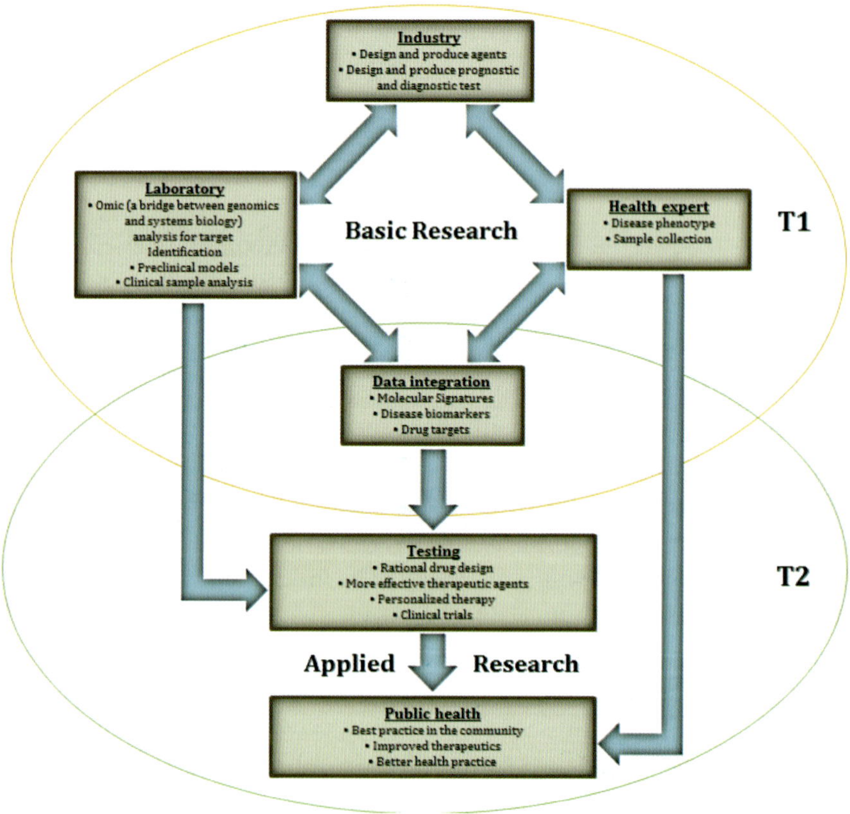

Fig. 2. The use of stem cells to treat several diseases. Stem cells can be assigned roles, and become part of any organ required. Stem cells can be used to repair damage in organs and tissue, treat neurodegenerative disease, heart disease, several cancers, diabetes, etc.

systems by using stem cells to study normal growth and identify the causes of birth defects.

20.2.2. The Unique Properties of Stem Cells

Stem cells have unique characteristics that differentiate them from other cells in the body. All stem cells are capable of dividing and renewing themselves for long periods (except blood cells, nerve cells and some muscles cells, which do not normally replicate themselves), they are unspecialized and they can give rise to specialized cell types. Many years have been spent in the laboratory learning how to derive and maintain stem cells without them spontaneously differentiating into specific cell types. It took two decades to learn how to grow human embryonic stem cells in the laboratory. One of the unique properties of a stem cell is that it does not have any tissue-specific structures that allow it to perform specialized functions. For example, a stem cell cannot work with its neighbors to pump blood through the body (like a heart muscle cell), and it cannot carry oxygen molecules through the bloodstream (like a red blood cell). However, unspecialized stem cells can give rise to specialized cells, including heart muscle cells, blood cells and nerve cells.

Adult stem cells typically generate the cell types of the tissue in which they reside. For example, a blood-forming adult stem cell in the bone marrow normally gives rise to the many types of blood cells. Thus, it is generally accepted that a blood-forming cell in the bone marrow, known as hematopoietic stem cells, cannot give rise to cells in a very different tissue, such as nerve cells in the brain. Research over the last several years has attempted to show that stem cells from one tissue may give rise to cell types of a completely different tissue (Fig. 1). This remains an area of great debate within the research community.

20.2.3. Clinical Application of Stem Cells

Stem cell-based therapies are already in clinical use and have been for decades. It is instructive to consider our experiences with these treatments, because it provides important insight into the challenging journey from proof-of-principle in the laboratory to real patient benefit in the clinic.[8] Hematopoietic stem cell transplantation has the longest history and is the most widely available stem cell therapy.[9] The stem cells used in treatment mainly come from bone marrow, peripheral blood or cord blood. For some applications, the patient's own cells are engrafted. However, allogeneic stem cell transplantation is now a common procedure for the treatment of bone marrow failure and hematological malignancies, such as leukemia. Donor stem cells are used to reconstitute immune function in such patients following radiation and/or chemotherapy.

Clinical studies over the last 10 years suggest that stem cell transplantation also has potential as a therapy for neurodegenerative diseases. Stem cell reprogramming has shown to treat Parkinsons's disease and brain related disorders.[10] Clinical trials have involved grafting brain tissue from aborted fetuses into patients with Parkinson's disease and Huntington's disease.[11,12] While some successes have been noted, the outcomes have not been uniform, and further clinical trials will involve more refined patient selection in an effort to predict who will benefit and who will not. Notably, aside from the opposition in many quarters to using fetal material, there are practical challenges associated with the availability and regularity of grafted cells. Thus, therapies with pure populations of stem cells are an important and achievable goal.[13,14] There is wide consensus that stem cells offer great potential to treat many human diseases and to repair tissue damage resulting from injury or aging.

20.2.4. Using Stem Cells to Treat Diseases

Stem cells are like blank paper: we can assign tasks to stem cells, and tell them to become part of any organ we require. The first step in using stem cells for disease treatment is to establish stem cell lines. Specific genes are then "switched on" so that the stem cell can differentiate into any cell required. Stem cell therapy has been successfully used for the treatment of several diseases in organs such as the liver, bladder, ear, lung, brain and heart (Table 1).[8,10] Stem cell therapy has also recently shown to provide a potential cure for AIDS.[15,16]

The first successful stem cell-based therapy treated leukemia by bone marrow transplantation,[17] allowing the patient's existing bone marrow

Table 1 Types of Stem Cells and Their Uses in Treating Diseases

No.	Type of Stem Cells	Source of Stem Cells	Uses in Treating Disease	References
1.	Blood stem cells	Adult blood tissues	Blood disorders, bone marrow transplantation	Ref. 54
2.	Cord blood stem cells	Umbilical cord	Leukemia, blood disorders in children	Refs. 54, 55
3.	Embryonic stem cells	Early stage embryo (blastocyst)	Eye disorders, heart diseases	Refs. 56, 57
4.	Induced pluripotent stem cells	Specialized adult cells	Various diseases	Ref. 58
5.	Limbal stem cells	Tissue from an area of the eye	Corneal damage	Ref. 56
6.	Mesenchymal stem cells	Bone marrow	Cartilage and bone repair, blood vessel repair, heart diseases, liver diseases	Ref. 59
7.	Skin stem cells	Adult skin tissue	Skin-related diseases, skin grafts	Ref. 60

to be destroyed by radiation and/or chemotherapy. In essence, donor bone marrow stem cells are injected into the patient and cells differentiate into the blood cells are required. Typically, medications prevent the patient's immune system from rejecting the new bone marrow.[18] Another limitation of this procedure is that it uses existing hematopoietic stem cells. To treat a failing heart, for example, stem cells could also be stimulated to differentiate into heart cells, and by injecting them into a patient's damaged heart, these new heart cells could grow and repair the damaged tissue.[8] As mentioned in Table 1, there are several other types of stem cells that can be used to treat different diseases. However, while stem cell treatment is being successfully used against certain diseases (bone marrow transplantation, heart related disease, skin grafting), there are major areas of medicine untouched by stem cell research.

20.2.5. Controversy in Stem Cell Research

Stem cell research has led to some of the biggest controversies involving scientific and religious communities. To obtain embryonic stem cells, scientists either have to use a donated embryo or clone an embryo using a cell from a patient's body and a donated egg. In either case, in order to harvest an embryo's stem cells, it must be destroyed, raising strong objections from religious groups, which see it as tantamount to taking a human life. As a consequence, research involving human embryonic stem cells remains highly controversial and alternatives are being keenly sought, partly due to these ethical concerns and also the limited availability of donor embryos.

20.2.6. Future Applications of Stem Cell Research

While stem cells have great potential to treat various human diseases,[8,10,19] there are many important considerations concerning the time and effort required to bring new therapies into the clinic. It is inspiring to be able to induce embryonic stem cells to differentiate into cardiomyocytes in a culture dish, but that is only one very small step towards effecting cardiac repair. There are a large number of human embryonic stem cell lines now available, and banking of clinical grade cells is underway, offering the opportunity for optimal immunological matching of donors and recipients. However, one of the attractions of transplanting induced pluripotent stem cells (iPSCs) is that the patient's own cells can be used, removing the need for immunosuppression. This breakthrough has helped us to understand an important goal: how the pluripotent state can be efficiently and stably induced and maintained by treating cells with pharmacologically active compounds rather than by genetic manipulation.[20] Recently, it has been shown that pancreatic exocrine cells in adult mice can be reprogrammed to become functional, insulin-producing beta-cells by expression of transcription factors that regulate pancreatic development.[19,21] The idea of repairing tissue through a process of cellular reprogramming *in situ* is an attractive paradigm to be explored further. A range of biomaterials are already in clinical use for tissue repair, in particular to repair defects in cartilage and bone.[22] Moreover, finding drugs that selectively target cancer stem cells offers the potential to develop cancer treatments that are not only more effective, but also cause less collateral damage to the patient's normal tissues than drugs currently in use. In addition, patient-specific iPSCs provide a new tool to identify underlying disease mechanisms.

20.3. TRANSLATIONAL RESEARCH

Translational research aims to simplify the translation of outcomes from basic science to practical applications that enhance human health and well-being. The primary goal of this new and fast-growing area is to integrate advancements in molecular biology with clinical trials, taking research from "bench to bedside." Translational research is practiced in the medical, behavioral, and social sciences.[23,24] In the field of medicine, it is used to translate the findings of basic research more quickly and efficiently into medical practice, and hence meaningful health outcomes. Applying the knowledge gained in basic science is a major stumbling block in science, partially due to the compartmentalization within science. Hence, translational research is seen as a key component to finding practical applications, especially within medicine.

Translational research includes two areas of translation. One is the process of applying discoveries generated during research in the laboratory, and in preclinical studies, to the development of trials and studies in humans, called "T1 translation." The second area of translation concerns research aimed at enhancing the adoption of best practices in the community, known as "T2 translation" (Fig. 3).

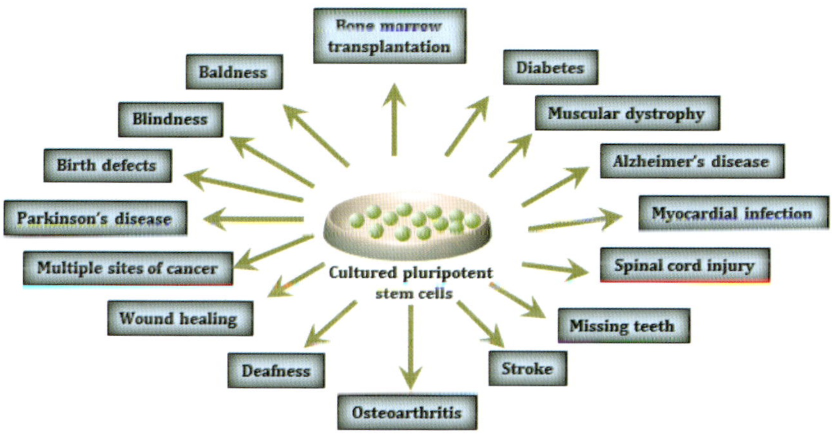

Fig. 3. The translational research cycle. Basic scientists, theoreticians, laboratory researchers, clinicians, and the pharmaceutical industry must work together to design rational drugs for improved therapeutic efficacy and best practice public health in the community.

Basic scientists are not generally trained to think about the clinical application of their work, clinicians are often not taught to formulate research studies based on clinical observations, and public health scientists may not have a strong background in basic or clinical research (but have the knowledge of the community the other two groups may lack). These three groups have long collaborated, but as our knowledge grows and research becomes more complicated, it has become apparent that new ways of approaching basic health problems are needed. Health organizations are addressing this issue through efforts aimed at accelerating both kinds of translation.

Translational research is traditionally broken down into two categories: basic and applied research. Basic research is necessary to further our understanding of normal versus disease states but does not directly translate this knowledge into clinically useful applications. Applied research advances the development of new diagnostic tests or drugs for patients based on our understanding of disease development and progression. In taking research from the "bench to bedside," the primary goal of translational research is to integrate these two categories of research.[23,25–28] Understanding and interpreting the molecular information gained through various laboratory techniques (microarrays, genome sequencing, and proteomics) requires that information be shared between laboratories and clinics.[29,30] Clinical researchers' observations about the nature and progression of a disease should drive basic science investigation. Basic scientists should then provide clinicians with new treatment strategies based on laboratory data. This constant feedback promotes the discovery of disease biomarkers and drug targets, resulting in more rational drug design, improved efficacy of therapeutic agents, and faster optimization of lead compounds for clinical use. One prime example of translational research in human disease is the study of cancer therapy, where extensive collaboration between basic researchers, clinicians, and industry has generated numerous novel targeted compounds with enhanced efficacy and decreased toxicity. In addition to the development of new anticancer agents, translational research can also be applied to predicting response to therapy and resistance and sensitizing cancer cells to current therapeutics.[23,25,29,31]

20.3.1. Basic Research

Basic science involves laboratory studies that provide the foundation for applied research. Basic research is performed without thought of practical ends. It results in general knowledge and an understanding of nature and its laws. This general knowledge provides the means of answering a large number of important practical problems, though it may not give a complete specific answer to any one of them. The function of applied research is to provide such complete answers.[24] Thus, the main objective of basic research is the acquisition of knowledge without the obligation to apply it to practical ends. Basic research training is ubiquitous in medical schools. Abilities within the basic sciences have been clearly defined, allowing for effective development and evaluation of educational programs.[24,32]

20.3.2. Applied Research

Applied research involves finding solutions to practical problems. It incorporates environmental factors and is designed to assess the effectiveness of interventions in real-world conditions.[33,34] Applied research differs from basic research in that it only considers interventions responsive to implementation in broad community contexts. In addition, it enrolls diverse study populations, it recruits from a variety of settings, and it measures a broad range of relevant health outcomes. For these reasons, applied research can be used to directly inform evidence-based practice.[35]

20.3.3. Basic Research Versus Applied Research

Translational research is an approach that facilitates the bridge between basic research and applied research. As such, it is applied in the domain of medicine but has more general applicability as a distinct research approach, and in practice is associated with the approaches of participative science and participatory action research. Conventionally, research is identified as basic research/fundamental research and applied research/clinical research.[36,37] Basic research is more theoretical and takes a long time to be applied in any practical context. Basic research often leads to breakthroughs or paradigm shifts in practice. On the other hand, applied research is considered as being capable of having an impact in practice within a relatively short time. Basic research lays down the foundation for the applied research that follows. Applied research is designed to solve practical problems, to improve human well-being, to improve clinical applications, and to improve cures for specific diseases.[36,37]

20.3.4. Importance of Translational Research

According to a report by the US National Institutes of Health (NIH), translational research includes two areas of translation. One is the process of applying discoveries generated during research in the laboratory, and in pre-clinical studies, to the development of trials and studies in humans. The second area of translation concerns research aimed at enhancing the adoption of best practices in the community.[24] Cost-effectiveness of prevention and treatment strategies is also an important part of translational science. According to the NIH report, translational research is part of a unidirectional continuum in which research findings are moved from the researcher's bench to the patient's bedside and the community. Along this continuum, the first stage of translational research (T1) transfers knowledge from basic research to clinical research, while the second stage (T2) transfers findings from clinical studies or clinical trials to practice settings and communities (Fig. 3), where the findings improve health.[24,37]

The importance of translational research (collaboration between basic science and clinical researchers) to determine the mechanisms responsible for epidemiological associations that cannot be underestimated. Once a clinically important association has been identified, translation to the basic science laboratory is often necessary to determine the actual causal pathway or mechanism. For example, basic science investigators developed a septic model to examine the effects of alcohol abuse in rats. The investigators determined that chronic ethanol ingestion in rats renders the lung susceptible to endotoxin-mediated edematous injury, a finding that was consistent with clinical epidemiological studies.[38]

Translational research may also allow more rapid development of potential therapeutics, thus reducing the time between drug target identification and clinically relevant therapeutic options. Currently, completion of all phases of pre-clinical and clinical testing of a single drug typically takes between 7 and 12 years. But with the new translational research being conducted around the world, there are encouraging signs that this time can be significantly reduced, providing real benefits for patients.[24,37]

20.3.5. Challenges in Translational Research

The current objective of translational research is to accelerate the translation of data into knowledge through collaboration, data sharing, data integration and the establishment of standards. Translational research requires information on causes and outcomes of illness, and effective prevention, early detection, and personalized treatments and data flow from hospitals, clinics and participants of studies in an organized and structured format to repositories and research-based facilities and laboratories.[39] The role of translational research in ensuring rapid progression of basic scientific knowledge to patient benefit has been emphasized for more than three decades.[40] The main challenges that have been repeatedly debated include cultural differences between basic scientists and clinicians, lack of resources in terms of workforce and infrastructure, and the complex regulatory environment.[41] Cultural differences between the two groups of investigators largely stem from differences in education, lack of communication, and training, different goals, and different reward mechanisms. Regulatory issues pose challenges for both basic scientists and clinicians, encompassing ethical questions relating to human research, tissue banking and material transfer regulations, intellectual property rights, toxicology and manufacturing regulations, approvals by bodies such as the Food and Drug Administration (US) and the Medicines and Healthcare Regulatory Agency (UK), study sponsorship and insurance, as well as trial and data monitoring. These are becoming even more complex with expanding work in the fields of cell and gene therapies and tissue engineering. Resource problems include lack of trained interdisciplinary staff to support investigations throughout the translational research cycle, protected time for research particularly for clinicians, as well as access to shared resources.[39] Together, these issues contribute to various checkpoints between the phases of translational research including the "valley of death" that exists between pre-clinical research and clinical trials.[32]

20.4. TRANSLATIONAL RESEARCH IN CANCER THERAPY

The conventional principle of chemotherapy is that the "ideal anti-cancer drug should be one that has a specific affinity for cancer cells without affecting normal cells."[42] During World War I, physicians hypothesized that mustard agents may be able to treat leukemia, which is a disease caused by abnormal proliferation of myeloid or lymphoid precursor cells. The next several decades saw a rapid increase in new therapeutic agents, including antimetabolites, DNA damaging agents, and taxanes, as well as the introduction of combination therapy. Indeed, most efforts at cancer therapy involve direct interference with cell proliferation by altering events that occur during the cell cycle, as cell growth is largely unregulated in cancer cells. Early chemotherapy focused on inhibiting cell growth through mitotic poisons to control tumor cell proliferation.[43–45] However, later research also exposed alterations in vasculature, growth regulation, and evasion of cell death as essential events in tumor growth.[23,43,46] Such changes present additional targets for anticancer strategies. In the following, we present a brief overview of cancer treatments and discuss how translational research has led to the development of targeted therapies.

Ionizing radiation and chemotherapy are both important types of cancer therapy that have been widely used since their efficacy was first demonstrated over a century ago. The former utilizes high-energy radiation to kill cancer cells by inducing lethal DNA damage and is often used in conjunction with either surgery or chemotherapy.[47,48] Although radiation therapy is generally well tolerated, secondary cancers, skeletal complications, radiation-induced heart disease, and lung disease are common side effects.[49,50] Due to the toxicity of radiation, much focus has been placed on improving its cancer cell specificity. This includes research into agents that sensitize cancer cells to radiation or protect normal cells from damage induced by radiation.[51–53] Chemotherapy involves the use of systemic drugs targeting various aspects of cell growth. Chemotherapy agents vary widely in their chemical composition, function, specificity, and toxicity. While generally effective, chemotherapeutic agents are highly toxic and damage normal cells as well as cancer cells, causing severe side effects. New varieties of chemotherapy medicines to be used in both solo and combination therapy are being developed to increase treatment efficacy. As some chemotherapy drugs are delivered through solvents that are not easily taken up by the body, research into novel drug delivery methods and on improved drug solubility is ongoing. Because the side effects of chemotherapy can be devastating to patients, chemoprotective and chemosensitizing agents are under development to increase drug efficacy without nonspecific toxicity.[44,45]

A key example of the translation of basic research into clinical application is the development of molecular targeted therapy, where cancer cell growth is inhibited by interfering with specific molecules that are necessary for tumor growth. Identification of specific molecular characteristics of tumors has facilitated rational drug development, and recognizing suitable targets has led to the generation of countless compounds that have been highly effective in both pre-clinical and clinical trials. These compounds are screened based on their effects on specific targets in tumor cells and the overall effect on cancer cell growth.[27]

20.5. CONCLUSION

The field of stem cell research has entered an inspiring translational phase that is paving the way for regenerative medicine to cure several diseases. The capacity to reprogram human adult somatic cells to a pluripotent state or a different cell type has opened the door to the development and study of disease-specific cells. These cells not only provide tools for understanding more about the mechanistic basis of disease, but also offer the possibility of drug testing in the laboratory. Although there is some way to go before we see clinical trials using reprogrammed patient-specific cells, other areas of stem cell research are closer to clinical application.

ACKNOWLEDGMENTS

The authors would like to thank all the laboratory members for their support during the production of this chapter.

REFERENCES

1. Lajtha LG. (1979) Stem cell concepts. *Nouv Rev Fr Hematol* **21**(1): 59–65.
2. Hall PA, Watt FM. (1989) Stem cells: The generation and maintenance of cellular diversity. *Development* **106**(4): 619–633.
3. Zhao C, Deng W, Gage FH. (2008) Mechanisms and functional implications of adult neurogenesis. *Cell* **132**(4): 645–660.
4. Zaret KS, Grompe M. (2008) Generation and regeneration of cells of the liver and pancreas. *Science* **322**(5907): 1490–1494.
5. Reya T, Morrison SJ, Clarke MF, Weissman IL. (2001) Stem cells, cancer, and cancer stem cells. *Nature* **414**(6859): 105–111.
6. Clarke MF, Dick JE, Dirks PB, *et al.* (2006) Cancer stem cells — Perspectives on current status and future directions: AACR Workshop on cancer stem cells. *Cancer Res* **66**(19): 9339–9344.
7. Dick JE. (2008) Stem cell concepts renew cancer research. *Blood* **112**(13): 4793–4807.
8. Maltais S, Joggerst SJ, Hatzopoulos A, *et al.* (2013) Stem cell therapy for chronic heart failure: An updated appraisal. *Expert Opin Biol Ther* **13**(4): 503–516.
9. Austin EB, Guttridge M, Pamphilon D, Watt SM. (2008) The role of blood services and regulatory bodies in stem cell transplantation. *Vox Sang* **94**(1): 6–17.
10. Ali F, Stott SR, Barker RA. (2013) Stem cells and the treatment of Parkinson's disease. *Exp Neurol.* Epub ahead of print.
11. Dunnett SB, Bjorklund A, Lindvall O. (2001) Cell therapy in Parkinson's disease — Stop or go? *Nat Rev Neurosci* **2**(5): 365–369.
12. Wright BLC, Barker RA. (2007) Established and emerging therapies for Huntington's disease. *Curr Mol Med* **7**(6): 579–587.
13. Conti L, Pollard SM, Gorba T, *et al.* (2005) Niche-independent symmetrical self-renewal of a mammalian tissue stem cell. *PLoS Biol* **3**(9): 1594–1606.
14. Lowell S, Benchoua A, Heavey B, Smith AG. (2006) Notch promotes neural lineage entry by pluripotent embryonic stem cells. *PLoS Biol* **4**(5): 805–818.
15. Hütter G, Nowak D, Mossner M, *et al.* (2009) Long-term control of HIV by CCR5 Delta32/Delta32 stem-cell transplantation. *N Engl J Med* **360**(7): 692–698.
16. Allers K, Hütter G, Hofmann J, *et al.* (2011) Evidence for the cure of HIV infection by CCR5Δ32/Δ32 stem cell transplantation. *Blood* **117**(10): 2791–2799.
17. Gluckman E, Broxmeyer HA, Auerbach AD, *et al.* (1989) Hematopoietic reconstitution in a patient with Fanconi's anemia by means of umbilical-cord blood from an HLA-identical sibling. *N Engl J Med* **321**(17): 1174–1178.

18. Rubinstein P, Carrier C, Scaradavou A, *et al.* (1998) Outcomes among 562 recipients of placental-blood transplants from unrelated donors. *N Engl J Med* **339**(22): 1565–1577.
19. Nostro MC, Keller G. (2012) Generation of beta cells from human pluripotent stem cells: Potential for regenerative medicine. *Semin Cell Dev Biol* **23**(6): 701–710.
20. Silva J, Barrandon O,Nichols J, *et al.* (2008) Promotion of reprogramming to ground state pluripotency by signal inhibition. *PLoS Biol* **6**(10): e253.
21. Zhou Q, Brown J, Kanarek A, *et al.* (2008) *In vivo* reprogramming of adult pancreatic exocrine cells to beta-cells. *Nature* **455**(7213): 627–632.
22. Kamitakahara M, Ohtsuki C, Miyazaki T. (2008) Review paper: Behavior of ceramic biomaterials derived from tricalcium phosphate in physiological condition. *J Biomater Appl* **23**(3): 197–212.
23. Chabner BA, Boral AL, Multani P. (1998) Translational research: Walking the bridge between idea and cure — Seventeenth Bruce F. Cain Memorial Award lecture. *Cancer Res* **58**(19): 4211–4216.
24. Rubio DM, Schoenbaum EE, Lee LS, *et al.* (2010) Defining translational research: Implications for training. *Acad Med* **85**(3): 470–475.
25. Gibbs JB. (2000) Mechanism-based target identification and drug discovery in cancer research. *Science* **287**(5460): 1969–1973.
26. Saijo N. (2002) Translational study in cancer research. *Intern Med* **41**(10): 770–773.
27. Saijo N, Nishio K, Tamura T. (2003) Translational and clinical studies of target-based cancer therapy. *Int J Clin Oncol* **8**(4): 187–192.
28. Woolf SH. (2008) The meaning of translational research and why it matters. *J Am Med Assoc* **299**(2): 211–213.
29. Toi M, Takebayashi Y, Chow LW. (2005) Translational research in breast cancer. *Breast Cancer* **12**(2): 86–90.
30. Mathew JP, Taylor BS, Bader GD, *et al.* (2007) From bytes to bedside: data integration and computational biology for translational cancer research. *PLoS Comput Biol* **3**(2): e12.
31. Hermiston TW, Kirn DH. (2005) Genetically based therapeutics for cancer: similarities and contrasts with traditional drug discovery and development. *Mol Ther* **11**(4): 496–507.
32. Butler D. (2008) Translational research: Crossing the valley of death. *Nature* **453**(7197): 840–842.
33. Tunis SR, Stryer DB, Clancy CM. (2003) Practical clinical trials: Increasing the value of clinical research for decision making in clinical and health policy. *J Am Med Assoc* **290**(12): 1624–1632.

34. Glasgow RE, Magid DJ, Beck A, *et al.* (2005) Practical clinical trials for translating research to practice: design and measurement recommendations. *Med Care* **43**(6): 551–557.
35. Fleming ES, Perkins J, Easa D, *et al.* (2008) The role of translational research in addressing health disparities: A conceptual framework. *Ethn Dis* **18**(2 Suppl 2): S2-155–160.
36. Tibayrenc M. (2002) Basic vs. applied research, field vs. bench work: the never-ending dialogues of the deaf. *Infect Genet Evol* **1**(4): 263–264.
37. Zinner DE, Campbell EG. (2009) Life-science research within US academic medical centers. *J Am Med Assoc* **302**(9): 969–976.
38. Holguin F, Moss I, Brown LA, Guidot DM. (1998) Chronic ethanol ingestion impairs alveolar type II cell glutathione homeostasis and function and predisposes to endotoxin-mediated acute edematous lung injury in rats. *J Clin Invest* **101**(4): 761–768.
39. Homer-Vanniasinkam S, Tsui J. (2012) The continuing challenges of translational research: Clinician-scientists' perspective. *Cardiol Res Pract* **10**(1155): 246710.
40. Wolf S. (1974) The real gap between bench and bedside. *N Engl J Med* **290**(14): 802–803.
41. Hait WN. (2005) Translating research into clinical practice: Deliberations from the American Association for Cancer Research. *Clin Cancer Res* **11**(12): 4275–4277.
42. Beumer HM, Porton WM. (1968) Morphologic effects of cytotoxic drugs on tumor cells. *Dis Chest* **53**(3): 252–256.
43. Leighton J. (1969) Propagation of cancer: Targets for future chemotherapy. *Cancer Res* **29**(12): 2457–2465.
44. Scott RB. (1970) Cancer chemotherapy — The first twenty-five years. *Br Med J* **4**(5730): 259–265.
45. DeVita VT Jr., Chu E. (2008) A history of cancer chemotherapy. *Cancer Res* **68**(21): 8643–8653.
46. Hanahan D, Weinberg RA. (2000) The hallmarks of cancer. *Cell* **100**(1): 57–70.
47. Bernier J, Hall EJ, Giaccia A. (2004) Radiation oncology: A century of achievements. *Nat Rev Cancer* **4**(9): 737–747.
48. Haffty BG, Kim JH, Yang Q, Higgins SA. (2006) Concurrent chemo-radiation in the conservative management of breast cancer. *Int J Radiat Oncol Biol Phys* **66**(5): 1306–1312.
49. Hirbe A, Morgan EA, Uluçkan O, Weilbaecher K. (2006) Skeletal complications of breast cancer therapies. *Clin Cancer Res* **12**(20 Pt 2): 6309s–6314s.

50. Munshi A. (2007) Breast cancer radiotherapy and cardiac risk: The 15-year paradox! *J Cancer Res Ther* **3**(4): 190–192.
51. Torres-Roca JF, Stevens CW. (2008) Predicting response to clinical radiotherapy: past, present, and future directions. *Cancer Control* **15**(2): 151–156.
52. Sofou S. (2008) Radionuclide carriers for targeting of cancer. *Int J Nanomedicine* **3**(2): 181–199.
53. van Meerbeeck JP, Meersschout S, De Pauw R, *et al.* (2008) Modern radiotherapy as part of combined modality treatment in locally advanced non-small cell lung cancer: Present status and future prospects. *Oncologist* **13**(6): 700–708.
54. Kiuru M, Itoh M, Cairo MS, Christiano AM. (2010) Bone marrow stem cell therapy for recessive dystrophic epidermolysis bullosa. *Dermatol Clin* **28**(2): 371–382, xii–xiii.
55. Liao Y, Itoh M, Yang A, *et al.* (2013) Human cord blood derived unrestricted somatic stem cells promote wound healing and have therapeutic potential for patients with recessive dystrophic epidermolysis bullosa. *Cell Transplant.* Epub ahead of print.
56. Osei-Bempong C, Figueiredo FC, Lako M. (2013) The limbal epithelium of the eye — A review of limbal stem cell biology, disease and treatment. *Bioessays* **35**(3): 211–219.
57. Ardehali R, Ali SR, Inlay MA, *et al.* (2013) Prospective isolation of human embryonic stem cell-derived cardiovascular progenitors that integrate into human fetal heart tissue. *Proc Natl Acad Sci USA* **110**(9): 3405–3410.
58. Tolar J, Xia L, Riddle MJ, *et al.* (2011) Induced pluripotent stem cells from individuals with recessive dystrophic epidermolysis bullosa. *J Invest Dermatol* **131**(4): 848–856.
59. Falavigna A, da Costa JC. (2013) Mesenchymal autologous stem cells. *World Neurosurg.* Epub ahead of print.
60. Sclafani AP. (2013) Stem cells and molecular advances in the treatment of facial skin. *Facial Plast Surg Clin North Am* **21**(1): 77–80.

CHAPTER 21

Stem Cells and Translational Research

*John R. Barbour**

21.1. INTRODUCTION

The traditional division of research was into one of two distinct categories: basic science and applied research. The primary goal of translational research is to meld the two paradigms together and bring the advancements from the laboratory to the clinical trial. Translational research requires that information and clinical findings flow from patient care outcomes and clinical studies to research-based facilities and basic science laboratories and *vice versa*. By removing traditional barriers to multidisciplinary alliances, translational research has the potential to drive the advancement of applied science for the future. An excellent example of how these two fields can work together in the treatment of disease is the usage of stem cell infusion and gene therapy.

The last 50 years have seen a focus on cellular alterations via pluripotent or omnipotent progenitor cells to interfere in disease processes such as heart failure, cancer and neuronal degeneration (Alzheimer's, multiple sclerosis, etc.). Stem cells represent an unheralded frontier in therapy for many disorders, but safe application merits a thorough evaluation of their effects on *in vitro* models. For this reason, bench scientists have become a valuable resource to the clinician researcher. This chapter will review

*Georgetown University School of Medicine, Washington, DC, USA

Full address: John R. Barbour, MD, Assistant Professor of Plastic Surgery, Georgetown University School of Medicine, Staff Surgeon, Washington DC VA Medical Center, Washington, DC 20007, USA; E-mail: *john.r.barbour@gunet.georgetown.edu* the pertinent current state of stem cell assisted translational research and prognosticate the future of the field of translational research and therapy.

21.2. HISTORY OF STEM CELL RESEARCH

Stem cells officially entered the scientific community when histologists postulated the existence of cells with hereditary characteristics of germ cells, developing the concept of pluripotency. The established fundamental characteristics of a stem cell include self-renewal and differentiation into somatic cells.[1] In the field of hematology, Pappenheim presented the notion of stem cells in describing a common cell origin that could produce both red and white blood cells.[2] Conheim and Pappenheim together proposed the idea of stem cells in the formation of tumors and leukemia. Thirty years later, evidence for single-cell self-renewal was demonstrated by the ability of leukemia cancer cells to transmit cancer from a single cell.

By the mid-20th century, identification of histocompatibility proteins and graft-versus-host disease provided the basis for immunologic tolerance. When the hematology and immunology fields converged in the 1950s through the study of the effects of radiation, it was shown that bone marrow reconstitution ensured successful skin grafts. It was through similar reconstitution experiments that the stem cell theory was proven in the early 1960s, when definitive evidence for the existence of hematopoietic stem cells (HSCs) was confirmed. Numerous tissue-specific or resident stem cells have also been described in the epidermis, intestine, brain, and to varying degrees in somatic tissue and solid organs.

Pioneering work involving pluripotent stem cells gained traction in the early 1980s with the successful isolation and culture of embryonic stem cells (ESCs) from the inner cell mass of blastocysts (pre-embryos). A scientific revolution for studying the embryonic to somatic cell transition was made possible for the first time, including the ability to study ESC self-renewal and differentiation outside the developing embryo. Despite this ability, it took 12 years to achieve proof of ESC self-renewal and pluripotency by generating living mice entirely from ESCs in 1993. In 1998, the ability to isolate human ESCs was described for the first time, revealing the possibility of a pluripotent stem cell as a source for new organs.[3]

In 2006, a major breakthrough was made when it was shown that somatic cells could revert to a pluripotent-like form through re-expression of key embryonic genes suppressed in the somatic state, and the concept of inducible pluripotent stem cells (iPSCs) was established.[4] It was also learned that a pluripotent cell could be produced by somatic cell nuclear transplantation into blastocysts. It was later discovered that ESCs could be isolated without destruction of the embryo.[5] These discoveries provided an opportunity to produce pluripotent stem cells while avoiding ethical objections and immunological rejection by using autologous cells.

As research emerged showing bone marrow stromal cells had many of the properties of multipotent mesenchymal stem cells (MSCs), scientists demonstrated that MSCs could differentiate into skeletal or cardiac muscle.[6] Scientists have transplanted bone marrow stem cells into the injured heart of rats and observed improvements in cardiac function. Bone marrow offers an attractive cell source due to its abundance and accessibility for autologous stem cell therapy. The past decade of basic and clinical studies have produced important findings, generated controversy, and raised new questions for the future of stem cell therapy.

21.3. EMBRYONIC STEM CELLS

Embryonic stem cells (ESCs) are pluripotent cells derived from the inner cell mass of a blastocyst. They contribute to all three germ layers: ectoderm, mesoderm and endoderm. A defining feature of ESCs is their ability to undergo prolonged symmetrical cell division in culture to produce identical pluripotent progeny. ESCs have evoked great interest, given their expected capacity to self-renew (resulting in an expansion of the cell population) and to differentiate into desired cell types (representing new sources for cell replacement therapy). Multiple signaling networks orchestrate the development and differentiation of ESCs and somatic stem cells into functional neuronal, hematopoietic, mesenchymal and epithelial lineages. There are active phase I trials with ESCs for cardiac disease, macular dystrophy, macular degeneration, and spinal cord injury. Assuming these demonstrate an acceptable safety profile, the number of clinical trials may grow at an unprecedented rate. They will likely expand the scope of stem cell therapy in traumatic injury, type-1 diabetes, muscular dystrophy, Parkinson's disease, or even multiple sclerosis and amyotrophic lateral sclerosis. Through translational studies, stem cell research and therapy have just begun to provide clinical answers.

21.4. MESENCHYMAL STEM CELLS

Mesenchymal stem cells (MSCs) are an attractive source for therapy: they provide reduced ethical concern, ease in expansion, and the potential for "off-the-shelf" stem cells. Adult MSCs can be isolated from a range of tissues including bone marrow and fat. The relatively accessible sources of MSCs combined with the ease with which the cells can be isolated and grown make them an attractive cell population for a range of therapeutic interventions. The differentiation of MSCs into different cell types is regulated by environmental cues. In general, MSCs differentiate along mesodermal lineages to form bone muscle and cartilage, although they have been suggested to be capable of differentiating into other lineages. One capacity of MSCs that is well established is their ability to release a wide range of signals that can modulate the host tissue responses. In a range of settings MSCs have been shown to exert a strong immune-modulatory effect on the host immune system.[7] This results in alterations in the relative expression levels of pro- and anti-inflammatory cytokines. Modulation of the immune system combined with the release of a range of trophic factors contributes to the capacity of MSCs to promote functional recovery in a number of settings. Clinical trials are currently ongoing or planned using MSCs in the treatment of graft-versus-host disease, heart failure, stroke, spinal cord injury, and multiple sclerosis.

MSCs exert immune suppressive properties, providing them with the potential for immune suppressive therapy such as autoimmunity, asthma, allergic rhinitis and graft versus host disease.[7] In addition, stem cells can be applied for bone and cartilage repair, cardiovascular disease, and neural repair/protection.

MSCs appear to be comprised of heterogeneous cell subsets, and a major advantage of studying MSCs is that they exhibit multilineage differentiation. However, it is unknown whether MSCs are indeed heterogeneous, or if differences in functions are attributed to the source and/or the method of culture. MSCs are ubiquitously present and can be isolated in both adult and fetal tissues, and they are in greatest concentration in bone marrow and adipose tissues. Human adipose tissue is a major source of MSCs, suggesting autologous lipoaspirate as a significant source of MSCs in future treatment.

MSCs differentiate along distinct lineages to generate stroma, adipocytes, chondrocytes, osteogenic cells, and cartilage. Expanded MSCs suggest that there are multiple subsets, and each subset might be primed to form a distinct specialized cell. This premise is based on the expression of specific differentiation genes. Studies suggest that it may be possible to select particular subsets of MSCs for specific cell therapy.

Morphologically, MSCs are symmetrical cells with fibroblastoid appearance. MSCs show structures comparable to smooth muscle and are generally classified as stem cells of mesodermal origin. The designation of neuroepithelial versus mesodermal is important to appreciate the limit of MSCs with regard to their ability to generate specialized cells. If the MSCs are of mesodermal origin, the ability to form neurons is significant, as this underscores the cells' plasticity to traverse germ layer: from mesoderm to ectoderm, generally referred as transdifferentiation. A concern for the clinical application of MSCs is their safety with regard to tumor formation and immune rejection. Limited data suggest that these stem cells could be safe, and importantly can be delivered across allogeneic barriers. If MSCs can be used as off-the-shelf sources, they are attractive for clinical application. In addition, MSCs can easily form other cell types, making them attractive for application to treat multiple disorders, as well as to repair and protect tissues.

The potential use of MSCs in clinical application is linked to their immune properties. Although currently considered immunosuppressive agents, MSCs can also exert immune-enhancing properties.[8] The results of early clinical trials for graft-versus-host disease with MSCs are mixed. Regardless of how MSCs behave in the laboratory, *in vivo* these cells will be exposed to a milieu of factors within any microenvironment. This will lead to functional crosstalk between the MSCs and mediators within the microenvironment. MSCs show functional plasticity with regard to their immune properties by exerting both immune suppressor and enhancer functions.[7] In addition, MSCs might be instructive cells to macrophages as a mechanism of tissue repair. MSCs produce varied cytokines that can mediate autocrine and/or paracrine stimulation.

MSCs offer the potential to treat complex disease for which no definitive solution has been obtained. These include neurological diseases such as Parkinson's disease, insulin-dependent diabetes, traumatic brain injury, Huntington's disease, and multiple sclerosis. Unlike *in vitro* conditions of the investigative laboratory, sites of injury and trauma present a vast number of proinflammatory mediators and cytokines. For example, if Interleukin-1 (IL-1) were produced in an inflammatory microenvironment, it would be able to interact with MSC-derived neurons. By placing MSCs in a microenvironment containing the appropriate cues, MSCs can give rise to functional myocardial tissue, allowing them to serve as a valuable source in regenerative medicine. MSCs can exert paracrine effects through secretion of various cytokines that lead to suppression of inflammation.[9]

Despite *in vitro* findings, the clinical significance in terms of treatment of patients remains to be tested. A major issue with treatment is MSCs' role in supporting and/or protecting tumors. Cancer stem cell therapy brings to the surface the safety of treating patients with MSCs, as the presence of cancer stem cells might not correlate with clinical detection of the cancer. As research in this area progresses, the future may see broad applications for MSCs in the treatment of cellular injury. In-depth experimental systems are required for defined animal models. The plastic properties of MSCs provide these cells the ability to interact with mediators at different microenvironments.

21.5. INDUCED PLURIPOTENT STEM CELLS

As viable human brain tissue is not available for use in studying disease development and creating therapies, researchers need an alternative cell source for this purpose. Embryonic stem cells fit this role but have disadvantages, especially for treatments, including immune rejection by the recipient. In 2006, Yamanaka made a landmark discovery: adult cells could be genetically engineered to revert back to a pluripotent, stem cell-like state.[4] These cells are referred to as inducible pluripotent stems cells (iPSCs).

As iPSC production has rapidly improved, the cells have served as an alternate source as compared to traditional fetal, embryonic and adult stem cells. The primary advantages of iPSCs compared to other stem cells are that iPSCs can be created from the tissue of the same patient that will receive the transplantation, avoiding immune rejection and the lack of ethical implications as cells are harvested from a consenting adult. These patient-specific cells can be used to study diseases *in vitro*, to test drugs on a human model without endangering anyone, and potentially act as tissue replacement for diseased and damaged cells.

Like other stem cells, iPSCs have the ability to proliferate indefinitely *in vitro*, creating a theoretically unlimited source of cells. Like embryonic stem cells, iPSCs can also differentiate into any cell of the body, regardless of the original tissue from which they are created. Scientists have found how to direct the differentiation of pluripotent stem cells into many types of target tissue, including neural tissue. iPSCs demonstrate that by the introduction of just four genes into somatic cells that normally cannot differentiate, cells can be created that can differentiate into every cell type in the body. The early results of iPSC differentiation studies look promising. Human fibroblasts have been successfully turned into iPSCs that then are differentiated into insulin-producing cells, a result that holds much potential for the treatment of diabetes. Mouse iPSCs have been differentiated into cardiovascular cells that show the contractile beating of myocardial tissue.[10]

There are issues that still must be addressed for iPSC technology, such as the tendency for tumors to evolve after iPSC transplantation and the low efficiency of the technology. Nonetheless, iPSCs could completely change how diseases are approached in biomedical research. iPSCs could create perfect models for the cells of the central nervous system that are harmed in disease. They demonstrate that specialized cells and tissue can be transformed into other types of cells, proving cells are more flexible than previously thought. However, establishing the safety and efficiency of inducing pluripotency in cells from older and diseased patients will require extensive research. An alternative to pluripotency could be direct cell reprogramming, such as turning fibroblasts directly into cardiomyocytes while avoiding a pluripotent stage. Alternatively, it has been suggested to store stem cells in advance from healthy young donors.

The issue of tissue compatibility remains one of the greatest unaddressed challenges. In consideration of the therapeutic paracrine effects from stem cells, it may not be necessary for stem cells to differentiate in order to be beneficial. It may be essential to either prolong the immune privilege or match histocompatibility profiles between the host and allogeneic donor. Since a pluripotent source is capable of nearly unlimited expansion, these cells could address both quantity and compatibility issues. An allogeneic stem cell source is an attractive option for overcoming quantity, age, and disease limitations, as stem cells can be harvested in sufficient quantity in advance and made available for widespread distribution. A cell bank of allogeneic stem cells representing all human histocompatibilities is an attractive possibility.

21.6. INFLAMMATORY MEDIATORS AND STEM CELLS

IL-1 is an inflammatory cytokine which regulates other cytokines with positive and negative effects. Transforming growth factor-β (TGF-β) is a separate cytokine that serves a role as both a pro- and anti-inflammatory mediator. An important characteristic of TGF-β is its role in oncogenesis. The oncogenic role of TGF-β is important if MSCs and other stem cells are introduced directly for therapy. The placement of stem cells within a milieu of inflammatory mediators will establish crosstalk between the cells and the microenvironment. This may alter the functions and also the biology of the implanted stem cells. The efficiency of MSCs or other stem cells in clinical application will depend on studies looking at the effects of cytokines on genes associated with pluripotency. Many of these genes are associated with oncogenesis and tumor suppression.

IL-1 is significant in an understanding of stem cell responses to tissue factors because of its ability to induce the expression of other inflammatory mediators. Since IL-1 can be induced by tissue insults such as infectious agents or hypoxia, it is likely that this cytokine can regulate the expression of inflammatory mediators at the sites of tissue injury. IL-1 can exert its effects on stem cells either directly or indirectly through other cytokines. In addition, IL-1 can affect neurons by inducing cytokines in the surrounding cells, which in turn can bind to neurons.

TGF-β receptors are ubiquitously expressed by various cell types, including malignant cells. TGF-β1 is an immune modulator, inhibits cell proliferation, and affects differentiation and apoptosis. TGF-β1 has also been reported to activate the differentiation of MSCs to myoblasts, which can support tumor growth.[11] This property of TGF-β on MSCs is critical to future therapy, as it would be dangerous if the recipient has an underlying/undiagnosed tumor.

Upon homing to target tissues, MSCs can secrete a variety of cytokines, including TGF-β, which has been shown to recruit immunosuppressive T-cell subsets. Through the secretion of TGF-β, MSCs may be able to enhance cardiac repair through recruitment of regulatory T lymphocytes.[12] It is critical to explore the effects of cytokines and MSCs within the cardiac tissue microenvironment in order to understand the benefits and limitations of stem cell therapy. The recruitment of T lymphocytes could be important for long-term engraftment of MSCs, as studies have shown immunogenic responses to differentiated MSCs in cardiac repair.

21.7. CURRENT TRANSLATIONAL DIRECTIONS

Translational research has proven to be a powerful process that drives the clinical research engine. However, a stronger research infrastructure could strengthen and accelerate this critical part of the clinical research enterprise. Growing barriers between clinical and basic research, along with the complexities involved in conducting clinical research, are making it more difficult to translate new knowledge to the clinic. Clinical trials are only initiated after extensive basic science and solid reproducible pre-clinical evidence supports their safety. Early clinical trials of stem cell therapy ultimately resulted in mixed results. However, new questions arise that can be explored or from which refined methods can be developed.

21.7.1. Cardiac Disease

As a result of improved patient management, survival following acute myocardial infarctions has increased dramatically. However, many of these survivors progress to heart failure because they lack functional recovery.

As the leading cause of mortality and morbidity in the developed world, cardiac disease has provided fertile ground for early translational stem cell research into clinical therapy. The ability to culture cells was established 60 years ago and was initially exclusive to cancer cell lines. In 1960, Harary and Farley cultured mammalian cardiomyocytes from rats.[13] It was 35 years later that the concept emerged of injecting cardiomyocytes into the heart to provide functional benefit following myocardial infarction.

Currently, cardiovascular disease ranks as the leading cause of death in the industrialized world, accounting for greater mortality than cancer, accidents and pulmonary disease. It is also a significant cause of morbidity worldwide. The incidence of myocardial ischemia increases with age and declining health. Over time, cardiomyocytes become susceptible to ischemia-induced death, leading to scar formation and diminished contractile function. Myocardial repair and regeneration has been a topic of interest in the field of stem cell biology, as MSCs have been shown to differentiate into functional myocytes when subjected to the proper microenvironment or chemical induction cocktail.[6] MSCs are an attractive stem cell agent in cardiac repair, showing potential differentiation to cardiac, vascular muscle, and endothelial cells.

At the dawn of the century, cardiac cell therapy merged with regenerative medicine. Researchers confirmed the therapeutic benefit of bone marrow stem cell transplantation following myocardial infarction and the ability of bone marrow cells to regenerate myocardium. Before optimization in pre-clinical models, the first human patient received bone marrow injections into their myocardium in 2001.

There have been significant therapeutic gains achieved through translational research and application of stem cell-based therapies in cardiac pathologies. It is acknowledged that unmanipulated bone marrow stem cell populations are unlikely to differentiate to cardiomyocytes to replace those lost from a myocardial infarction. From long-term studies and meta-analyses, it has been demonstrated that stem cell therapy provides significant benefit to some patients, just not all patients. Inconsistencies in clinical protocols can partially explain the early failure to deliver the functional improvements observed in young, healthy animals. The age and the effect of disease on the stem cell source are likely the most significant detractions on measured outcomes.

Unlike traditional therapeutic agents, stem cell therapy is currently limited by the availability of biological substrate from the patient. This presents a unique problem: an afflicted patient population could be depleted of stem cells in the organ most in need of therapy, or in the bone marrow as a consequence of chronic disease or age. Adjuvant therapy can combine stem cells with pharmacology, bioengineering or gene therapy to enhance the therapeutic utility of stem cells for expansion or function. A system of standardized protocols for producing or combining stem cells and adjuvant therapy for clinical intervention should be formulated.

A balanced approach in the basic and clinical sciences is needed to determine the most effective stem cell source and protocol for intervention to address pathologies we do not fully understand. It is important to acknowledge that the only way to know whether a protocol for stem cell delivery is effective is to conduct a clinical trial. For future successes in stem cell therapy, it will be important to build collaborations to achieve genuine clinical translation. Extensive interaction will be required between disciplines, such as the engineering and biological sciences, to develop novel techniques for functional monitoring of stem cells and the recipient organs. There are several conditions that require cardiac cell remodeling, which is likely to be achieved only from a pluripotent source.

Prior to the administration of MSCs for cardiac repair, the hurdle of delivery must be overcome. Intravenous administration is an attractive strategy because it is not invasive and also allows for repeated administration. The migratory ability of MSCs to cardiac tissue is one of the reasons why these cells may be efficient for cardiac repair. However, a significant obstacle posed by MSC therapy is the low percentage of MSCs that ultimately migrate to the injured heart. Co-administration of MSCs and granulocyte colony-stimulating factor in rats with myocardial infarction has been shown to result in improved efficiency.[14] Research into optimization interactions may lead to facilitation of MSC delivery to ischemic cardiac tissue.

Another significant drawback of stem cell therapy using MSCs for cardiovascular disease is that MSCs have fastidious growth conditions, leading to cell death if the stem cells are not properly maintained. MSCs may be engineered to express chemokines to improve the cells' functions in cardiac repair. Contact-independent factors play important roles in maintaining

MSC viability in the context of stem cell therapy for cardiovascular disease.

Within the next decade, it is likely that at least one or more stem cell therapy protocols will become an accepted standard for cardiac patients. However, it is unlikely that pluripotent stem cell sources will enter standard practice in the immediate future. There will be a high burden of proof to show that a pluripotent source is safe, necessary, and superior to current autologous cell therapy.

21.7.2. Neurological Disease

The capacity for self-renewal sets stem cells apart from other precursor or progenitor cells and implies that stem cells have the potential for the generation of unlimited numbers of progeny. This characteristic presents both a strength as well as a liability for stem cell-based therapies in the central nervous system (CNS). There are multiple types of stem cells that arise at different stages in development and become increasingly restricted in the types of progeny they generate. While ESCs can generate a wide range of different tissue cell types during early development, tissue-specific stem cells are retained in many tissues in the adult. The retention of tissue-specific stem cells in some tissues is self-evident. Tissues in which there is continuous cell turnover, such as blood and skin, require a constant source of cells to replenish those lost. What was less anticipated was that tissues such as the nervous system, where it was thought there was relatively little cell turnover, would also contain stem cells in the adult. Studies over the last two decades have, however, demonstrated the presence of neural stem cells in both the developing and adult CNS.[15,16] These cells are found in specific regions of the CNS and have the potential to generate a wide range of neurons as well as astrocytes and oligodendrocytes. Under non-pathological conditions, endogenous neural stem cells generate new neurons that populate the hippocampus and the olfactory bulb.

One of the first diseases to be the focus of cell therapies was Parkinson's disease. The initial attraction of Parkinson's disease was that the functional deficits in this disease result from the loss of dopaminergic neurons located in the substantia nigra. The unique specificity of the type of cells and their defined location were originally thought to be an advantage for cell-based therapies. However, it has become evident that more widespread neural diseases, particularly those with a significant immunological involvement, are better targets for stem cell therapy.

In studies where the goal is the development of clinical applications of stem cell therapies, a key step should be to define the mechanisms by which stem cell therapies enhance functional recovery. Understanding the mode of action of stem cells will then inform the selection of cell type and route of application. ESCs have been extensively studied in models of neural injury and disease. While ESCs have the advantage of being the most plastic and therefore capable of generating the most diverse cell populations, in most therapeutic situations this is unnecessary and may be detrimental. Early application of human ESC-derived oligodendrocyte precursor cells (OPCs) to treat patients with spinal cord injury has been halted because of expense and questionable efficacy.[17] In general, in pathologies where specific populations of cells are lost, a primary goal of stem cell therapies is functional replacement of the lost neurons and functional integration into the host CNS. In such cases, a logical option would be neural stem cells.

MSCs may be ideal candidates for therapeutic treatment in the adult CNS. Damage to the CNS through either disease or injury leads to areas of ischemia that result in neuronal cell loss, and oligodendrocyte death.[18] Contusion or penetrating lesions to the CNS cause bleeding, neuronal and oligodendrocyte loss, and glial scar formation. Even diffuse conditions such as Alzheimer's disease or multiple sclerosis (MS) generate regions characterized by neuronal cell death as well as glial scarring. In most cases of neurological disease, there is loss of neurons and/or oligodendrocytes and astrocyte activation. The activation of astrocytes occurs in response to a local proinflammatory stimulus, indicating that therapies which promote the genesis of neurons and oligodendrocytes while both reducing astrocyte activation and suppressing immune responses may be beneficial.[18] Several studies support the notion that treatment with MSCs regulates neural injury.

A potential mechanism of function of neural stems cells (NSCs) is that they are home to areas of damage, and proliferate and differentiate into the missing cell type, resulting in cell replacement. The class of neural precursors that is most easily isolated and grown in large quantities is OPCs. These cells share many of the characteristics of stem cells and have been tested in models of MS. In MS, auto reactive T cells attack the myelin sheath surrounding axons in the CNS, leading to a blockade of signal transduction along the damaged axon and death of the oligodendrocytes that are the source of the myelin sheath. Replacement of damaged oligodendrocytes by new OPCs has been shown to have benefit in MS as well as spinal cord injury and stroke.[19,20]

Many stem cell populations including NSCs and MSCs have strong immunosuppressive properties. In animal models of MS, treatment with MSCs suppresses T-cell activation consistent with an immune-regulatory role.[21] The significance of this immune-modulatory action has been demonstrated through adoptive transfer studies in which T cells were taken from animals with autoimmune encephalitis (EAE) that had been treated with NSC-derived neurospheres. These T cells had a greatly reduced capacity to induce disease when transferred to naive animals compared to T cells derived from untreated EAE animals.[22] The cellular and molecular mechanisms mediating these changes are not well defined and may reflect both cell-to-cell interactions as well as the release of immune-modulatory cytokines.

Neural stem cells are found in the developing and adult CNS of virtually all mammals, including humans. These cells or their progeny are capable of migrating long distances through the CNS and replacing neurons and oligodendrocytes lost to injury or insult. Studies demonstrate that MSCs promote the responsiveness of endogenous NSCs. Transplantation of bone marrow MSCs stimulates the proliferation of stem cells in the neurogenic regions of the hippocampus. These effects likely reflect the release of bioactive signals from the transplanted MSCs.

21.7.3. Endocrine Disease

Type-1 diabetes results from autoimmune destruction of pancreatic islet β cells, with insulin deficiency and complete dependence on exogenous insulin treatment. The paucity of donors for pancreas or islet allograft transplantation has prompted the search for alternative sources for β-cell replacement therapy. Pluripotent stem cells induced to differentiate into β cells can be used to overcome the shortage of therapeutically effective material to transplant. Studies have shown that β-cell mass is dynamically regulated like other tissues.[23,24] The interplay of cell expansion and reduction mechanisms determines the amount of β-cell mass. Expansion can occur through β-cell hypertrophy, self-replication, transdifferentiation and neogenesis. In contrast, reduction can result from β-cell atrophy, death or loss of stability. The development of strategies to avoid β-cell mass reduction or enhance β-cell mass expansion could provide a promising avenue for therapy of both type-1 and type-2 diabetes. The microenvironmental cures required for differentiation of stem cells into pancreatic β cells will promote the regeneration of large cells required for therapy of the disease.[24] Several sources of stem/precursor cells have been suggested that can repopulate the damaged β cells, and those include ESCs, HSCs, MSCs, resident stem cells, and iPSCs. MSCs have been used to achieve this goal and to mitigate the effect of hyperglycemia by regenerating β cells.

Numerous studies have suggested the existence of stem cells within the pancreas that can give rise to insulin-producing β cells. There is additional evidence suggesting that transdifferentiation of liver cells can generate β cells.[25] Several studies have reported that bone marrow-derived stem cells can be differentiated into insulin-expressing cells.[26,27] Neural progenitor cells from the brain also have the capacity to differentiate into insulin-expressing cells. ESCs have the ability to differentiate into cells with an insulin-expressing phenotype.[28] Other sources for β-cell regeneration include pancreas-derived multipotent progenitor cells, pancreatic duct cells, and umbilical cord blood cells.[29] MSCs have suppressive effects on T-cell response to antigens and offer a novel cell-based approach for the prevention of autoimmune diabetes and for islet cell transplantation. Translational studies looking at the effect in human patients at controlling hyperglycemia have focused on all these progenitor cells and may hold the key to therapeutic management and cure for diabetes. Transplantation of adult human bone marrow-derived MSCs could be a promising source to replenish insulin-producing cells.

21.7.4. Cancer/Cancer Syndromes

Although the existence of cancer stem cells (CSCs) was first proposed over four decades ago, only in the past decade have these cells been identified in hematological malignancies and solid tumors in areas such as the breast, prostate, brain and colon. Exploration of the difference between CSCs and normal stem cells is crucial not only for the understanding of tumor biology but also for the development of specific therapies that target these cells in patients.[30] Yet the origin of CSCs and the mechanisms by which they arise remain elusive. For tumors containing a subpopulation of CSCs, there are at least two proposed mechanisms for how the CSCs could have arisen: oncogenic mutations that inactivate the constraints on normal stem cell expansion or, alternatively, oncogenic mutations that generate continual proliferation of cells in the cell cycle that no longer enter a postmitotic differentiated state. This would effectively create a pool of self-renewing cells in which further mutations can accumulate.[31,32]

Signaling mechanisms activated by TGF-β family proteins have emerged as key players in the self-renewal and maintenance of stem cells in their undifferentiated state. This includes the selection of a differentiation lineage and the progression of differentiation along individual lineage.[30] Through gene knockout experiments and observation of ESCs, TGF-β-family proteins have emerged as regulators of the maturation of cells and as suppressors of carcinogenesis.[33] When TGF-β signaling is disrupted, the imbalance can result in an undifferentiated phenotype, and cancer may ensue.[34]

Stem cells share some characteristics of cancer cells, including their ability to proliferate by a similar self-renewal process and the loss of contact inhibition.[35] Furthermore, tumor growth and cancer progression are thought to be driven by a cancer stem cell population. Thus, studies of stem cells may provide guidance for our understanding of cancer development, and *vice versa.* Hepatocellular carcinoma (HCC) is a highly complex disease that is generally resistant to commonly used chemotherapeutics and radiation therapy. As a virus-associated and inflammation-associated cancer, both host immune response and tumor microenvironment have crucial roles in HCC pathogenesis. Early molecular classification of HCCs has occurred through transcriptomic, genetic and epigenetic profiling of tumors, and novel molecular and cellular targets in HCC have been pursued, including cancer stem cells.[36,37]

An approach to colorectal cancer (CRC) stem cell therapy involves targeting of disrupted pathways essential to stem cell self-renewal in CRC. These include the Wnt, Hedgehog, Notch, and TGF-β pathways.[38] Such an approach requires specific identification and delineation of the molecular pathways used by CRC stem cells and identification of agents that can either block the pathways or propel CRC stem cells to differentiate, thereby enhancing their sensitivity to chemotherapeutic agents. One such proposed agent is oral calcium supplementation. Dietary calcium has been extensively shown to reduce colon cell proliferation, the extent of the crypt's proliferative zone, and colon carcinogenesis in animal models as well as humans.[39] Malignant transformation of colon cells, however, leads to decreased sensitivity of these cells to calcium and disruption of their apoptotic mechanisms. Paradoxically, calcium supplementation is reported to stimulate colon cell proliferation in adenomatous polyps. This apparent antagonistic response likely is mediated by disrupted Wnt signaling in colorectal tumors and demonstrates the tightly linked and regulated process of colonic stem cell self-renewal, proliferation and differentiation.[39] Targeting of Wnt-driven stem cell proliferation, along with dietary calcium loading to restrain APC and CaSR and promote adherens junctions, may prove an effective strategy. This highlights the necessity of novel combinations of therapy targeting the multifaceted nature of CRC stem cells.[40] The stem cell niche is essential to modulate the capacity of colonic stem cells to proliferate, migrate or invade. Strategies targeting the CRC stem cell niche also are an attractive option and may prove effective as CRC therapy.[41]

Lastly, hereditary cancer syndromes can provide powerful insight into our understanding of somatic mutations in sporadic cancers, as well as implicated cell signaling pathways.[30,42,43] Beckwith–Wiedemann syndrome (BWS) is a hereditary stem cell cancer syndrome currently linked to deregulation of an imprinted cluster on human chromosome 11p15.[44–46] It has been observed that β2SP$^{+/-}$ mice are born with many phenotypic characteristics observed in BWS patients. These include dramatic visceromegaly, macroglossia, abnormal ear folds, and mid-face dysmorphology. This is followed by the development of multiple cancers, including carcinomas of the gastrointestinal tract (liver, stomach, intestine and pancreas), as well as renal and adrenal adenocarcinomas.[47–49] It has been theorized that loss of β2SP is one of the causal factors leading to the syndrome.[30,50] Thus, mutations of β2SP in cancers could lead to new diagnostic, prognostic insights and new therapeutic strategies into difficult to manage subsets of CRC and HCCs.[51,52] Epigenetic regulation of β2SP expression in human BWS and the $\beta 2SP^{+/-}$ mouse phenotype could offer valuable models for further genetic studies of this disease, as well as sporadic cancers associated with this stem cell disorder.[53–55]

21.8. FUTURE DIRECTIONS

Most investigators agree that the best combination of cells and adjunctive therapies has not been identified. Tissue engineering has not yet found its place in cardiac regeneration owing to the limited knowledge of cardiac remodeling. Stem cell therapy alone will be insufficient and will require adjuvants such as gene therapy, cell-based gene therapy, or tissue engineering techniques to stimulate and complement the intervention. Until these restrictions are better understood, the ability to translate stem cell therapy universally is limited.

The vast majority of our understanding comes from studies on animal models, and before stem cell therapies can be widely utilized for the treatment of disease, there are challenges that must be overcome. One question is whether human stem cell populations have similar functional properties to their animal counterparts. Encouraging early studies suggest this is to be expected. Treatment of mice with EAE with human MSCs results in a dramatic reduction in functional deficits, improved histological appearance and reduction in the levels of pro- and anti-inflammatory cytokines. These data suggest that knowledge gained from animal models may be applicable to human cells.

An additional challenge in moving stem cell therapies into the clinic is to identify the most suitable source of stem cells for therapeutic purposes. Several aspects contribute to defining a suitable source of cells. These include the ease with which the original stem cells can be obtained, the efficacy with which those cells can be expanded to generate cells required for treatments, the efficiency with which stem cells can be converted to the appropriate precursor or product, and long-term outcomes in functional recovery. Spinal cord injury may require relatively few cells in a specific location adjacent to the area of damage, while more diffuse conditions such as MS may require multiple systemic infusions of large numbers of cells. While it may be feasible to generate sufficient NSCs for spinal cord injuries, MSCs may be a better cellular source for MS.

The advent of stem cell therapy, other than the well-established therapy with hematopoietic stem cells, brings us the question of how the cells should be applied: as pluripotent cells versus partially or fully differentiated cells. Another fundamental issue is defining the heterogeneity in the transplanted populations of cells. While the majority of therapeutic stem cells are induced to differentiate along a particular lineage, residual stem cells may have the capacity to generate unwanted cell types or act as a future source for tumor formation. Currently, there is little evidence from animal studies that stem cell therapies lead to tumor formation; however, these studies are short lived and patients may survive many decades following stem cell therapies.

A final issue with developing stem cell therapies is their labor-intensive nature. In most ongoing and proposed clinical trials of MSCs in MS, there is a tendency to use autologous cells that are derived from the patient's bone marrow. These cells have to be harvested by a skilled physician, expanded under at least GLP-like conditions, and then infused at the initiation of therapy. These steps are time and labor intensive and each step adds risk of failure and expense. For experimental studies in animals or humans this is not a major concern, but if stem cell therapies are widely implemented then the process will need to be reduced and the uniformity of growth conditions established.

Given the early stage at which the field of stem cell therapies exists, there is little insight into potential complications. Although MSCs have been used as an adjunct therapy in graft-versus-host disease for a number of years, they have yet to be widely used in other clinical trials. Studies in spinal cord injury models in the rodent highlight the potential for unexpected outcomes. Transplantation of OPCs or a subset of astrocytes results in some functional recovery, but this is complicated by an unfortunate increase in allodynia. The mechanisms responsible for these symptoms are unknown and compromise the use of these cells for this condition. The temptation to move rapidly forward with clinical trials of multiple varieties of stem cells for different clinical indications is very strong; however, this should be tempered. A realization should be that our current understanding of the mechanisms of stem cell therapies is limited and the ability to control stem cells once they are introduced into the patient is non-existent.

Identification of the molecular mechanisms mediating the therapeutic effects of stem cells will provide opportunities to enhance their efficacy. It is an attractive concept that once critical signaling pathways are identified, the therapeutic capacity of stem cells may be enhanced through increasing their expression of the relevant molecules. The half-life of transplanted cells or their progeny is relatively short and the stem cells are lost over a period of days even though their effects are prolonged. The development of inducible suicide mechanisms in stem cell populations developed for clinical use will likely be an important advance for the future.

The possibility that there may be commercially available, well-characterized stem cell populations available for clinical use could be a major step forward. An alternative source of autologous stem cells for clinical applications may be derived from the emerging induced iPSC field. Animal studies have developed protocols that allow the directed differentiation of iPSC-derived neural cells down specified lineages and have shown functional capabilities. Studies on human neural precursors and iPSCs are quickly gaining similar momentum.

21.9. CONCLUSION

Within the next decade, it is likely that at least one or more stem cell therapy protocols will become the standard of care for cardiac patients. However, it is unlikely that pluripotent stem cell sources will enter standard practice in the immediate future. There are active investigations looking at stem cell effects on cardiac disease, macular dystrophy, macular degeneration, and spinal cord injury. These studies will likely expand the scope of stem cell therapy in trauma, type-1 diabetes, muscular dystrophy, Parkinson's disease, multiple sclerosis, and amyotrophic lateral sclerosis. Through translational studies, stem cell research and therapy have the potential to provide important clinical answers.

Once critical signaling pathways are identified, the therapeutic capacity of stem cells may be focused. The temptation to move rapidly forward with clinical trials of multiple varieties of stem cells for different clinical indications is strong; however, clinicians should be cautious. Understanding of the mechanisms of stem cell therapies is limited and the ability to control stem cells after implantation into the patient is inadequate. The potential for oncogenesis or tumor formation exists. There will be a high burden of proof based on quality clinical trials to show that a pluripotent source is safe, necessary, and superior to current autologous cell therapy.

REFERENCES

1. Morrison SJ, Kimble J. (2006) Asymmetric and symmetric stem-cell divisions in development and cancer. *Nature* **441**: 1068–1074.
2. Pappenheim A. (1917) Prinzipien der neueren morphologischen Haematozytologie nach zytogenetischer Grundlage. *Folia Haematologica* **21**: 91.
3. Thomson JA. (1998) Embryonic stem cell lines derived from human blastocysts. *Science* **282**: 1145–1147.
4. Takahashi K, Yamanaka S. (2006) Induction of pluripotent stem cells from mouse embryonic and adult fibroblast cultures by defined factors. *Cell* **126**: 663–676.
5. Martin GR. (1981) Isolation of a pluripotent cell line from early mouse embryos cultured in medium conditioned by teratocarcinoma stem cells. *Proc Natl Acad Sci USA* **78**: 7634–7638.
6. Pittenger MF. (1999) Multilineage potential of adult human mesenchymal stem cells. *Science* **284**: 143–147.
7. Chen PM. (2011) Immunomodulatory properties of human adult and fetal multipotent mesenchymal stem cells. *J Biomed Sci* **18**: 49.
8. Newman RE. (2009) Treatment of inflammatory diseases with mesenchymal stem cells. *Inflamm Allergy Drug Targets* **8**: 110–123.
9. Gnecchi M. (2008) Paracrine mechanisms in adult stem cell signaling and therapy. *Circ Res* **103**: 1204–1219.
10. Mauritz C. (2008) Generation of functional murine cardiac myocytes from induced pluripotent stem cells. *Circulation* **118**: 507–517.
11. Li Y. (2004) Transforming growth factor-beta1 induces the differentiation of myogenic cells into fibrotic cells in injured skeletal muscle: A key event in muscle fibrogenesis. *Am J Pathol* **164**: 1007–1019.
12. Burchfield JS, Dimmeler S. (2008) Role of paracrine factors in stem and progenitor cell mediated cardiac repair and tissue fibrosis. *Fibrogenesis Tissue Repair* **1**: 4.

13. Harary I, Farley B. (1960) *In vitro* studies of single isolated beating heart cells. *Science* **131**: 1674–1675.
14. Cheng Z. (2008) Mobilization of mesenchymal stem cells by granulocyte colony-stimulating factor in rats with acute myocardial infarction. *Cardiovasc Drugs Ther* **22**: 363–371.
15. Song HJ, Stevens CF, Gage FH. (2002) Neural stem cells from adult hippocampus develop essential properties of functional CNS neurons. *Nat Neurosci* **5**: 438–445.
16. Weiss S. (1996) Multipotent CNS stem cells are present in the adult mammalian spinal cord and ventricular neuroaxis. *J Neurosci* **16**: 7599–7609.
17. All AH. (2012) Human embryonic stem cell-derived oligodendrocyte progenitors aid in functional recovery of sensory pathways following contusive spinal cord injury. *PLoS One* **7**: e47645.
18. Amor S. (2010) Inflammation in neurodegenerative diseases. *Immunology* **129**: 154–169.
19. Tai YT, Svendsen CN. (2004) Stem cells as a potential treatment of neurological disorders. *Curr Opin Pharmacol* **4**: 98–104.
20. Lindvall O, Kokaia Z. (2006) Stem cells for the treatment of neurological disorders. *Nature* **441**: 1094–1096.
21. Ghannam S. (2010) Immunosuppression by mesenchymal stem cells: Mechanisms and clinical applications. *Stem Cell Res Ther* **1**: 2.
22. Pluchino S. (2003) Injection of adult neurospheres induces recovery in a chronic model of multiple sclerosis. *Nature* **422**: 688–694.
23. Bouwens L, Rooman I. (2005) Regulation of pancreatic beta-cell mass. *Physiol Rev* **85**: 1255–1270.
24. Bonner-Weir S. (1994) Regulation of pancreatic beta-cell mass *in vivo. Recent Prog Horm Res* **49**: 91–104.
25. Banga A. (2012) *In vivo* reprogramming of Sox9+ cells in the liver to insulin-secreting ducts. *Proc Natl Acad Sci USA* **109**: 15336–15341.
26. Milanesi A. (2012) beta-Cell regeneration mediated by human bone marrow mesenchymal stem cells. *PLoS One* **7**: e42177.
27. Zanini C. (2011) Differentiation of mesenchymal stem cells derived from pancreatic islets and bone marrow into islet-like cell phenotype. *PLoS One* **6**: e28175.
28. Schroeder IS (2006) Insulin-producing cells. *Methods Enzymol* **418**: 315–333.
29. Reddi AS, Kuppasani K, Ende N. (2010) Human umbilical cord blood as an emerging stem cell therapy for diabetes mellitus. *Curr Stem Cell Res Ther* **5**: 356–361.

30. Mishra L, Derynck R, Mishra B. (2005) Transforming growth factor-beta signaling in stem cells and cancer. *Science* **310**: 68–71.
31. Pardal R, Clarke MF, Morrison SJ. (2003) Applying the principles of stem-cell biology to cancer. *Nat Rev Cancer* **3**: 895–902.
32. Tang Y. (2008) Progenitor/stem cells give rise to liver cancer due to aberrant TGF-beta and IL-6 signaling. *Proc Natl Acad Sci USA* **105**: 2445–2450.
33. Massague J, Blain SW, Lo RS. (2000) TGF-beta signaling in growth control, cancer, and heritable disorders. *Cell* **103**: 295–309.
34. Mishra L. (2005) The role of TGF-beta and Wnt signaling in gastrointestinal stem cells and cancer. *Oncogene* **24**: 5775–5789.
35. Mishra L. (2009) Liver stem cells and hepatocellular carcinoma. *Hepatology* **49**: 318–329.
36. Ji J, Wang XD. (2012) Clinical implications of cancer stem cell biology in hepatocellular carcinoma. *Semin Oncol* **39**: 461–472.
37. Tanaka S, Arii S. (2012) Molecular targeted therapies in hepatocellular carcinoma. *Semin Oncol* **39**: 486–492.
38. Li L, Neaves WB. (2006) Normal stem cells and cancer stem cells: The niche matters. *Cancer Res* **66**: 4553–4557.
39. Whitfield JF. (2009) Calcium, calcium-sensing receptor and colon cancer. *Cancer Lett* **275**: 9–16.
40. Abdul Khalek FJ, Gallicano GI, Mishra L. (2010) Colon cancer stem cells. *Gastrointest Cancer Res*(Suppl 1): S16–S23.
41. Boman BM, Huang E. (2008) Human colon cancer stem cells: A new paradigm in gastrointestinal oncology. *J Clin Oncol* **26**: 2828–2838.
42. Massague J. (2008) TGF-beta in Cancer. *Cell* **134**: 215–230.
43. Radtke F, Clevers H. (2005) Self-renewal and cancer of the gut: Two sides of a coin. *Science* **307**: 1904–1909.
44. Feinberg AP, Ohlsson R, Henikoff S. (2006) The epigenetic progenitor origin of human cancer. *Nat Rev Genet* **7**: 21–33.
45. Feinberg AP. (2007) Phenotypic plasticity and the epigenetics of human disease. *Nature* **447**: 433–440.
46. Weksberg R, Shuman C, Smith AC. (2005) Beckwith–Wiedemann syndrome. *Am J Med Genet C Semin Med Genet* **137C**: 12–23.
47. Miles HL, Hofman PL, Cutfield WS. (2005) Fetal origins of adult disease: A paediatric perspective. *Rev Endocr Metab Disord* **6**: 261–268.
48. Wiedemann HR. (1964) Familial malformation complex with umbilical hernia and macroglossia — A "new syndrome"? *J Genet Hum* **13**: 223–232.

49. Combs JT, Grunt JA, Brandt IK. (1966) New syndrome of neonatal hypoglycemia. Association with visceromegaly, macroglossia, microcephaly and abnormal umbilicus. *N Engl J Med* **275**: 236–243.
50. Ying BW. (2003) Allele frequencies for two STR loci D11S1977 and D22S444 in Chinese population. *J Forensic Sci* **48**: 219.
51. Tang Y. (2005) Transforming growth factor-beta suppresses nonmetastatic colon cancer through Smad4 and adaptor protein ELF at an early stage of tumorigenesis. *Cancer Res* **65**: 4228–4237.
52. Lin L. (2009) The STAT3 inhibitor NSC 74859 is effective in hepatocellular cancers with disrupted TGF-beta signaling. *Oncogene* **28**: 961–972.
53. Halliday J. (2004) Beckwith–Wiedemann syndrome and IVF: A case-control study. *Am J Hum Genet* **75**: 526–528.
54. Gosden R. (2003) Rare congenital disorders, imprinted genes, and assisted reproductive technology. *Lancet* **361**: 1975–1977.
55. Gosden RG, Feinberg AP. (2007) Genetics and epigenetics — Nature's pen-and-pencil set. *N Engl J Med* **356**: 731–733.

IX. The Role of Translational Research in Public Health and Behavioral Sciences

Tobacco Use and the Cancer Patient: Missing the Translation of Effective Therapy

Graham W. Warren[*,†,||] *and Erica N. Peters*[‡,§]

22.1. INTRODUCTION

Tobacco use remains the leading preventable cause of premature death in the US, accounting for over 440,000 deaths each year.[1] According to the 2010 Surgeon General Report, smoking has been causally linked to multiple types of cancer, including cancer of the lung, head and neck, stomach, pancreas, kidney, cervix, and bladder, as well as acute myeloid leukemia.[2] Smoking has a particularly robust relationship with cancer, as smoking been shown to cause 30 percent of all cancers and 80 percent of mortality from head and neck and lung cancer.[1] In spite of the pernicious effects of tobacco use on cancer development and course, upward of 50 percent of patients with cancer who were smokers before their diagnosis continue to smoke.[4–7] Even for patients who are able to quit after their diagnosis, relapse rates are

*Department of Radiation Oncology, Hollings Cancer Center, Medical University of South Carolina, Charleston, South Carolina, USA
†Department of Cell and Molecular Pharmacology and Experimental Therapeutics, Hollings Cancer Center, Medical University of South Carolina, Charleston, South Carolina, USA
‡Friends Research Institute, Baltimore, Maryland, USA
§Yale University School of Medicine, New Haven, Connecticut, USA
||Corresponding author: Graham W. Warren, MD, PhD, Associate Professor, Vice Chairman for Radiation Oncology, Department of Radiation Oncology, Department of Cell and Molecular Pharmacology and Experimental Therapeutics, Medical University of South Carolina, 169 Ashley Ave., Charleston, SC 29425, USA; Tel:+1-843-876-2295; E-mail: *warrengw@musc.edu*

substantial[8] and relapse will often occur within just a few weeks or months of quitting.[9–11] Thus, further knowledge on how to most effectively address tobacco use in patients with cancer is needed to reduce the prevalence and impact of tobacco use in this vulnerable population.

Although attention has increasingly focused on the need to effectively address tobacco use in oncology research and practice, multiple barriers to tobacco use assessment, smoking cessation, and tobacco use treatment still exist. These barriers may prevent evidence on the deleterious effects of tobacco use on cancer treatment response from being translated into standard oncology research and practice. These barriers may spread across several domains, from characteristics of patients to systemic attitudes regarding cancer research funding, and may hinder further progress in reducing tobacco use in cancer patients. Identification of barriers is a necessary step before determining specific, targeted strategies to most effectively promote tobacco use assessment and smoking cessation interventions in oncology research and practice.

In this chapter, we summarize existing literature on how tobacco use affects treatment outcomes in patients with cancer and how tobacco use is currently addressed in oncology research and practice. First, we examine how tobacco use affects treatment outcomes in patients with cancer by describing effects of tobacco use on outcomes for cancer treatment. Second, we provide the current status of tobacco use assessment in oncology research and practice and of smoking cessation treatment options available to patients with cancer. Third, because tobacco use assessment and smoking cessation interventions are not universal in oncology research and practice, we report on barriers to implementing evidence-based tobacco use assessment and treatment among cancer patients. Fourth, we offer strategies for overcoming the challenges these implementation barriers present, in the hopes of translating scientific findings on tobacco use in cancer patients into improved cancer treatment outcomes.

22.2. EFFECTS OF TOBACCO USE ON OUTCOMES IN CANCER PATIENTS

A full review of the effects of smoking in cancer patients is beyond the scope of this chapter. The objective of this section is to review some of the breadth of clinical effects of smoking on outcomes for cancer treatment as related to survival, toxicity, risk of second malignancies, and other health effects. In addition, a few studies are mentioned that present some of the evidence that smoking cessation may improve outcomes in cancer patients.

22.2.1. Survival

The deleterious effects of tobacco smoking on cancer treatment response, as indicated by survival outcomes, have been consistently observed in both tobacco-related and non-tobacco-related disease sites. In a cohort of 5,185 cancer patients from 13 disease sites, current tobacco smoking at diagnosis increased overall mortality as compared with recent quitters (within 12 months prior to diagnosis), former smokers (quitting 12 months or more prior to diagnosis), and never-smokers.[12] Current smoking increased disease-specific mortality as compared with former and never-smokers in the overall cohort, and also increased disease-specific mortality as compared with recent quitters in patients with head/neck and lung cancer. In other studies of patients with cancer in traditional tobacco-related disease sites, such as lung or head/neck, tobacco use has been associated with decreased overall survival and progression-free survival.[13–15] The effect of tobacco smoking on overall survival and progression-free survival in head/neck cancer patients has been estimated to be about 1 percent per pack year.[16] Though nasopharyngeal cancers are not necessarily associated with tobacco use, smoking has also been associated with decreased overall survival in nasopharyngeal cancer patients.[17]

The negative effects of tobacco on survival outcomes have also been noted in cancer patients with traditionally non-tobacco-related cancers. Among patients with breast cancer, tobacco smoking increases the risk of overall mortality[12,18–20] and breast cancer mortality.[12,18,20] Among patients with gynecological malignancies (i.e., cancer of the ovary, cervix or endometrium), current tobacco smoking decreases overall, disease-specific and progression-free survival[21–27]; however, former smoking, duration of tobacco use, and cigarette packs per day may not be significantly related to survival.[22,24–25] Among patients with gastrointestinal malignancies, ever-smoking and smoking at cancer treatment follow-up have been shown to decrease overall and cause-specific survival.[28–30] In one study, the adverse effects of smoking on survival have been observed specifically in patients treated with chemoradiotherapy but not surgery.[31] Among patients with prostate and genitourinary cancer, current smoking increases the risk of high-risk disease, increases the rate of progression to hormone refractory prostate cancer, and decreases cancer-specific and overall survival.[32–39] Results from these individual studies have been supported by the conclusion of a meta-analysis of 24 cohort studies including 21,759 prostate cancer patients in which current smoking increased the risk of fatal prostate cancer with higher risks in heavier smokers.[40] Finally, among patients with non-solid malignancies (i.e., acute myeloid leukemia or non-Hodgkin's lymphoma), smoking decreases progression-free, disease-specific and overall survival[41–46] with effects noted primarily in current smokers rather than former smokers.[44]

The effect of smoking on decreased cancer survival may be facilitated by the effect of smoking on increased risk of cancer recurrence after treatment. Among patients with cancer of the head/neck,[15] bladder,[47,48] and prostate,[36,49] current or former smoking increases the risk of recurrence after treatment with medication, surgery or radiation. Among patients with chronic myelogenous leukemia treated with stem cell transplant, ever-smoking increased the risk of cancer recurrence by 1.7 percent per pack year of smoking.[50] Overall, smoking appears to decrease the effectiveness of cancer treatment as well as increase the aggressiveness of cancer, both contributing to decreased cancer-related survival.

Smoking is further associated with poor cancer treatment outcome as indicated by decreased survival patterns as well as adverse non-cancer-related outcomes such as heart disease. Among breast cancer patients or survivors, smoking is associated with increased risk of cardiomyopathy, myocardial infarction, coronary artery disease requiring intervention, congestive heart failure, and death due to acute myocardial infarction.[34,51–54] Furthermore, risk of heart disease may be significantly increased when radiotherapy for breast cancer is combined with current smoking.[51] Smoking at or following cancer diagnosis is associated with increased risk for cardiovascular disease in testicular cancer survivors[55] and survivors of non-Hodgkin's lymphoma.[56] Due to the fact that the net effect of increased cardiovascular risks is an increased risk of death, the non-cancer-related effect due to cardiovascular outcomes may dominate overall cancer survival patterns in diseases such as prostate cancer.[32] As a consequence, clinicians and patients should be aware of the cancer-related and non-cancer-related mortality risks of tobacco use in cancer patients.

22.2.2. Toxicities

Another cancer treatment outcome influenced by tobacco smoking is prevalence of cancer treatment-related toxicities. Among patients with lung cancer, tobacco smoking is associated with decreased lung function.[57] In breast cancer patients, smoking is associated with increased nausea, depression, migraines, telangiectasia, skin necrosis, infections, reconstructive failure, and overall complications, as well as decreased hip bone mineral density.[58–63] Smoking increases surgical complications such as risk for wound failure in sarcoma patients[64] and active smoking increases the risk of developing anastomotic leak, pneumonia, and pulmonary morbidity in esophageal cancer patients.[65–67] Current smoking increases clinically-relevant chemotherapy-induced mucositisin patients with solid tumors.[68] In leukemia patients treated with hematopoietic stem cell transplant, current smoking increases the number of days for hospitalization and pulmonary and respiratory deaths.[44] Current smoking increases the risk of complications related to the rectum, bladder, small bowel, and overall pelvis, as well as the risk of comorbidity and postoperative infections in cervical cancer patients.[30,69] Current smoking also increases overall complications, 30-day mortality, and wound healing[70] in colorectal cancer patients. Among patients with prostate cancer, current smoking decreases urinary function recovery and utility, but former smoking has no effect on recovery.[71]

22.2.3. Second Malignancies

Smoking increases the risk of second malignancy in cancer patients. Among testicular cancer patients with at least five years of survival, smoking at or following cancer diagnosis increases risk for second malignancy.[55] Among breast cancer patients, current smoking at diagnosis and at most recent follow-up interview increases risk of contralateral breast cancer.[72] In gastric cancer patients treated with curative surgery, current smoking increases the risk of developing second primary cancers, with no increased risk in former smokers,[73] suggesting that the effects of smoking on risk of second malignancy may be reversible with cessation.

Several studies suggest that smoking may enhance the carcinogenic effects of cancer treatment. Current smoking at diagnosis in Hodgkin's disease patients increases the risk of developing lung cancer, with a lesser effect in former smokers.[74] Notably, the addition of smoking to radiotherapy or to chemoradiotherapy appears to have a synergistic effect on the risk of developing lung cancer.[74] Among breast cancer patients with a primary lung cancer ten or more years after diagnosis, never-smokers with postmastectomy radiotherapy have no significant increase in the risk of lung cancer, but smoking with no radiotherapy increases the risk of lung cancer 5.9 fold; when smoking is combined with radiotherapy, the risk of any lung cancer increases 18.9 fold, and the risk of ipsilateral breast cancer increases 37.6 fold.[75] The synergistic effects of radiotherapy and smoking have also been observed in patients with prostate cancer treated with radiotherapy. Current smoking alone significantly increases bladder cancer risk, and current smoking combined with radiotherapy further increases risk.[76]

22.2.4. Other Health-related Effects

Smoking negatively impacts the quality of life and health behaviors of cancer patients. Among female patients with cancer of the breast, colon or rectum, or endometrium participating in the longitudinal Women's Health Study, persistent smokers have a lower quality of life as measured by higher incidence of stroke, higher rate of hypertension, lower physical activity, lower mental health, and lower emotional health.[77] Current smoking is associated with increased depressive symptoms in testicular cancer survivors.[78] Lung cancer patients appear to feel more shame than breast or prostate cancer patients[79]; however, people with a history of smoking have higher feelings of guilt and shame in all patients regardless of disease site, suggesting that social and emotional health may be related to a "guilt by association" phenomenon. In terms of health behaviors, current smoking is associated with decreased breast, cervical and gastric cancer screening among cancer survivors.[80] Current smoking is also a significant risk factor for poor adherence to cancer-related therapy.[81] In a trial of medication to prevent breast cancer, smoking decreases medication adherence by 25 percent.[82]

22.2.5. Smoking Cessation and Cancer Outcomes

In spite of the widespread effects of tobacco on cancer treatment response, there are limited studies evaluating the effects of tobacco cessation on cancer treatment outcomes. However, in these studies, data suggest that smoking cessation may improve outcomes for cancer patients. Among patients with oral cavity cancer treated with surgery, smoking reduction and cessation after diagnosis improves three-year and five-year survival.[83] In men with non-muscle invasive bladder cancer treated with transurethral resection, current smoking increases risk of recurrence 2.2 fold as compared with quitters.[84] In prostate cancer patients treated with radiotherapy, current smoking increases diarrhea, cramps, defecation urgency, sudden emptying, and incomplete emptying, while patients who quit after radiotherapy only have increased sudden emptying.[85] Among prostate cancer patients treated with prostatectomy, current smoking five years prior to surgery increases the risk of diagnosis at a younger age, advanced stage at diagnosis, and positive surgical margins; however, only current smoking at one year after diagnosis is associated with increased recurrence.[86] These data suggest that smoking cessation may prevent the adverse effects of smoking in cancer patients, but considerable work is needed to improve our understanding of the potential benefits of smoking cessation after a diagnosis of cancer.

22.2.6. Limitations in the Current Evidence

Unfortunately, most studies that have demonstrated an effect of tobacco use on cancer treatment outcomes have either relied on retrospective reviews of medical records or have only minimally assessed tobacco use (i.e., assessed any former or current use with a categorical index, without assessing amount of former and current use). Categories of smoking status generally include current, recent quitter, former, ever, never, and unknown smoking status. However, there is no standard method to categorize smoking status. For example, current smoking in the published literature has been defined as any smoking at diagnosis, smoking within one month of diagnosis, smoking within six months of diagnosis, smoking within one year of diagnosis, smoking within five years of diagnosis, smoking with a 20 pack-year history, smoking one year after diagnosis, etc. As a result, it is difficult to standardize published analyses based upon smoking status. Analyses that include prior tobacco use are also non-standard and include definitions based upon pack-year history, duration of smoking, age of smoking initiation, time since quitting, and a broad diversity of exposure history (e.g., 1, 3, 7, 10, 13, 20 and 31 pack-years). This limitation has been observed by others[87–91] who collectively note that these methodological limitations make it difficult to accurately gauge or quantify the direct impact of tobacco use on cancer treatment outcomes. However, these limitations also confer some strength in the association between smoking and negative outcomes in cancer patients because most studies support a negative association regardless of tobacco use definition. Currently, major oncology groups, including the American Association for Cancer Research and the American Society of Clinical Oncology, maintain policy statements about the importance of tobacco control.[92,93] Additional work is clearly needed to standardize assessments and tobacco use definitions.

22.3. TOBACCO USE ASSESSMENT AND TREATMENT FOR PATIENTS WITH CANCER

Tobacco use is such a critical factor for an individual's medical condition that smoking status has been called a "vital sign."[94] Accordingly, standards for tobacco use assessment in all individuals (i.e., all general patients) have been issued.[95] These standards include asking every patient who presents to a healthcare facility if they use tobacco, advising all tobacco users to quit, and assessing the willingness of all tobacco users to make a quit attempt; these comprise the first three of the five As (Ask, Advise, Assess, Assist and Arrange) model for treating tobacco use and dependence.[95]

Specific to individuals with cancer, recommendations for standardized tobacco use assessment in cancer clinical trials have been proposed.[96] These include assessment of lifetime smoking status and secondhand smoke exposure for all patients with cancer, amount of tobacco exposure (i.e., cigarettes plus other forms of tobacco) for former and current smokers, nicotine dependence, and readiness to quit for current smokers. Tobacco status should be collected at cancer diagnosis, at treatment intake, and throughout treatment and follow-up.[96]

Despite evidence-based standards and recommendations, routine assessment of tobacco use has not been fully integrated into cancer research protocols or practice. An examination of clinical trials in one US state for non-tobacco-related cancer malignancies showed that only three of 46 trials assessed tobacco status at treatment intake, and none assessed tobacco status through follow-up.[97] Additionally, a recent study of 155 actively accruing clinical trials in the National Cancer Institute Cooperative Group Program revealed that only 29 percent and 5 percent of trials assessed any tobacco use at enrollment and during follow-up, respectively.[90] Although a search of hospital records in the cancer registry of one US state suggested that tobacco use assessment may be more prevalent in clinical practice (83.3 percent) than in cancer research protocols, not all current and former smokers were assessed for key information on tobacco exposure, such as cigarettes per day or duration of quitting.[98] Thus, both oncology research and practice appear to suffer from a lack of complete information on tobacco use history in patients with cancer.

A diagnosis of cancer often motivates patients to spontaneously stop smoking.[4] Indeed, patients with cancer report that they are motivated to quit smoking[9,10,96,99] and believe that quitting smoking would be beneficial to their health.[11,100] Efficacious smoking cessation interventions have been shown to significantly increase the odds of quitting among all smokers.[95] These interventions include behavioral counseling and pharmacotherapy, such as nicotine replacement therapy (i.e., gum, patch, lozenge, nasal spray), bupropion (Zyban), and varenicline (Chantix). Among patients with cancer, these same interventions have documented efficacy, and their use is strongly encouraged.[4,101–107] The importance of successful smoking cessation in patients with cancer cannot be understated; stopping smoking is associated with fewer post-operative complications, fewer tobacco-related second primary cancers, increased survival time, and improved quality of life.[62,89,101,108–117] Therefore, promoting the use of efficacious interventions in patients with cancer is critical for increasing the likelihood of successful smoking cessation and improving cancer treatment outcomes.

22.4. BARRIERS TO TOBACCO USE ASSESSMENT AND TREATMENT IN PATIENTS WITH CANCER

A strong evidence base has consistently supported the need to integrate tobacco use assessment, emphasize the importance of smoking cessation, and promote the use of efficacious smoking cessation interventions in oncology research and practice. However, these aims have not yet been fully realized. Below, we describe domains of barriers to complete implementation of tobacco control strategies among patients with cancer.

22.4.1. Patient-Level Barriers

Few barriers to prospective, comprehensive assessment of tobacco use have been identified that relate to characteristics of cancer patients. One patient-level barrier that has been mentioned in the literature is patients' reluctance to admit persistent smoking with a diagnosis of a malignancy, especially if the malignancy is a tobacco-related cancer.[96] Another patient-level barrier is variability in cancer patients' smoking patterns over time. Cancer patients will often report high quit rates at cancer diagnosis or the beginning of treatment but later show high relapse rates.[118] However, smoking relapse is delayed in cancer patients relative to non-cancer patients.[119,120] Failure to assess tobacco use at all patient encounters may miss clinically meaningful changes in smoking status that can dramatically influence cancer treatment outcome. Other patient-level barriers to tobacco use assessment have not been identified, likely because integrating tobacco use assessment into oncology research and practice is often initiated by providers, health systems, and policy makers rather than patients themselves.

Several patient-level barriers to smoking cessation and use of smoking cessation interventions have been identified. Demographic characteristics that are associated with poor smoking cessation outcomes after cancer diagnosis, either with or without treatments, are male gender,[121] younger age,[122–125] less education,[121,126] and lower income.[120] Smoking-related patient characteristics that relate to poor cessation outcomes include high rates of nicotine dependence,[119,127–128] more intense cravings,[120,129,130] lower self-efficacy to quit,[129,130] lower perceived risk of smoking,[127,130] no prior smoking quit attempts,[102] and having relatives who smoke in the home.[122,131] For cancer patients who do quit smoking, shorter quit duration before surgery is associated with smoking relapse.[120,132]

Patient-level barriers to successful smoking cessation also arise from biopsychosocial factors that may be either premorbid or directly related to cancer diagnosis and treatment. These include poorer health,[9] elevated symptoms of psychological and physical distress,[119,121,122,131,133–136] and alcohol abuse.[133] Patients who smoke and have a tobacco-related malignancy may be aware of the robust relationship between tobacco use and cancer and, thus, experience guilt and responsibility for their disease, fear being stigmatized, and feel it might be too late for them to quit.[118,137–140] These negative reactions may contribute to patients' reluctance to discuss their smoking with their providers and consequent failure to receive information about cessation resources.[140] Other patients may not be aware of the relationship of their smoking to their cancer or may have misperceptions about their vulnerability to smoking-related illnesses, potentially making them less likely to change their smoking.[136,141]

Efficacious interventions are available to assist cancer patients in quitting smoking, but patients with cancer appear to underutilize these interventions. Although unaided quit attempts are significantly less successful than aided attempts,[95] cancer patients frequently report that they have quit "cold turkey," i.e., without the aid of treatment.[11,121,129,131,142–144] To our knowledge, reasons for the high frequency of unaided quit attempts in patients with cancer have not been elucidated. One possible explanation is that some patients may be overwhelmed with information at the time of cancer diagnosis and are not able to absorb provider messages about efficacious smoking cessation strategies.[136] Collectively, much work remains to integrate the diversity of potential patient-level barriers into more effective tobacco cessation strategies for cancer patients.

22.4.2. Provider-Level Barriers

Although the majority of cancer patients who smoke report that their healthcare providers (i.e., oncology physicians, nurses, and staff) have advised them to quit smoking,[142,143,145,146] there may be barriers to universal tobacco use assessment and provision of smoking cessation interventions that can be attributed to providers' behavior or attitudes. Most of the barriers detailed below have arisen from studies on smoking cessation interventions in cancer patients; however, they may also have relevance for tobacco use assessment.

Research on provider-level barriers to addressing tobacco use in cancer patients has consistently cited time constraints as a reason to not assess tobacco use or provide smoking cessation resources.[104,143,147–151] In the face of competing time demands, providers may miss opportunities to identify smokers, encourage them to quit, and facilitate a quit attempt.[104,151] As a way of managing time constraints, providers may provide targeted smoking cessation advice to those cancer patients who are more vulnerable to continued smoking and relapse due to multiple comorbid illnesses, high psychological distress, lack of healthcare insurance, or heavy smoking.[143] This means that cancer patients who are perceived as less vulnerable may receive less clinical attention, even though they may equally benefit from tobacco use assessment and smoking cessation intervention. As another way of managing time constraints, providers may partially implement evidence-based cessation advice, which has unknown effects on the likelihood of successful cessation.[152]

Another consistently cited provider-level barrier to addressing tobacco use in cancer patients is lack of tobacco-related knowledge or training. Although efforts to include tobacco in medical curricula have grown in recent years,[153] providers may have limited training or experience in working with patients who smoke.[154] They may also lack skills and knowledge about the benefits of smoking cessation in patients with cancer[150,155] and may have uncertainty regarding the delivery of smoking cessation medication or appropriate health behavior messages.[104,147,149,156] Even when providers do assess and treat smoking cessation, there may be important variability in the advice and type of assistance they supply.[140]

Providers' attitudes about the relative importance of tobacco use in cancer patients stand as potential barriers to adequately addressing tobacco use. Providers may be reluctant to add to patients' stress level and guilt about tobacco use,[149,150] and they may misperceive that patients are not interested in smoking cessation.[104,149] In spite of evidence that smoking cessation after cancer diagnosis is associated with improved cancer treatment response, providers may believe that it is too late to stop smoking once diagnosed with cancer.[149,150,157] It is unclear what contributes to unfavorable attitudes about the role of tobacco use assessment and smoking cessation interventions in cancer patients, although it is possible that providers being current smokers themselves may make delivery of cessation interventions less likely.[154]

There are few studies evaluating perceptions of tobacco assessment and cessation by oncology providers. A recent survey was completed by over 1,500 members of the International Association for the Study of Lung Cancer (IASLC) comprised primarily of thoracic oncology providers to evaluate tobacco assessment and cessation practice patterns, perceptions and barriers to implementation.[158] Importantly, over 90 percent of respon dents reported that tobacco was important to cancer outcomes and that tobacco cessation should be a standard part of cancer care. However, only approximately 40 percent of MD-level practitioners provided cessation support. Respondents reported that inadequate education and inability to get patients to quit were the dominant barriers to providing cessation support. These data demonstrate that even motivated practitioners (who believe that tobacco cessation is an important part of cancer care) do not routinely provide tobacco cessation support. Increasing assessment and cessation support, increasing provider education, and increasing the efficacy of cessation are potentially dominant mechanisms to improve tobacco control in cancer patients.[158]

22.4.3. Disease-Level Barriers

In comparison to research on patient- and provider-level barriers, research on disease-level barriers to tobacco use assessment and smoking cessation interventions is scarce. The studies that are available indicate that type of cancer and the inherent nature of cancer as a potentially life-threatening illness may influence the likelihood of addressing tobacco use in cancer patients.

In the aforementioned examination of 155 actively accruing clinical trials in the National Cancer Institute Cooperative Group Program, frequency of assessing any tobacco use at treatment intake varied by type of cancer, with assessment occurring more often in trials of lung or head and neck cancer (i.e., tobacco-related cancer sites) than trials of any other cancer type.[90] According to a recent population-based survey of US cancer survivors and non-cancer individuals, smoking cessation also varies across type of cancer, with cervical cancer (22.5 percent) and melanoma (23.3 percent) having the lowest smoking quit rates.[125] Smoking cessation may vary by stage of cancer diagnosis[3] and type of cancer treatment received.[113]

Several inherent aspects of the disease may impede adequate implementation of tobacco use assessment and smoking cessation in oncology research and practice. For example, addressing tobacco use in the face of a life-threatening illness may seem like a low priority.[119] However, a longer time duration between cancer diagnosis and assessment of smoking status seems to make cessation less likely.[131] Even when tobacco use is addressed, some smoking cessation treatment options may be limited by medical contraindications, such as trouble swallowing or depression.[118] It appears that addressing tobacco use within the context of cancer treatment is also important to increase the likelihood of adhering to medical treatment.[131]

22.4.4. System-Level Barriers

Finally, system-level factors may impact tobacco use assessment and smoking cessation interventions among cancer patients. Pertaining to a broad array of institutions, these barriers may be found in systems related to training oncology providers, treating cancer patients, and conducting and funding oncology research. System-level barriers may be conceptualized as surrounding some other barriers; for instance, the attitudes and behaviors conveyed by systems that provide medical treatment to cancer patients may have direct bearing on the practices of oncology providers.

System-level barriers that impede tobacco use assessment in oncology research and practice may overlap with ones that have characterized providers, such as perceived lack of relevance of smoking to cancer treatment outcome and lack of training in tobacco use assessment and smoking cessation outcomes. Besides occurring among providers, these barriers could be evident among administrators of oncology settings who have decision-making authority to mandate tobacco use assessment and the provision of smoking cessation resources in their systems. Even if systems dictate that tobacco use be addressed in oncology settings, sustained maintenance may be difficult due to changes in other parts of the system or to decreased funding (e.g., fewer oncology staff members).[104] The lack of systemic support for tobacco use assessment and treatment is even apparent in National Cancer Institute cancer centers: the provision of tobacco use treatment is not considered a "core service" at most centers, and less than half of them have designated personnel to offer tobacco use treatment.[118] Moreover, less than half of these cancer centers even assess smoking status as a vital sign.[118]

Within the research domain, system-level barriers may arise from the belief that smoking must significantly affect cancer treatment outcomes in order to justify inclusion in research objectives.[96] However, without accurate assessment of tobacco use in research studies, statistical examination of the effect of smoking on cancer treatment cannot be undertaken, and the lack of accurate assessments will further limit the development of an evidence-based precedence that would justify inclusion of smoking status in future studies. Another example of a system-level barrier in the research domain may explain the reluctance of investigators to include tobacco use assessment in oncology studies: there may be a lack of adequate research support (e.g., funding, available staff) for the collection and storage of desired tobacco use data.[96] Also contributing to barriers in the research system are underfunding of research, especially with regard to lung cancer research, and historical conflict and perception of different goals among institutes that would fund cancer research.[159] With the anticipated merger of some institutes within the National Institutes of Health, it is unclear how funding of research on tobacco use and cancer will be affected.

22.5. OVERCOMING BARRIERS TO TOBACCO USE ASSESSMENT AND TREATMENT IN PATIENTS WITH CANCER

To overcome the challenges that the aforementioned barriers represent, the following topics warrant attention in future research.

22.5.1. Improving and Increasing Tobacco Use Assessment

Not all patients with cancer are assessed for former and current tobacco use. In fact, a minority of patients in cancer clinical trials are assessed for any tobacco use at treatment enrollment, and even fewer are assessed throughout cancer treatment.[90] Those patients who are assessed for tobacco use in the context of clinical practice may not be asked to provide essential information on patterns of former and current use. Underscoring the need for improved quality of tobacco use assessment in patients with cancer, several studies have emphasized the need for prospective, repeated tobacco use assessment that gathers details of smoking beyond categorical distinction of individuals as former, current or non-smokers.[90,96] To avoid redundancy with these studies, we do not explicitly detail all tobacco-related items that should be assessed in cancer patients; we refer readers to Table 1 in Ref. 96 for a more thorough articulation of recommended assessment items. However, we do reiterate the rationale for the assessment strategy provided in Ref. 96 as a way of highlighting the need for improved tobacco use assessment through standardized assessments at cancer diagnosis, during treatment, and at follow-up and to include tobacco cessation support as a standard part of cancer care.

Prospective assessment is needed in order to minimize recall biases,[160] and because recall may be less accurate for some tobacco use variables, such as cigarettes per day, relative to others.[161] Repeated assessment is needed because smoking patterns in cancer patients tend to show variability over time,[118–120] and consistently inquiring as to tobacco use status at all patient encounters may detect clinically meaningful changes that can dramatically influence cancer treatment outcomes. Importantly, assessment of tobacco use in patients with cancer may be easier than in the general population because most patients with cancer often follow a rigorous medical schedule for 6 to 18 months during and following cancer treatment. This schedule promotes opportunities to address tobacco use through repeated assessments and cessation counseling for appropriate patients.[90]

To further enhance the validity of data collected from prospective, repeated tobacco use assessment, biochemical verification of tobacco use (e.g., breath carbon monoxide, urine or serum cotinine) can be employed. Data show that cancer patients will be compliant with biochemical verification, and biochemical verification may be essential for confirming or refuting self-report of smoking abstinence.[162] Furthermore, biochemical verification is standard practice in smoking clinical trials[163] and may be a cost-effective mechanism of potentially improving cancer treatment outcomes.[162]

With a clear rationale for and a strong evidence base to support improved tobacco use assessment in patients with cancer, the frequency of tobacco use assessment stands to increase in oncology research and practice. Barriers to tobacco use assessment can be overcome by relying on established assessment guidelines that can be easily incorporated into most clinical trial designs without altering primary or secondary trial objectives, clinical evaluations, stratification, drug administration, or outcomes analysis. Relevant to both researchers and providers, accurate assessments can be completed rapidly (i.e., in a few minutes) and with minimal demand on staff or financial resources.

A potential strategy for overcoming barriers to tobacco use assessment may involve incentivizing providers for demonstrating compliance with evidence-based tobacco use assessment. Incentivizing procedures, such as pay-for-performance systems, deliver monetary incentives to an individual or group of providers, or even to institutions, contingent on the performance of a target behavior or achievement of performance milestones. Pay-for-performance systems are increasingly being adopted as a means of improving the quality of healthcare and reducing public health risks in healthcare settings.[164] Future research, especially with the use of randomized controlled trials, can investigate whether or not incentivizing procedures can effectively stimulate universal integration of tobacco use assessment into oncology settings.

22.5.2. Promoting Smoking Cessation and Use of Smoking Cessation Interventions

Stopping smoking has beneficial effects on cancer treatment outcomes, and efficacious smoking cessation treatments can be safely applied in patients with cancer. Nonetheless, not all cancer patients initiate smoking cessation at the time of cancer diagnosis, and those that do quit usually relapse. Only a minority of cancer patients take advantage of stop-smoking aids that could significantly enhance their likelihood of successfully quitting smoking. Barriers to successful smoking cessation and utilization of smoking cessation interventions include demographic and smoking history characteristics of patients, reluctance or difficulty in advising best practices for smoking cessation among providers, type and stage of cancer, beliefs about the importance of smoking cessation relative to other aspects of cancer treatment, and lack of institutional support for smoking cessation. As a way of informing potential future research, we offer strategies that have been identified, but not yet fully developed, as potential ways to overcome these multiple barriers to successful smoking cessation. Rigorous future research will be essential for developing effective strategies to promote smoking cessation and use of smoking cessation interventions in patients with cancer.

22.5.3. Tailoring Smoking Cessation Treatments

Tailoring existing smoking cessation treatments to individuals' needs has been offered as a strategy for optimizing the efficacy of treatments in all smokers,[95] and this strategy may be even more important in patients with cancer. As Gritz *et al.*[119] state, challenges of tailoring cessation interventions to meet the particular needs of individuals with cancer include: "(1) high levels of nicotine dependence, (2) pressure for abrupt and immediate smoking cessation to enhance cancer treatment efficacy, (3) elevated levels of psychological distress, which are known to impede smoking cessation efforts, (4) the delayed nature of relapse compared to smokers in the general population, (5) physical limitations imposed by disease and treatment which can affect recommendations regarding exercise regimens and dietary change, and (6) medical contraindications to certain types of NRT and other pharmacotherapy." In light of these challenges, careful consideration of matching smoking cessation treatment to individuals' clinical needs appears necessary. One way of ensuring a good match of treatments to individuals is by soliciting patients' perceptions of treatments they are likely to use and find beneficial.[140,152] Another way of effectively matching treatments to individuals may come from pharmacogenetics: identifying genetic variants that are predictive of therapeutic response may boost smoking cessation treatment uptake and efficacy.[165]

Related to the topic of tailoring smoking cessation interventions is determining patients' preferred channel of intervention delivery. In various research studies, smokers have reported that they prefer individualized versus group smoking cessation programs[142] and were more interested in mailed health interventions as compared with in-person or phone- or computer-based interventions.[166] Patient factors (e.g., age, presence of a partner who smokes)[142] may be associated with preferred channel of intervention delivery or likelihood of quitting after receiving an intervention, suggesting that matching of interventions to individuals' needs is critical.

Finally, treatments may need to be tailored by gender. In the aforementioned study of 5,185 cancer patients from 13 disease sites, tobacco smoking decreased survival in head/neck cancer and lung cancer more in men than women.[12] Among bladder cancer patients treated with radical cystectomy, tobacco smoking decreased overall survival, but the effect of tobacco on disease specific survival was noted only in men.[167] In colon and rectal cancer patients, tobacco smoking increased the risk of diabetes and ischemic heart disease, but the effects were noted specifically in men.[168] These studies raise interesting questions regarding potential gender-specific effects of tobacco on cancer outcomes and the relevance of tailoring tobacco cessation treatments to gender. Also, these studies suggest a potential necessity to include gender-specific effects of tobacco on cancer outcomes, as well as considerations for potential differences in cessation efficacy based upon gender.

22.5.4. Consistent Delivery of Smoking Cessation Interventions

Patients with cancer tend to receive cancer-related care from multiple providers, such as oncology physicians, nurses and staff. They may receive follow-up care and management of general medical issues from providers in community oncology and internal medicine settings.[169–171] They may also have encounters during and after cancer treatment from tobacco treatment specialists. The question therefore arises as to which of these providers should advise smoking cessation and deliver smoking cessation interventions. Patients have reported smoking cessation advice as being more help ful when provided by physicians versus staff,[152] and researchers have made the case for various providers being ideally positioned to deliver smoking cessation interventions.[143,149,154]

For all smokers, advice from multiple healthcare providers is considered more effective than advice from a single provider.[95,172] Because patients with cancer will interact with multiple different providers at different stages of their cancer treatment, the question of who should deliver smoking cessation interventions might be overruled by the question of how to make delivery of smoking cessation interventions consistent across all providers who have contact with cancer patients.[143] That is, all providers who interact with cancer patients, either in the context of acute oncology treatment or after cancer treatments are completed, will likely be called upon to address tobacco use. Consistency in the delivery of smoking cessation interventions may be increased by major healthcare groups and organizations promoting and reinforcing evidence-based standards for tobacco use assessment and treatment. Notably, whereas multiple care providers should be involved in reinforcing the importance of tobacco cessation, all providers can rely on a consistency of need for intervention in all cancer patients.

22.5.5. Optimal Timing of Smoking Cessation Interventions

Some controversy exists about the optimal time for patients with cancer to quit smoking,[173,174] perhaps due to questions about when individuals are most receptive to health behavior interventions[175] or to providers' preferences to wait until the initiation of medical treatment or until patients are hospitalized.[136] However, patients themselves have stated that the ideal timing for smoking cessation intervention is early in cancer treatment: at either the first medical consultation or when decisions about cancer treatment have been finalized.[176] Smoking cessation interventions appear effective when delivered shortly after initial cancer diagnosis,[177] plus evidence suggests that it is safe and important to quit smoking as soon as possible before cancer treatment.[9,156] In fact, a recent review indicated that a preoperative smoke-free period of more than 10 weeks produced post-operative pulmonary complication rates similar to those of patients who had never smoked.[178] Thus, promoting smoking cessation interventions early in cancer treatment may avoid or circumvent some barriers to addressing tobacco use that may arise later in treatment. In addition, early effective cessation interventions may ultimately improve the efficacy of cancer treatment.

Other questions that future research can answer include whether or not it is appropriate to delay cancer treatment in order to allow time for sustained smoking cessation[88] and how long smoking cessation interventions should last. The latter question is important to examine because providers may stop assessing smoking status after a cancer patient reports that he has quit,[140] even though this would potentially miss critical changes in tobacco use. Cancer patients tend to be older, and perhaps smoking cessation treatment ought to be extended in length, as it has been for older smokers without cancer.[179] Regardless, consideration for altering cancer treatment based upon smoking status in hopes that a more efficacious cancer treatment will occur is a very intriguing concept that will require substantial detailed investigation prior to implementation.

22.5.6. Incorporating Family Members in Smoking Cessation Interventions

The presence of a family member who smokes, especially one who smokes in the home, is a robust correlate of difficulty quitting smoking in cancer patients.[180] Family members who continue to smoke may themselves be impacted by cancer diagnosis (i.e., through increased depression and anxiety or decreased quality of life).[181] Unfortunately, only a minority of relatives of cancer patients may quit smoking.[182] It has been long recognized that integrating family members into smoking cessation interventions for patients with cancer is essential, as family members may be in a unique position to provide more helpful coping skills to cancer patients,[136] and group processes in the family setting may influence health behavior changes of individuals.[183] The feasibility and utility of family-based smoking cessation interventions have been investigated,[139,184] but to our knowledge family-based interventions have not been routinely implemented among patients with cancer. Further research on effective strategies for incorporating both smoking and non-smoking family members in smoking cessation interventions have yet to be elucidated.

22.5.7. Determining the Cost-Effectiveness of Smoking Cessation Interventions

As healthcare costs have increased exponentially in recent years, calculating and improving the cost-effectiveness of medical interventions in healthcare systems has become critical. The only evidence that we could locate on the cost-effectiveness of tobacco use assessment and treatment in cancer patients indicates that a smoking cessation program initiated before surgical lung resection in cancer patients is cost-effective at both one and five years postsurgery.[185] Although favoring the utility of addressing tobacco use among cancer patients, this evidence would be strengthened by additional research across a wide range of patients with cancer receiving different treatment modalities. Reliable evidence on the cost-effectiveness of smoking cessation interventions in cancer patients may motivate systems and institutions to change policies on addressing tobacco use in oncology settings. Importantly, tobacco assessment and cessation has the potential to be a single medical guideline that may improve the cost effectiveness of cancer treatment through decreased toxicity, decreased hospitalization, decreased medical comorbidity, increased quality of life, increased efficacy of cancer treatment (with subsequent reductions in the utilization of second line therapy after primary cancer treatment failure), and ultimately increased survival.

22.6. CONCLUSION

There are several potential incentives for including tobacco assessment and cessation into standard clinical practice for cancer patients including:

(i) improved cancer treatment outcomes,
(ii) improved non-cancer-related health benefits,
(iii) improved quality of life,
(iv) decreased treatment-related toxicity, and
(v) decreased healthcare costs.

Notably, these incentives are likely relevant to virtually all cancer disease sites and treatments. As a consequence, a single intervention may yield significant health-related benefits for all cancer patients.

There are several actions that must occur to realize the potential benefits of tobacco cessation in cancer patients including:

(i) standardizing tobacco assessments and tobacco use definitions for cancer patients;

(ii) mandatory assessment of tobacco at diagnosis, during treatment, and during follow-up;
(iii) mandatory referral to dedicated tobacco cessation resources and/or structured cessation support by educated providers for cancer patients at risk for continued tobacco use;
(iv) increasing research emphasis to improve cessation efficacy in cancer patients with consideration of health-related effects, level of addiction, social environment, behavioral comorbidity, and continuity of care; and
(v) improving access to care through improved reimbursement and coordination between providers, cancer centers, insurers, and community resources.

Fundamentally, system-level changes are necessary to make tobacco assessment and cessation a critical component of cancer care. However, even relatively simple changes may result in substantial healthcare benefits for cancer patients.

22.7. DISCLOSURES

The authors have no financial disclosures to report.

REFERENCES

1. Adhikari B, Kahende J, Malarcher A, *et al.* (2008) Smoking-attributable mortality, years of potential life lost, and productivity losses — United States, 2000–2004. *Morb Mortal Wkly Rep* 57: 1226–1228.
2. US Department of Health and Human Services. (2010) *How Tobacco Smoke Causes Disease: The Biology and Behavioral Basis for Smoking-Attributable Disease: A Report of the Surgeon General* US Department of Health and Human Services, Centers for Disease Control and Prevention, National Center for Chronic Disease Prevention and Health Promotion, Office on Smoking and Health, Atlanta, GA.
3. Ostroff JS, Hay JL, Schantx SP, Maher MM. (2000) A survey of smoking status and cancer risk perceptions among participants attending a hospital-based head and neck screening program. *Psychol Health* 14: 979–990.

4. Cox LS, Africano NL, Tercyak KP, Taylor KL. (2003) Nicotine dependence treatment for patients with cancer: Review and recommendations. *Cancer* **98**: 632–644.
5. Tsivian M, Moreira DM, Caso JR, *et al.* (2011) Cigarette smoking is associated with advanced renal cell carcinoma. *J Clin Oncol* **29**: 2027–2031.
6. Vilensky D, Lawrentschuk N, Hersey K, Fleshner NE. (2012) A smoking cessation program as a resource for bladder cancer patients. *Can Urol Assoc J* **6**: E167–E173.
7. Waggoner SE, Darcy KM, Tian C, Lanciano R. (2010) Smoking behavior in women with locally advanced cervical carcinoma: A Gynecologic Oncology Group study. *Am J Obstet Gynecol* **202**: 283.e1–7.
8. Schnoll RA, James C, Malstrom M, *et al.* (2003) Longitudinal predictors of continued tobacco use among patients diagnosed with cancer. *Ann Behav Med* **25**: 214–222.
9. Gritz ER, Nisenbaum R, Elashoff RE, Holmes EC. (1991) Smoking behavior following diagnosis in patients with stage I non-small cell lung cancer. *Cancer Causes Control* **2**: 105–112.
10. Gritz ER, Carr CR, Rapkin D, *et al.* (1993) Predictors of long-term smoking cessation in head and neck cancer patients. *Cancer Epidemiol Biomarkers Prev* **2**: 261–270.
11. Ostroff JS, Jacobsen PB, Moadel AB, *et al.* (1995) Prevalence and predictors of continued tobacco use after treatment of patients with head and neck cancer. *Cancer* **75**: 569–576.
12. Warren GW, Kasza KA, Reid ME, *et al.* (2013) Smoking at diagnosis and survival in cancer patients. *Int J Cancer* **132**: 401–410.
13. Browman GP, Wong G, Hodson I, *et al.* (1993) Influence of cigarette smoking on the efficacy of radiation therapy in head and neck cancer. *N Engl J Med* **328**: 159–163.
14. Gillison ML, Zhang Q, Jordan R, *et al.* (2012) Tobacco smoking and increased risk of death and progression for patients with p16-positive and p16-negative oropharyngeal cancer. *J Clin Oncol* **30**: 2102–2111.
15. Hoff CM, Grau C, Overgaard J.(2012) Effect of smoking on oxygen delivery and outcome in patients treated with radiotherapy for head and neck squamous cell carcinoma: A prospective study. *Radiother Oncol* **103**: 38–44.
16. Ang KK, Harris J, Wheeler R, *et al.* (2010) Human papillomavirus and survival of patients with oropharyngeal cancer. *N Engl J Med* **363**: 24–35.
17. Shen GP, Xu FH, He F, *et al.*(2012) Pretreatment lifestyle behaviors as survival predictors for patients with nasopharyngeal carcinoma. *PLoS One* **7**: e36515.

18. Dal Maso L, Zucchetto A, Talamini R, *et al.*; Prospective Analysis of Case-control studies on Environmental factors and health (PACE) study group. (2008) Effect of obesity and other lifestyle factors on mortality in women with breast cancer. *Int J Cancer* **123**: 2188–2194.
19. Dragun AE, Huang B, Tucker TC, Spanos WJ. (2011) Disparities in the application of adjuvant radiotherapy after breast-conserving surgery for early stage breast cancer: Impact on overall survival. *Cancer* **117**: 2590–2598.
20. Sagiv SK, Gaudet MM, Eng SM, *et al.* (2007) Active and passive cigarette smoke and breast cancer survival. *Ann Epidemiol* **17**: 385–393.
21. Coker AL, DeSimone CP, Eggleston KS, *et al.* (2009) Smoking and survival among Kentucky women diagnosed with invasive cervical cancer: 1995–2005. *Gynecol Oncol* **112**: 365–369.
22. Kjærbye-Thygesen A, Frederiksen K, Høgdall EV, *et al.* (2006) Smoking and overweight: Negative prognostic factors in stage III epithelial ovarian cancer. *Cancer Epidemiol Biomarkers Prev* **15**: 798–803.
23. Modesitt SC, Huang B, Shelton BJ, Wyatt S. (2006) Endometrial cancer in Kentucky: The impact of age, smoking status, and rural residence. *Gynecol Oncol* **103**: 300–306.
24. Nagle CM, Bain CJ, Webb PM. (2006) Cigarette smoking and survival after ovarian cancer diagnosis. *Cancer Epidemiol Biomarkers Prev* **15**: 2557–2560.
25. Ngô C, Alran S, Plancher C, *et al.*; Institut Curie Gynaecological Cancer Study Group coordinated by P. Cottu. (2011) Outcome in early cervical cancer following pre-operative low dose rate brachytherapy: A ten-year follow up of 257 patients treated at a single institution. *Gynecol Oncol* **123**: 248–252.
26. Schlumbrecht MP, Sun CC, Wong KN, *et al.* (2011) Clinicodemographic factors influencing outcomes in patients with low-grade serous ovarian carcinoma. *Cancer* **117**: 3741–3749.
27. Waggoner SE, Darcy KM, Fuhrman B, *et al.*; Gynecologic Oncology Group. (2006) Association between cigarette smoking and prognosis in locally advanced cervical carcinoma treated with chemoradiation: A Gynecologic Oncology Group study. *Gynecol Oncol* **103**: 853–858.
28. Munro AJ, Bentley AH, Ackland C, Boyle PJ. (2006) Smoking compromises cause-specific survival in patients with operable colorectal cancer. *Clin Oncol, (R Coll Radiol)* **18**: 436–440.
29. Phipps AI, Baron J, Newcomb PA. (2011) Prediagnostic smoking history, alcohol consumption, and colorectal cancer survival: The Seattle Colon Cancer Family Registry. *Cancer* **117**: 4948–4957.
30. Roxburgh CS, Platt JJ, Leitch EF, *et al.* (2011) Relationship between preoperative comorbidity, systemic inflammatory response, and survival in patients

undergoing curative resection for colorectal cancer. *Ann Surg Oncol* **18**: 997–1005.

31. Shitara K, Matsuo K, Hatooka S, *et al.* (2010) Heavy smoking history interacts with chemoradiotherapy for esophageal cancer prognosis: A retrospective study. *Cancer Sci* **101**: 1001–1006.
32. Bittner N, Merrick GS, Galbreath RW, *et al.* (2008) Primary causes of death after permanent prostate brachytherapy. *Int J Radiat Oncol Biol Phys* **72**: 433–440.
33. Gong Z, Agalliu I, Lin DW, *et al.* (2008) Cigarette smoking and prostate cancer-specific mortality following diagnosis in middle-aged men. *Cancer Causes Control* **19**: 25–31.
34. Kenfield SA, Stampfer MJ, Chan JM, Giovannucci E. (2011) Smoking and prostate cancer survival and recurrence. *J Am Med Assoc* **305**: 2548–2555.
35. Kroeger N, Klatte T, Birkhäuser FD, *et al.* (2012) Smoking negatively impacts renal cell carcinoma overall and cancer-specific survival. *Cancer* **118**: 1795–1802.
36. Oefelein MG, Resnick MI. (2004) Association of tobacco use with hormone refractory disease and survival of patients with prostate cancer. *J Urol* **171**: 2281–2284.
37. Parker A, Lohse C, Cheville J, *et al.* (2008) Evaluation of the association of current cigarette smoking and outcome for patients with clear cell renal cell carcinoma. *Int J Urol* **15**: 304–308.
38. Richey SL, Culp SH, Jonasch E, *et al.* (2011) Outcome of patients with metastatic renal cell carcinoma treated with targeted therapy without cytoreductive nephrectomy. *Ann Oncol* **22**: 1048–1053.
39. Taira AV, Merrick GS, Butler WM, *et al.* (2011) Long-term outcome for clinically localized prostate cancer treated with permanent interstitial brachytherapy. *Int J Radiat Oncol Biol Phys* **79**: 1336–1342.
40. Huncharek M, Haddock KS, Reid R, Kupelnick B. (2010) Smoking as a risk factor for prostate cancer: A meta-analysis of 24 prospective cohort studies. *Am J Public Health* **100**: 693–701.
41. Archimbaud E, Maupas J, Lecluze-Palazzolo C, *et al.* (1989) Influence of cigarette smoking on the presentation and course of chronic myelogenous leukemia. *Cancer* **63**: 2060–2065.
42. Battaglioli T, Gorini G, Costantini AS, *et al.* (2006) Cigarette smoking and alcohol consumption as determinants of survival in non-Hodgkin's lymphoma: A population-based study. *Ann Oncol* **17**: 1283–1289.
43. Chelghoum Y, Danaila C, Belhabri A, *et al.* (2002) Influence of cigarette smoking on the presentation and course of acute myeloid leukemia. *Ann Oncol* **13**: 1621–1627.

44. Ehlers SL, Gastineau DA, Patten CA, *et al.* (2011) The impact of smoking on outcomes among patients undergoing hematopoietic SCT for the treatment of acute leukemia. *Bone Marrow Transplant* **46**: 285–290.
45. Talamini R, Polesel J, Spina M, *et al.* (2008) The impact of tobacco smoking and alcohol drinking on survival of patients with non-Hodgkin lymphoma. *Int J Cancer* **122**: 1624–1629.
46. Varadarajan R, Licht AS, Hyland AJ, *et al.* (2012) Smoking adversely affects survival in acute myeloid leukemia patients. *Int J Cancer* **130**: 1451–1458.
47. Fleshner N, Garland J, Moadel A, *et al.* (1999) Influence of smoking status on the disease-related outcomes of patients with tobacco-associated superficial transitional cell carcinoma of the bladder. *Cancer* **86**: 2337–2345.
48. Lammers RJ, Witjes WP, Hendricksen K, *et al.* (2011) Smoking status is a risk factor for recurrence after transurethral resection of non-muscle-invasive bladder cancer. *Eur Urol* **60**: 713–720.
49. Moreira DM, Antonelli JA, Presti JC Jr, *et al.* (2010) Association of cigarette smoking with interval to biochemical recurrence after radical prostatectomy: Results from the SEARCH database. *Urology* **76**: 1218–1223.
50. Chang G, Orav EJ, McNamara T, *et al.* (2004) Depression, cigarette smoking, and hematopoietic stem cell transplantation outcome. *Cancer* **101**: 782–789.
51. Hooning MJ, Botma A, Aleman BM, *et al.* (2007) Long-term risk of cardiovascular disease in 10-year survivors of breast cancer. *J Natl Cancer Inst* **99**: 365–375.
52. Jagsi R, Griffith KA, Koelling T, *et al.* (2007) Rates of myocardial infarction and coronary artery disease and risk factors in patients treated with radiation therapy for early-stage breast cancer. *Cancer* **104**: 650–657.
53. Paszat LF, Vallis KA, Benk VM, *et al.* (2007) A population-based case-cohort study of the risk of myocardial infarction following radiation therapy for breast cancer. *Radiother Oncol* **82**: 294–300.
54. Wadhwa D, Fallah-Rad N, Grenier D, *et al.* (2009) Trastuzumab mediated cardiotoxicity in the setting of adjuvant chemotherapy for breast cancer: A retrospective study. *Breast Cancer Res Treat* **117**: 357–364.
55. van den Belt-Dusebout AW, de Wit R, Gietema JA, *et al.* (2007) Treatment-specific risks of second malignancies and cardiovascular disease in 5-year survivors of testicular cancer. *J Clin Oncol* **25**: 4370–4378.
56. Moser EC, Noordijk EM, Carde P, *et al.* (2005) Late non-neoplastic events in patients with aggressive non-Hodgkin's lymphoma in four randomized European Organisation for Research and Treatment of Cancer trials. *Clin Lymphoma Myeloma* **6**: 122–130.
57. Haugnes HS, Aass N, Fossa SD, *et al.* (2009) Pulmonary function in long-term survivors of testicular cancer. *J Clin Oncol* **27**: 2779–2786.

58. Goodwin SJ, McCarthy CM, Pusic AL, *et al.* (2005) Complications in smokers after postmastectomy tissue expander/implant breast reconstruction. *Ann Plast Surg* **55**: 16–20.
59. Lilla C, Ambrosone CB, Kropp S, *et al.* (2007) Predictive factors for late normal tissue complications following radiotherapy for breast cancer. *Breast Cancer Res Treat* **106**: 143–150.
60. Pinsolle V, Grinfeder C, Mathoulin-Pelissier S, Faucher A. (2006) Complications analysis of 266 immediate breast reconstructions. *J Plast Reconstr Aesthet Surg* **59**: 1017–1024.
61. Woerdeman LA, Hage JJ, Hofland MM, Rutgers EJ. (2007) A prospective assessment of surgical risk factors in 400 cases of skin-sparing mastectomy and immediate breast reconstruction with implants to establish selection criteria. *Plast Reconstr Surg* **119**: 455–463.
62. Zaman M, Bilal H, Mahmood S, Tang A. (2012) Does getting smokers to stop smoking before lung resections reduce their risk? *Interact Cardiovasc Thorac Surg* **14**: 320–323.
63. Zhan M, Flaws JA, Gallicchio L, *et al.* (2007) Profiles of tamoxifen-related side effects by race and smoking status in women with breast cancer. *Cancer Detect Prev* **31**: 384–390.
64. Peat BG, Bell RS, Davis A, *et al.* (1994) Wound-healing complications after soft-tissue sarcoma surgery. *Plast Reconstr Surg* **93**: 980–987.
65. Cooke DT, Lin GC, Lau CL, *et al.* (2009) Analysis of cervical esophagogastric anastomotic leaks after transhiatalesophagectomy: Risk factors, presentation, and detection. *Ann Thorac Surg* **88**: 177–185.
66. Wright CD, Kucharczuk JC, O'Brien SM, *et al.* (2009) Predictors of major morbidity and mortality after esophagectomy for esophageal cancer: A Society of Thoracic Surgeons General Thoracic Surgery Database risk adjustment model. *J Thorac Cardiovasc Surg* **137**: 587–596.
67. Zingg U, Smithers BM, Gotley DC, *et al.* (2011) Factors associated with postoperative pulmonary morbidity after esophagectomy for cancer. *Ann Surg Oncol* **18**: 1460–1468.
68. Wuketich S, Hienz SA, Marosi C. (2012) Prevalence of clinically relevant oral mucositis in outpatients receiving myelosuppressive chemotherapy for solid tumors. *Support Care Cancer* **20**: 175–183.
69. Eifel PJ, Jhingran A, Bodurka DC, *et al.* (2002) Correlation of smoking history and other patient characteristics with major complications of pelvic radiation therapy for cervical cancer. *J Clin Oncol* **20**: 3651–3657.
70. Nickelsen TN, Jorgensen T, Kronborg O. (2005) Lifestyle and 30-day complications to surgery for colorectal cancer. *Acta Oncol* **44**: 218–223.

71. Ku J, Krahn M, Trachtenberg J, *et al.* (2009) Changes in health utilities and health-related quality of life over 12 months following radical prostatectomy. *Can Urol Assoc J* **3**: 445–452.
72. Li CI, Daling JR, Porter PL, *et al.* (2009) Relationship between potentially modifiable lifestyle factors and risk of second primary contralateral breast cancer among women diagnosed with estrogen receptor-positive invasive breast cancer. *J Clin Oncol* **27**: 5312–5318.
73. Kinoshita Y, Tsukuma H, Ajiki W, *et al.* (2000) The risk for second primaries in gastric cancer patients: Adjuvant therapy and habitual smoking and drinking. *J Epidemiol* **10**: 300–304.
74. Travis LB, Gospodarowicz M, Curtis RE, *et al.* (2002) Lung cancer following chemotherapy and radiotherapy for Hodgkin's disease. *J Natl Cancer Inst* **94**: 182–192.
75. Kaufman EL, Jacobson JS, Hershman DL, *et al.* (2008) Effect of breast cancer radiotherapy and cigarette smoking on risk of second primary lung cancer. *J Clin Oncol* **26**: 392–398.
76. Boorjian S, Cowan JE, Konety BR, *et al.*; Cancer of the Prostate Strategic Urologic Research Endeavor Investigators. (2007) Bladder cancer incidence and risk factors in men with prostate cancer: Results from Cancer of the Prostate Strategic Urologic Research Endeavor. *J Urol* **177**: 883–888.
77. Jang S, Prizment A, Haddad T, *et al.* (2011) Smoking and quality of life among female survivors of breast, colorectal and endometrial cancers in a prospective cohort study. *J Cancer Surviv* **5**: 115–122.
78. Shinn EH, Basen-Engquist K, Thornton B, *et al.* (2007) Health behaviors and depressive symptoms in testicular cancer survivors. *Urology* **69**: 748–753.
79. LoConte NK, Else-Quest NM, Eickhoff J, *et al.* (2008) Assessment of guilt and shame in patients with non-small-cell lung cancer compared with patients with breast and prostate cancer. *Clin Lung Cancer* **9**: 171–178.
80. Cho J, Guallar E, Hsu YJ, *et al.* (2010) A comparison of cancer screening practices in cancer survivors and in the general population: The Korean national health and nutrition examination survey (KNHANES) 2001–2007. *Cancer Causes Control* **21**: 2203–2212.
81. Lin JH, Zhang SM, Manson JE. (2011) Predicting adherence to tamoxifen for breast cancer adjuvant therapy and prevention. *Cancer Prev Res* **4**: 1360–1365.
82. Land SR, Cronin WM, Wickerham DL, *et al.* (2011) Cigarette smoking, obesity, physical activity, and alcohol use as predictors of chemoprevention adherence in the national surgical adjuvant breast and bowel project p-1 breast cancer prevention trial. *Cancer Prev Res* **4**: 1393–1400.

83. Jerjes W, Upile T, Radhi H, *et al.* (2012) The effect of tobacco and alcohol and their reduction/cessation on mortality in oral cancer patients. *Head Neck Oncol* **4**: 6.
84. Chen CH, Shun CT, Huang KH, *et al.* (2007) Stopping smoking might reduce tumour recurrence in non-muscle-invasive bladder cancer. *BJU Int* **100**: 281–286.
85. Alsadius D, Hedelin M, Johansson KA, *et al.* (2011) Tobacco smoking and long-lasting symptoms from the bowel and the anal-sphincter region after radiotherapy for prostate cancer. *Radiother Oncol* **101**: 495–501.
86. Joshu CE, Mondul AM, Meinhold CL, *et al.* (2011) Cigarette smoking and prostate cancer recurrence after prostatectomy. *J Natl Cancer Inst* **103**: 835–838.
87. Aveyard P, Adab P, Cheng KK, *et al.* (2002) Does smoking status influence the prognosis of bladder cancer? A systematic review. *BJU Int* **90**: 228–239.
88. Land SR. (2012) Methodologic barriers to addressing critical questions about tobacco and cancer prognosis. *J Clin Oncol* **30**: 2030–2032.
89. Parsons A, Daley A, Begh R, Aveyard P. (2010) Influence of smoking cessation after diagnosis of early stage lung cancer on prognosis: Systematic review of observational studies with meta-analysis. *Br Med J* **340**: b5569.
90. Peters EN, Torres E, Toll BA, *et al.* (2012) Tobacco assessment in actively accruing National Cancer Institute Cooperative Group Program Clinical Trials. *J Clin Oncol* **30**: 2869–2875.
91. Zu K, Giovannucci E. (2009) Smoking and aggressive prostate cancer: A review of the epidemiologic evidence. *Cancer Causes Control* **20**: 1799–1810.
92. American Society of Clinical Oncology. (2003) American Society of Clinical Oncology Policy Statement Update: Tobacco Control —Reducing Cancer Incidence and Saving Lives. *J Clin Oncol* **21**: 1–10.
93. Viswanath K, Herbst RS, Land SR, *et al.*; Writing Committee for the AACR Task Force on Tobacco and Cancer. (2010) Tobacco and cancer: An American Association for Cancer Research policy statement. *Cancer Res* **70**: 3419–3430.
94. Fiore MC, Jorenby DE, Schensky AE, *et al.* (1995) Smoking status as the new vital sign: Effect on assessment and intervention in patients who smoke. *Mayo Clin Proc* **70**: 209–213.
95. Fiore MC, Jaen CR, Baker TB, *et al.* (2008) *Treating Tobacco Use and Dependence: 2008 Update*, Clinical Practice Guideline. US Department of Health and Human Services. Public Health Service, Rockville, MD.
96. Gritz ER, Dresler C, Sarna L. (2005) Smoking, the missing drug interaction in clinical trials: Ignoring the obvious. *Cancer Epidemiol Biomarkers Prev* **14**: 2287–2293.

97. Gregorio DI, Hollenbeck M, Samociuk H. (2009) Who's assessing tobacco use in cancer clinical trials? *Nicotine Tob Res* **11**: 1354–1358.
98. Polednak AP. (2006) Obtaining smoking histories for population-based studies on multiple primary cancers: Connecticut, 2002. *Int J Cancer* **119**: 233–235.
99. Cox LS, Patten CA, Ebbert JO, *et al.* (2002) Tobacco use outcomes among patients with lung cancer treated for nicotine dependence. *J Clin Oncol* **20**: 3461–3469.
100. Demark-Wahnefried W, Peterson B, McBride C, *et al.* (2000) Current health behaviors and readiness to pursue life-style changes among men and women diagnosed with early stage prostate and breast carcinomas. *Cancer* **88**: 674–684.
101. Gritz ER, Fingeret MC, Vidrine DJ, *et al.* (2006) Successes and failures of the teachable moment: Smoking cessation in cancer patients. *Cancer* **106**: 17–27.
102. de Bruin-Visser JC, Ackerstaff AH, Rehorst H, *et al.* (2012) Integration of a smoking cessation program in the treatment protocol for patients with head and neck and lung cancer. *Eur Arch Otorhinolaryngol* **269**: 659–665.
103. Emmons KM, Puleo E, Park E, *et al.* (2005) Peer-delivered smoking counseling for childhood cancer survivors increases rate of cessation: The partnership for health study. *J Clin Oncol* **23**: 6516–6523.
104. Gosselin MH, Mahoney MC, Cummings KM, *et al.* (2011) Evaluation of an intervention to enhance the delivery of smoking cessation services to patients with cancer. *J Cancer Educ* **26**: 577–582.
105. Jonsdottir H, Jonsdottir R, Geirsdottir T, *et al.* (2004) Multicomponent individualized smoking cessation intervention for patients with lung disease. *J Adv Nurs* **48**: 594–604.
106. Schnoll RA, Rothman RL, Wielt DB, *et al.* (2005) A randomized pilot study of cognitive-behavioral therapy versus basic health education for smoking cessation among cancer patients. *Ann Behav Med* **30**: 1–11.
107. Sharp L, Johansson H, Fagerström K, Rutqvist LE. (2008) Smoking cessation among patients with head and neck cancer: Cancer as a "teachable moment". *Eur J Cancer Care* **17**: 114–119.
108. Baser S, Shannon VR, Eapen GA, *et al.* (2006) Smoking cessation after diagnosis of lung cancer is associated with a beneficial effect on performance status. *Chest* **130**: 1784–1790.
109. Do KA, Johnson MM, Doherty DA, *et al.* (2003) Second primary tumors in patients with upper aerodigestive tract cancers: Joint effects of smoking and alcohol (United States). *Cancer Causes Control* **14**: 131–138.

110. Ebbert JO, Yang P, Vachon CM, *et al.* (2003) Lung cancer risk reduction after smoking cessation: Observations from a prospective cohort of women. *J Clin Oncol* **21**: 921–926.
111. Fox JL, Rosenzweig KE, Ostroff JS. (2004) The effect of smoking status on survival following radiation therapy for non-small cell lung cancer. *Lung Cancer* **44**: 287–293.
112. Fujisawa T, Iizasa T, Saitoh Y, *et al.* (1999) Smoking before surgery predicts poor long-term survival in patients with stage I non-small-cell lung carcinomas. *J Clin Oncol* **17**: 2086–2091.
113. Garces YI, Yang P, Parkinson J, *et al.* (2004) The relationship between cigarette smoking and quality of life after lung cancer diagnosis. *Chest* **126**: 1733–1741.
114. Johnson BE. (1998) Second lung cancers in patients after treatment for an initial lung cancer. *J Natl Cancer Inst* **90**: 1335–1345.
115. Lippman SM, Lee JJ, Karp DD, *et al.* (2001) Randomized phase III intergroup trial of isotretinoin to prevent second primary tumors in stage I non-small-cell lung cancer. *J Natl Cancer Inst* **93**: 605–618.
116. Rice D, Kim HW, Sabichi A, *et al.* (2003) The risk of second primary tumors after resection of stage I non-small cell lung cancer. *Ann Thorac Surg* **76**: 1001–1008.
117. Richardson GE, Tucker MA, Venzon DJ, *et al.* (1993) Smoking cessation after successful treatment of small-cell lung cancer is associated with fewer smoking-related second primary cancers. *Ann Intern Med* **119**: 383–390.
118. Morgan G, Schnoll RA, Alfano CM, *et al.* (2011) National Cancer Institute Conference on Treating Tobacco Dependence at Cancer Centers. *J Oncol Pract* **7**: 178–182.
119. Gritz ER, Vidrine DJ, Fingeret MC. (2007) Smoking cessation: A critical component of medical management in chronic disease populations. *Am J Prev Med* **33**: S414–S422.
120. Walker MS, Vidrine DJ, Gritz ER, *et al.* (2006) Smoking relapse during the first year after treatment for early-stage non-small-cell lung cancer. *Cancer Epidemiol Biomarkers Prev* **15**: 2370–2377.
121. Cooley ME, Sarna L, Kotlerman J, *et al.* (2009) Smoking cessation is challenging even for patients recovering from lung cancer surgery with curative intent. *Lung Cancer* **66**: 218–225.
122. Cooley ME, Sarna L, Brown JK, *et al.* (2007) Tobacco use in women with lung cancer. *Ann Behav Med* **33**: 242–250.
123. Frobisher C, Winter DL, Lancashire ER, *et al.*; British Childhood Cancer Survivor Study. (2008) Extent of smoking and age at initiation of smoking

among adult survivors of childhood cancer in Britain. *J Natl Cancer Inst* **100**: 1068–1081.

124. Hentrich M, Fegg MJ, Meiler S, *et al.* (2006) Smoking cessation in long-term survivors of germ cell tumour. *J Cancer Res Clin Oncol* **132**: 557–560.
125. Tseng TS, Lin HY, Martin MY, *et al.* (2010) Disparities in smoking and cessation status among cancer survivors and non-cancer individuals: A population-based study from National Health and Nutrition Examination Survey. *J Cancer Surviv* **4**: 313–321.
126. Walker M, Larsen R, Zona D, *et al.* (2004) Smoking urges and relapse among lung cancer patients: Findings from a preliminary retrospective study. *Prev Med* **39**: 449–457.
127. Schnoll RA, Zhang B, Rue M, *et al.* (2003) Brief physician-initiated quit-smoking strategies for clinical oncology settings: A trial coordinated by the Eastern Cooperative Oncology Group. *J Clin Oncol* **21**: 355–365.
128. Garces YI, Schroeder DR, Nirelli LM, *et al.* (2007) Second primary tumors following tobacco dependence treatments among head and neck cancer patients. *Am J Clin Oncol* **30**: 531–539.
129. Cooley ME, Wang Q, Johnson BE, *et al.* (2012) Factors associated with smoking abstinence among smokers and recent-quitters with lung and head and neck cancer. *Lung Cancer* **76**: 144–149.
130. Schnoll RA, Subramanian S, Martinez E, Engstrom PF. (2011) Correlates of continued tobacco use and intention to quit smoking among Russian cancer patients. *Int J Behav Med* **18**: 325–332.
131. Schnoll RA, Malstrom M, James C, *et al.* (2002) Correlates of tobacco use among smokers and recent quitters diagnosed with cancer. *Patient Educ Couns* **46**: 137–145.
132. Dresler CM, Bailey M, Roper CR, *et al.* (1996) Smoking cessation and lung cancer resection. *Chest* **110**: 1199–1202.
133. Blalock JA, Lam C, Minnix JA, *et al.* (2011) The effect of mood, anxiety, and alcohol use disorders on smoking cessation in cancer patients. *J Cogn Psychother* **25**: 82–96.
134. Daniel M, Keefe FJ, Lyna P, *et al.* (2009) Persistent smoking after a diagnosis of lung cancer is associated with higher reported pain levels. *J Pain* **10**: 323–328.
135. Ditre JW, Gonzalez BD, Simmons VN, *et al.* (2011) Associations between pain and current smoking status among cancer patients. *Pain* **152**: 60–65.
136. Gritz ER. (2000) Facilitating smoking cessation in cancer patients. *Tob Control* **9**: I50.
137. Chapple A, Ziebland S, McPherson A. (2004) Stigma, shame, and blame experienced by patients with lung cancer: Qualitative study. *Br Med J* **328**: 1470.

138. Lebel S, Devins GM. (2008) Stigma in cancer patients whose behavior may have contributed to their disease. *Future Oncol* **4**: 717–733.
139. Ozakinci G, Wells M, Williams B, *et al.* (2010) Cancer diagnosis: An opportune time to help patients and their families stop smoking? *Public Health* **124**: 479–482.
140. Simmons VN, Litvin EB, Patel RD, *et al.* (2009) Patient-provider communication and perspectives on smoking cessation and relapse in the oncology setting. *Patient Educ Couns* **77**: 398–403.
141. Emmons KM, Butterfield RM, Puleo E, *et al.* (2003) Smoking among participants in the childhood cancer survivors cohort: The Partnership for Health Study. *J Clin Oncol* **21**: 189–196.
142. Cooley ME, Emmons KM, Haddad R, *et al.* (2011) Patient-reported receipt of and interest in smoking-cessation interventions after a diagnosis of cancer. *Cancer* **117**: 2961–2969.
143. Coups EJ, Dhingra LK, Heckman CJ, Manne SL. (2009) Receipt of provider advice for smoking cessation and use of smoking cessation treatments among cancer survivors. *J Gen Intern Med* **24**: S480–S486.
144. Schnoll RA, Rothman RL, Newman H, *et al.* (2004) Characteristics of cancer patients entering a smoking cessation program and correlates of quit motivation: Implications for the development of tobacco control programs for cancer patients. *Psychooncology* **13**: 346–358.
145. Barnhill D, O'Connor D, Farley J, *et al.* (1992) Clinical surveillance of gynecologic cancer patients. *Gynecol Oncol* **46**: 275–280.
146. Burke L, Miller LA, Saad A, Abraham J. (2009) Smoking behaviors among cancer survivors: An observational clinical study. *J Oncol Pract* **5**: 6–9.
147. Demark-Wahnefried W, Pinto BM, Gritz ER. (2006) Promoting health and physical function among cancer survivors: Potential for prevention and questions that remain. *J Clin Oncol* **24**: 5125–5131.
148. Sabatino SA, Coates RJ, Uhler RJ, *et al.* (2007) Provider counseling about health behaviors among cancer survivors in the United States. *J Clin Oncol* **25**: 2100–2106.
149. Sarna LP, Brown JK, Lillington L, *et al.* (2000) Tobacco interventions by oncology nurses in clinical practice: Report from a national survey. *Cancer* **89**: 881–889.
150. Sharp L, Tishelman C. (2005) Smoking cessation for patients with head and neck cancer: A qualitative study of patients' and nurses' experiences in a nurse-led intervention. *Cancer Nurs* **28**: 226–235.

151. Strope SA, Montie JE. (2008) The causal role of cigarette smoking in bladder cancer initiation and progression, and the role of urologists in smoking cessation. *J Urol* **180**: 31–37.
152. Simmons VN, Litvin EB, Unrod M, Brandon TH. (2012) Oncology healthcare providers' implementation of the 5A's model of brief intervention for smoking cessation: Patients' perceptions. *Patient Educ Couns* **86**: 414–419.
153. Richmond R, Zwar N, Taylor R, *et al.* (2009) Teaching about tobacco in medical schools: A worldwide study. *Drug Alcohol Rev* **28**: 484–497.
154. Sarna L, Wewers ME, Brown JK, *et al.* (2001) Barriers to tobacco cessation in clinical practice: Report from a National Survey of Oncology Nurses. *Nurs Outlook* **49**: 166–172.
155. Bjurlin MA, Goble SM, Hollowell CM. (2010) Smoking cessation assistance for patients with bladder cancer: A national survey of American urologists. *J Urol* **184**: 1901–1906.
156. Cooley ME, Sipples RL, Murphy M, Sarna L. (2008) Smoking cessation and lung cancer: Oncology nurses can make a difference. *Semin Oncol Nurs* **24**: 16–26.
157. Cataldo JK. (2007) Clinical implications of smoking and aging: Breaking through the barriers. *J Gerontol Nurs* **33** :32–41.
158. Warren GW, Marshall JR, Cummings KM, *et al.*, on behalf of the IASLC Tobacco Control and Smoking Cessation Committee. (2013) Practice patterns and perceptions of thoracic oncology providers on tobacco use and cessation in cancer patients *J Thorac Oncol* **8**: 543–548.
159. Gritz ER, Sarna L, Dresler C, Healton CG. (2007) Building a united front: Aligning the agendas for tobacco control, lung cancer research, and policy. *Cancer Epidemiol Biomarkers Prev* **16**: 859–863.
160. Hammersley R. (1994) A digest of memory phenomena for addiction research. *Addiction* **89**: 283–293.
161. Donato F, Boffetta P, Fazioli R, *et al.* (1998) Reliability of data on smoking habit and coffee drinking collected by personal interview in a hospital-based case-control study. *Eur J Epidemiol* **14**: 259–267.
162. Warren GW, Arnold SM, Valentino JP, *et al.* (2012) Accuracy of self-reported tobacco assessments in a head and neck cancer treatment population. *Radiother Oncol* **103**: 45–48.
163. SRNT Subcommittee on Biochemical Verification. (2002) Biochemical verification of tobacco use and cessation. *Nicotine Tob Res* **4**. 149–159.
164. Greene SE, Nash DB. (2009) Pay for performance: An overview of the literature. *Am J Med Qual* **24**: 140–163.

165. Patterson F, Schnoll RA, Wileyto EP, *et al.* (2008) Toward personalized therapy for smoking cessation: A randomized placebo-controlled trial of bupropion. *Clin Pharmacol Ther* **84**: 320–325.
166. Demark-Wahnefried W, Aziz NM, Rowland JH, Pinto BM. (2005) Riding the crest of the teachable moment: Promoting long-term health after the diagnosis of cancer. *J Clin Oncol* **23** :5814–5830.
167. Bostrom PJ, Alkhateeb S, Trottier G, *et al.* (2012) Sex differences in bladder cancer outcomes among smokers with advanced bladder cancer. *BJU Int* **109**: 70–76.
168. Hawkes AL, Lynch BM, Owen N, Aitken JF. (2011) Lifestyle factors associated concurrently and prospectively with co-morbid cardiovascular disease in a population-based cohort of colorectal cancer survivors. *Eur J Cancer* **47**: 267–276.
169. Hewitt M, Greenfield S, Stovall E, eds. (2006) *From Cancer Patient to Cancer Survivor: Lost in Transition* National Academies Press, Washington, DC.
170. McCabe MS, Jacobs L. (2008) Survivorship care: Models and programs. *Semin Oncol Nurs* **24**: 202–207.
171. Oeffinger KC, McCabe MS. (2006) Models for delivering survivorship care. *J Clin Oncol* **24**: 5117–5124.
172. An LC, Foldes SS, Alesci NL, *et al.* (2008) The impact of smoking-cessation intervention by multiple health professionals. *Am J Prev Med* **34**: 54–60.
173. Barrera RS, Amar W, Thaler D, *et al.* (2005) Smoking and timing of cessation: Impact on pulmonary complications after thoracotomy. *Chest* **127**: 1977–1983.
174. Caporciyan A, Merriman KW, Ece F, *et al.* (2002) Incidence of major pulmonary morbidity after pneumonectomy: Association with timing of smoking cessation. *Ann Thorac Surg* **73**: 420–426.
175. Demark-Wahnefried W, Jones LW. (2008) Promoting a healthy lifestyle among cancer survivors. *Hematol Oncol Clin North Am* **22**: 319–342.
176. Hsu CC, Kwan GN, Chawla A, *et al.* (2011) Smoking habits of radiotherapy patients: Did the diagnosis of cancer make an impact and is there an opportunity to intervene? *J Med Imaging Radiat Oncol* **55**: 526–531.
177. Garces YI, Schroeder DR, Nirelli LM, *et al.* (2004) Tobacco use outcomes among patients with head and neck carcinoma treated for nicotine dependence: A matched-pair analysis. *Cancer* **101**: 116–124.
178. Zaman K, Thürlimann B, Huober J, *et al.*; on behalf of the Swiss Group for Clinical Cancer Research (SAKK). (2012) Bone mineral density in breast cancer patients treated with adjuvant letrozole, tamoxifen, or sequences of

letrozole and tamoxifen in the BIG 1-98 study (SAKK 21/07). *Ann Oncol* **23**: 1474–1481.
179. Hall SM, Humfleet GL, Muñoz RF, *et al.* (2009) Extended treatment of older cigarette smokers. *Addiction* **104**: 1043–1052.
180. Hymowitz N, Cummings KM, Hyland A, *et al.* (1997) Predictors of smoking cessation in a cohort of adult smokers followed for five years. *Tob Control* **6**: S57–S62.
181. Weaver KE, Rowland JH, Augustson E, Atienza AA. (2011) Smoking concordance in lung and colorectal cancer patient-caregiver dyads and quality of life. *Cancer Epidemiol Biomarkers Prev* **20**: 239–248.
182. Sarna L. (1995) Smoking behaviors of women after diagnosis with lung cancer. *Image* **27**: 35–41.
183. Bottorff JL, Robinson CA, Sullivan KM, Smith ML. (2009) Continued family smoking after lung cancer diagnosis: The patient's perspective. *Oncol Nurs Forum*, **36**: E126–E132.
184. Schilling A, Conaway MR, Wingate PJ, *et al.* (1997) Recruiting cancer patients to participate in motivating their relatives to quit smoking. A cancer control study of the Cancer and Leukemia Group B (CALGB 9072). *Cancer* **79**: 152–160.
185. Schilling A, Conaway MR, Wingate PJ, *et al.* (1997) Recruiting cancer patients to participate in motivating their relatives to quit smoking. A cancer control study of the Cancer and Leukemia Group B (CALGB 9072). *Cancer* **79**: 152–160.
186. Slatore CG, Au DH, Hollingworth W. (2009) Cost effectiveness of a smoking cessation program implemented at the time of surgery for lung cancer. *J Thorac Oncol* **4**: 499–504.

CHAPTER 23

The Role of Translational Research in Behavioral Science and Public Health

Maria E. Fernandez[*,‡], *L. Kay Bartholomew*[*], *Jennifer I. Vidrine*[†], *Belinda Reininger*[*], *Sarah Krasny*[*] *and David W. Wetter*[†]

23.1. INTRODUCTION

This chapter describes translational research in behavioral science, and more generally, in public health, and provides examples of contributions of these fields along the translational science continuum. The chapter begins with a review of the history of translational research within the disciplines of biomedical science, public health and behavioral sciences. This is followed by a discussion and examples of: (i) how behavioral science and public health approaches can accelerate the translation of both biomedical discoveries and public health interventions, and (ii) how dissemination and implementation research can inform translation processes to accelerate and improve translation across the continuum.

*University of Texas Health Science Center at Houston, School of Public Health, Division of Health Promotion and Behavioral Sciences, Houston, Texas, USA.

†University of Texas, MD Anderson Cancer Center, Department of Health Disparities Research, Houston, Texas, USA.

‡Corresponding author: Maria E. Fernandez, PhD, School of Public Health, University of Texas Health Science Center at Houston, 7000 Fannin Suite 2558, Houston, TX 77030, USA; E-mail: *maria.e.fernandez@uth.tmc.edu*; Tel: +1-713-500-9626; Fax: +1-713-500-9750.

23.1.1. A Historical Perspective

The term *translational research* was first coined in the early 1990s when researchers and clinicians discussed ways to better transfer biomedical discoveries to new methods in cancer diagnosis and treatment.[1] Following the Institute of Medicine Report, *Crossing the Quality Chasm: A New Health System for the 21st Century*,[2] Elias Zerhouni, former NIH Director, issued the NIH "Roadmap," a cross-institute initiative aimed at accelerating biomedical research translation to improve the nation's clinical research system and its impact on health outcomes.[3] Among its priorities, the Roadmap called for the establishment of Regional Translation Research Centers to increase interactions between basic and clinical scientists and accelerate the translational development of new drugs, biomarkers, and treatment strategies from the laboratory bench to clinical settings.[4] The types of research laid out in the Roadmap have been labeled as T1 and T2 research. Through T1, discoveries from basic science research are translated for clinical applications, whereas in T2, clinical applications are tested. Since this early conceptualization, many scientists have viewed translational research as exclusively focused on the transfer of biomedical innovations to clinical settings,[5] a process also referred to as "bench-to-bedside."[6,7]

Despite a tendency over the past two decades to focus on biomedical translation,[7] early descriptions of translational research underscored the importance of behavioral sciences as a way to move basic biomedical findings to clinical practice and wider dissemination. For example, in 1994, Morrow and Bellg described the potential contribution of behavioral science in translational research and cancer control to identify problems that obstruct efforts to translate research findings into clinical practice.[8] Recently, the importance of public health, including the social and behavioral sciences, has received renewed attention as a way of accelerating the translation of basic biomedical discoveries for the benefit of patient care.[7] While it is encouraging that public health and behavioral science contributions have been recently emphasized as an essential part of the translational science endeavor, there seems to be little recognition that translational research within the two disciplines — biomedical sciences and behavioral sciences — have developed in parallel.

The term *translational research* had been used in behavioral and social sciences preceding its inclusion in the 2003 NIH Roadmap.[7] For example, in 1998 the National Institute of Mental Health (NIMH) convened the Behavioral Science Workgroup to identify better strategies to translate basic behavioral research findings into medical innovations.[1] Released in 2000, the Workgroup's report, *Translating Behavioral Science into Action*, highlighted the importance of translating basic behavioral processes in mental illness to clinical care and of considering contextual influences on mental illness and treatment. In the same year, the NIMH and the National Institute on Drug Abuse (NIDA) released a Request for Application (RFA) called *Developing Translational Research in Behavioral Sciences*. The purpose of the RFA was to "encourage the development of collaborative partnerships between scientists who study basic behavioral processes (e.g., cognition, emotion, decision making, social networks, culture) and those who study the etiology, diagnosis, treatment, and prevention of mental and behavioral disorders (including drug abuse and addiction) and the delivery of services to those suffering from those disorders."[9]

The history of translational research reveals that research paradigms in biomedical sciences and behavioral sciences have evolved along separate trajectories, with little or no dialogue between the two. In fact, each discipline has its own translational research journal that until recently have had primarily non overlapping manuscript topics. The Association for Clinical and Translational Science began a journal in 2008, *Clinical and Translational Science*, to provide a forum for researchers working to bridge the gap between discovery and improved population outcomes.[10] The Society of Behavioral Medicine established in 2011, *Translational Behavioral Medicine*, to "engage, inform, and catalyze dialogue among the research, practice, and policy communities about behavioral medicine."[11] Over the past two years, *Clinical and Translational Science* has published articles from a wider range of translational research topics including participatory methods for engaging communities in research, translating research to the community through controlled community-based efficacy trials, and the theory behind training scientists to engage in translational research. This may indicate that scientists are beginning to recognize that biomedical science, behavioral science, and public health all have much to offer translational research.

23.2. TRANSLATIONAL RESEARCH IN BIOMEDICINE AND PUBLIC HEALTH — ALIKE AND DIFFERENT

Translation is the process of ensuring effective dissemination of knowledge or interventions while translational research encompasses research that leads to usable diagnostic tools, treatments and interventions, as well as research to explain and improve processes to promote translation. Translation in both biomedical and public health applications (including behavioral science) can be thought of as having four distinct phases, each with unique types of research and outcomes (see Fig. 1).[12] Although these phases are the same in public health and biomedical disciplines, the types of problems studied and the processes within each phase may vary between disciplines, as illustrated in Fig. 1. Translation includes not only the processes of discovering new knowledge and translating that knowledge to initial studies in humans (T1), but also the movement of new treatments and other interventions into later stage research studies and evidence-based guidelines to reach the clinical and community populations for whom they are intended (T2).[6,13] Some authors also propose T3 and T4 phases to depict later stages of translation to promote optimal health impact.[12] The T3 phase establishes practice guidelines and explores active dissemination to promote wide adoption, while T4 translation assures the widest adoption of treatments and interventions to achieve the predicted health outcomes among the population at large. As shown in Fig. 1, both translational processes and outcomes occur within a phase and can include what is referred to by Woolf as translational roadblocks.[6] It has been estimated that efficacious interventions take 17 years to be well-integrated into common medical practice[14] and the full impact of public health knowledge and interventions (e.g., smoking prevention and cessation) can take decades. The purpose of focusing on translational science is ultimately to develop usable research products and to increase understanding required by researchers and policy-makers to plan for and overcome barriers to the

Discovery	T1 Translation to Health Applications → Health Applications in Humans	T2 Translation to Patients & Populations → Interventions to Intended Patients & Populations	T3 Translation to Practice → Wide Adoption in Medical Practice & Communities	T4 Translation to Health Impact → Improvement in Patient & Population Health
Biological and Medical Sciences				
• Basic biologic discovery • Disease mechanisms	• Definition of health outcomes • Clinical intervention development • Initial human testing • Phase 1 and 2 trials	• Establishing clinical utility • Identifying stakeholders • Effectiveness testing (Phase 3 trials) • Synthesize evidence/Develop guidelines	• Active dissemination to health systems • D&I research • Policy analysis • Routine adoption in health care	• Reach, maintenance and institutionalization for optimal clinical effects
e.g. Discovery of role of adrenalin in artery constriction and coronary artery disease	e.g. Drug to block the effects of adrenalin tested in Phase 1 and 2 trials	e.g. Phase 3 drug trial; Incorporation of Beta-blockers into post-myocardial infarction treatment guidelines	e.g. Wide dissemination and proliferation of hypertension medications and clinical guidelines, but wide control of hypertension not achieved	e.g. Optimal clinical effects from hypertension medication not achieved
Public Health Sciences				
• Discovery of population sciences • Risk factor associations • Intervention development	• Initial human testing • Human population and behavioral research • Interventnion efficacy testing	• Establishing public health and/or behavioral utility • Effectiveness testing (Phase 3 community or behavioral trials) • Evidence synthesis/Guideline development	• Active dissemination in communities • D&I research • Routine adoption in populations • Public knowledge, awareness and behavior change	• Reach, maintenance and institutionalization for optimal population health effects
e.g. Discovery of relation of hypertension to stroke and the role of salt in hypertension	e.g. Testing of low salt diet and hypertension	e.g. Guideline development for blood pressure control in hypertension; Community/population diet and lifestyle trials	e.g. NHLBI National High Blood Pressure Program improves treatment uptake; Lifestyle interventions/approaches not widely adopted; Continued controversies in when and what to treat, classes of medication	e.g. Continuing roadblocks to blood pressure control
Behavioral Sciences				
• Basic behavioral processes	• Behavioral processes interventions • Human pop./behavioral research • Intervention efficacy testing (Phase 2 clinical trials)	• Effectiveness testing (Phase 3 community or behavioral trials • Synthesize evidence/Develop guidelines	• Active dissemination • D&I research	• Health effects
e.g. Self-efficacy and use of coping skills identified as determinants of smoking cessation outcomes	e.g. Randomized controlled trial to demonstrate the efficacy of behavioral treatments for smoking cessation in clinic-based settings	e.g. Evaluated the efficacy of delivering behavioral treatments for smoking cessation via state telephone Quitlines to the general population	e.g. Ask-Advise-Connect links smokers with Quitline-delivered treatment via the Electronic Health Record system. AAC trials in primary care settings resulted in a 13-32 fold increase in smoking cessation treatment enrollment.	e.g. Widespread adoption and implementation of Ask-Advise-Connect in community health centers, hospitals and private practice; increases in smoking cessation improve health

Fig. 1. Translational science continuum in biomedicine, public health and behavioral sciences.

progression of new knowledge along the research continuum from discovery to delivery.[3]

Figure 1 presents examples of the research and translation progression in biomedical science, public health and behavioral science. Since this type of figure is often used within the context of biomedical science, we will give only a brief summary of the translational research example within this discipline, and provide a more extensive description of the translational research examples within public health and behavioral science. The biomedical sciences row is a typical biological mechanism and drug development example. The discovery of the role of adrenalin in artery constriction and coronary artery disease illustrates how biomedical discoveries move along the translational research continuum. Following the discovery of the biological mechanism (T0), a drug was developed to block the effects of adrenalin. The discovery was then translated to humans and tested in phase 1 and 2 trials (T1) followed by phase 3 drug trials which incorporated beta-blockers into treatment guidelines for post-myocardial infarction patients (T2). Although the new clinical guidelines for coronary artery disease treatment were widely disseminated and there was a significant increase in the use of the corresponding medications (T3), there was not a significant decrease in the control of hypertension among the general population.

Cardiovascular disease has also been a source of concern among public health researchers engaged in translational research. Within the field of public health, the translational research continuum for cardiovascular disease spans the discovery of the relation of hypertension to health outcomes such as stroke and the role of salt in inducing hypertension (T1); testing of low salt diets in order to reduce hypertension (T2); the development of guidelines to control blood pressure and reduce hypertension (T3); attempts to disseminate adequate blood pressure control in population contexts (T4); and roadblocks in the later stages of dissemination (T4). Further examination of the last two phases of translation within this example reveals the difficulties of translating interventions to medical practices and communities and to populations (T4). One effort to disseminate antihypertensive trial results was the National High Blood Pressure Education Program (NHBEP) of the National Heart, Lung, and

Blood Institute (NHLBI), a consortium of professional and voluntary associations participating in a long-term program to disseminate results from major multicenter clinical trials of antihypertensive treatment.[15–18] The NHBEP influenced the relatively steady progress in awareness, treatment and control of hypertension, and may have contributed to declines in mortality from cardiovascular diseases.[19,20] Nevertheless, progress in translating findings from hypertension research advances into practice has fallen short of Healthy People blood pressure goals.[21] Over the last three decades, the NHLBI has attempted to stimulate and direct innovative methods to accelerate this kind of translation, especially in the period immediately following additional major research in this area.[22–24]

A clinical trial with major implications for public health was the Antihypertensive and Lipid-Lowering Treatment to Prevent Heart Attack Trial (ALLHAT). This large, randomized, double-blind, practice-based, multicenter clinical trial was designed to determine whether the occurrence of fatal coronary heart disease or nonfatal myocardial infarction, stroke, heart failure, renal disease and others cause mortality varied for patients treated with different classes of medication.[25] In part, this research effort was developed to solve some of the barriers related to optimal dissemination of hypertension treatment, namely controversies among providers about drug choice. The final results showed that first-step treatment based on an inexpensive thiazide type diuretic was superior to treatment based on other widely prescribed drug classes in preventing one or more major forms of cardiovascular disease.[26,27]

The resulting publication (a typical science dissemination method) produced some initial increase in prescriptions based on the ALLHAT results; however, this trend did not continue. As a result, the NHLBI funded the development and implementation of a more active dissemination plan. The theory and evidence-based dissemination intervention used peer outreach to primary care providers, also called academic detailing.[28–31] Academic detailing reached 18,550 physicians in 1,698 venues via 147 investigator-educators.[32] The results of the dissemination project suggested that academic detailing may modestly increase physicians' implementation of clinical trial results thereby making prescribing more consistent with evidence. However, one of the lessons learned in this endeavor was that it is possible that fairly limited dissemination efforts on the part of clinical trials may not be able to offset environmental pressures on prescribing practices such as the vested interests and resources of pharmaceutical companies. Another lesson learned was the need to consider stakeholders early in the translation process. A consideration of who might be available, effective and willing, at both the individual and organizational levels, to diffuse trial results should not wait until the evidence is generated. Glasgow and colleagues[33,34] suggested the need for dissemination planning early in the planning of the original trial so that partners who could participate in the dissemination have a stake in evidence generation from the beginning. More about the theory and evidence-based development of the ALLHAT dissemination is included under behavioral science approaches.

The third row of the figure shows a very robust example of the translational process within the field of behavioral science. Unlike the ALLHAT example above, which depicts a targeted dissemination project in a trajectory full of roadblocks, this tobacco cessation example depicts a strong research trajectory that has spanned the entire translational research continuum. Behavioral theory and research have identified self-efficacy and the use of coping skills as important determinants of smoking cessation outcomes (T0).[35–37] Behavioral treatments for smoking cessation have been largely based upon a skills training approach derived from social learning theory.[38] Key elements of such treatments are typically coping skills training, self-efficacy enhancement, and modeling/observational learning. The overarching focus of these treatments is on the acquisition of skills that can be utilized in high-risk situations to prevent relapse.[39] Randomized controlled trials at T1 initially demonstrated the efficacy of behavioral treatments for smoking cessation in clinic-based settings,[40–42] but the reach of these interventions was inherently limited given their intensive, in-person, and group-based nature.[40] Based on these findings, T2 research has evaluated the efficacy of behavioral treatments for smoking cessation that have been adapted for delivery via telephone quitlines. Quitline-delivered smoking cessation treatment has demonstrated impressive efficacy and real-world effectiveness,[42–46] and quitlines are available in most states (*www.naquitline.org*). Using T3 research, a new approach designed to facilitate linking smokers in primary care settings with quitline-delivered behavioral smoking cessation treatment was recently evaluated in a large group-randomized trial. The approach, called Ask Advise Connect (AAC), involved using an automated link in the electronic health record (EHR) to directly send the names and phone numbers of smokers interested in treatment to the state quitline. Compared to the current recommend standard of care in the field, Ask Advise Refer, AAC resulted in a 13-fold increase in smoking cessation treatment enrollment.[47] Based on the efficacy of AAC demonstrated in this large group-randomized trial, the implementation of AAC in two separate healthcare systems is currently being supported by grants from the Cancer Prevention and Research Institute of Texas. Studies are also underway to develop and test strategies for broad dissemination (T4) of AAC in Federally Qualified Health Centers.

As the previous examples illustrate, translational research within each of the three disciplines presents different opportunities and challenges. At the same time, there is a common thread that ties together translational researchers who operate in these distinct fields: the desire to ensure that lifesaving drugs, treatments, and methods of disease prevention are quickly and effectively moved into practical applications to benefit the public. The task for current and future translational science researchers is to critically analyze the shortcomings of the translation process and to find new ways to collaborate and make use of approaches across disciplines to overcome these roadblocks.

23.3. BEHAVIORAL SCIENCE AND PUBLIC HEALTH APPROACHES TO ADVANCE TRANSLATIONAL SCIENCE

Despite the focus on translation of evidence-based approaches by funders including foundations and federal grantmakers such as the Centers for Disease Control and Prevention (CDC) and the National Institutes of Health (NIH), the proliferation of new technologies, treatments and interventions is generally not accompanied by increased use of effective medical innovations, practices, programs and policies. Several authors have described barriers and challenges to effective translation, which include researcher focused studies and designs with little or no input from practitioners and communities, little consideration of external validity,[48] pro-innovation bias, and an overemphasis on the "push" of research products out from developers without considering the need to increase "pull" from potential users — practitioners and communities.[49]

The following section proposes a number of approaches from public health, and more specifically from behavioral science, that can be used to address the challenges mentioned above and to accelerate the translation of biomedical and public health discoveries. These approaches include the ecological model of influence including the use of ecological logic modeling for intervention development, the use of theory to better understand adoption of new knowledge and behavior, community-based participatory research, community-academic partnerships including the formation of strategic alliances, and team science.

23.3.1. The Ecological Model

The ecological paradigm, first introduced in the 1970s by Urie Bronfenbrenner, a developmental psychologist, challenged the restricted view that the study of human development should revolve around an individual's psychology.[50–53] Bronfenbrenner believed that, "environmental events and conditions outside any immediate setting containing the person can have a profound influence on behavior and development" (Ref. 53, p. 18). Building on Lewin's theory of psychological fields,[54] Bronfenbrenner conceptualized the environment as a set of nested structures that comprised five systems: micro, meso, exo, macro and chrono (see Table 1).

Table 1 The Five Systems of Bronfenbrenner's Ecological Model[53]

System Level	Definition
Microsystem	Patterns of activities, social roles and interpersonal relations experienced by the developing person
Mesosystem	The linkages and processes taking place between two or more settings that contain the developing person
Exosystem	The linkages and processes taking place between two or more settings, at least one of which does not contain the developing person
Macrosystem	The belief systems, bodies of knowledge, and customs that are part of a given culture or subculture
Chronosystem	The change or consistency over time in relation to the characteristics of the developing person and the environment in which the person lives

Following Bronfenbrenner's contribution, there was a gradual shift within public health away from an emphasis on individual health behaviors and towards an environmentally based and community-oriented approach to health promotion and disease prevention. The shift, however, did not come without its critics. Even today, there is still a tension between practitioners, policymakers and researchers who view health status as a result of personal lifestyle choices and those who consider health behaviors to be influenced primarily by the environmental structures in which the individual is embedded. The ecological approach, however, strikes a balance between these two viewpoints by recognizing that health behavior is a result of the dynamic and reciprocal interactions between an individual and the environment.[55,56]

In 1986, the Ottawa Charter for Health Promotion (the culmination of the First International Conference on Health Promotion sponsored by the World Health Organization) paved the way for the ecological approach to take on a prominent role within the fields of health education and health promotion.[57] Specific to the field of health promotion, McLeroy and colleagues[58] proposed an ecological model that defined five levels of influence for health behaviors and conditions: (i) intrapersonal or individual, (ii) interpersonal, (iii) institutional or organizational, (iv) community, and (v) public policies. Figure 2 provides an illustration and brief description of each level of influence. Subsequently, the ecological model has been refined, analyzed and applied by other researchers engaged in planning and evaluating health promotion programs.[59–62] In recent years, there have been excellent reviews of the evolution of the ecological model since its inception.[63,64]

Bronfenbrenner's and McLeroy's models have primarily been used for the development and translation of health promotion and disease prevention interventions into real-world settings.[60] As such, they have had a profound effect on the way that we approach behavior change in many disciplines within the behavioral and social sciences.[6]

There are numerous examples of public health and behavioral research that have applied the ecological model in translational science phases T1 through T4, from the assessment of health risks to the development of dissemination interventions for complex public health issues. For example,

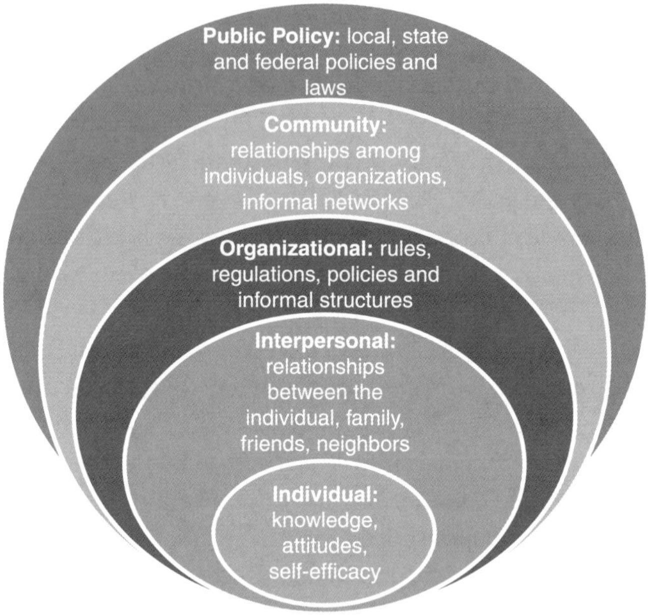

Fig. 2. Ecological levels of influence.[58]

the model has been used to investigate factors associated with adolescent cigarette smoking at the individual, family, peer, school, neighborhood and state policy level.[65] In another tobacco study, researchers found that African American adult smokers living in neighborhoods where there are perceived problems (e.g., vandalism, street litter) and that require high levels of vigilance exhibited greater tobacco dependence than those living in neighborhoods with fewer perceived problems and warranting less vigilance.[66] The ecological model has also been used to develop effective interventions to increase fruit and vegetable intake among African Americans.[67] For older adults living in retirement communities, it has been used to design a multilevel intervention to increase physical activity by addressing individual, interpersonal and community influences on behavior change.[68] Fernandez and colleagues[69] conducted a review of factors influencing HPV vaccination and organized these according to several ecological levels of influence to develop a multilevel conceptual model of HPV vaccination. These examples illustrate that the ecological model can be useful for conceptualizing and identifying factors that influence both disease risk and health behaviors among diverse populations and for planning multilevel interventions which address both behavioral and environmental conditions that influence health outcomes.

The ecological model can have important implications for translational research in biomedical science even in early phases. In the last decade of his life, Bronfenbrenner, who continued to revise the model until his death in 2005, reconceptualized the relevance of biological and genetic aspects of the person in human development and renamed it the bioecological model.[70,71] Within this new framework, he posited that interactions and processes between the individual and the environment represent explanatory mechanisms through which genotypes are transformed into phenotypes, and that heritability is greatly influenced by the individual's environment.[70] Currently, the accepted view is that neither genetics nor environments are solely responsible for producing individual variation, and that gene–environment interactions are commonplace.[72–74] The revision to the model underscores the importance of considering environmental influences when translating basic science research into clinical applications during T1 translational research.

23.3.2. Theory- and Evidence-based Interventions to Promote Translation

Combining an understanding of the ecological model with theory and evidence-based health promotion planning can help researchers address behavioral and environmental influences that must be taken into account when planning research with an eye to translation or when planning active dissemination. Too often, researchers may see dissemination as a process of translating knowledge rather than a process of promoting adoption *behavior*. We suggest a systematic approach to both designing interventions with an eye to disseminabilty in the first place and using an ecological, systematic approach to planning translation in the second place.[62] For translation, the approach we suggest is to follow a process of: (i) development of an ecological causal model of behavioral and environmental factors (and their determinants) related to a stage of translation, and in particular, related to barriers to translation (i.e., the logic model of the problem: why do clinicians prescribe less than optimal hypertension drugs; why do patients fail to adopt lifestyle changes); (ii) development of a causal model that includes theoretical constructs for producing change in the behavior and environmental factors of interest (i.e., the logic model of change: how can the determinants of translational behaviors be changed at multiple levels of influence); (iii) selection of effective intervention methods and delivery of practical applications to achieve changes in health behavior.

In our view, the use of theory is necessary for behavior change research to ensure that researchers identify relevant causal factors of the behavior (i.e., the logic model of the problem, or as MacKinnon and Leuken referred to it,[75] concept theory) and identify change methods that address the concept theory and maximize intervention effectiveness (i.e., the logic model of change, or as MacKinnon and Leuken referred to it,[75] action theory).[76] Further, use of theory helps researchers measure and describe the pathways through which change occurs or the points where change breaks down, making the findings even of failed trials useful in informing subsequent research. Importantly, the use of theory must go beyond mere lip service and should be embedded throughout intervention development and testing.

Effective development, testing and reporting of interventions often requires approaching theory in a way that is fundamentally different from either the generation of theory, testing single theories, or comparing theory effectiveness for explaining or changing behavior. Researchers seeking a perspective on how to promote translation have a behavior change problem to solve. This is a different task than that of a behavioral or social scientist whose main concern may be testing theory. A researcher looking for solutions to translational roadblocks should be encouraged to consider one or multiple theories, empirical evidence, and new research both to assess a problem and to solve or prevent a problem. By theory, we mean a cohesive explanation for a set of specific causal relations among constructs, and between these constructs and target behaviors. For instance, Social Cognitive Theory views behavior as a result of causal, reciprocal interactions among individual cognition, behavior, and the environment.[77] A model is a hypothesized set of relations between constructs and target behaviors, and models can help a researcher identify the full range of factors that may influence translation.

For example, in the development of the dissemination of ALLHAT trial results described above, the team modeled hypothesized determinants of physician prescribing behavior working from a Social Cognitive Theory (SCT) perspective.[32] This theory focuses on both individual cognitive influences on behavior and on social environmental influences.[77] The team combined detailed descriptions of the targeted healthcare provider behavioral change with cognitive and affective factors such as awareness of, or familiarity with, guidelines, behavioral capability and skills (knowing what to do and how to do it), self-efficacy and outcome expectations for practice change as well as social influences such as patient adherence and follow-up for re-evaluation, commercial marketing, and presence of guidelines and standards of care.

The ecological perspective can be immensely helpful to translational science researchers through its conceptualization of the various levels of influence over processes affecting the entire translational science continuum including studies of early clinical applications of biomedical advances to the design, implementation and scale-up of evidence-based treatments and interventions in clinical settings, practices, and communities. Additionally, this perspective can function to bring biomedical, behavioral and public health scientists together in efforts to influence programs and policies that impact these environmental factors at multiple phases of the translational research continuum.

23.3.3. CBPR Methods to Enhance Translational Science

Community-based participatory research (CBPR) is an approach to research that prioritizes and fosters equitable relationships between community members and scientists to build research capacity and address community needs through action.[78–80] With this approach, the community and researchers jointly define the problem, choose the study design, determine methods, collect, analyze, and interpret data, disseminate findings and create actions resulting in policy, programs or practices. CBPR emphasizes community and academic dialogue and co-ownership of research early on and throughout the translational process. With a CBPR approach, the needs, interests and values of the community can be better addressed in the research process.[78] Participatory models typically advocate the inclusion of stakeholders such as community organizations, social service agencies, community leaders, faith-based organizations, community health centers, and lay health worker programs.

CBPR has been used to carry out epidemiologic, intervention, evaluation and policy studies[81] for many issues including alcohol and drug prevention among youth,[82] cancer screening,[83] HPV vulnerabilities and prevention,[84] environmental justice,[85] injury prevention,[86,87] and obesity prevention.[88,89] CBPR has also been posited as a method for improving primary healthcare in practice-based research networks by promoting translation of research into practice.[81,90]

Interest in CBPR methods among public health and clinical practice researchers is growing as results continue to demonstrate that it can improve dissemination and the sustainability of interventions leading to improvements in healthcare delivery and community health.[79,80] Both CBPR and translational science have as their ultimate focus a research process that creates practical innovations and applications to improve population health.[91–93] CBPR can help ensure relevance and external validity of research findings because potential beneficiaries of the research identify problems to be addressed,[94] assist in planning usable and feasible interventions, and help influence factors that may be important for adoption and implementation. CBPR approaches can help close the gap between research and practice.

Community-engaged research is an integral part of the translational science process, particularly when researchers seek improvements to health outcomes in populations experiencing health-related disparities. Translation can begin with identifying unsolved health problems for exploration in biomedical "bench" research (T0), from bench research to clinical trials (T1), from clinical trials into practice (T2), from limited application into widespread adoption (T3), and from broad adoption into population outcomes (T4) and requires bidirectional communication and engagement between researchers and the potential end users or consumers of health-related advances. The community partners for CBPR should represent multiple sectors of the community to more fully account for diversity of opinions and potential uses of the innovation, but also to set the stage for stronger engagement and sustainability of advances.[95] Depending on the nature of the research, community representatives could come from not-for-profit organizations, government, schools, faith-based organizations, healthcare providers, business, law enforcement, and so on. Also, depending on the research, constituents should represent broad diversity by ethnicity, age, gender, socioeconomic status, and cultural background so that the dialogue between community and academic researchers is more robust regarding the research being proposed and its uses.

During the translational research process, community members and academic researchers have complementary roles. Figure 3 illustrates multiple points where CBPR can enhance research activities at various points along the translational research continuum.

During the discovery phase, sometimes referred to as T0 translation, CBPR approaches could reduce the time for identifying unexamined health problems or salient determinants of these problems, particularly among populations facing health disparities. This type of contribution is possible when researchers and community members have trusting relationships where dialogue about relevant health issues or observations in clinical or community settings occurs. Community members express priorities and relevance of health in their lives; researchers express whether there is scientific value and funding for undertaking the research endeavor. For example, Hebert and colleagues described a previously unconsidered association between a chemical compound and cancer that was identified because both the community and the researchers agreed on its relevance and scientific merit. In T1, community members can help enhance enrollment of populations typically reluctant to participate in clinical trials. They can ensure that the trial aligns with health issues of importance for the marginalized population, work with community health workers to advise and assist on recruitment and retention approaches to more effectively reach desirable populations, and voice support for the trial within their social networks. A community member's role is to express concerns over safety of, and barriers to, participation while a researcher's role is commitment to safe and scientifically appropriate recruitment approaches and trial procedures. In T2, CBPR approaches could enhance dialogue about

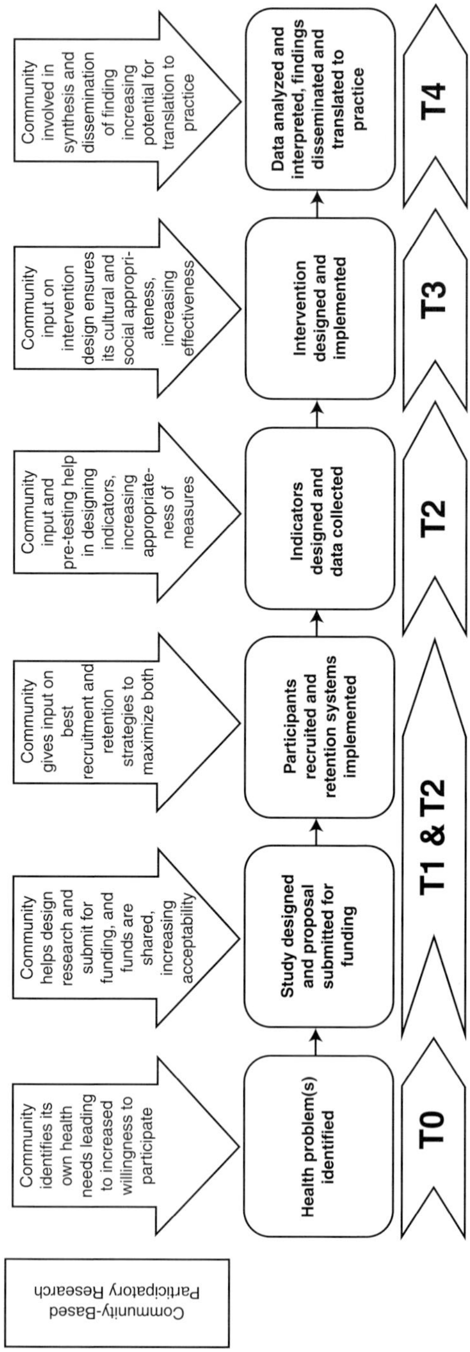

Fig. 3. Contribution of CBPR at various points in the research process. (Adapted from AHRQ Evidence Report/Technology Assessment No. 99.[213])

context that should be considered in the development and rigorous examination of interventions based on trial results to maximize relevance, reach and sustainability. When community members are partners in intervention development, they may also assist in a pilot testing and modification phase. Community members often express the need for culturally appropriate and low burden data collection and intervention methods; researchers express the need for scientific rigor to draw conclusions. The community-engaged pilot testing conducted during T2 can bring "street credibility" in T3 to market the benefits of the intervention and overcome the barriers to adoption. Additionally, during T3 science, community partners could assist in dissemination through their networks and accelerate dissemination and implementation research efforts, particularly if partners include potential adopters and implementers of the effective treatment, practice change, program or policy. Community members can serve as role models to other communities considering adoption of the innovation (T4).

While CBPR can accelerate the translational science process, there are issues that should be considered. Researchers have discussed several challenges to CBPR including the longer timeframe needed to conduct CBPR, conflicts that can arise due to differing cultural viewpoints (e.g., culture, social class, financial), the need to find a balance on issues of scientific rigor, tensions about issue selection and framing, and the willingness to share power, resources and rewards.[96,97] A common problem contributing to the perspective that CBPR approaches have limited utility occurs when research is labeled as CBPR when it is not. CBPR is not a community advisory board "rubber-stamping" research agendas previously determined by researchers, or community advisory boards being nominally involved in selected elements of the research process when it is advantageous to the researchers.[94] While community participation with academic researchers can range along a continuum from networking, coordination and cooperation to full collaboration,[98] "less than full" applications of CBPR truncates the potential for continued documentation of the impact CBPR can have in translational science.

23.3.4. Community–Academic Partnerships

Related to CBPR, the development of formal and informal partnerships between researchers and community organizations is important for extending the reach of effective interventions.[99,100] Public health professionals have been using the approach of forming community–academic partnerships for many years.[101] In their chapter titled "If translational research is the answer, what's the question and who gets to ask it?" Wandersman and Lesesne point out that consumer and practitioner perspectives are critical for understanding what information practitioners need and what consumers desire and understand.[48] These authors further described limitations to the "research-to-practice" models and propose a multidimensional framework for bridging research and practice. This framework illustrates the existing push of innovations for translation from funders and researchers to practitioners and consumers and highlights the limited and needed interactions between consumers/practitioners and researchers/funders.[48] They posited that funders and researchers should consider a consumer–practitioner perspective so that research evidence and products that are developed are relevant, will be supported and implemented by practitioners, and accepted by consumers. They also propose collaborations with national advocacy organizations, such as the American Cancer Society, that periodically assess information needs from a variety of groups, monitor trends in media use, and track practitioner behavior.[48] This information can be useful in planning comprehensive translation efforts that take consumer–practitioner perspectives into account for the design and implementation of interventions that are acceptable, feasible and sustainable.[48] As Wandersman and Lesesne point out, while researchers have adequate methods to address questions related to how to address health problems, they often do not ask the necessary questions related to acceptability, feasibility, sustainability and value of key stakeholders in their translation efforts.[48]

Challenges with academic, community and practice partnerships include differences not only in perspectives about what is important, but also the differences that often exist between researchers and practitioners in assessing and using evidence.[102] Practitioners, often working under severe time and resource constraints, require immediate solutions to problems and may make early judgments about the value of a particular program or strategy. Researchers, on the other hand, are trained to avoid making premature conclusions about scientific findings and intervention effectiveness.

Another challenge is that even when there is sufficient evidence or guidelines, researchers often lack the skills needed to communicate in commonsense terms the findings from research and apply these to practical problems. Kerner recommended that, "to close the philosophical gap between research, practice, and policy, investments of time and energy need to be made by scientists, practitioners, and policymakers to help create a new 'culture' of trans-disciplinary collaboration" (Ref. 103, p. 94).

The National Cancer Institute's (NCI) Community Networks Program (CNP) is a cooperative U54 agreement among 25 academic sites across the U.S. that funds community–academic partnerships that represent this type of transdisciplinary collaboration.[103] CNP centers (CNPCs) aim to reduce cancer-related disparities through community-based education, training and research. The CNPCs establish local partnerships with practitioners and community organizations to help define, implement and interpret findings related to cancer control. Each CNPC has a community outreach core that encourages researchers and partners to engage in CBPR to create interventions that benefit from the perspectives of users and community partners. These centers also engage in efforts that could aid in translational science endeavors at earlier (T1 and T2) stages of the translation continuum. For instance, the Tampa Bay Community Cancer Network conducted a qualitative study to assess the knowledge, attitudes, beliefs and informational needs about cancer-related biospecimen collection among mostly Hispanic and African American community members. The findings were used to inform the design of Spanish and English communication tools to present biobanking educational content through print and visual media.[104]

Another example, the Cancer Prevention and Control Research Network (CPCRN) was established in 2002 with funding from the CDC and the NCI. Comprising 10 centers in nine states, the CPCRN is a thematic research network that is part of the Prevention Research Centers, CDC's flagship program designed to prevent and control chronic diseases.[105] Each center has a variety of academic, healthcare provider and community organization partners who work together to accelerate the use of evidence-based programs in communities and to fill in evidence gaps about "what works" in cancer prevention and control and on dissemination and implementation research, especially among minorities and the medically underserved.[106]

In 2008, the CPCRN conducted a survey of 282 cancer control planners to capture knowledge, attitudes, behaviors and training needs of cancer control practitioners for translating research evidence into practice. These planners represented government agencies, health service providers, and community-based organizations and coalitions. The survey results indicated that less than half of respondents (48 percent) had ever used online resources that provide access to and resources for implementing evidence-based programs for cancer control such as R-TIPS or Cancer Control P.L.A.N.E.T.[107] In addition, nearly all respondents (97 percent) expressed the need for training. These results led to other CPCRN efforts aimed at providing guidance to network partners for finding, adapting and implementing evidence-based programs, practices and policies in communities[107] including: (i) the development of an online decision support system to assist health program planners adapt evidence-based programs;[108] (ii) the development of a CPCRN Capacity Building Technical Assistance and Training workgroup which develops and provides training on finding, using and adapting evidence-based approaches (EBAs) for cancer control;[109] and (iii) several CPCRN regional networks have provided mini-grants and technical assistance to community partners implementing and adapting EBAs.[110,111]

Establishing community–academic partnerships increases the likelihood that research products will be relevant, acceptable, feasible and sustainable in communities and practice settings. These partnerships can contribute to decision-making across the stages of translations from discovery to delivery. Although there can be notable differences between the perspectives, motivations and goals of researchers and practitioners/consumers of health innovations, these differences are not insurmountable and ultimately enrich products of research. The Community Networks Program and the Cancer Prevention and Control Research Network provide real examples of the kind of infrastructure, institutional support and resources that are needed to facilitate sustainable connections between the community and academic institutions to accelerate the use of effective treatments, practices, programs and policies to improve health.

23.3.4.1. *Strategic alliances to advance translation and address health disparities*

Translational research has an important role in the elimination of health disparities and is a major priority for the CDC, DHHS and Affordable Care Act. It is widely understood that innovations, when they are first diffused in populations, can actually increase disparities;[112,113] innovative treatments, diagnostic tools and preventive measures are no exception. This is largely because those individuals who have access to resources including comprehensive health insurance coverage, access to hospitals and academic health centers have greater possibilities for receiving state-of-the-art services while those living in poverty, who have no insurance or are underinsured, may not have access to the same types or quality of services.[114] Thus, even when we have been successful in increasing reach through T3 translation efforts, we may be unwittingly increasing health disparities. If we are to avoid the pitfalls inherent in attempts to disseminate innovations to benefit those most in need, we must forge strategic alliances that can best make use of translational research products. While the types of community–academic partnerships described above, an approach used by public health professionals for many years,[101] can provide a mechanism for ensuring that important perspectives are taken into consideration as researchers and stakeholders make decisions across the translational science continuum, strategic alliances with social service and health service partners show particular promise for speedy delivery of research evidence to those in need.[115–118] One approach for alleviating this problem is to form alliances with existing service systems that have large reach, particularly among populations that experience the greatest health disparities — for example, housing programs, child maltreatment services, and juvenile justice.

These strategic alliances must be forged through a CBPR approach rather than through the lens of a unidirectional research "pipeline" where researchers are delivering innovations to service agencies. Instead, information, research products, and tacit knowledge about needs and contextual factors affecting health should flow in both directions between researchers and social service agencies. This type of alliance can accomplish several synergistic goals: (i) advance translation while avoiding a concurrent increase in health disparities, (ii) assist social service agencies in fulfilling their main functions, and (iii) help their clients achieve social and health well-being.[119]

To date, translation efforts in social service systems have been mostly focused on implementing complex protocols for difficult-to-treat psychiatric conditions, such as substance abuse, conduct disorder, depression and post-traumatic stress disorder. And there has been little translation of effective prevention programs such as primary and secondary prevention interventions that address behavioral risk factors (e.g., healthy eating, physical activity, tobacco cessation, and cancer screenings).[119] However, few studies have been conducted in public housing settings using the community-based participatory research approach. For example, McNeil and colleagues conducted a community-based randomized controlled trial in public housing and showed the effectiveness of a peer-led colorectal cancer prevention program.[120] Andrews *et al.* partnered with public housing services to inform a culturally situated, ecologically based, multi-level tobacco cessation intervention to help African American women living in urban, high poverty, public housing neighborhoods to quit smoking.[121]

An excellent example of the type of strategic partnership we refer to was established between researchers in social and behavioral science and the 2-1-1 system to bridge the gap between research and practice particularly to benefit the underserved. In 2010, a national 2-1-1 Research Consortium was established with members from the United Way, 2-1-1 U.S., individual 2-1-1 systems across the nation, NCI, CDC, and university-based researchers.[122] More detail about the products of this partnership is included elsewhere.[123]

The 2-1-1 system is a three-digit telephone information and referral service that connects people to health and social services available in their communities. There are more than 200 2-1-1 centers operating in all 50 states, the District of Columbia, and Puerto Rico. In 2011, there were nearly 17 million calls to 2-1-1.[124] When callers dial 2-1-1, they talk with compassionate and professionally trained information specialists who are skilled in resource identification, matching and referral, and who provide concrete information about places to go and agencies to call to get help. Callers can also be transferred directly to services where previous arrangements have been made with participating agencies. Callers to 2-1-1 are often racial or ethnic minorities with lower income and educational levels than the general population, and who suffer higher rates of unemployment or job insecurity.[122] Typically, callers are seeking assistance to alleviate basic needs such as lack of food, shelter or electricity when their unemployment benefits run out, and during (or in the aftermath of) natural disasters or disease outbreaks. 2-1-1 callers represent populations that suffer from a wide range of health disparities and are often considered "hard to reach" (i.e., they are less likely to have a primary care provider, get preventive health services, or have access to innovative treatments or opportunities to participate in clinical trials).[123]

Various research collaborations highlighted in the recent supplement of the *American Journal of Preventive Medicine* have demonstrated that 2-1-1 is an innovative and effective system for screening, recruiting and/or intervening in health issues with disadvantaged populations beyond a response to callers' immediate service requests.[123] Eddens *et al.* have found that 2-1-1 callers are willing and able to complete a cancer risk assessment tool when they seek help from 2-1-1 information specialists.[122] Other studies have shown significant cancer control needs among 2-1-1 callers through similar assessments[125–127] and statistical modeling.[128] Savas *et al.* found that the HPV vaccine uptake among daughters of Hispanic and African American parents is lower than other low-income minority groups in Texas and identified factors that influence their HPV vaccination decisions.[126] Moving beyond assessment to interventions, Kreuter *et al.*'s randomized controlled trial is the first to show that proactive referrals for preventive services motivated callers to follow up with cancer control services such as mammograms, Pap tests, and smoking cessation treatments.[129] Currently, Fernandez and colleagues are also implementing and evaluating navigation services and referrals for preventive services for 2-1-1 callers in Texas.[127] A partnership with the Los Angeles 2-1-1 system screened callers for developmentally disabled and/or autistic children in the household and connected them with free or low-cost services in the community. Follow-up care coordination was also provided to facilitate completion of referrals for diagnostic evaluation, early childhood education, and other developmental needs among low-income children who might not have received the care otherwise.[130] Rodgers *et al.* partnered with 2-1-1 San Diego and community members to build the Healthcare Navigation Program to assist low-income callers in applying for social and health programs such as health insurance coverage, prescription assistance, food assistance, as well as overcoming other barriers to healthcare such as transportation, scheduling appointments, and child/elder care.[131] Given the extensive reach of 2-1-1 systems, even a modest response to these screenings, referrals and/or intervention programs could have a meaningful impact on population health and health disparities.[123]

The tremendous reach of 2-1-1 systems could be expanded when combined with other social service systems. For example, Bennett partnered with the Federal Communication Commission's LifeLine Assistance program, which provides millions of low-income Americans in 38 states with a free mobile phone, service and texting plan.[115] His study suggested that the 2-1-1 systems, when connected with mobile or eHealth technology, could reduce health disparities to a greater degree and on a larger scale.[115] Another example was a partnership between the 2-1-1 system and the Centers for Medicaid and Medicare Services to help callers undergo preliminary screening for Medicaid eligibility and provide assistance in completing Medicaid applications, especially for uninsured children who are eligible but not yet enrolled. These studies have laid the foundation for larger dissemination efforts of health-related programs, policies and interventions to the 2-1-1 systems across the country. Creating partnerships between the 2-1-1 systems and other social service systems represents a promising approach to advance translation efforts to improve the health of disadvantaged populations. In sum, the strategic partnership approach, which makes use of researcher knowledge and experience of innovative interventions and leverages existing social service resources, strategies and delivery channels, shows a strong potential to accelerate translation efforts while simultaneously reducing health disparities.

23.3.5. Team Science Approaches to Enhance Translational Science

Recently, there has been an emphasis on the importance of *team science* for translational research. Team science seeks to bring together scientists from diverse disciplines who are able to integrate a variety of concepts, approaches and methods in order to tackle complex, real-world health problems.[132] Since its inception, public health has benefited from teams of researchers and professionals from many different fields to understand and combat disease.[133,134] Interdisciplinary teams in public health including epidemiologists, sociologists, physicians, biological scientists, health educators, bioethicists and environmental health specialists create comprehensive, integrated solutions to complex problems.[135–138] These collaborations enable consideration of the public health impact of solutions and make decisions that ultimately lead to treatments, programs and policies that can be readily translated to improve public health.[139,140] In *Research for the Public Good*, Wethington and Dunifon note that a common theme among contributed chapters is the multi-method approaches to translation.[141] Team science offers wide expertise in methodology including mixed methods approaches, CBPR, and practice and policy.[141] The team science approach can be used both to address the challenges of conducting translational research in the behavioral and social sciences and in using public health and behavioral science approaches to advance research translation in biomedical fields.[141]

Largely led by public health and behavioral scientists, and funded by the NIH and the National Center for Advancing Translational Science, the Science of Team Science (SciTC) field has recently emerged to provide evidence-based understanding of the characteristics of effective team-based research and to document what team-based research contributes to scientific progress.[142–144] For example, Hall and colleagues[145] found that transdisciplinary research center-initiated grants had a higher rate of scientific publication and greater collaboration (as indicated by higher average number of coauthors on the publications) than investigator-initiated grants, indicating that team science approaches can accelerate scientific output and progress.

23.4. DISSEMINATION AND IMPLEMENTATION RESEARCH CONTRIBUTIONS TO TRANSLATIONAL SCIENCE

The growing evidence-to-practice movement in public health and medicine has underscored gaps that exist not only in our evidence base, but also in the processes and factors that affect the adoption, implementation and maintenance of effective health innovations.[146–148] Although the definitions and parameters are still evolving,[6] for many public health and behavioral science researchers and practitioners, translational research is synonymous with dissemination and implementation (D&I) research.

D&I research focuses on understanding and intervening in the processes that influence the translation of health innovations including treatments, practice guidelines, and behavioral interventions into real-world settings to improve health. Several terms are used interchangeably to describe D&I research: knowledge translation, knowledge exchange, and knowledge utilization.[149] According to Rabin and colleagues, "Dissemination is the active approach of spreading evidence-based interventions to the target audience via determined channels using planned strategies. Implementation is the process of putting to use or integrating evidence-based interventions within a setting."[150] Dissemination and implementation of research findings are necessary to achieve a return on investment within the larger research enterprise and to improve population health and well-being.[151] Numerous studies have shown that passive dissemination (e.g., publications, mass mailings) of evidence-based interventions has been ineffective, resulting in small impact in the new settings.[152] Therefore, more targeted, proactive approaches to D&I of evidence-based interventions are needed that take into account the characteristics of the potential users, evidence-based interventions, implementation processes, and the inner and outer settings in which the intervention is implemented.[151,153] As Colditz argued, there is no shortage of research; the real problem is figuring out how to sift through studies and draw inferences to disseminate and implement effective programs and policies more broadly.[151] In the current healthcare and public heath landscape, several factors point to the urgency for D&I research, including (i) the underperforming healthcare system with unsatisfactory population health outcomes, (ii) ever-growing healthcare expenses, (iii) inequities in health conditions and access to care, and (iv) the prevalence of balkanized approaches to both clinical and public health interventions.[154] These issues have raised important questions to be answered by D&I research (adapted from Ref. 152):

(i) How do we gather information on effective interventions to form the evidence base?

(ii) How will research-tested interventions be applicable in different settings?
(iii) What methods should we use to decide what to disseminate or implement?
(iv) Which dissemination and implementation strategies will yield the greatest impact on population health?
(v) What outcomes should be tracked to know if we are making progress?
(vi) What will it take to maintain or sustain evidence-based practices?

The following sections will introduce the contemporary theoretical frameworks, research designs, and measurement methods in D&I research to address these questions.

23.4.1. Dissemination and Implementation Frameworks

Although D&I science is a relatively young discipline,[155] there is a wide range of theories and frameworks used by researchers to inform D&I study designs[156] that seek to understand how to effectively translate evidence-based approaches (i.e., guidelines, treatments, programs, policies) into everyday practice.

23.4.1.1. *Diffusion of Innovations Theory*

For over a century, there has been a rich history of theorizing about the diffusion of innovations — new ideas, beliefs, knowledge, practices, programs and technologies.[157] It was not until 1962, however, when Everett Rogers published his book *Diffusion of Innovations* that the theory became widely recognized. Rogers defines diffusion as the process by which an innovation is communicated through certain channels over time among the members of a social system.[158] Rogers was concerned with understanding why, how, by whom, and the rate at which innovations are adopted over time. He identified five attributes of an innovation that are positively related to the rate of adoption: relative advantage, compatibility, complexity, trialability and observability. Table 2 provides a brief description of each attribute.[158]

Table 2 The Five Innovation Attributes of Rogers' Diffusion of Innovations Theory

Attribute	Description
Relative advantage	The degree to which an innovation is perceived by potential adopters as being better than the idea or the practice that it is replacing
Compatibility	The degree to which the innovation is compatible with accepted socio-cultural, economic and philosophical values
Complexity	The degree to which an innovation is perceived by potential adopters as relatively difficult to understand or use
Trialability	The degree to which an innovation may be tried out for a limited time by potential adopters
Observability	The degree to which the results of an innovation are easily observable by others and easy to communicate

Glanz and Oldenburg summarize the importance of these innovation attributes along with the characteristics of individuals that are potential adopters and the role of the setting in which the innovation is diffused.[159] Rogers' classical diffusion model was later applied to health promotion by Orlandi and colleagues[160] and by Green *et al.*[161] Orlandi proposes that the diffusion process is most successful when it involves a collaborative partnership between the resource system (i.e., group or individual promoting the program) and the user system (i.e., the potential users of the program). He also suggests that linkage agents can then be used to enhance the transfer of knowledge between the actors of the two systems. As Dearing points out, this transfer of knowledge, the key to translational research, represents the balance between dissemination and diffusion.[162] On one hand, members of the resource system are disseminating or transmitting information about the innovation. On the other hand, the knowledge is diffusing through members of the user system as a result of social processes that may or may not occur with great force or strength. Dearing also describes advances in dissemination theory beyond the Diffusion of Innovations Theory, and emphasizes the importance of considering organizational factors and "networks of influence" between organizations to create strategies that influence program use.[157]

23.4.1.2. *RE-AIM*

Over a decade ago, Glasgow and colleagues[33] challenged the conventional view that public health promotion interventions should be evaluated based on an efficacy paradigm.[163] This paradigm, they said, was an over simplification because performing experiments in a controlled environment ensuring internal validity and eliminating all confounding variables was of little use to researchers concerned with improving the health of populations in the real world, particularly in understaffed public health clinics, large health systems, or community settings.[164] Recognizing the complexity of operating in real-world settings, public health researchers began to incorporate behavioral and environmental components into their interventions consistent with the ecological model perspective.

Expanding on the work of Abrams and colleagues,[165] who had defined the impact of an intervention as the product of a program's reach and efficacy ($I = R \times E$), Glasgow and colleagues[33] added three new dimensions, namely: adoption, implementation and maintenance (AIM). The resulting model, RE-AIM, provides a comprehensive framework to evaluate the new generation of multilevel public health and community-based interventions. The five dimensions of the model are described in Table 3.[166] The RE-AIM framework has become widely used among researchers, funders, policymakers and public health program planners who are engaged in translational research work.

The RE-AIM framework has been used to address questions related to the dissemination and implementation of interventions to reduce health disparities.[167] Because of the focus on considering parameters such as reach, implementation and maintenance, it is well suited to guiding both the development of interventions as well as their evaluation.[168,169] Glasgow and colleagues propose that RE-AIM can help bridge the gap between efficacy and effectiveness trials to improve external validity and consequently improve acceptance, adoption, implementation and maintenance.[33] Research across the translational science continuum should

Table 3 The Five Dimensions of the RE-AIM Model

Dimension	Definition
Reach	The participation rate within the target population and the barriers that it faces in attempting to participate in the intervention (e.g., transportation, cost)
Efficacy	The impact of an intervention regarding specific outcome criteria
Adoption	The proportion and diversity of organizations that adopt an intervention and the factors that affect the decision to adopt (e.g., expertise of adopters, institutional requirements)
Implementation	The level of fidelity and the quality of the intervention as it is replicated in real-world settings
Maintenance	Whether or not the intervention lasts over time and the extent to which it becomes institutionalized within the delivery setting

consider such dimensions as potential reach, impact and sustainability in making decisions about research focus, clinical applications, recommendations for practice and broad scale up and use.

23.4.1.3. *The Consolidated Framework for Implementation Research (CFIR)*

Beyond RE-AIM, there are a number of published frameworks that strengthen the field of implementation by providing guidelines and constructs that help explain implementation, provide frameworks for exploring possible mediators and moderators of successful translation, and provide targets for intervening to improve implementation and maintenance of effective interventions. For example, Damschroder and colleagues[153] used a snowballing sampling approach to identify the various dissemination and implementation theories, and to unify and consolidate the key constructs into a meta-theoretical framework: the Consolidated Framework for Implementation Research (CFIR). CFIR is composed of five domains: (i) intervention characteristics, (ii) outer setting, (iii) inner setting, (iv) individuals, and (v) process. Within each domain there are a number of constructs that facilitate the development, planning and evaluation of health innovations aimed at creating behavior change (see Table 4). Overall, CFIR enhances

Table 4 The Five Domains of the Consolidated Framework for Implementation Research

Dimension	Definition
Intervention characteristics	The intervention may be complex and multifaceted but can be thought of as having indispensable "core components" and an "adaptable periphery" that can be modified according to the implementing organization
Outer setting	The economic, political and social context within which the implementing organization is embedded
Inner setting	The structural, cultural and political context and climate through which the implementation process will be executed
Individuals	The mindsets, norms, interests and affiliations of adopters and decision makers involved in the intervention
Process	Planning, engaging and executing the implementation

translational research by emphasizing the importance of understanding the characteristics of health innovations and proposing factors that influence implementation.

Implementation research that explores the relationship between these constructs and adoption and implementation outcomes can elucidate those factors that can be targets of dissemination intervention efforts to increase adoption and implementation. For example, using the CFIR framework as a guide to identify and develop measurement instruments, the CPCRN is currently conducting both qualitative and quantitative studies to assess the influence of various inner setting constructs on implementation of colorectal cancer screening practices in Federally Qualified Health Centers. This research will be used to develop interventions aimed at addressing those changeable factors to improve implementation outcomes.[170]

23.4.1.4. *The Interactive Systems Framework*

In 2008, Wandersman and colleagues[171] proposed the Interactive Systems Framework (ISF) for dissemination and implementation. The ISF is extremely useful for translational researchers who seek to bridge the gap between research and practice. The framework incorporates the perspectives and dynamic interactions between multiple actors such as practitioners, funding agencies, support agencies and researchers. The ISF recognizes how crucial it is to understand the needs and interests of each set of actors in order to systematically influence the widespread adoption and implementation of health innovations.[48] Specifically, the ISF describes the key systems, functions and relationships involved in dissemination and implementation of health prevention innovations.

The ISF is comprised of three systems: (i) the Prevention Synthesis and Translation System, which helps make research products more easily accessible and usable for practitioners; (ii) the Prevention Support System, which provides general and intervention-specific support to build capacity for implementation in adopting organizations; and (iii) the Prevention Delivery System, which executes the activities needed to implement evidence-based programs. The authors suggest that the ISF can: (a) help identify potential partners and understand how they interact with other systems, (b) allow different people within the various systems to better understand the perspectives of individuals in other systems, and (c) help funders identify the types of support they need to provide for synthesis, translation, support and delivery. Translational research, which takes into account interactions across the three systems, can lead to a better understanding of the needs of key stakeholders, enhance the development of more useful prevention products, and develop strategies that can be used to increase the capacity of organizations involved in adoption and implementation.

23.4.2. Dissemination and Implementation Research Methods

As previously noted, there is a significant gap between science and practice, which prevails in clinical practice, public health programs and health policy. Many researchers argue that this gap exists due to the overemphasis on internal validity (i.e., the causal relationships) of explanatory trials at the expense of external validity (i.e., compromising the relevance, applicability and generalizability of research findings).[172,173] Most traditional explanatory trials test average effects within conditions among "ideal" participants, with an assumption that the effects, often characterized in a dose-response linear relationship, can apply universally.[175] However, practitioners who operate in the real world often view such research as irrelevant, which is the most cited barrier to evidence-based practice.[173,176] Therefore, practical and pragmatic approaches with more emphasis on external validity are highly desired and needed.[177–180]

Glasgow and Chambers summarized the methodological characteristics of such approaches to achieve both rigor and relevance, including (i) engaging practitioners, patients and policy makers to form research questions that can inform real-world decision-making; (ii) recruiting a variety of participants that represent the population to which the intervention would apply; (iii) comparing interventions to real-world conditions; (iv) using flexible designs to fit the questions relevant to stakeholders; and (v) reporting transparently on recruitment, implementation processes, contextual issues and outcomes across multiple levels.[175] Since few studies are completely pragmatic or explanatory, they argued that there is no dichotomy between pragmatic trials and traditional explanatory trials, but rather a continuum.[181] The CONSORT Statement on pragmatic trials also concurs with that assertion.[182] As Kessler and Glasgow pointed out, such approaches include a broader range of research designs that can be considered the "gold standard" based on the specific context.[173] Some novel designs in D&I research are briefly introduced below. Common to all of them is the aim to accelerate the translation process from research discoveries to routine practice.

23.4.2.1. *Hybrid designs*

The traditional dominant research approach also encourages delimited, step-wise progressions of research on clinical efficacy, followed by research on clinical effectiveness, and finally implementation research. Curran *et al.* proposed a typology of three types of effectiveness-implementation hybrid designs, including (i) testing effects of a clinical intervention on relevant outcomes while observing and gathering information on implementation; (ii) dual testing of clinical and implementation interventions and strategies, and (iii) testing of an implementation strategy while observing and gathering information on the clinical intervention's impact on relevant outcomes.[183]

23.4.2.2. *Mixed method approaches*

Mixed methods research approaches that utilize both quantitative and qualitative methods have been widely used in D&I research. In such designs, qualitative methods are used to obtain depth of understanding of the reasons for success or failure in implementation. Quantitative methods are used to test and confirm hypotheses and obtain understanding of predictors of implementation. Mixed methods designs can allow researchers to conduct both exploratory and confirmatory research, to examine both intervention content and context, and to incorporate the perspectives of practitioners and clients of evidence-based practices.[184]

23.4.2.3. *Alternative designs*

Currently, randomized designs constitute the majority of D&I studies. However, randomization in D&I research is faced with many challenges due to the multilevel nature of D&I processes (levels of change include individual, group/team, organization, and larger system/environment).[185] For example, random assignment can be done at levels higher than the individual depending on the focus of the intervention and context, but this might lead to insufficient power as the number of units of analysis diminishes when moving to higher levels. In addition, a "wait-list" design is often utilized in D&I studies with communities, but the data from the second half of the study when the wait-list group receives the intervention are weak or of little use in answering the research questions.[184] One example of a solution to such problems is the dynamic wait-listed designs. These designs randomly assign units, which may be schools, clinics or even counties, to different times of intervention, with a small number of units receiving the intervention at different time points and eventually all of the units receiving the intervention. Such designs often render substantially greater statistical power, enable researchers to focus on a manageable number of units of intervention in a given time period, and provide more robustness given multiple times of measurement that offset the influences of potential exogenous factors, such as sudden economic downturns or natural disasters.[186]

Some researchers recommend considering quasi-experimental designs without randomization, such as before-after, interrupted time series, nonequivalent group and regression-discontinuity designs for D&I research.[177] Some recent studies suggested that observational studies (cohort or case-control) may also be considered for D&I research since the results of observational studies do not systematically overestimate the magnitude of the effects of treatment as compared to those in randomized controlled trials on the same topic.[187]

23.4.2.4. *Measurement in D&I research*

Measurement tools for D&I research are still underdeveloped. Key issues to be addressed include methodological challenges to measurement such as the level of analysis for D&I outcomes, construct validity and criterion-related validity,[188] inconsistent conceptualization and terminology of D&I strategies and outcomes. D&I processes and strategies reflect "how" to disseminate and implement research findings or evidence-based interventions. A challenge related to the evaluation and measurement of D&I strategies is that they are often "bundled" or "packaged" approaches in which the effect of specific components is not known.[188] As Michie *et al.* noted, this lack of theoretical understanding of D&I processes and strategies has thwarted D&I research. Therefore, advancing the definition, categorization and operationalization of D&I processes and strategies should be a high priority.[189]

The measurement of D&I outcomes, though still under development, has advanced in clarity as Proctor and colleagues developed a taxonomy of implementation outcomes with conceptually distinct definitions: acceptability, adoption, appropriateness, feasibility, fidelity, implementation cost, penetration and sustainability.[190] Fidelity, defined as the degree to which an intervention is implemented as it was prescribed in the original protocol, is the most commonly measured implementation outcome.[150] Careful measurement of fidelity can help researchers distinguish whether the success or failure of an intervention is due to the intervention itself or other factors.[191] However, in a rigorous and relevant study design, fidelity should not be a sole marker of implementation.[175] Other implementation outcomes are also important in understanding the implementation processes and the context. Numerous studies have proved that D&I outcomes influence intervention outcomes, but researchers have only begun to explore the ways in which D&I outcomes are interrelated. Important work remains to model these interrelationships, which will likely inform the definitions of D&I processes and strategies.[188]

The success of D&I efforts largely rests on their congruence with the preferences and priorities of the stakeholders who fund, shape, deliver, participate in or receive the interventions. As noted before, stakeholders such as community partners should be engaged in practice-based D&I research in forming the research questions, D&I outcomes to be measured, and how the resulting knowledge can most benefit broad scale up and use of health-related innovations.[172,175] Their perspectives should also be systematically assessed and integrated to ensure the applicability of D&I outcomes across different settings.

Although D&I research is critical to population health, the proportion of resources dedicated to translating research products into practice and policy is small compared to the amount invested in developing interventions (i.e., new drugs and technologies) to prevent and treat disease.[14] One example of an NIH award mechanism that encourages investigators to pursue D&I research is the Dissemination and Implementation Research in Health R01. This mechanism seeks proposals that will "identify, develop, and refine effective and efficient methods, structures, and strategies to disseminate and implement research-tested health behavior change interventions and evidence-based prevention, early detection, diagnostic, treatment, and quality of life improvement services into public health and clinical practice settings."[193]

The field of dissemination and implementation research has already provided much insight about what can be done to improve research translation. As the field continues to gain momentum and increase the scientific understanding of processes involved in research translation and the best methods and strategies for affecting change, we must ensure that this knowledge is applied to speed the use of biomedical, public health and behavioral science findings for the benefit of patient care and community health.

23.4.3. Examples of Dissemination and Implementation Research in Public Health

23.4.3.1. *AAC: An example of translational research in public health*

Using T3 translational research (i.e., research that assesses the value of an application for health practice leading to the development of evidence-based guidelines), Irvin-Vidrine and colleagues tested and evaluated an innovative conceptual model designed to change the way tobacco control interventions are delivered within heathcare systems.[193] This approach, called Ask Advise Connect (AAC), was designed to link smokers in healthcare settings with evidence-based tobacco cessation treatment. Vidrine and colleagues initially conducted a pair-matched, two-treatment-arm group randomized trial in 10 family practice clinics that were part of a large private healthcare system. Clinics were randomized to AAC or to a standard of care control condition called Ask Advise Refer (AAR). Smoking status was assessed and recorded in the electronic health record (EHR) at every patient visit by licensed vocational nurses and medical assistants, and all smokers were given brief advice to quit. In AAC, the names and phone numbers of smokers who agreed to be connected to the quitline were sent electronically to the quitline daily through an automated link in the EHR, and patients were proactively called by the quitline within 48 hours. Smokers in AAR clinics were handed a referral card and encouraged to call the quitline on their own for assistance. Both approaches were implemented for a period of nine months, and results indicated a 13-fold difference in treatment enrollment between AAC and AAR.[194] That is, 7.8 percent of identified smokers at AAC clinics enrolled in quitline-delivered treatment, whereas 0.6 percent of identified smokers at AAR clinics enrolled in the same treatment.

Vidrine and colleagues also conducted a parallel pair-matched, two-treatment-arm group randomized trial in 10 community health centers that were part of a large safety-net healthcare system.[194] Within this healthcare system, 90 percent of patients were racial/ethnic minorities, nearly half lived below the poverty line, and all were uninsured or underinsured. As in the initial trial, clinics were randomized to AAC or AAR. All other study procedures were identical to those in the initial trial. AAC and AAR were implemented for a period of 18 months, and results indicated that 14.7 percent of identified smokers at AAC clinics enrolled in treatment, whereas 0.5 percent of identified smokers at AAR clinics enrolled in the same treatment. This represented a 32-fold increase in treatment enrollment, and the nearly 15 percent treatment uptake rate in the AAC condition is the highest rate reported to date. Results provided strong support for AAC and indicated that the approach could be easily adopted and maintained in the real world.

Based on the demonstrated efficacy of AAC in the two large randomized trials, the research team was awarded funding to conduct T4 translational research (i.e., research that seeks to evaluate the "real-world" health outcomes of an application in practice) to implement and evaluate AAC in real-world clinical practice. Specifically, the funding has provided support to implement AAC within a single Federally Qualified Health Center, and throughout the same safety-net healthcare system in which AAC was initially evaluated. Through these projects, Vidrine and colleagues will carefully attend to and address factors that may attenuate or enhance implementation of AAC within the real world.

These studies have tremendous potential to increase smoking cessation rates at the population level, and AAC has implications for the dissemination of other cancer prevention strategies. Furthermore, the systems-level changes implemented in these studies can be immediately implemented in the clinics and are easily adapted for use with other cancer prevention and control strategies. The potential public health impact of this work is also supported by a recent meta-analysis published in the *Journal of the National Cancer Institute*,[195] which evaluated the impact of active versus passive recruitment approaches to quitline-delivered treatment. Active recruitment resulted in point estimates of treatment effects that were equivalent to passive recruitment, which strongly supports the importance of expanding the reach of quitlines through active recruitment. Dr. Vidrine co-authored an editorial that described the importance of the findings.[196]

23.4.3.2. *Coordinated Approach to Child Health (CATCH)*

The dissemination of the CATCH program provides an example of a systematic effort to increase adoption and implementation of an evidence-based program to improve cardiovascular health. Formally titled the Child and Adolescent Trial for Cardiovascular Health, the Coordinated Approach to Child Health (CATCH) is a school-based health promotion program targeting school-age children to promote healthy behaviors. CATCH uses a systematic and coordinated approach among the various change agents within schools and in children's lives to promote healthy eating and physical activity among school-age children.[198] The randomized clinical trial to test the effectiveness of CATCH was conducted in 96 schools throughout four states. The program focused on improving cardiovascular health by decreasing fat, saturated fat, and sodium in children's diets, increasing physical activity, and preventing tobacco use among elementary school children. The program used an ecological approach with components targeting various levels of influence: school physical education (PE), school classrooms, families, and school food service.[199] The CATCH PE component aimed to increase moderate to vigorous physical activities during PE class. The classroom curricula included skills training for the children focused on healthy eating and physical activity, while the family-based component was intended to develop home-based skills and assist parents in supporting children's healthy behavior. The Eat Smart component was designed to make the cafeteria food healthier, through menu, purchasing and preparation changes as well as promotion of those changes.[197,199] Evaluation of this trial indicated that the intervention was effective in decreasing fat consumption and increasing physical activity, and in maintaining these positive health behaviors three years later.[198,199]

Later iterations of the program (1) have focused on preventing obesity through the promotion of physical activity and healthy eating, (2) have been adapted for various age-groups and settings, and (3) have been updated to reflect new national guidelines for physical activity and nutrition, among other changes.[197,200] CATCH remains a coordinated, multilevel intervention with the same core components. Components such as the CATCH Campus Team and CATCH Social Marketing, additional trainings, and ongoing external support for schools, have been added to increase school and community involvement, school-environmental changes to support healthy behaviors, and fidelity and sustainability of the program. These components have led to improved behavioral outcomes in children.[197,200]

Due to the success of the original trial, the Texas Department of Health Diabetes Council approached the CATCH investigators to disseminate the program to public elementary schools in Texas. The initial dissemination strategy was ineffective in reaching the 3,000 targeted elementary schools; it involved mass mailing of order forms for subsidized CATCH materials to Texas public elementary schools, which garnered six schools, and presentations by the Diabetes Council to school districts, which garnered an additional 120 schools.[197]

Following the limited adoption of the CATCH program, a targeted dissemination effort was launched between 1998 and 2001. At this juncture, the CATCH program rebranded itself, took on its new name and formed a theoretical framework for dissemination. This framework includes theoretical constructs from Social Cognitive Theory, social marketing, and diffusion theory.[77,201,202] The team focused its strategies on the factors that influence the extent to which the program is diffused, namely attributes of the innovation from Rogers' diffusion theory,[159] characteristics of the adopter, the type of decisions required to implement the program, channels of communication, the social context of the system into which the innovation is introduced, and the efforts of change agents.[195]

Attributes of an innovation which affect its dissemination include relative advantage, compatibility, complexity, trialability, and observability.[203] CATCH had relative advantage, that is, it was one of the most innovative, reasonably priced programs that resulted in demonstrated positive behavioral changes. The program also offered compatibility with the needs of the state and teachers, as well with the national guidelines for school meal menus. The CATCH program was designed with minimal complexity, so that it would be easy for teachers to use and integrate into the classroom curriculum and activities. The program also offered trialability, with CATCH materials made available to potential adopters before purchase. Lastly, presentations, training videotapes, and hands-on training sessions throughout the state gave the CATCH program observability, allowing potential adopters to see how the various program components worked.[197]

Characteristics of the adopter are also critical for effective dissemination.[203] Early adopters, especially individuals with a wide range of influence and power at the local or state level, were targeted for CATCH dissemination. Relationships were formed with these individuals and partnerships were established with critical government and other organizations at the state and national levels, which would provide opportunities for funding and furthering dissemination efforts. The level of authority in which the decision for adopting an innovation is made influences dissemination. Since school curricula adoption can be made at various levels, school district administrators (authoritative type of innovation decision), schools within the districts and teachers (collective type), and individual teachers (optional type) were targeted through professional meetings or tailored trainings.[197]

Various communication channels were used to disseminate CATCH. Interpersonal networking efforts with decision makers and stakeholders were time-consuming and costly, but they were crucial to getting change agents on board for adoption of CATCH. These efforts were paired with dissemination through various media channels, such as training and recruitment videos, brochures, cover letters and a website detailing the attributes of the program, testimonials from other adopters, successful implementation stories and the ease of use. The social system into which each of the CATCH components was introduced differed; although PE teachers had a strong and established network in Texas, classroom teachers did not. This made dissemination through the PE teachers' professional network effective, whereas efforts to disseminate to classroom teachers have been limited.[197] Lastly, the efforts of change agents in advocating CATCH and sharing information about it through their own networks worked to further the dissemination efforts in the state.

More recently, CATCH Middle School disseminated its program throughout Central Texas through direct contact with school districts and support from Texas Education Agency Educational Service Centers (ESCs). However, a restricted state budget made obtaining support from ESCs difficult and limited dissemination.[199] Despite minor dissemination setbacks, CATCH is well recognized in the Texas public school system and is now used in its various formats within 8,500 schools around the US and overseas.[205]

The AAC and CATCH studies provide illustrations of both research translation and translational research. The translational strategies employed in these studies resulted in increased adoption and implementation of effective programs. The results of these studies have also served to increase our understanding of the processes that can accelerate translation in both biomedical and behavioral science.

23.5. CONCLUSIONS AND RECOMMENDATIONS

The use of innovations always requires behavior change in addition to knowledge transfer; therefore, behavioral science can plan a critical role in all translational efforts. Researchers in public health and biomedical fields should consider the use of behavior change strategies and findings from dissemination and implementation research as they design their studies with an eye toward active dissemination, and as they plan translational efforts.

Public health and behavioral science have played an important role in the history of translational research. Both of these disciplines have their own T1–T4 trajectory with unique approaches, research designs, and methods to measure outcomes which provide significant contributions to improving health. An important lesson that can be observed across translation efforts is that there are common roadblocks encountered along the pathway from discovery to delivery, yet these can be overcome with careful planning using theory to guide translational efforts.

Perspectives and methods commonly used in public health and behavioral science can be used to accelerate the translation of research findings. For example, the ecological model can be used to identify factors that influence, interact with, mediate, or moderate disease risk and/or health behaviors. It can also provide a valuable perspective to guide the development of multilevel interventions to address these issues. Community-based participatory research (CBPR) methods were also discussed as an approach to ensure that research topics, applications and products are relevant, feasible and sustainable in practice. An important point to consider in applying CBPR approaches is that the "community" should be defined broadly and should include individuals who play important roles along the translation continuum including community stakeholders, practitioners, hospital administrators, and community leaders. The development of community–academic partnerships was another approach recommended to improve research translation and translational research. Such partnerships provide a platform for true community engagement that can contribute to decision-making across the stages of translation from discovery to delivery and increase effective and sustainable treatments, interventions, and other health-related innovations in communities and practice settings. Strategic alliances with community partners such as social service agencies can assist in reaching large numbers of people experiencing health disparities to ensure that as we speed the discovery-to-delivery trajectory we are not simultaneously increasing disparities among those without ready access to services and new technologies. Research-practice-service and policy partnerships can ultimately lead to a shared decision-making model that integrates the best science with clinic practice, service delivery and policy initiatives that can effectively improve health.

The chapter also reviewed the basics of dissemination and implementation research and described both the major frameworks used in advancing D&I science as well as the methods that may differ from traditional research paradigms. Current D&I research has already improved and could further advance the translation of research into practice to address health disparities by (i) providing a better understanding of the disadvantaged population, community, organizational and environmental context, as well as why an evidence-based intervention is effective in a particular setting or not; and (ii) developing dissemination strategies to increase the adoption, implementation, maintenance and impact of evidence-based interventions in the continuum of care for disadvantaged populations.[206] As such, D&I research is perhaps one of the most important types of translational research in that it elucidates the mechanisms influencing the pathway from discovery to delivery and broad scale use and identifies strategic approaches to accelerate this pathway.

23.5.1. Training Translational Researchers

All of the recommended approaches used in public health and behavioral science that can advance translational science can only be done well through a team science approach. This type of transdisciplinary collaboration maximizes the potential for multiple views and skills to be brought to bear to address the complex and multilevel influences on health in patient populations and community settings. Researchers and practitioners trained in translational research and implementation and dissemination science are greatly needed to facilitate the translation of evidence into practice.[207–209] While translational research fosters the multidirectional integration of basic research, patient-oriented research, and population-based research, collaboration among disciplines through transdisciplinary teams is required to facilitate the generation of novel concepts and approaches for translational efforts. Therefore, it is imperative for translational researchers to develop the competencies needed to thrive in a transdisciplinary collaborative environment, which includes basic understanding of some of the principles of behavioral science and public health.[209] The recent emergence of "T3" translational research, which builds on T2 and involves the translation of research findings into actual dissemination, implementation and policy, has expanded and reinforced the interdisciplinary imperative inherent in translational research and called for new paradigms of cooperation that also require such competencies. On the other hand, failure of existing dissemination and implementation programs to translate evidence-based findings into actual behavior or practice changes implies ineffective or incomplete use of behavioral theories and methods.[211,212] Further training for translational researchers in behavioral science and public health approaches that can enhance translational efforts is needed.

REFERENCES

1. Perlstadt H. (2009) Translational research: Enabling the biomedical and social behavioral sciences to benefit society. *Humboldt J Social Relat* **32**(1): 4–34.
2. Institute of Medicine. (2001) *Crossing the Quality Chasm: A New Health System for the 21st Century*. National Academy Press, Washington, DC.
3. Zerhouni E. (2003) Medicine. The NIH roadmap. *Science* **302**(5642): 63–72.
4. Zerhouni EA. (2013) NIH roadmap — Themes, implementation groups, and initiatives. *Science* **302**: 63–72. Available from: *www.sciencemag.org/content/suppl/2003/10/03/302.5642.63.DC1/Zerhouni.SOM.Table.pdf*.

5. Breckler SJ. (2008) The NIH Roadmap: Are psychologists in or out? *J Clin Psychol Med Settings* **15**(1): 60–64.
6. Woolf SH. (2008) The meaning of translational research and why it matters. *J Am Med Assoc* **299**(2): 211–213.
7. Wethington E, Herman H, Pillemer K. (2012) Introduction: Translational research in the social and behavioral sciences. In: Wethington E, Dunifon RE (eds), *Research for the Public Good: Applying the Methods of Translational Research to Improve Human Health and Well-Being.* American Psychological Association, Washington, DC, pp. 3–19.
8. Morrow GR, Bellg AJ. (1994) Behavioral science in translational research and cancer control. *Cancer* **74**: 1409–1417.
9. National Institute of Mental Health, National Institute on Drug Abuse. (2013) Developing Translational Research in Behavioral Sciences — RFA.
10. Association for Clinical and Translational Sciences. (2013) Research Purpose. Available from: *www.ctssociety.org/?page=Purpose.*
11. Society of Behavioral Medicine. (2013) Translational Behavioral Medicine Mission. Available from: *www.sbm.org/publications/translational-behavioral-medicine.*
12. Khoury MJ, Gwinn M, Yoon PW, *et al.* (2007) The continuum of translation research in genomic medicine: How can we accelerate the appropriate integration of human genome discoveries into health care and disease prevention? *Genet Med* **9**(10): 665–674.
13. Westfall JM, Mold J, Fagnan L. (2007) Practice-based research — "Blue Highways" on the NIH roadmap. *J Am Med Assoc* **297**(4): 403–406.
14. Balas EA, Boren SA. (2000) Managing clinical knowledge for health care improvement. In: Bemmel J, McCray A (eds), *Yearbook of Medical Informatics 2000: Patient-Centered Systems.* Schattauer Verlagsgesellschaft, Stuttgart, pp. 65–70.
15. Veterans Administration Cooperative Study Group on Anti hypertensive Agents. (1967) Effects of treatment on morbidity in hypertension. Results in patients with diastolic blood pressures averaging 115 through 129 mm Hg. *J Am Med Assoc* **202**: 1028–1034.
16. Veterans Administration Cooperative Study Group on Antihypertensive Agents. (1970) Effects of treatment on morbidity in hypertension. II. Results in patients with diastolic blood pressure averaging 90 through 114 mm Hg. *J Am Med Assoc* **213**: 1143–1152.
17. Hypertension Detection and Follow-up Program Cooperative Group, NHLBI, NIH. (1979) Five-year findings of the hypertension detection and

follow-up program. I. Reduction in mortality of persons with high blood pressure, including mild hypertension. *J Am Med Assoc* **242**: 2562–2571.

18. SHEP Cooperative Research Group. (1991) Prevention of stroke by antihypertensive drug treatment in older persons with isolated systolic hypertension: Final results of the Systolic Hypertension in the Elderly Program (SHEP). *J Am Med Assoc* **265**: 3255–3264.
19. Rodriguez T, Malvezzi M, Chatenoud L, *et al.* (2006) Trends in mortality from coronary heart and cerebrovascular diseases in the Americas: 1970–2000. *Heart* **92**(4): 453–460.
20. Thom T, Roccella E. (1999) Trends in blood pressure control and mortality. In: Izzo J, Black H (eds), *Hypertension Primer: The essentials of High Blood Pressure.* American Heart Association, Dallas, pp. 268–270.
21. US Department of Health and Human Services. (2012) Healthy People 2010 Final Review. Available from: *www.cdc.gov/nchs/data/hpdata2010/hp2010_final_review.pdf.*
22. Expert Panel on Detection, Evaluation, and Treatment of High Blood Cholesterol in Adults. (2001) Executive Summary of The Third Report of The National Cholesterol Education Program (NCEP) Expert Panel on Detection, Evaluation, and Treatment of High Blood Cholesterol in Adults (Adult Treatment Panel III). *J Am Med Assoc* **285**(19): 2486–2497.
23. Sacks FM, Svetkey LP, Vollmer WM, *et al.* (2001) Effects on blood pressure of reduced dietary sodium and the Dietary Approaches to Stop Hypertension (DASH) diet. DASH-Sodium Collaborative Research Group. *N Engl J Med* **344**(1): 3–10.
24. Gershlick AH, Stephens-Lloyd A, Hughes S, *et al.* (2005) Rescue angioplasty after failed thrombolytic therapy for acute myocardial infarction. *N Engl J Med* **353**(26): 2758–2768.
25. Davis BR, Cutler JA, Gordon DJ, *et al.* (1996) Rationale and design for the Antihypertensive and Lipid Lowering Treatment to Prevent Heart Attack Trial (ALLHAT). ALLHAT Research Group. *Am J Hypertens* **9**(4 Pt 1): 342–360.
26. ALLHAT Collaborative Research Group. (2002) Major outcomes in high-risk hypertensive patients randomized to angiotensin-converting enzyme inhibitor or calcium channel blocker vs diuretic: The Antihypertensive and Lipid-Lowering Treatment to Prevent Heart Attack Trial (ALLHAT). *J Am Med Assoc* **288**(23): 2981–2997.
27. ALLHAT Collaborative Research Group. (2003) Diuretic versus alpha-blocker as first-step antihypertensive therapy: Final results from the Antihypertensive and Lipid-Lowering Treatment to Prevent Heart Attack Trial (ALLHAT). *Hypertension* **42**(3): 239–246.

28. Simon SR, Majumdar SR, Prosser LA, *et al.* (2005) Group versus individual academic detailing to improve the use of antihypertensive medications in primary care: A cluster-randomized controlled trial. *Am J Med* **118**(5): 521–528.
29. Thomson O'Brien MA, Oxman AD, *et al.* (2000) Educational outreach visits: Effects on professional practice and health care outcomes. *Cochrane Database Syst Rev* **2000**(2):CD000409.
30. Soumerai SB, Avorn J. (1990) Principles of educational outreach ('academic detailing') to improve clinical decision making. *J Am Med Assoc* **263**(4): 549–556.
31. Bartholomew LK, Cushman WC, Cutler JA, *et al.* ALLHAT Collaborative Research Group. Getting clinical trial results into practice: Design, implementation, and process evaluation of the ALLHAT Dissemination Project. *Clin Trials* **6**(4): 329–343.
32. Stafford RS, Bartholomew LK, Cushman WC, *et al.* (2010) Impact of the ALLHAT/JNC7 Dissemination Project on thiazide-type diuretic use. *Arch Intern Med* **170**(10): 851–858.
33. Glasgow RE, Vogt TM, Boles SM. (1999) Evaluating the public health impact of health promotion interventions: The RE-AIM framework. *Am J Public Health* **89**(9): 1322–1327.
34. Glasgow RE, Marcus AC, Bull SS, Wilson KM. (2004) Disseminating effective cancer screening interventions. *Cancer* **101**(Suppl 5): 1239–1250.
35. DiClemente CC, Fairhurst SK, Piotrowski NA. (1995) Self-efficacy and addictive behaviors. In: Maddux J (ed), *Self-efficacy, Adaptation, and Adjustment: Theory, Research, and Application.* Plenum Press, New York, pp. 109–141.
36. Fiore MC, Bailey WC, Cohen SJ, *et al.* (2000) *Treating Tobacco Use and Dependence: A Clinical Practice Guideline* (No. 1-58763-007-9). US Department of Health and Human Services, Rockville, MD.
37. Shiffman S. (1984) Cognitive antecedents and sequelae of smoking relapse crises. *J Appl Soc Psychol* **14**: 296–309.
38. Bandura A. (1977) *Social Learning Theory.* Prentice Hall, Englewood Cliffs, NJ.
39. Marlatt GA, Donovan DM, eds. (2005) *Relapse Prevention: Maintenance Strategies in the Treatment of Addictive Behaviors*, 2nd ed. The Guilford Press, New York.
40. Vidrine JI, Cofta-Woerpel L, Daza P, *et al.* (2006) Smoking cessation 2: Behavioral treatments. *Behav Med* **32**(3). 99–109.
41. Irvin JE, Bowers CA, Dunn ME, Wang MC. (1999) Efficacy of relapse prevention: A meta-analytic review. *J Consult Clin Psychol* **67**(4): 563–570.

42. Fiore MC, Jaen CR, Baker TB, *et al.* (2008) Treating Tobacco Use and Dependence: 2008 Update. Available from: *www.ahrq.gov/professionals/clinicians-providers/guidelines-recommendations/tobacco/clinicians/treating_tobacco_ use08.pdf.*
43. Fiore MC. (2000) Treating tobacco use and dependence: An introduction to the US Public Health Service Clinical Practice Guideline. *Respir Care* **45**(10): 1196–1199.
44. Stead LF, Perera R, Lancaster T. (2006) Telephone counseling for smoking cessation. *Cochrane Database Syst Rev* **2006**(3): CD002850.
45. Ossip-Klein DJ, McIntosh S. (2003) Quitlines in North America: Evidence base and applications. *Am J Med Sci* **326**(4): 201–205.
46. Rabius V, McAlister AL, Geiger A, *et al.* (2004) Telephone counseling increases cessation rates among young adult smokers. *Health Psychol* **23**(5): 539–541.
47. Vidrine JI, Shete S, Cao Y, *et al.* (2013) Ask-Advise-Connect: A new approach to smoking treatment delivery in health care settings. *J Am Med Assoc Intern Med* **173**(6): 458–464.
48. Wandersman A, Lesesne CA. (2012) If translational research is the answer, what's the question? Who gets to ask it? In: Wethington E, Dunifon RE (eds), *Research for the Public Good: Applying the Methods of Translational Research to Improve Human Health and Well-Being.* American Psychological Association, Washington, DC, pp. 33–52.
49. Orleans CT. (2007) Increasing the demand for and use of effective smoking-cessation treatments reaping the full health benefits of tobacco-control science and policy gains — in our lifetime. *Am J Prev Med* **33**(6 Suppl): S340–S348.
50. Bronfenbrenner U. (1974) Developmental research, public policy, and the ecology of childhood. *Child Dev* **45**(1): 1–5.
51. Bronfenbrenner U. (1976) The experimental ecology of education. *Teach Coll Rec* **78**(2): 157–204.
52. Bronfenbrenner U. (1977) Toward an experimental ecology of human development. *Am Psychol* **32**: 515–531.
53. Bronfenbrenner U. (1979) *The Ecology of Human Development: Experiments by Nature and Design.* Harvard University Press, Cambridge, MA.
54. Lewin K. (1951) *Field Theory in Social Science: Selected Theoretical Papers.* Harper & Row, New York.
55. Minkler M. (1999) Personal responsibility for health? A review of the arguments and the evidence at century's end. *Health Educ Behav* **26**(1): 121–140.
56. National Cancer Institute. (2005) Theory at a Glance. Available from: *www.cancer.gov/cancertopics/cancerlibrary/theory.pdf.*

57. World Health Organization. (1986) The Ottawa Charter for Health Promotion: First International Conference on Health Promotion, November 21, Ottawa. Available from: *www.who.int/healthpromotion/conferences/previous/ottawa/en/index1.html.*
58. McLeroy KR, Bibeau D, Steckler A, Glanz K. (1988) An ecological perspective on health promotion programs. *Health Educ Q* **15**(4): 351–377.
59. Richard L, Potvin L, Kishchuk N, *et al.* (1996) Assessment of the integration of the ecological approach in health promotion programs. *Am J Health Promot* **10**(4): 318–328.
60. Stokols D. (1996) Translating social ecological theory into guidelines for community health promotion. *Am J Health Promot* **10**(4): 282–298.
61. Green LW, Richard L, Potvin L. (1996) Ecological foundations of health promotion. *Am J Health Promot* **10**(4): 270–281.
62. Bartholomew LK, Parcel GS, Kok G, *et al.* (2011) *Planning Health Promotion Programs: An Intervention Mapping Approach*, 3rd ed. Jossey-Bass, San Francisco.
63. Kok G, Gottlieb NH, Commers M, Smerecnik C. (2008) The ecological approach in health promotion programs: A decade later. *Am J Health Promot* **22**(6): 437–442.
64. Richard L, Gauvin L, Raine K. (2011) Ecological models revisited: Their uses and evolution in health promotion over two decades. *Annu Rev Public Health* **32**: 307–326.
65. Wen M, Van DH, Olson LM. (2009) Social contexts of regular smoking in adolescence: Towards a multidimensional ecological model. *J Adolesc* **32**(3): 671–692.
66. Reitzel LR, Vidrine JI, Businelle MS, *et al.* (2012) Neighborhood perceptions are associated with tobacco dependence among African American smokers. *Nicotine Tob Res* **14**(7): 786–793.
67. Robinson T. (2008) Applying the socio-ecological model to improving fruit and vegetable intake among low-income African Americans. *J Community Health* **33**(6): 395–406.
68. Kerr J, Rosenberg DE, Nathan A, *et al.* (2012) Applying the ecological model of behavior change to a physical activity trial in retirement communities: Description of the study protocol. *Contemp Clin Trials* **33**(6): 1180–1188.
69. Fernandez ME, Allen JD, Mistry R, Kahn JA. (2010) Integrating clinical, community, and policy perspectives on human papillomavirus vaccination. *Annu Rev Public Health* **31**: 235–252.
70. Bronfenbrenner U. (2005) The bioecological theory of human development. In: Bronfenbrenner U (ed), *Making Human Beings Human: Bioecological*

Perspectives on Human Development. Sage Publications, Thousand Oaks, pp. 3–15.
71. Bronfenbrenner U, Morris P. (2006) The bioecological model of human development. In: Lerner RM, Damon W (eds), *Handbook of Child Pyschology: Volume 1, Theoretical Models of Human Development,* 6th ed. John Wiley, New York, pp. 793–828.
72. Rutter M. (2006) *Genes and Behavior: Nature–Nurture Interplay Explained.* Blackwell, Oxford.
73. Khoury MJ, Davis R, Gwinn M, *et al.* (2005) Do we need genomic research for the prevention of common diseases with environmental causes? *Am J Epidemiol* **161**(9): 799–805.
74. Willet WC. (2002) Balancing lifestyle and genomic research for disease prevention. *Science* **269**(5568): 695–698.
75. Mackinnon DP, Luecken LJ. (2011) Statistical analysis for identifying mediating variables in public health dentistry interventions. *J Public Health Dent* **71**(Suppl 1):S37–S46.
76. Bartholomew LK, Mullen PD. (2011) Five roles for using theory and evidence in the design and testing of behavior change interventions. *J Public Health Dent* **71**(Suppl 1): S20–S33.
77. Bandura A. (1986) *Social Foundations of Thought and Action: A Social Cognitive Theory.* Prentice Hall, Englewood Cliffs, NJ.
78. Morello-Frosch R, Pastor M, Sadd JL, *et al.* (2005) Citizens, science, and data judo: Leveraging secondary data analysis to build a community-academic collaborative for environmental justice in southern California. In: Israel BA, Eng E, Schulz AJ, Parker EA (eds), *Methods in Community-Based Participatory Research.* Jossey-Bass, San Francisco, pp. 371–392.
79. Israel BA, Schulz AJ, Parker EA, Becker AB. (1998) Review of community-based research: Assessing partnership approaches to improve public health. *Annu Rev Public Health* **19**: 173–202.
80. Minkler M, Wallerstein N. (2003) *Community Based Participatory Research for Health.* Jossey-Bass, San Francisco.
81. Viswanathan M, Ammerman A, Eng E, *et al.* (2004) Community-Based Participatory Research: Assessing the Evidence: Summary. AHRQ Evidence Report Summaries 2004. Available from: *www.ncbi.nlm.nih.gov/books. NBK11852.*
82. Wallerstein N, Martinez L. (1994) Empowerment evaluation: A case study of an adolescent substance abuse prevention program in New Mexico. *Am J Eval* **15**(2): 131–138.

83. Shiramizu B, Milne C, Terada K, *et al.* (2012) A community-based approach to enhancing anal cancer screening in Hawaii's HIV-infected ethnic minorities. *J AIDS Clin Res* 3(6): 162.
84. DiStefano A, Peters R, Tanjasiri SP, *et al.* (2013) A community-based participatory research study of HIV and HPV vulnerabilities and prevention in two pacific islander communities: Ethical challenges and solutions. *J Empir Res Hum Res Ethics* **8**(1): 68–78.
85. Minkler M, Vasquez VB, Tajik M, Petersen D. (2008) Promoting environmental justice through community-based participatory research: The role of community and partnership capacity. *Health Educ Behav* **35**(1): 119–137.
86. Forst L, Ahonen E, Zanoni J, *et al.* (2013) More than training: Community-based participatory research to reduce injuries among hispanic construction workers. *Am J Ind Med.*
87. Arcury TA, Quandt SA, Dearry A. (2001) Farmworker pesticide exposure and community-based participatory research: Rationale and practical applications. *Environ Health Perspect* **109**(Suppl 3): 429–434.
88. Reininger BM, Barroso CS, Mitchell-Bennett L, *et al.* Process evaluation and participatory methods in an obesity-prevention media campaign for Mexican Americans. *Health Promot Pract* **11**(3): 347–357.
89. Davis DS, Goldmon MV, Coker-Appiah DS. (2011) Using a community-based participatory research approach to develop a faith-based obesity intervention for African American children. *Health Promot Pract* **12**(6): 811–822.
90. Tapp H, Dulin M. (2010) The science of primary health-care improvement: Potential and use of community-based participatory research by practice-based research networks for translation of research into practice. *Exp Biol Med* **235**(3): 290–299.
91. Hebert JR, Brandt HM, Armstead CA, *et al.* (2009) Interdisciplinary, translational, and community-based participatory research: Finding a common language to improve cancer research. *Cancer Epidemiol Biomarkers Prev* **18**(4): 1213–1217.
92. U.S. Department of Health and Human Services: National Institutes of Health. (2008) NIH Roadmap for Medical Research. Available from: *http://nihroadmap.nih.gov*.
93. Hawk E, Viner JL. (2006) What is the future of oncology? National Cancer Institute initiatives to improve research, development, and implementation in cancer prevention and treatment. *Semin Oncol* **33**(6 Suppl 11): S6–S9.

94. Trickett EJ. Community-based participatory research as worldview or instrumental strategy: Is it lost in translation(al) research? *Am J Public Health* **101**(8): 1353–1355.
95. Wallerstein NB, Duran B. (2006) Using community-based participatory research to address health disparities. *Health Promot Pract* 7(3): 312–323.
96. Minkler M. (2005) Community-based research partnerships: Challenges and opportunities. *J Urban Health* **82**(2): ii3–ii12.
97. Horowitz CR, Robinson M, Seifer S. (2009) Community-based participatory research from the margin to the mainstream: Are researchers prepared? *Circulation* **119**(19): 2633–2642.
98. Himmelmann AT. (2002) Collaboration for a Change: Definitions, Decision-Making Models, Roles, and Collaboration Process Guide. Available from: *http://depts.washington.edu/ccph/pdf_files/4achange.pdf.*
99. Wallerstein N, Duran B. (2010) Community-based participatory research contributions to intervention research: The intersection of science and practice to improve health equity. *Am J Public Health* **100**(Suppl 1): S40–S46.
100. Proctor EK, Landsverk J, Aarons G, *et al.* (2009) Implementation research in mental health services: An emerging science with conceptual, methodological, and training challenges. *Adm Policy Ment Health* **36**(1): 24–34.
101. Roussos ST, Fawcett SB. (2000) A review of collaborative partnerships as a strategy for improving community health. *Annu Rev Public Health* **21**: 369–402.
102. Kerner J. (2010) Integrating science with service in cancer control: Closing the gap between discovery and delivery. In: Elwood JM, Sutcliffe SB (eds), *Cancer Control.* Oxford University Press, Oxford.
103. National Cancer Institute. (2009) Community Networks Program (CNP) Program Information. Available from: *http://crchd.cancer.gov/cnp/program-information.html.*
104. Luque JS, Quinn GP, Montel-Ishino FA, *et al.* (2012) Formative research on perceptions of biobanking: What community members think. *J Cancer Educ* **27**(1): 91–99.
105. Cancer Prevention and Control Research Network. (2013) Cancer Prevention and Control Research Network. Available from: *http://cpcrn.org/.*
106. Harris JR, Brown PK, Coughlin S, *et al.* (2005) The cancer prevention and control research network. *Prev Chronic Dis* **2**(1): A21.
107. Hannon PA, Fernandez ME, Williams RS, *et al.* (2010) Cancer control planners' perceptions and use of evidence-based programs. *J Public Health Manag Pract* **16**(3): E1–E8.

108. Mullen PD, Fernandez ME. (2013) Increasing Reach and Implementation of Evidence Based Programs for Cancer Control 5R01CA163526-02. Available from: *http://projectreporter.nih.gov/project_info_description.cfm?aid=8473834&icde=16020223&ddparam=&ddvalue=&ddsub=&cr=5&csb=default&cs=ASC.*
109. Ekwenugo L, Benard V, Vinson C. (2013) News from the CDC: Collaborations to build capacity at the community level in cancer prevention and control. *Transl Behav Med* **3**(1): 3–5.
110. Honeycutt S, Carvalho M, Glanz K, *et al.* (2012) Research to reality: A process evaluation of a mini-grants program to disseminate evidence-based nutrition programs to rural churches and worksites. *J Public Health Manag Pract* **18**(5): 431–439.
111. Carvalho M, Honeycutt S, Escoffery C, *et al.* (2013) Balancing fidelity and adaptation: Implementing evidence-based chronic disease prevention programs. *J Public Health Manag Pract* [Epub ahead of print].
112. Gibbons CM. (2011) Use of health information technology among racial and ethnic underserved communities. *Perspect Health Inf Manag* **8** (Winter).
113. Glied S, Lleras-Muney A. (2008) Technological innovation and inequality in health. *Demography* **45**(3): 741–761.
114. Yancey AT. (2012) Creating a healthy milieu for all. Essay on the current state and future of preventive medicine. *Prev Med* **55**(6): 571–572.
115. Bennett GG. (2012) Connecting eHealth with 2-1-1 to reduce health disparities. *Am J Prev Med* **43**(6 Suppl 5): S509–S511.
116. Kreuter MW. (2012) Reach, effectiveness, and connections: The case for partnering with 2-1-1 to eliminate health disparities. *Am J Prev Med* **43**(6 Suppl 5): S420–S421.
117. Hall KL, Stipelman BA, Eddens KS, *et al.* (2012) Advancing collaborative research with 2-1-1 to reduce health disparities: Challenges, opportunities, and recommendations. *Am J Prev Med* **43**(6 Suppl 5): S518–S528.
118. Eddens KS. (2012) Guiding principles for collaborative research with 2-1-1. *Am J Prev Med* **43**(6 Suppl 5): S512–S517.
119. McMillen C. Dissemination and implementation in social service settings. In: Brownson RC, Colditz GA, Proctor EK (eds), *Dissemination and Implementation Research in Health.* Oxford University Press, New York, pp. 384–399.
120. McNeill LH, Coeling M, Puleo E, *et al.* (2009) Colorectal cancer prevention for low-income, sociodemographically-diverse adults in public housing: Baseline findings of a randomized controlled trial. *BMC Public Health* **9**: 353.

121. Andrews JO, Tingen MS, Jarriel SC, *et al.*(2012) Application of a CBPR framework to inform a multi-level tobacco cessation intervention in public housing neighborhoods. *Am J Community Psychol* **50**(1–2): 129–140.
122. Eddens KS, Kreuter MW. (2011) Proactive screening for health needs in United Way's 2-1-1 information and referral service. *J Soc Serv Res* **37**(2): 113–123.
123. Linnan LA. Research collaboration with 2-1-1 to eliminate health disparities: An introduction. *Am J Prev Med* **43**(6 Suppl 5): S415–S419.
124. Daily LS. (2012) Health research and surveillance potential to partner with 2-1-1. *Am J Prev Med* **43**(6 Suppl 5): S422–S424.
125. Purnell JQ, Kreuter MW, Eddens KS, *et al.* (2012) Cancer control needs of 2-1-1 callers in Missouri, North Carolina, Texas, and Washington. *J Health Care Poor Underserved* **23**(2): 752–767.
126. Savas LS, Fernandez ME, Jobe D, Carmack CC. (2012) Human papillomavirus vaccine: 2-1-1 helplines and minority parent decision-making. *Am J Prev Med* **43**(6 Suppl 5): S490–S496.
127. Fernandez ME, Ball-Ricks KA, Vernon SW, Savas L. (2012) *Advancing Dissemination and Implementation Research and Practice: A Collaboration Between the CPCRN and 2-1-1.* Oral presentation at Cancer Prevention and Research Institute of Texas.
128. Alcaraz KI, Arnold LD, Eddens KS, *et al.* (2012) Exploring 2-1-1 service requests as potential markers for cancer control needs. *Am J Prev Med* **43**(6 Suppl 5): S469–S474.
129. Kreuter MW, Eddens KS, Alcaraz KI, *et al.* (2012) Use of cancer control referrals by 2-1-1 callers: A randomized trial. *Am J Prev Med* **43**(6 Suppl 5): S425–S434.
130. Roux AM, Herrera P, Wold CM, *et al.* (2012) Developmental and autism screening through 2-1-1: Reaching underserved families. *Am J Prev Med* **43**(6 Suppl 5): S457–S463.
131. Rodgers JT, Purnell JQ. (2012) Healthcare navigation service in 2-1-1 San Diego: Guiding individuals to the care they need. *Am J Prev Med* **43**(6 Suppl 5): S450–S456.
132. Hall KL, Feng AX, Moser RP, *et al.* (2008) Moving the science of team science forward: Collaboration and creativity. *Am J Prev Med* **35**(2 Suppl): S243–S249.
133. Brandt AM, Gardner M. (2000) Antagonism and accommodation: Interpreting the relationship between public health and medicine in the United States during the 20th century. *Am J Public Health* **90**(5): 707.

134. Gebbie K, Rosenstock L, Hernandez LM. (2003) *Who Will Keep the Public Healthy?: Educating Public Health Professionals for the 21st Century.* National Academies Press, Washington, DC.
135. Awofeso N. (2004) What's new about the "new public health"? *Am J Public Health* **94**(5): 705–709.
136. Axelsson R, Axelsson SB. (2006) Integration and collaboration in public health — A conceptual framework. *Int J Health Plann Manag* **21**(1): 75–88.
137. Gebbie KM, Turnock BJ. (2006) The public health workforce, 2006: New challenges. *Health Aff (Millwood)* **25**(4): 923–933.
138. Levin BW, Fleischman AR. (2002) Public health and bioethics: The benefits of collaboration. *Am J Public Health* **92**(2): 165–167.
139. Choi BC, Pak AW. (2006) Multidisciplinarity, interdisciplinarity and transdisciplinarity in health research, services, education and policy: 1. Definitions, objectives, and evidence of effectiveness. *Clin Invest Med* **29**(6): 351.
140. Glanz K, Rimer BK, Viswanath K. (2008) *Health Behavior and Health Education: Theory, Research, and Practice.* 4th ed. Jossey-Bass, San Francisco, CA.
141. Wethington E, Dunifon RE. Afterword. (2012) In: Wethington E, Dunifon RE (eds), *Research for the Public Good: Applying the Methods of Translational Research to Improve Human Health and Well-Being.* American Pyschological Association, Washington, DC, pp. 191–198.
142. Croyle RT. (2008) The National Cancer Institute's transdisciplinary centers initiatives and the need for building a science of team science. *Am J Prev Med* **35**(2): S90.
143. Hall KL, Olster DH, Stipelman BA, Vogel AL. (2012) News from NIH: Resources for team-based research to more effectively address complex public health problems. *Transl Behav Med* **2**(4): 373–375.
144. Stokols D, Hall KL, Taylor BK, Moser RP. (2008) The science of team science: Overview of the field and introduction to the supplement. *Am J Prev Med* **35**(2): S77–S89.
145. Hall KL, Stokols D, Stipelman BA, *et al.* (2012) Assessing the value of team science: A study comparing center-and investigator-initiated grants. *Am J Prev Med* **42**(2): 157.
146. Shriver M, de BR, Brown C, *et al.* (1998) Bridging the gap between science and practice: Insight to researchers from practitioners. *Public Health Rep* **113**(Suppl 1): 189–193.
147. Scharff DP, Rabin BA, Cook RA, *et al.* (2008) Bridging research and practice through competency-based public health education. *J Public Health Manag Pract* **14**(2): 131–137.

148. Brownson RC, Kreuter MW, Arrington BA, True WR. (2006) Translating scientific discoveries into public health action: How can schools of public health move us forward? *Public Health Rep* **121**(1): 97–103.
149. Rabin BA, Brownson RC. (2012) Developing the terminology for dissemination and implementation research. In: Brownson RC, Colditz G, Proctor EK (eds), *Dissemination and Implementation Research in Health: Translating Science to Practice.* Oxford University Press, New York.
150. Rabin BA, Brownson RC, Haire-Joshu D, *et al.* (2008) A glossary for dissemination and implementation research in health. *J Public Health Manag Pract* **14**(2): 117–123.
151. Colditz G. (2012) The promise and challenges of dissemination and implementation research. In: Brownson RC, Colditz G, Proctor EK (eds), *Dissemination and Implementation Research in Health: Translating Science to Practice.* Oxford University Press, New York, pp. 3–22.
152. Bero LA, Grilli R, Grimshaw JM, *et al.* (1998) Closing the gap between research and practice: An overview of systematic reviews of interventions to promote the implementation of research findings. The Cochrane Effective Practice and Organization of Care Review Group. *Br Med J* **317**(7156): 465–468.
153. Damschroder LJ, Aron DC, Keith RE, *et al.* (2009) Fostering implementation of health services research findings into practice: A consolidated framework for advancing implementation science. *Implement Sci* **4**: 50.
154. Glasgow RE, Babcock-Parziale J. (2012) Rationale for "D&I" Research. Presentation at Training Institute for Dissemination and Implementation Research in Health. Available from: *http://conferences.thehillgroup.com/OBSSRinstitutes/TIDIRH2012/presentations/Day1_Babcock&Glasgow_Rationale%20 for%20D&I%20Research.pdf.*
155. Stamatakis KA, Norton WE, Stirman SW, *et al.* (2013) Developing the next generation of dissemination and implementation researchers: Insights from initial trainees. *Implement Sci* **8**(1): 29.
156. Tabak RG, Khoong EC, Chambers DA, Brownson RC. (2012) Bridging research and practice: Models for dissemination and implementation research. *Am J Prev Med* **43**(3): 337–350.
157. Dearing JW. (2008) Evolution of diffusion and dissemination theory. *J Public Health Manag Pract* **14**(2): 99–108.
158. Rogers EM. (1995) *Diffusion of Innovations.* 4th ed. Free Press, New York.
159. Oldenburg B, Glanz K. (2008) Diffusion of innovations. In: Glanz K, Rimer BK, Lewis FM (eds), *Health Behavior and Health Education: Theory, Research, and Practice.* 4th ed. Jossey-Bass, San Francisco, pp. 313–333.

160. Orlandi MA, Landers C., Weston R, Haley N. (1990) Diffusion of health promotion interventions. In: Glanz K, Lewis FM, Rimer BK (eds), *Health Behavior and Health Education: Theory, Research, and Practice.* Jossey-Bass, San Francisco, pp. 288–313.
161. Green LW, Gottlieb NH, Parcel GS. (1991) Diffusion theory extended and applied. In: Ward WB, Lewis FM (eds), *Advances in Health Education and Promotion.* Jessica Kingsley Publishers, pp. 91–117.
162. Dearing JW, Kreuter MW. (2010) Designing for diffusion: How can we increase uptake of cancer communication innovations? *Patient Educ Couns* **81**(Suppl): S100–S110.
163. Flay BR. (1986) Efficacy and effectiveness trials and other phases of research in the development of health promotion programs. *Prev Med* **15**(5): 451–474.
164. Starfield B. (1998) Quality-of-care research: Internal elegance and external relevance. *J Am Med Assoc* **280**(11): 1006–1008.
165. Abrams DB, Orleans CT, Niaura RS, *et al.* (1996) Integrating individual and public health perspectives for treatment of tobacco dependence under managed health care: A combined stepped-care and matching model. *Ann Behav Med* **18**(4): 290–304.
166. Glasgow RE, McKay HG, Piette JD, Reynolds KD. (2001) The RE-AIM framework for evaluating interventions: What can it tell us about approaches to chronic illness management? *Patient Educ Couns* **44**(2): 119–127.
167. Glasgow RE, Askew S, Purcell P, *et al.* (2013) Use of RE-AIM to address health inequities: Application in a low-income community health center-based weight loss and hypertension self-management program. *Transl Behav Med.*
168. Glasgow RE, Lichtenstein E, Marcus AC. (2003) Why don't we see more translation of health promotion research to practice? Rethinking the efficacy-to-effectiveness transition. *Am J Public Health* **93**(8): 1261–1267.
169. Gaglio B, Glasgow R. (2012) Evaluation approaches for dissemination and implementation research. In: Brownson RC, Colditz G, Proctor EK (eds). *Dissemination and Implementation Research in Health: Translating Science to Practice.* Oxford University Press, New York, pp. 327–358.
170. Fernandez M. (2012) *Factors Influencing Implementation of Evidence-based Cancer Prevention and Control Practices in FQHCs: A Qualitative Study.* Oral Presentation at Centers for Disease Control National Cancer Conference. Washington, DC.
171. Wandersman A, Duffy J, Flaspohler P, *et al.* (2008) Bridging the gap between prevention research and practice: The interactive systems framework for dissemination and implementation. *Am J Community Psychol* **41**(3): 171–181.

172. Green LW, Glasgow RE, Atkins D, Stange K. (2009) Making evidence from research more relevant, useful, and actionable in policy, program planning, and practice slips "twixt cup and lip". *Am J Prev Med* **37**(6 Suppl 1): S187–S191.
173. Kessler R, Glasgow RE. (2011) A proposal to speed translation of healthcare research into practice: Dramatic change is needed. *Am J Prev Med* **40**(6): 637–644.
174. Zwarenstein M, Treweek S. (2009) What kind of randomised trials do patients and clinicians need? *Evid Based Med* **14**(4): 101–103.
175. Glasgow RE, Chambers D. (2012) Developing robust, sustainable, implementation systems using rigorous, rapid and relevant science. *Clin Transl Sci* **5**(1): 48–55.
176. Rothwell PM. (2005) External validity of randomised controlled trials: "To whom do the results of this trial apply?". *Lancet* **365**(9453): 82–93.
177. Glasgow RE, Magid DJ, Beck A, *et al.* (2005) Practical clinical trials for translating research to practice: Design and measurement recommendations. *Med Care* **43**(6): 551–557.
178. Tunis SR, Stryer DB, Clancy CM. (2003) Practical clinical trials: Increasing the value of clinical research for decision making in clinical and health policy. *J Am Med Assoc* **290**(12): 1624–1632.
179. Glasgow RE, Emmons KM. (2007) How can we increase translation of research into practice? Types of evidence needed. *Annu Rev Public Health* **28**: 413–433.
180. Glasgow RE, Vinson C, Chambers D, *et al.* (2012) National Institutes of Health approaches to dissemination and implementation science: Current and future directions. *Am J Public Health* **102**(7): 1274–1281.
181. Thorpe KE, Zwarenstein M, Oxman AD, *et al.* (2009) A pragmatic-explanatory continuum indicator summary (PRECIS): A tool to help trial designers. *Can Med Assoc J* **180**(10): E47–E57.
182. Zwarenstein M, Treweek S, Gagnier JJ, *et al.* (2008) Improving the reporting of pragmatic trials: An extension of the CONSORT statement. *Br Med J* **337**: a2390.
183. Curran GM, Bauer M, Mittman B, *et al.* (2012) Effectiveness-implementation hybrid designs: Combining elements of clinical effectiveness and implementation research to enhance public health impact. *Med Care* **50**(3): 217–226.
184. Landsverk J, Brown CH, Chamberlain P, *et al.* (2012) Design and analysis in dissemination and implementation research. In: Brownson RC, Colditz G, Proctor EK (eds), *Dissemination and Implementation in Health: Translating Science to Practice*. Oxford University Press, New York, pp. 225–260.

185. Shortell SM. (2004) Increasing value: A research agenda for addressing the managerial and organizational challenges facing health care delivery in the United States. *Med Care Res Rev* **61**(3 Suppl): S12–S30.
186. Brown CH, Wyman PA, Guo J, Pena J. (2006) Dynamic wait-listed designs for randomized trials: New designs for prevention of youth suicide. *Clin Trials* **3**(3): 259–271.
187. Concato J, Shah N, Horwitz RI. (2000) Randomized controlled trials, observational studies, and the hierarchy of research designs. *New Engl J Med* **342**(25): 1887–1892.
188. Proctor EK, Brownson RC. (2012) Measurement issues in dissemination and implementation research. In: Brownson RC, Colditz G, Proctor EK (eds), *Dissemination and Implementation Research in Health.* Oxford University Press, New York, pp. 261–280.
189. Michie S, Johnston M, Abraham C, *et al.* (2005) Making psychological theory useful for implementing evidence based practice: A consensus approach. *Qual Saf Health Care* **14**(1): 26–33.
190. Proctor E, Silmere H, Raghavan R, *et al.* (2011) Outcomes for implementation research: Conceptual distinctions, measurement challenges, and research agenda. *Adm Policy Ment Health* **38**(2): 65–76.
191. Carroll C, Patterson M, Wood S, *et al.* (2007) A conceptual framework for implementation fidelity. *Implement Sci* **2**: 40.
192. Eccles MP, Armstrong D, Baker R, *et al.* (2009) An implementation research agenda. *Implement Sci* **4**: 18.
193. National Institutes of Health. (2013) Dissemination and Implementation Research in Health (R01). Available from: *http://grants.nih.gov/grants/guide/pa-files/PAR-10-038.html.*
194. Vidrine JI, Shete S, Cao Y, *et al.* (2013) Ask-advise-connect: A new approach to smoking treatment delivery in health care settings. *JAMA Intern Med* **173**(6): 458–464.
195. Vidrine JI, Shete S, Li Y, *et al.* (2013) Efficacy of ask advise connect in a safety net healthcare system. Unpublished work.
196. Tzelepis F, Paul CL, Walsh RA, *et al.* (2011) Proactive telephone counseling for smoking cessation: Meta-analyses by recruitment channel and methodological quality. *J Natl Cancer Inst* **103**(12): 922–941.
197. Vidrine DJ, Vidrine JI. (2011) Active vs passive recruitment to quitline studies: Public health implications. *J Natl Cancer Inst* **103**(12): 909–910.
198. Hoelscher DM, Kelder SH, Murray N, *et al.* (2001) Dissemination and adoption of the Child and Adolescent Trial for Cardiovascular Health (CATCH): A case study in Texas. *J Public Health Manag Pract* **7**(2): 90–100.

199. Perry CL, Stone EJ, Parcel GS, *et al.* (1990) School-based cardiovascular health promotion: The child and adolescent trial for cardiovascular health (CATCH). *J Sch Health* **60**(8): 406–413.
200. Kelder SH, Springer A, Hoelscher DM, *et al.* (2013) Central Texas CATCH Middle School Project.University of Texas School of Public Health, Austin Regional Campus.
201. Luepker RV, Perry CL, McKinlay SM, *et al.* for the CATCH Collaborative Group. (1996) Outcomes of a field trial to improve children's dietary patterns and physical activity: The Child and Adolescent Trial for Cardiovascular Health. *J Am Med Assoc* **275**(10): 768–776.
202. Nader PR, Stone EJ, Lytle LA, *et al.* (1999) Three-year maintenance of improved diet and physical activity: The CATCH cohort. *Arch Pediatr Adolesc Med* **153**(7): 695.
203. Hoelscher DM, Springer AE, Ranjit N, *et al.*(2010) Reductions in child obesity among disadvantaged school children with community involvement: The Travis County CATCH Trial. *Obesity* **18**: S36–S44.
204. Rogers EM. (1995) Lessons for guidelines from the diffusion of innovations. *Jt Comm J Qual Improv* **21**(7): 324–328.
205. Siegel M, Doner L. (2004) *Marketing Public Health: Strategies to Promote Social Change.* Aspen Pub.
206. University of Texas School of Public Health. (2013) CATCH Overview. Available from: *https://sph.uth.edu/research/centers/dell/catchproject/.*
207. Bennett GG. (2012) D&I science and health disparities: Research gaps. Presentation at Training Institute for Dissemination and Implementation Research in Health, July 9. Available from: *http://conferences.thehillgroup.com/OBSSRinstitutes/TIDIRH2012/presentations/Day3_Bennett_Health%20Dispa- rities%20and%20Health%20Inequities.pdf.*
208. Gonzales R, Handley MA, Ackerman S, O'sullivan PS. (2012) A framework for training health professionals in implementation and dissemination science. *Acad Med* **87**(3): 271–278.
209. Dougherty D, Conway PH. (2008) The "3T's" road map to transform US health care: The "how" of high-quality care. *J Am Med Assoc* **299**(19): 2319–2321.
210. Pfund C, House S, Spencer K, *et al.* (2013) A research mentor training curriculum for clinical and translational researchers. *Clin Transl Sci* **6**(1): 26–33.
211. Avorn J, Fischer M. (2010) "Bench to behavior": Translating comparative effectiveness research into improved clinical practice. *Health Aff (Millwood)***29**(10): 1891–1900.

212. Avorn J. (2010) Transforming trial results into practice change: The final translational hurdle: Comment on "Impact of the ALLHAT/JNC7 Dissemination Project on thiazide-type diuretic use". *Arch Intern Med* **170**(10): 858–860.

213. Viswanathan M, Ammerman A, Eng E, *et al.* (2004) Community-based Participatory Research: Assessing the Evidence. Evidence Report/Technology Assessment No. 99. Available from: *http://archive.ahrq.gov/downloads/pub/evidence/pdf/cbpr/cbpr.pdf.*

X. Translational Epidemiology, Biostatistics and Informatics

CHAPTER 24

Translational Epidemiology, Biostatistics and Informatics

Tor D. Tosteson, Christopher I. Amos† and Jason H. Moore*

24.1. INTRODUCTION

This chapter discusses the unique contributions of biostatistics, epidemiology and bioinformatics to translational science. The first two of these closely interrelated quantitative disciplines have histories of a century or more. The third, bioinformatics, developed more recently in response to the dramatic development of computing and genetics in recent decades.

Biostatistics is the mathematical and quantitative science devoted to the study of techniques for the analysis and collection of data in support of scientific inference in biomedical research. The need for such a discipline derives from realization that the biological sciences and medicine rely on imperfect quantitative measurements. Our understanding of the determinants of human diseases and effective strategies for their treatment cannot progress without incorporating proper "statistical thinking" at every stage of the research process.

Epidemiology is the study of the etiology of human disease through population-based methods, including the study of related quantitative

*Corresponding author: The Geisel School of Medicine at Dartmouth, Section of Biostatistics & Epidemiology, Dartmouth College, One Medical Center Drive, 7927 Rubin Building, Lebanon, NH 03756, USA; E-mail: *tor.devin.tosteson@dartmouth.edu*; Tel: +1-603-653-3677; Fax: +1-603-653-9094

†The Geisel School of Medicine at Dartmouth, Dartmouth College, Lebanon, New Hampshire, USA

methodologies. Epidemiology and biostatistics share many common interests in study design and clinical applications. Epidemiology is oriented towards the development of biological and medical hypotheses about the causes of disease. In contrast, biostatistics is oriented towards the development of mathematical and computational approaches for evaluating hypotheses. Both disciplines share an interest in causal inference and the philosophy of science.

Bioinformatics got its start after the development of high-throughput DNA sequencing technologies in the 1970s,[1] and became a formal discipline concurrently with the momentum of the Human Genome Project and the availability of the Internet. The word *bioinformatics* did not start appearing in the biomedical literature until around 1990 but quickly caught on as the descriptor of this important new field. An important goal of bioinformatics is to facilitate the management, analysis and interpretation of data from biological experiments and observational studies. Thus, much of bioinformatics can be categorized as database development and implementation, data analysis and data mining, and biological interpretation.

The sections that follow examine in greater detail the broad themes within and between the three disciplines. The focus is on the unique features of translational research and associated issues related to the practice and theory of biostatistics, epidemiology and bioinformatics.

24.2. BIOSTATISTICS

By common definitions, translational research spans two or more scientific disciplines that have evolved within distinct intellectual environments and traditions. Cross-disciplinary differences in the scientific cultures often lead to separation in the traditions of statistical practice. Fortunately, statisticians and statistical science have historically thrived in the conditions typically encountered in translational research. In fact, the challenges of translation often stimulate seminal developments within statistics itself. Thus, the process of such research is both familiar and invigorating for statistical scientists.

Data comes in many forms depending on the disciplines involved. In some instances, translation will consist of juxtaposing data collected via the methods of one discipline against data collected via methods from another discipline in a conceptually simple analysis, but one that may demand interdisciplinary innovation. Consider the impact of mass genotyping and gene expression technologies in the post-human genome era. Molecular genetic researchers were confronted with exceptionally detailed data demanding sophisticated analytic methodologies seldom used in this context. Statisticians have been able to adapt their theories and analyses for this purpose, although the challenges continue to multiply.

Accompanying the demands for new methods of data analysis are corresponding demands for improved study designs that make the most efficient use of the scarce resources used in translational research. Research design is a very broad, cross-disciplinary topic, and is not uniquely the province of biostatistics. However, because of the focus on data analysis as the culmination of the process of experimental and observational research, statistical design has become an essential component of the scientific process. At the core of the design exercise are the planned statistical data analyses, the "bottom line" of the experiment or study. This can be as simple as a difference in means, or as complex as a joint analysis of millions of separate data points with many targeted parameters.

Increasingly, the publication and dissemination of research data has led to opportunities and challenges in reinterpretation and synthesis of scientific data. This process is often inherently translational, as it allows the direct incorporation of data developed within narrow investigations to place them quantitatively into the context of a broader collection of experiments in the same field. Similarly, the wide availability of data from many fields allows the construction of extended theoretical quantitative models connecting the several stages of translation.

24.2.1. Statistical Methods and Data Analysis

At the core of biostatistics is a formal mathematical and philosophical theory of statistical inference. In this theory, probability distributions are used to model experimental and sampling variability. Probabilistic statements can be made about the properties (parameters) of the distributions, including optimal estimates, associated confidence intervals, and hypothesis tests. The process of statistical inference is closely linked to the scientific method and serves as a focal point for many translational research studies.

The primary motivation for new research in biostatistics derives from the need to adapt statistical principles to new forms of data, typically at the scientific boundaries characteristic of translational science. The highly developed theory of linear regression and least squares dates back more than 200 years to the work of C.F. Gauss and A.M. Legendre, and includes many related statistical procedures such as analysis of variance and analysis of covariance. This theory was a product of the demands of the most important scientific data analyses of the era in which it was conceived, including calculations for celestial orbits and navigation.

The needs of translational research have continued to drive development in biostatistics. For example, quantal bioassay data,[2] linking a continuous measure of dose of a toxic substance to the binary vital status of experimental animals, led statisticians such as Berkson and Cornfield[3,4] to study and apply the principles underlying logistic regression. Here the challenge of a new type of a data and experimental design led to a major development in the theory of biostatistics, a general theory of regression for binary and counted outcomes.[5] This theory has allowed statisticians to benefit from key conceptual approaches developed for linear regression with continuous dependent outcomes.

In a related development, D.R. Cox united actuarial methods for construction of life tables and regression theory to create more sophisticated models for continuous survival data subject to censoring.[6] His work built on the previous advances[7] allowing the estimation of distributions in the presence of censoring. Censoring is a form of missing data that usually occurs in clinical trials as well as many longitudinal studies where unequal lengths of survival and maximum observation time vary on an individual basis. The result is that the actual survival time may not be observed, only the time at which the study period ended without an event, a process called censoring. Cox's model prompted a major advance in biostatistics, leading to an entire field of theoretical and applied work that extended the useful techniques for binary and linear regression to censored survival data. Ultimately the theory expanded to include interval censoring in which the knowledge of the survival times is limited to knowledge of an interval containing the actual time, and regression predictors varying as a function of time. The Kaplan–Meier estimator and the Cox model remain today among the most commonly used and referenced techniques developed in biostatistics. It is notable that, as with many advances in biostatistics, development of censored data methods have involved "translation" from within the mathematical sciences, particularly the use of stochastic process theory to prove the advanced features of the Cox model,[8] such as those that allow modeling effects from covariates or predictors whose effects vary over time.

Data involving repeated measurements and clustered data are frequently encountered in many areas of translational science, ranging from *in vitro* experiments to animal studies to human cohorts in clinical trials and epidemiology. The central issue of concern for statistical theory is the dependence structure imposed on the observed data. For example, repeated measurements of a biomarker over time may vary systematically by animal, and observations may be made on families that have correlated exposures or on bilateral organs in the same person. Correlations within observational units can alter the results of statistical procedures. Early developments to deal with this type of data included applications of "random effects" in analysis of variance and linear models (see Ref. 9 for a review). More recently, these models have been expanded to include binary and counted data, and censored survival models.[10] A major advance in this regard has been the development of models that require fewer assumptions about the precise structure of the dependencies among the clustered observations, allowing wider and more valid applications of regression procedures for all types of clustered data.[11]

A major challenge for biostatistics in translational science has been the adoption of direct measurement of genetic data and the advent of genomics. Statistics and genetics developed together during the pre-human genome era. The English geneticist and statistician R.A. Fisher is often credited with a historical role in the development of both fields. The interpretation of familial modes of inheritance and linkage analysis played a central role in establishing the genetic basis of human disease.

The emergence of genomic technologies has offered opportunities as well as great challenges. The most fundamental of these relates to the extremely high dimensional data subjected to statistical analysis. This has accelerated research on the topics of "multiple comparisons" for hypothesis testing and variable selection methods for regression analysis.[12] Important cross-fertilization is now evident from machine learning methodologies and computer science. As the era of "big data" has progressed, computational issues have become increasingly important. The effects on biostatistics have been both theoretical, in terms of the types of models and procedures that can now be contemplated, and practical, as tools have been developed that can allow statistical analyses of more advanced translational measurement methodologies in fields such as genomics and medical imaging.

24.2.2. Study Design

The translational research process — from bench to bedside and finally to medical systems and populations — is closely associated with a progression in statistical designs. Pre-clinical studies may include a wide variety of *in vivo* and *in vitro* assays, each with unique characteristics, and increasingly involving "big data" issues historically encountered only later (if at all) in the research progression.

Any discussion of statistical design would be incomplete without mention of the important role of randomization. This method was popularized by statisticians such as R.A. Fisher as a means for designing studies to yield estimates for treatment or experimental effects which are unbiased by differences of characteristics among the experimental groups that might affect the outcomes. Randomized experiments and trials are thus considered the gold standard for research design, especially when combined with techniques such as "masking" of study participants and researchers so that subjective and observational biases are minimized.

When direct randomization is not feasible, other methods to control for confounding have been developed. These include the use of regression models that incorporate terms that adjust for the effect of confounding. For instance, an epidemiological study of alcohol use and cancer might employ a survival regression model with a term for alcohol use and a term for smoking exposure. The technique of regression adjustment has been reconsidered from the perspective of causal inference,[13] the theory of which suggests the use of propensity score adjustments based on estimates of the probability of treatment exposures given the observed values of confounding variables. When the confounders are not observed, methods based on instrumental variables that simulate the conditions of randomized studies have been explored.[14]

Early phase clinical trials are typically sequential, and often incorporate "correlative" studies aimed at assessing the biological mechanisms underlying the new treatment or intervention. Because of the small numbers of subjects, a specialized area of trial design research has emerged for these phase I studies primarily intended to establish safety for novel therapeutics. Phase II studies are modestly sized trials aimed at establishing preliminary estimates of efficacy, whereas phase III are large multicenter trials involving randomization and other techniques such as treatment masking to achieve the highest levels of scientific evidence that a proposed intervention is an improvement over standard care.[15] The increased emphasis on rapid translation has led to recent innovations in statistical designs. Phase I and II designs are increasingly combined so that there will be a faster transition to efficacy determination following determination of safe doses. Accelerated dose-escalation and other improvements towards a more rapid process for selecting optimal doses are also being explored. Adaptive randomization methods offer the opportunity to maximize the impact of targeted therapies by incorporating individual characteristics[16] and may serve as a primary tool in the future development of personalized medicine.

An important contribution by statisticians to translational and clinical research has been a theory of optimal statistical design. At the core of this process are the planned analyses based on the key design features of the study. Often it is a calculation involving the "operating characteristics" of a simple hypothesis test comparing means or proportions between two groups, with the focus on the sample size required to achieve a given "power" (probability of the test correctly selecting the alternative hypothesis) for a given significance level (probability of incorrectly rejecting the null hypothesis). However, many translational research study designs do not result in simple comparisons of means. For instance, phase II trials can involve sequential designs where the sample size is allowed to vary according to the accumulating results of the trial. Studies involving genomics may entail comparisons of highly dimensional array data. For these and other more elaborate designs, special methods are used.[17]

24.3. EPIDEMIOLOGY

The insights gained from epidemiology rank historically among the most influential scientific findings directly affecting public health. Early epidemiologic studies were essential to understanding and effectively intervening to prevent infectious diseases such as cholera.[18] For chronic diseases, the linkages established between tobacco consumption, cancer and cardiovascular disease have had a profound influence in more recent times. Even more recently, epidemiologic methods have been central to the fight against HIV, which has aspects of both an infectious and a chronic disease.

Traditionally, population-based research was conducted by investigators who established areas of individual expertise to identify the specific exposures that influenced regional disease burden. This approach to disease causality requires careful observation, interaction with the community, and can provide valuable local guidance on controlling exposures. Regional and local studies were highly effective at identifying exposures that dramatically increase disease risks, starting with the landmark study by John Snow that identified water-born pathogens as the source of the London cholera epidemics of the 1800s,[18] and proceeding through the discovery that bladder cancer risks are higher among aniline dye workers,[19] attributable to exposure to aromatic arylamines.[20]

Community engagement is a key requirement for translating findings from population-based studies for implementation and behavior change, and requires the adoption of individualized or regionalized approaches to intervention. However, for characterizing and controlling causes of most chronic diseases, extensive and careful characterization of large populations is necessary. The discovery that tobacco smoke causes lung cancer and many other common chronic diseases required a paradigm shift in the collection and analysis of data. Providing enough evidence to support a causal relationship between cumulative exposures to tobacco and increasing risk for lung cancer required the development of new epidemiological designs and biostatistical methods. Major criticisms of the causal link between tobacco smoke and lung cancer risk proposed by Doll and Hill (1950)[21] led to the development of modern epidemiological designs, by requiring that incident rather than prevalent cases be studied to avoid survival bias, and by recognizing that controls need to be collected from the same sampling frame as the cases to avoid ascertainment biases. Similarly, the need to quantitate the relationship between the extent of exposure and risk for lung cancer development was an important application of logistic regression analysis, a method that is still the primary tool used in epidemiological studies for evaluating the impact that exposures have on risk for disease development.[4] These seminal developments were needed to evaluate the complex relationships between an exposure with strong effects on disease risk but for which there was a lag between the exposure and disease development and for which large numbers of individuals had to be studied (given the low incidence of lung cancer in the general population), and the incomplete association between smoking exposure and subsequent lung cancer development.

The development of many new advanced biotechnologies has provided opportunities for characterizing risk factors with previously unimaginable precision and depth. As we enter the era of application of these technologies in epidemiology, new challenges will arise, requiring innovative designs, analytical approaches and methods for translating our findings for use in the community. Applications will include evaluating exposure patterns, disease characteristics and individualized risks for disease development. At a population level, risks for disease from many exposures may appear limited, but variations in susceptibility can result in individualized risks being substantively higher. Therefore, increasingly large studies are needed to assure the availability of enough individuals who have a range of exposure patterns that are sufficient to evaluate the combinations of exposure and individual characteristics that have the strongest impact on disease risk.

Developing large populations for study has required a cultural shift in the conduct of epidemiological research, which had previously focused on aggregated regional observations using tools developed to address questions specific to particular and limited populations. To assist in improving standardization of data collection processes, particularly application of questionnaires and consenting of patients and management of samples, several initiatives were spawned, including the P3G project[22] and PhenX.[23,24] The P3G project states that its goals are to "[e]ncourage collaboration between researchers and biobankers, promote harmonization of data, [and] optimize the design, set-up and research activities of studies, biobanks, research databases and other similar health and social research infrastructures" (see *http://p3g.org/resources*). P3G makes available to the research community information about a large number of studies that have collected biological material and phenotypic information, most of which is derived from questionnaires. Questionnaires for many large studies are provided as a means to assist researchers in harmonizing their own data collection activities with those at other sites. Finally, information to assist in establishing biorepositories, including consenting and sample processing protocols that have been accumulated from many studies, are freely available.

PhenX (*www.phenx.org*) is a consortium established by the National Human Genome Research Institute that consolidates and disseminates approaches for collecting data with an emphasis on facilitating coordinated analysis of large-scale genome-wide association studies. To facilitate interactions, PhenX collaborators were tasked with reaching a consensus for presentation of up to 15 questionnaires to assess phenotypes, and harmonization procedures to allow linking across questionnaires.

Given the concerted effort that has been adopted by many investigators to assemble common panels of questionnaires, one may ask why there are such a large number of different questionnaires and study designs in place. The heterogeneity in data collection and processing methods across institutions and studies presents major hurdles to investigators. Part of the range in methods reflects the history of epidemiological investigation, which was often driven by individual investigators or approaches, and it also reflects the longevity of research on human populations. Once a study has been initiated, investigators are reluctant to change the study collection process, because that makes analyses within the study more difficult, even though it facilitates across-study analyses. An additional challenge to integrating data across resource centers is the need to obtain releases that allow data to be shared. The consent process by which data are collected also needs to state that data sharing may be involved. Further allowing individuals to indicate which data can be shared and for what purposes (for example individuals may not want to share sensitive genetic data) protects individual rights, but also introduces complexities in data management because the release of information has to be limited.

All of these challenges suggest that epidemiologically derived data needs to be collected in a more sophisticated manner. Reflecting the complexity in harmonizing data across ongoing studies, many integrative genetic analyses only incorporate the most basic epidemiological data, such as age at onset of disease. To overcome this challenge, the Genetic Associations and Mechanisms in Oncology Study (*http://epi.grants.cancer.gov/gameon*) was formed to perform genomic studies across diverse populations while integrating epidemiological information among studies. Because of the challenges of collecting epidemiologically relevant information, the Tumor Cancer Genome Atlas, as an example, decided against collecting data from questionnaires and only collected information derived from medical records. While this strategy for facilitating rapid data acquisition was effective, it also reduced the value of the resulting data for identifying the role that epidemiological exposures have in disease development.

The analysis of extensive data derived from genetic and other biomarker studies, such as RNA expression arrays or large-scale proteomic studies, also requires a paradigm shift in the epidemiological process. Epidemiologists follow a biological model of inquiry in which specific hypotheses are stated about the populations under study and the causes for disease or the influences on a biomarker of disease. When a very large number of hypotheses can be tested simultaneously, it is no longer scientifically appropriate to test all null hypotheses (such as that a genetic marker does not associate with disease risk), and accept tests as rejecting the null unless a correction for multiple testing is applied or a very well-developed validation approach is included in the study design. For example, if one were testing association of the one million markers that are typically queried by application of a genomic single nucleotide polymorphism (SNP) array and employed a 5 percent critical value, there would be 50,000 false positive tests that arise during the testing process even if all one million markers were not associated with the outcome. To deal with concerns about excess false positive results, several approaches have been developed. For association studies of genetic predisposition to disease, analysis of SNP arrays includes only a very small proportion (typically less than 0.5 percent) of true associations, and therefore applying standard corrections that adjust the critical value for rejecting the null hypothesis to account for multiple tests such as a Bonferroni or Sidak correction provides an acceptable strategy for reducing false positive findings, although at some cost to the power to detect associations. Procedures for up-weighting some tests according to prior evidence that specific regions or genetic regions are likely to be associated can help to recover power while preserving scientific validity by limiting the number of false positive findings.[25]

Studies of expression arrays and biomarker studies of disease often lead to studies in which a larger proportion of true positive findings are expected (e.g., greater than 5 percent true positive findings). When sample sizes are limited and further studies are planned to confirm the findings, an alternative approach to deciding which results to pursue further is warranted. For these situations, approaches to control the proportion of false discoveries have been effective. In these approaches, the observed distribution of test statistics is used to assess the threshold for a positive result (i.e., rejection of the null hypothesis), and test results exceeding that threshold.

In either approach, the entire set of hypotheses that will be tested is established at the beginning of the analysis and a paradigm for deciding which results warrant further study is specified. As a result, findings from large-scale genetic or genomic studies can provide reliable inferences about biomarkers associated with disease and can subsequently be validated by replication.

In summary, when a very large number of hypotheses are evaluated and no approach is taken to jointly analyze findings, a plethora of false positive results can be anticipated. Without a suitably structured approach to the testing procedure, it is likely that subsequent researchers will be unable to confirm results. Providing information about the full set of hypotheses that have been tested in epidemiological or biomarker studies provides the scientific community with information that can be used for a full appraisal of the statistical validity of such studies. Approaches for data sharing and documentation of studies are discussed below.

Even when studies are appropriately designed and associations have been identified between epidemiological or genomic factors with disease risks, significant barriers must be overcome to bring a novel test to widespread use for characterizing individual risk. Research findings are often obtained by broad-scale analysis of hundreds of tests, most of which are not informative. In order for a new test to be worthy of broad-scale application, it must be defined with thresholds known to have acceptable cost, while maintaining validity when used within specified quality control metrics. New tests that are considered for application for screening or diagnosis in a target population should undergo additional validation analyses in a population distinct from the one used for the initial discovery. Test performance is graded by calibration, discrimination and accuracy. Calibration determines a model's ability to predict the number of events within specified subgroups of the population and is assessed by the goodness-of-fit test. Discrimination measures whether or not a model can differentiate between those individuals who will develop disease versus those who will not, and is commonly estimated using the area under the receiver-operator characteristic (ROC) curve (AUC, also known as the concordance statistic). The positive predictive value (PPV) and negative predictive value (NPV) measure a model's ability to accurately categorize affected and non-affected individuals, respectively. These characteristics are important to assess model performance for estimating disease burden or for clinical decision-making or screening (good discrimination and good accuracy).

There are tremendous new opportunities in translational research for identifying predictors of many diseases, and we highlight here approaches for studying cancer development and its successful treatment. These opportunities for understanding cancer development are being provided by new technological advancements in several areas. First, there has been a revolution in the "omic" area that is allowing us to comprehensively profile genomes at low cost for germ line variants and somatic changes, and also for epigenetic alterations often due to risky behaviors like smoking. Second, methods for assessing individual environments are improving dramatically. Third, improvements in biobanking and sample management are allowing us to more effectively retrieve and use samples from large collections of individuals. Last, decreasing computational costs are allowing ever more precise approaches for individualized risk assessment to be possible.

Genetic mutations influence cancer progression and outcomes. We can anticipate that cancer outcomes may be largely determined by the genetic and epigenetic changes that occur in a tumor. Genetic analysis of tumors will provide important determinants for allocating cancer therapies. In addition, dose limiting toxicity depends, to some currently unknown extent, on an individual's genotype as well as host-specific susceptibility, which is determined by demographic factors such as age, sex and ethnicity, and risk behaviors such as smoking history. Further phenotyping to evaluate individual susceptibility to cancer development and sensitivity to its treatment would provide valuable information to better characterize causes of cancer and its prognosis. Several assays for DNA repair capacity and susceptibility to DNA damage have been developed though not yet deployed systematically, but are amenable to analysis using cell-based nanotechnologies.

Finally, improving technologies are affecting risk prediction and management. For example, the recent National Lung Screening Trial[26] showed a 20 percent reduction in cause-specific mortality from helical CT, but with only a 4 percent positive predictive value for this relatively healthy population of current and former smokers. These findings raise concerns about the potential financial burden of population-level implementation of spiral CT among the large number of at-risk ever-smokers, although the costs have not been reported as of the date of this review. Newer approaches for individualized risk assessment that take advantage of microRNA profiling, genetic analysis, and host-specific measures of response to DNA damage may allow us to provide more precise risk estimates so that only a subset of highest risk individuals are evaluated, increasing the positive predictive value.

24.4. BIOINFORMATICS

The need to interpret information from whole-genome sequencing projects in the context of biological information acquired during decades of research studies prompted the establishment, in November 1988, of the National Center for Biotechnology Information (NCBI) as a division of the National Library of Medicine (NLM) at the National Institutes of Health (NIH) in the US. When the NCBI was established, it was charged with (i) creating automated systems for storing and analyzing knowledge about molecular biology, biochemistry and genetics; (ii) performing research into advanced methods of computer-based information processing for analyzing the structure and function of biologically important molecules and compounds; (iii) facilitating the use of databases and software by biotechnology researchers and medical care personnel; and (iv) coordination of efforts to gather biotechnology information worldwide.[27] Since 1988, the NCBI has fulfilled many of these goals and has delivered a set of databases and computational tools that are essential for modern biomedical research in a wide range of disciplines, including molecular epidemiology. The NCBI and other international efforts such as the European Bioinformatics Institute (EBI), which was established in 1992,[28] have played a very important role in inspiring and motivating the establishment of research groups and centers around the world that are dedicated to providing bioinformatics tools and expertise.

24.4.1. Databases for Translational Research

One of the most important pre-study activities is the design and development of one or more databases that can accept, store and manage molecular epidemiology data. Haynes and Blach (2006)[29] list eight steps for establishing an effective information management system. The first step is to develop the experimental plan for the laboratory, molecular, and sample information that will be collected. What are the specific needs for the database? The second step is to establish the information flow. That is, how does the information find its way from the laboratory to the database? The third step is to create a model for information storage. How are the data related? The fourth step is to determine the hardware and software requirements. How much data needs to be stored? How quickly will investigators need to access the data? What operating system will be used? Will a freely available database such as mySQL (*www.mysql.com*) serve the needs of the project or will a commercial dataset solution such as Oracle (*www.oracle.com*) be needed? The fifth step is to implement the database. The important consideration here is to define the database structure so that data integrity is maintained. The sixth step is to choose the user interface to the database. Is a web page portal to the data sufficient or does a specialized software application for the desktop need to be created? The seventh step is to determine the security requirements. Do HIPAA regulations (*www.hhs.gov/ocr/privacy*) need to be followed? Most databases need to be password protected at a minimum. The eighth and final step outlined by Haynes and Blach[29] is to select the software tools that will interface with the data for summary and analysis. Some of these tools will be reviewed below.

Although most investigators choose to develop and manage their own database for security and confidentiality reasons, there are an increasing number of public databases for depositing data and making it widely available to other investigators. The tradition of making data publicly available soon after it has been analyzed and published can largely be attributed to the community of investigators using gene expression microarrays. Microarrays[30] represent one of the most revolutionary applications that derived from the knowledge of whole genome sequences and expression levels of RNA. The extensive use of this technology has led to the need to store and search expression data for all the genes in the genome acquired in different genetic backgrounds or in different environmental conditions. This has resulted in a number of public databases such as the Stanford Microarray Database (*http://genome-www5.stanford.edu*),[31] the Gene Expression Omnibus or GEO (*www.ncbi.nlm.nih.gov/geo*),[32,33] Array Express (*www.ebi.ac.uk/arrayexpress*)[34,35] and others, which anyone can use to upload or download data. The nearly universal acceptance of the data-sharing culture in this area has yielded a number of useful tools that might not otherwise have been developed. The need to define standards for the ontology and annotation of microarray experiments has led to proposals such as the Minimum Information About a Microarray Experiment (MIAME) (*www.mged.org/Workgroups/MIAME/miame.html*)[36,37] that provided a standard that greatly facilitates the storage, retrieval and sharing of data from microarray experiments. The MIAME standards provide an example for other types of data such as SNPs and protein mass spectrometry spectra. See Ref. 38 for a comprehensive review of standards for data sharing in genetics, genomics, proteomics and systems biology. The success of the different databases then depends on the availability of methods for easily depositing data and tools for searching the databases often after data normalization.

Despite the acceptance of data sharing in the genomics community, the same culture does not yet exist in many areas of the population sciences. One of the few such examples is the Pharmacogenomics Knowledge Base of PharmGKB (*www.pharmgkb.org*).[39,40] PharmGKB was established with funding from the NIH to store, manage and make available molecular data in addition to phenotype data from pharmacogenetic and pharmacogenomic experiments and clinical studies. It is anticipated that similar databases for a variety of different disciplines will appear and gain acceptance over the next few years as the NIH and various journals start to require data from public research be made available to the public. In an effort to encourage data sharing and particularly given the high cost of many population-based genetic and genomic studies, researchers funded by NIH initiatives are required to deposit their data into the NCBI-sponsored database of genotypes and phenotypes (dbGaP). In order to protect individuals who have participated in these studies, IRB approval is required in order to retrieve data.

In addition to the need for a database to store and manage molecular data collected from experimental or observational studies, there are a number of database resources that can be very helpful for planning a study. A good starting point for database resources are those maintained at the NCBI (*www.ncbi.nlm.nih.gov*).[41] The NCBI maintains the PubMed literature database with more than 22 million indexed abstracts from published papers in more than 5,000 life science journals. The PubMed Central database (*www.pubmedcentral.nih.gov*) is quickly becoming an indispensable tool. Rapid and free access to the complete text of published papers significantly enhances the planning, execution and interpretation phases of any scientific study. The new Bookshelf database (*www.ncbi.nlm.nih.gov/books*) provides free access for the first time to electronic versions of many textbooks and other resources such as the *NCBI Handbook*, which serves as a guide to the resources that NCBI has to offer. This is a particularly important resource for students and investigators that need to learn a new discipline such as genomics. One of the oldest databases provided by the NCBI is the GenBank DNA sequence resource (*www.ncbi.nlm.nih.gov/genbank*).[42,43] DNA sequence data for more than 250,000 species has been deposited in GenBank for more than two decades now. GenBank is a common starting point for the design of PCR primers and other molecular assays that require specific knowledge of gene sequences. Curated information about genes, their chromosomal location, their function, their pathways, and so on can be accessed through the Entrez Gene database (*www.ncbi.nlm.nih.gov/gene*), for example.

Important emerging databases include those that store and summarize DNA sequence variations. NCBI maintains the dbSNP (*www.ncbi.nlm.nih.gov/projects/SNP*)[44,45] database for SNPs. dbSNP provides a wide range of different information about SNPs including the flanking sequence primers, the position, the validation methods, and the frequency of the alleles in different populations. As with all NCBI databases, it is possible to link to a number of other datasets, such as PubMed.

In addition to databases for storing raw data, there are a number of databases that retrieve and store knowledge in an accessible form. For example, the Kyoto Encyclopedia of Genes and Genomes (KEGG) database stores knowledge on genes and their pathways (*www.genome.jp/kegg*).[46,47] The Pathway component of KEGG currently stores knowledge on more than 43,000 pathways. While the Pathway component documents molecular interaction in pathways, the KEGG Brite database stores knowledge on higher-order biological functions. One of the most useful knowledge sources is the Gene Ontology (GO) project, which has created a controlled vocabulary to describe genes and gene products in any organism in terms of their biological processes, cellular components and molecular functions (*www.geneontology.org*).[48] GO descriptions and KEGG pathways are both captured and summarized in the NCBI databases. For example, the description of p53 in Entrez Gene includes KEGG pathways such as cell cycle and apoptosis. It also includes GO descriptions such as protein binding and cell proliferation.

In general, a good place to start for information about available databases is the annual Database issue and the annual Web Server issue of the journal *Nucleic Acids Research* (*http://nar.oxfordjournals.org*). These special issues include annual reports from many of the commonly used databases.

24.4.2. Bioinformatics Analysis

Once the data is collected and stored in a database, an important goal is to identify biomolecular patterns that are associated with an observed phenotypic outcome. Data analysis in the biological sciences has moved away from traditional univariate statistical methods such as the t-test towards data mining and machine learning methods such as cluster analysis and support vector machines as the size and complexity of molecular datasets have grown. Machine learning and data mining methods can detect nonlinear patterns in high-dimensional data that might more closely reflect the underlying hierarchical complexity of biological systems. Although powerful research tools, these methods are typically more difficult to implement because they require knowledge of computer science and often require more computing power than is available using a single processor on a desktop or laptop computer. An important development in the last few years is the availability of open-source and user-friendly software that brings many of these advanced computer science methods to the biologist.

R is perhaps the one software package that everyone should have in their bioinformatics arsenal. R is an open-source and freely available programming language and data analysis and visualization environment that can be downloaded from *www.r-project.org*. According to the web page, R includes (i) an effective data handling and storage facility; (ii) a suite of operators for calculations on arrays, particularly matrices; (iii) a large, coherent, integrated collection of intermediate tools for data analysis; (iv) graphical capabilities for data analysis and display either on-screen or on hardcopy; and (v) a well-developed, simple and effective programming language that includes conditionals, loops, user-defined recursive functions, and input and output facilities. A major strength of R is the enormous community of developers and users that ensure just about any analysis method you need is available. Perhaps the most useful contribution to R for bioinformatics is the Bioconductor project (*www.bioconductor.org*).[49] According to the Bioconductor web page, the goals of the project are to (i) provide access to a wide range of powerful statistical and graphical methods for the analysis of genomic data; (ii) facilitate the integration of biological metadata (e.g., PubMed, GO) in the analysis of experimental data; (iii) allow the rapid development of extensible, scalable and interoperable software; (iv) promote high-quality and reproducible research; and (v) provide training in computational and statistical methods for the analysis of genomic data. Many of the available tools are specific to microarray data but some are more generally applicable to genetics and epidemiology. For example, there are tools in Bioconductor for accessing data from the KEGG database mentioned above.

There are numerous packages for machine learning and data mining that are either part of the base R software or can be easily added. For example, the *neural* package includes routines for neural network analysis. Others include *arules* for association rule mining, *cluster* for cluster analysis, *genalg* for genetic algorithms, *som* for self-organizing maps, and *tree* for classification and regression trees. Many others are available. A full list of contributed packages for R can be found at *http://cran.r-project.org/*.

The primary advantages of using R as your data mining software package are programmability and open source contributions. However, the learning curve can be challenging at first since some computer programming in the R language is usually necessary. Fortunately, there is plenty of documentation available on the Web and in published books.

24.4.3. Translational Bioinformatics

Our brief review of bioinformatics above provides some context for the analysis of "omics" data. This is in contrast to biomedical informatics, which focuses much more on the management, retrieval and analysis of clinical data from an electronic health record (EHR). An emerging discipline called "translational bioinformatics" attempts to tie the bioinformatics approaches described above to methods and applications that have been developed for biomedical informatics in the clinical realm.

One of the first uses of the term *translational bioinformatics* can be found in a published paper by Butte and Chen[50] that attempted to find gene expression data stored in the NCBI GEO database that are related to human diseases. This study tied GEO data to diseases by linking them with PubMed identifiers from papers that described the original experiments. In doing so, the authors were able to associate 35 percent of publically available gene expression data in GEO to more than 270 human diseases and phenotypes. This was one of the first studies to use informatics methods to link genomics data with human disease keywords.

This idea of linking genomics data with clinical data has taken off with efforts to formalize the discipline of translational bioinformatics. Butte[51] provided a viewpoint piece highlighting the call to formally recognize translational bioinformatics as a third major arm of informatics as defined by the American Medical Informatics Association (AMIA). The AMIA definition of translational bioinformatics is tied to the creation of new tools for medicine from the integration of biological data such as that from genomics. Butte[51] goes on to call for increased funding in this area and to increase the number of trained translational bioinformaticists. Both are needed if we are to fully integrate large-scale biological data for the improvement of medicine.

The translational bioinformatics movement is gaining momentum. For example, Shortliffe *et al.*[52] announced a special issue of the *Journal of Biomedical Informatics* on this topic that was realized in 2010.[53] This special issue was concurrent with the new annual AMIA Summit on Translational Bioinformatics, which is now planning its sixth meeting. There is now a Translational Bioinformatics Conference (TBC) in Asia that will be held for the third time in South Korea in 2013. This conference publishes its best papers in the *Journal of the American Medical Informatics Association* (JAMIA). There was even a special issue of *PLoS Computational Biology* that covered a wide range of topics on translational bioinformatics.[54]

Bioinformatics has traditionally been a very basic discipline focused on DNA sequence analysis, gene expression analysis and other application areas such as proteomics and structural biology. The computational demands of these emerging disciplines were very real, and bioinformatics was created to meet that demand with new expertise, education, training and software. However, we now live in a reality whereby it is increasingly important to tie research to medicine and human health. Funding agencies such as the NIH are increasingly awarding grants to those research studies with a translational component. It is not surprising that the natural progression from basic research to clinical and translational research has given rise to translational bioinformatics.

24.5. CONCLUSION

Biostatistics, epidemiology and bioinformatics are highly dynamic disciplines that play a crucial role in translational research. In turn, translational research has transformed these fields by introducing new scientific concepts and technologies demanding interdisciplinary collaborations throughout the quantitative biomedical sciences. This development and synergy is not unexpected given the origins of the fields on the boundaries of scientific disciplines where translation is taking place.

Acknowledgments

This work was supported by Dartmouth SYNERGY: The Clinical and Translational Science Institute; and grants from the National Institutes of Health, CA23108, AR062799, LM010098, AI59694, and LM009012.

REFERENCES

1. Boguski MS. (1994) Bioinformatics. *Curr Opin Genet Dev* **4**: 383–388.
2. Finney DJ. (1952) *Statistical Methods in Biological Assay.* Hafner Publishing, New York, NY.
3. Berkson J. (1953)A statistically precise and relatively simple method of estimating the bioassay with quantal response based on the logistic function. *J Amer Stat Assoc* **48**: 565–599.
4. Cornfield J, Gordon T, Smith W. (1961) Quantal response curves for experimentally uncontroled variables. *Bull Int Stat Inst* **38**: 97–115.
5. Mucullagh P, Nelder JA. (1989) *Generalized Linear Models,* 2nd ed. Chapman and Hall, London, UK.
6. Cox DR. (1972) Regression models and life-tables. *J Royal Stat Soc* **34**: 187–220.
7. Kaplan EL, Meier P. (1958) Nonparametric estimation from incomplete observations. *J Amer Stat Assoc* **53**: 457–481.
8. Andersen PK, Gill RD. (1982) Cox's regression model for counting processes: A large sample study. *Ann Statist* **10**: 1100–1120.
9. Demidenko E. (2004) *Mixed Models: Theory and Applications.* John Wiley & Sons, Hoboken, NJ.
10. Diggle PJ, Heagerty P, Liang K-Y, Zeger SL. (2002) *Analysis of Longitudinal Data.* Oxford University Press, Oxford, UK.
11. Liang K-Y, Zeger SL. (1986) Longitudinal data analysis using generalized linear models. *Biometrika* **73**: 13–22.
12. Hastie T, Tibshirani R, Friedman J. (2001) *The Elements of Statistical Learning.* Springer, New York, NY.
13. Rosenbaum PR, Rubin DB. (1983) The central role of the propensity score in the observational studies for causal effects. *Biometrika* **70**: 41–55.
14. Angrist JD, Imbens GW, Rubin DB. (1996) Identification of causal effects using instrumental variables, *J Amer Stat Assoc* **91**: 444–455.
15. Friedman LM, Furberg CD, DeMets DL. (2010) *Fundamentals of Clinical Trials.* Springer, New York, NY.

16. Kim ES, *et al.* (2011) The battle trial: Personalizing therapy for lung cancer. *Cancer Discov* **1**: 44–53.
17. Chow S-C, Wang H, Shao J. (2008) *Sample Size Calculations in Clinical Research*. Chapman & Hall/CRC, Boca Raton, FL.
18. Snow J. (1855) *On the Mode of Communication of Cholera in London*. John Churchill, London, England.
19. Rehn L. (1895) Blasengeschwulste bei Fuchsinarbeitern. *Arch Klin Chir* **50**: 588–600.
20. Hueper WCW, Wiley FH, Wolfe HD. (1938) Experimental production of bladder tumors in dogs by administration of beta-naphthylamine. *J Ind Hyg Toxicol* **20**: 40–84.
21. Doll R, Hill AB. (1950) Smoking and carcinoma of the lung: Preliminary report. *Br Med J* **2**: 739–748.
22. Knoppers BM, Fortier I, Legault D, Burton P. (2008) The Public Population Project in Genomics (P3G): A proof of concept? *Eur J Hum Genet* **16**: 664–665.
23. Schad PA, Mobley LR, Hamilton CM. (2011) Building a biomedical cyberinfrastructure for collaborative research. *Am J Prev Med* **40**: S144–S150.
24. Stover PJ, Harlan WR, Hammond JA, *et al.* (2010) Phenx: A toolkit for interdisciplinary genetics research. *Curr Opin Lipidol* **21**: 136–140.
25. Roeder K, Wasserman L. (2009) Genome-wide significance levels and weighted hypothesis testing. *Stat Sci* **24**: 398–413.
26. Aberle DR, Adams AM, Berg CD, *et al.* (National Lung Screening Trial Research Team). (2011) Reduced lung-cancer mortality with low-dose computed tomographic screening. *N Engl J Med* **365**: 395–409.
27. Benson D, Boguski M, Lipman D, Ostell J. (1990) The National Center for Biotechnology Information. *Genomics* **6**: 389–391.
28. Robinson C. (1994) The European Bioinformatics Institute (EBI) — Open for business, *Trends Biotechnol* **12**: 391–392.
29. Haynes C, Blach C. (2006) Information management. In: Haines JL, Pericak-Vance M. (eds). *Genetic Analysis of Complex Disease*. John Wiley & Sons, Hoboken, NJ.
30. Schena M, Shalon D, Davis RW, Brown PO. (1995) Quantitative monitoring of gene expression patterns with a complementary DNA microarray. *Science* **270**: 467–470.
31. Sherlock G, Hernandez-Boussard T, Kasarskis A, *et al.* (2001) The Stanford Microarray Database. *Nucleic Acids Res* **29**: 152–155.
32. Barrett T, Troup DB, Wilhite SE, *et al.* (2005) NCBI GEO: Mining millions of expression profiles — Database and tools. *Nucleic Acids Res* **33**: D562–D566.

33. Barrett T, Wilhite SE, Ledoux P, *et al.* (2013) NCBI GEO: Archive for functional genomics data sets — Update. *Nucleic Acids Res* **41**: D991–D995.
34. Brazma A, Parkinson H, Sarkans U, *et al.* (2003) Array Express — A public repository for microarray gene expression data at the EBI. *Nucleic Acids Res* **31**: 68–71.
35. Rustici G, Kolesnikov N, Brandizi M, *et al.* (2013) Array express Update — Trends in database growth and links to data analysis tools. *Nucleic Acids Res* **41**: D987–D990.
36. Ball CA, Brazma A. (2006) MGED standards: Work in progress. *OMICS* **10**: 138–144.
37. Brazma A, Hingamp P, Quackenbush J, *et al.* (2001) Minimum information about a microarray experiment (MIAME) — Toward standards for microarray data. *Nat Genet* **29**: 365–371.
38. Brazma A, Krestyaninova M, Sarkans U. (2006) Standards for systems biology. *Nat Rev Genet* **7**: 593–605.
39. Altman RB. (2007) PharmGKB: A logical home for knowledge relating genotype to drug response phenotype. *Nat Genet* **39**: 426.
40. Hewett M, Oliver DE, Rubin DL, *et al.* (2002) PharmGKB: The pharmacogenetics knowledge base. *Nucleic Acids Res* **30**: 163–165.
41. NCBI Resource Coordinators. (2013) Database resources of the National Center for Biotechnology Information. *Nucleic Acids Res* **41**: D8–D20.
42. Benson D, Lipman DJ, Ostell J. (1993) Genbank. *Nucleic Acids Res* **21**: 2963–2965.
43. Benson DA, Cavanaugh M, Clark K, *et al.* (2013) Genbank. *Nucleic Acids Res* **41**: D36–D42.
44. Sherry ST, Ward M, Sirotkin K. (1999) dbSNP — Database for single nucleotide polymorphisms and other classes of minor genetic variation. *Genome Res* **9**: 677–679.
45. Sherry ST, Ward MH, Kholodov M, *et al.* (2001) dbSNP: The NCBI database of genetic variation. *Nucleic Acids Res* **29**: 308–311.
46. Kanehisa M. (1997) A database for post-genome analysis. *Trends Genet* **13**: 375–376.
47. Ogata H, Goto S, Sato K, *et al.* (1999) Kegg: Kyoto encyclopedia of genes and genomes. *Nucleic Acids Res* **27**: 29–34.
48. Ashburner M, Ball CA, Blake JA, *et al.* (2000) Gene ontology: Tool for the unification of biology. The gene ontology consortium. *Nat Genet* **25**: 25–29.
49. Reimers M, Carey VJ. (2006) Bioconductor: An open source framework for bioinformatics and computational biology. *Methods Enzymol* **411**: 119–134.

50. Butte AJ, Chen R. (2006) Finding disease-related genomic experiments within an international repository: First steps in translational bioinformatics. *AMIA Annu Symp Proc* 106–110.
51. Butte AJ. (2008) Translational bioinformatics: Coming of age. *J Am Med Inform Assoc* **15**: 709–714.
52. Shortliffe EH, Califano A, Hunter L. (2009) New JBI emphasis on translational bioinformatics. *J Biomed Inform* **42**: 199–200.
53. Lussier YA, Butte AJ, Hunter L. (2010) Current methodologies for translational bioinformatics. *J Biomed Inform* **43**: 355–357.
54. Altman RB. (2012) Introduction to translational bioinformatics collection. *PLoS Comput Biol* **8**: e1002796.

CHAPTER 25

Research Methods for Clinical Trials in Personalized Medicine: A Systematic Review

*Zheng Ren**, *Marie Davidian*[†,§], *Stephen L. George*[‡,§], *Richard M. Goldberg*[‖], *Fred A. Wright**, *Anastasios A. Tsiatis*[†,§] and *Michael R. Kosorok*[*,¶,**]

25.1. INTRODUCTION

The emerging field of personalized medicine has been the focus of vigorous recent research. Since the initiation of the Human Genome Project 20 years ago,[1] researchers have successfully identified tens of thousands of genes and studied their protein products and functions, and advances in genetic typing and sequencing techniques have revolutionized our understanding of individual genetic variation,[2,3] spurring research on new therapeutic agents that can target genetic differences across individuals. Differences

*Department of Biostatistics, University of North Carolina at Chapel Hill, Chapel Hill, North Carolina, USA.
†Department of Statistics, North Carolina State University, Raleigh, North Carolina, USA.
‡Cancer Center Biostatistics, Duke University Medical Center, Durham, North Carolina, USA.
§Department of Biostatistics and Bioinformatics, Duke University Medical Center, Durham, North Carolina, USA.
‖Comprehensive Cancer Center, The Ohio State University Medical Center, Columbus, Ohio, USA.
¶Department of Statistics and Operations Research, University of North Carolina at Chapel Hill, Chapel Hill, North Carolina, USA.
**Corresponding author: Michael R. Kosorok, PhD, Department of Biostatistics and Department of Statistics and Operations Research, University of North Carolina at Chapel Hill, 3101 McGavran-Greenberg Hall, CB 7420, Chapel Hill, NC 27599-7420; E-mail: *kosorok@unc.edu*

in therapeutic response among individuals may arise from a number of other sources, such as cumulative environmental exposures, which may be difficult to assess. The genetic revolution has thus provided a measurable basis for personalized medicine and has placed the field in the international spotlight. The goal of the Genomics and Personalized Medicine Act of 2010 (GPMA), introduced in the United States (US) House of Representatives in May 2010, is to encourage genomics research and the application of personalized medicine[4]; a similar act was introduced previously in the US Senate by then-Senator Barack Obama. As public awareness and interest in genetic testing continues to heighten, research on the use of genomic and other patient information to improve the prevention, diagnosis and treatment of disease is likely to accelerate.

The ultimate goal of personalized medicine is to make the optimal decisions on a patient's care based on all of the information from the patient, including not only genetic information but also age, gender, other clinical factors, current disease status, and other characteristics. Methods for exploiting very large quantities of data, integrated with biological knowledge, and innovative study designs are critical to this goal.

In this chapter, we report on a systematic review of methodologic approaches that have been applied in published studies to use patient genomic information as the basis for improving the efficacy of treatments and reducing toxicity. Issues and challenges in the design and analysis of personalized medicine studies are also discussed, and new approaches are proposed.

25.2. BACKGROUND

There is no single definition of "personalized medicine," and differing terminology has been used in the literature by various stakeholders to describe the concept, including personalized medicine,[5–8] personalized therapy,[9,10] personalized drugs[11] and tailored therapy.[12,13] The US National Institutes of Health (NIH), for example, defines personalized medicine as "an emerging practice of medicine that uses an individual's genetic profile to guide decisions made in regard to the prevention, diagnosis, and treatment of disease. Knowledge of a patient's genetic profile can help doctors select the proper medication or therapy and administer it using the proper dose or regimen." For the US Food and Drug Administration (FDA), the goal of personalized medicine is "to get the best medical outcomes by choosing treatments that work well with a person's genomic profile or with certain characteristics in the person's blood proteins or cell surface proteins."[14] In the GPMA, personalized medicine is defined as "any clinical practice model that emphasizes the systematic use of preventive, diagnostic, and therapeutic interventions that use genome and family history information to improve health outcomes." Recently, Margaret A. Hamburg, Commissioner of the FDA, and Francis S. Collins, Director of NIH, shared their joint opinion about the concept,[15] proposing that the goal of personalized medicine is to identify the best treatment strategy to achieve the optimal clinical outcome based on a patient's individual profile. Note that the definitions encompass variation in constitutional genetic profile, which is stable for an individual, as well as more variable genomic or other biomarkers that may be specific to a disease state, tumor or tissue.

Personalized medicine has demonstrated the potential to lead to enhanced treatment effect in clinical studies of already-approved therapies within gene-profile stratified subgroups,[16] to avoid unnecessary toxicity associated with treatments[17] and to minimize the rate of adverse events.[18] In many settings, it is likely that some subgroups of patients will have a better response to a new treatment and others will have a worse response. If the population is considered as a whole, the overall difference would be attenuated by those with poorer responses, and no significant improvement would be detected for the population (Fig. 1). Therefore, personalized medicine has the potential to improve the performance of therapy for individual patients through recognizing and capitalizing on patient heterogeneity. Note that the very concept of personalized medicine represents a profound shift in the interpretation of treatment data, especially in the context of controlled clinical trials, for which subgroup analysis has often been viewed with suspicion as a potential source of spurious findings.

A striking example of meaningful subgroup analysis occurred in a randomized prospective phase III clinical trial in patients with advanced non-small cell lung cancer that confirmed the benefit of first-line gefitinib, an epidermal growth factor receptor (EGFR) tyrosine kinase inhibitor, to chemotherapy. In subjects with EGFR mutation-positive tumors, PFS was significantly improved for gefitinib versus chemotherapy (median PFS,

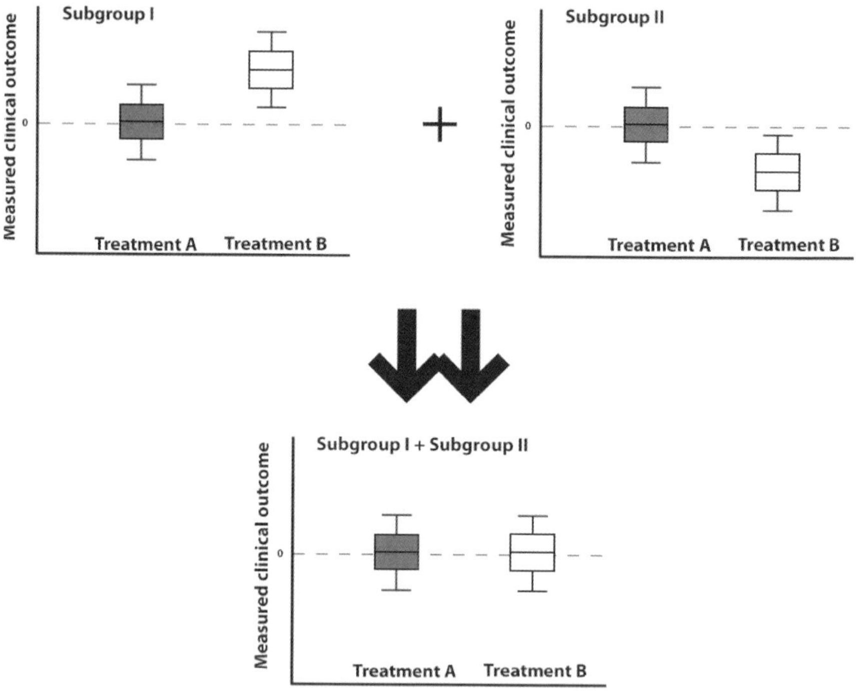

Fig. 1. Comparisons among subgroups. Subgroup I has a better response to treatment B, but subgroup II has a worse response. The overall efficacy of treatment B in the whole population may not be statistically significant.

9.5 months versus 6.3 months), suggesting that the presence of EGFR positive mutation should be used as a criterion for determining first-line therapy for patients with advanced non-small cell lung cancer.[19]

25.3. SYSTEMATIC REVIEW

In this review, we summarize studies related to personalized medicine that were published in six high-impact journals — *Journal of the American Medical Association*, *Journal of the National Cancer Institute*, *The Lancet*, *Nature*, *Nature Medicine*, and the *New England Journal of Medicine* — from 2006 to 2011. All papers were manually selected and reviewed. The inclusion criteria were: (i) papers published between January 1, 2006 and December 31, 2011; (ii) papers reporting the results of original clinical studies using genetic information obtained from DNA, RNA, protein or tumor mutations to stratify the study population; and (iii) papers reporting the association between biomarkers and patient clinical outcomes. Exclusion criteria were (i) papers focused mainly on the association between genetic profile and incident disease; (ii) papers focused on identifying biomarkers for disease diagnosis; and (iii) papers reporting systematic reviews and meta-analysis. Ninety articles (15 papers published in the *Journal of the American Medical Association*, 20 papers published in the *Journal of the National Cancer Institute*, 9 papers published in *The Lancet*, 6 papers published in *Nature*, 7 papers published in *Nature Medicine*, and 33 papers published in the *New England Journal of Medicine*) were selected meeting the above criteria.[16,20–108] As discussed shortly, two of these[74,87] have since been retracted and are not included in the summaries in Table 1 or elsewhere in this chapter. The predominance of cancer studies reflects the fact that cancer inherently involves genetic dysregulation, increasing the likelihood that suitable biomarkers and targeted therapies may be identified. The genomic data in most of the reviewed studies consisted of transcriptional expression, profiled by microarray or polymerase chain reaction (PCR).

25.4. LITERATURE ANALYSIS

25.4.1. Approaches to Finding Biomarkers for Personalized Medicine

A complete process leading to effective personalized medicine will typically include the following five key elements: obtaining patient genetic/genomic data using array and other high-throughput technology[109]; identifying one or more biomarkers (as discussed shortly)[110]; developing new or selecting available therapies[111]; measuring the relationship between biomarkers and clinical outcomes, including prognosis and response to therapy; and verifying the relationship in a prospective randomized clinical trial.[112]

A biomarker is an indicator that can potentially stratify patients into subgroups with common features. Biomarkers can consist of DNA, RNA, proteins and types of tumors. Because of the so-called "curse of dimensionality,"[113] where there are vast numbers of genes relative to patient samples, identifying a potential biomarker from patient genomic profiles is a tremendous challenge for geneticists and statisticians. Many techniques

Table 1 Summary of Personalized Medicine Studies Published between 2006 and 2011 in Six Journals

Number of Genes or Proteins in Each Biomarker	Greater than 100 genes	6 (7%)
	Between 10 and 100 genes	9 (10%)
	Between 2 and 10 genes	11 (13%)
	Only 1 gene	62 (70%)
Sample Size	Larger than 1,000 patients	21 (24%)
	between 500 and 1,000 patients	15 (17%)
	between 100 and 500 patients	42 (48%)
	Less than 100	10 (11%)
Cancer	Breast cancer[16,20,28,33,35,37,38,41,43,45,52,54,55,62,66,75,76,83–85,91,94,96,104,108]	25 (28%)
	Lung cancer[26,44,58,60,61,67,70,81,88,98,105]	11(14%)
	Leukemia[22,31,39,46,65,69,71,80]	8 (9%)
	Colorectal cancer and adenomas[21,27,30,36,42,59,64,103]	8 (9%)
	Melanoma[48,75,101]	3 (3%)
	Ovarian carcinomas[92,106]	2 (2%)
	Gastric cancer[49]	1 (1%)
	Liver cancer[63]	1 (1%)
	Lymphomas[93]	1 (1%)
	Mesothelioma[40]	1 (1%)
	Neuroblastomas[34]	1 (1%)
	Prostate cancer[47]	1 (1%)
	Sarcomas[82]	1 (1%)
Non-cancer	Cardiovascular[23,24,29,51,56,72,79,80,107]	9 (10%)
	Asthma[50,57,95]	3 (3%)
	Hepatitis C virus[89,90,102]	3 (3%)
	Adverse event[99,100]	2 (3%)
	Thrombosis and anti-coagulation[32,78]	2 (3%)
	Autoimmune disease[86]	1 (1%)
	Cystic fibrosis[97]	1 (1%)
	Diabetes[53]	1 (1%)
	HIV[68]	1 (1%)
	Kidney transplant[25]	1 (1%)

for the development and validation of biomarkers are available.[114,115] In the studies reviewed, two main approaches were taken: a data-driven approach[116] and a knowledge-driven approach[117] (Fig. 2).

In the data-driven approach, extensive genetic information is collected on each participant, and an analysis is conducted to select those genes or sets of genes that are most strongly associated with the targeted

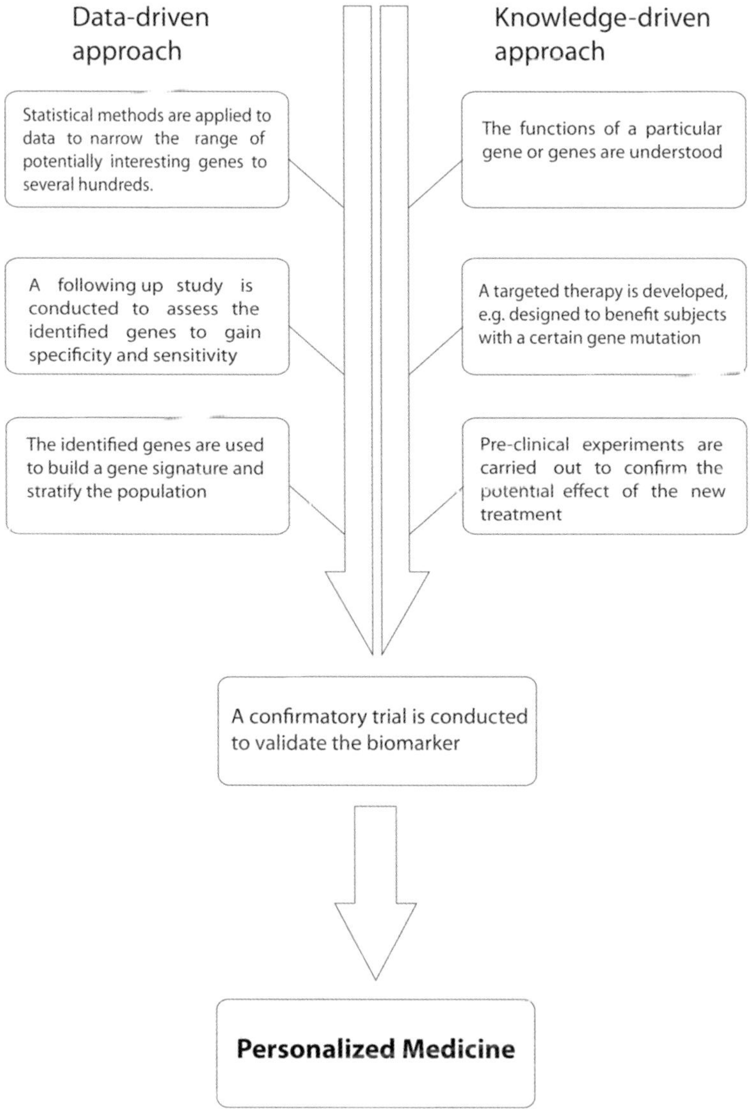

Fig. 2. Two approaches for identifying genetic biomarkers for personalized medicine.

clinical outcome. The strength of this approach is that it is unbiased in the sense that all genes are considered and their relationship to clinical outcome is tested. During the selection process, new genes or gene functions can potentially be identified as involved in disease. For example, in one simple data-driven approach, information on response to a therapy and gene expression data is collected on each patient. Each gene's expression is compared between the response and non-response groups, and p-values are calculated using t-tests; then the p-value for each gene is adjusted upward to account for multiple comparisons via the Bonferroni method and based on the number of genes used in the tests.[118] Genes with significant adjusted p-values are considered to be potential biomarkers for the response to the therapy, which can be verified in follow-up trials.[35]

A typical data-driven approach attempts to identify a potential biomarker profile constructed from one or more genes from among tens of thousands, a process complicated by the correlation structure and multiplicity of high-dimensional data. Many statistical methods have been used to identify promising genetic patterns from numerous genes, including the correlation coefficient,[12] t-tests,[82] hierarchical clustering,[119] significance analysis of microarrays (SAM),[120] prediction analysis for microarrays (PAM),[121] and principal component analysis (PCA).[122] Once the number of candidate genes is narrowed down to several hundred, other statistical techniques can be applied, such as the proportional hazards model[123] or a receiver operator characteristic (ROC)[124] analysis. In one microarray study, the expression of 25,000 genes was measured in 78 lymph-node-negative breast cancers, and 5,000 genes expressed in more than 3 of 78 tumors were selected. The correlation coefficient of the expression for each gene with disease outcome was calculated and the 5,000 genes were further narrowed to 231 (correlation coefficient less than −0.3 or greater than 0.3). This group of 231 genes was rank-ordered on the basis of the magnitude of the correlation coefficient. A subset of five genes was subsequently added to the prognosis classifier until the accuracy was maximized. Seventy genes were identified to constitute a signature based on correlation coefficients for predicting clinical outcome of breast cancer.[12] The signature was validated in a follow-up study, and it outperformed the current standard method in predicting all endpoints.[37]

Data quality is a key issue for the data-driven approach and, indeed, for any approach. Several studies with similar experimental designs generated different gene signatures from similar populations based on this approach, possibly owing to varying data quality.[117,125,126] Moreover, gene signatures identified by this approach are difficult to interpret because the genes may not be causal but may result instead from correlation with some underlying causal mechanism. In addition, large sets of genes are highly correlated, and additional follow-up studies are usually required to refine the gene signature. New statistical methods and software continue to be proposed to identify gene signatures in a more efficient and precise way. Several articles have systematically reviewed such statistical methods,[117,127,128] but there is no clear consensus in the statistics and data-mining community about which methods should be used for data-driven gene signature identification.

The knowledge-driven approach is based on existing knowledge of the biological functions of certain genes or proteins that may arise, for example, through a pathway analysis to establish a mechanism for growth inhibition in tumor cells.[8] A targeted inhibitor that may benefit patients with a specific gene mutation can be designed using this approach, as with cetuximab and panitumumab, approved by the FDA and targeting the epidermal growth factor receptor in multiple cancers.[129] The knowledge-driven approach can also help limit the number of candidate genes investigated. For example, only predetermined single nucleotide polymorphisms (SNPs) or proteins might be considered as biomarkers. This was illustrated in a recent metastatic colorectal cancer study, where 15 candidate genes were investigated as predictors of adverse events and response to chemotherapy. Finally, four genes showed significant association with adverse events.[130] This method avoids the issues associated with interpreting high-dimensional data that arise in the data-driven approach and improves the accuracy of the analysis; however, the drawback is that the results are only as good as the existing state of knowledge: genes that are not already known to be involved in a process are not considered.

Some studies in our sample combined the two approaches to develop a gene signature. The data-driven approach is employed first to reduce the number of available genes from tens of thousands to several hundred, and then the knowledge-driven approach employs a pathway analysis. Only the genes that appear on both lists are included in the final gene signature.[82] Grouping genes according to different biological pathways is another way to combine the two approaches and reduce the dimension of available information efficiently.[108]

Overall, 62 of 88 studies in our sample explored new biomarkers and 26 studies validated the biomarkers discovered in previous studies. Among 62 exploratory studies, 19 of them used primarily a data-driven approach, 38 studies used a knowledge-driven approach, and five studies used a combined approach. Across the 88 studies, 73 used a gene signature comprising fewer than 10 genes, mutations or SNPs as the biomarker to stratify the study population, perhaps because biomarkers with fewer genes are easier to analyze and interpret.

25.4.2. Prognostic and Predictive Biomarkers

In the studies reviewed, two types of relationships between biomarkers and clinical out comes were investigated: association between biomarkers and patient prognosis and association between biomarkers and response to treatment. In common parlance, the first type of analysis refers to "prognostic" biomarkers and the second to "predictive" biomarkers. In the study of potential prognostic biomarkers, patient information is pooled and a prognostic indicator is generated based on patient clinical outcomes without considering the different treatments or perhaps restricting to some standard treatment. The prognostic indicator is expected to predict patient survival without regard to the treatments the patients received. A good example would be the 70-gene signature for breast cancers mentioned above. This kind of investigation can be conducted by pooling available data sets from several similar studies. The results can help clinicians predict patient performance but cannot be used to assign the proper treatment to patients based on their genetic profiles and clinical factors. In the study of potential predictive biomarkers, responses to different treatments are compared within biomarker strata and between patients with different biomarkers. These studies require well-designed clinical trials to verify the hypotheses and to show efficacy in and between biomarker groups. In the study conducted by Amado *et al.*, the effectiveness of panitumumab was compared between patients with wild type and mutations of KRAS in colorectal cancers in a phase III clinical trial. Panitumumab was shown to significantly improve the survival of patients with wild-type KRAS as compared to the best supportive care alone, but there was no significant improvement for mutation carriers. KRAS mutations showed resistance to panitumumab treatment, and this finding was confirmed in several follow-up studies.[130] Results obtained from both types of investigations are important for clinical practice, but knowledge that a specific treatment elicits different outcomes across subgroups is more valuable for personalized medicine, because it can guide an optimal treatment plan based on biomarker information. For example, it has been shown that patients with human epidermal growth factor receptor 2 (HER2)-positive breast cancer have a worse prognosis than other subgroups, but have a better response to trastuzumab, which is designed to interfere with the HER2 receptor.[131] According to these results, a patient with HER2-positive breast cancer would be given trastuzumab to maximize treatment benefit.

In the reviewed literature, 19 studies compared the efficacy of different treatments for one group of patients; 33 investigated the effect of the same therapy among different subgroup populations; and 16 made both types of comparisons.

25.5. CURRENT AND FUTURE CHALLENGES

25.5.1. Reliability and Reproducibility of Personalized Medicine

A continuing controversy of personalized medicine focuses on its reliability and reproducibility. Some personalized medicine studies have been reported as non-replicable, and the related clinical trials have been suspended and scrutinized[132,133]; indeed, two of the papers reviewed were retracted on this basis.[74,87] The complexity of the data and statistical analyses involved in personalized medicine make study of reproducibility of results essential. Hence, the associated datasets must be made publicly available for verification of results. The obtained biomarkers need to be validated in a different group of patients to avoid potential selection bias from the study population. Because extensive high-dimensional data are involved in many personalized medicine studies, data management is another important issue. Some recommendations for improved data management in genetics research and personalized medicine have been made.[2,134–136]

25.5.2. Perspectives on Personalized Medicine

A recurrent theme in the literature on personalized medicine summarized here is the goal of identification and verification of biomarkers that can be used to define subgroups of patients likely to benefit from a new treatment. That is, much of the work on personalized medicine discovery has been on subgroup identification and targeting treatment to subgroups and on clinical trial designs focused on this objective, such as the biomarker-adaptive threshold design and Bayesian designs,[137] including the Investigation of Serial Studies to Predict Your Therapeutic Response with Imaging and molecular Analysis (I-SPY 2) trial, which involves an adaptive design to investigate biomarkers for women with breast cancer (Fig. 3).[138] These designs allow comparison of several different biomarkers with different treatments in the same clinical trial. Bayesian designs have also been implemented in ongoing phase III clinical trials to find the best treatment for patients with different biomarkers.[137]

Under the foregoing perspective on personalized medicine, the goal is to identify subgroups of patients who can be treated successfully with a specific treatment or treatments through identification of biomarkers that characterize the subgroup. An alternative perspective that is gaining traction is to instead focus on the development of decision rules that specify how to treat optimally any patient from the population using the feasible treatment options available based on all information available on the patient. One general approach relies on standard regression models of clinical outcomes given treatment and other covariates. Interactions between treatment and covariates are included in such regression models, and the optimal decision rules are obtained by identifying the treatment leading to the largest mean clinical outcome based on the model for any combination of covariate values. Methods for discovery of optimal decision rules from existing databases have been proposed, as have clinical trial designs to collect data with this objective in mind.[139,140] Another approach is to use machine learning techniques rather than conventional regression models to determine the relationship between clinical outcomes and treatment plus characteristics such as age, gender and biomarkers.[141] These methods, used extensively in artificial intelligence, lead to models for these relationships that are more flexible than those in standard

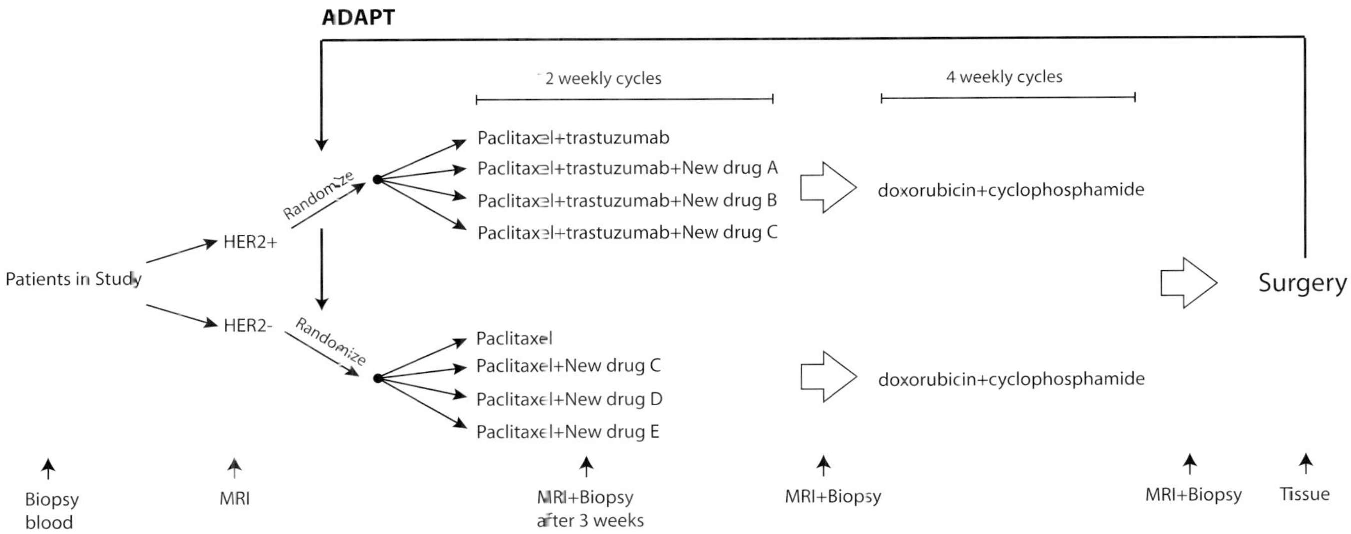

Fig. 3. The overall trial design for I-SPY 2: MRI and blood sample draw is used to determine biomarker signature and eligibility; patients are randomized to seven treatment groups including two control groups and five new treatment groups. After three weeks of the assigned treatment, patients receive a repeat MRI and core biopsy and finish treatment over nine additional weeks. A third MRI and core biopsy are performed before initiating standard chemotherapy with doxorubicin and cyclophosphamide. Another blood sample draw and a fourth MRI are given prior to surgery. Tumor tissue is collected at surgery to assess whether the patient has pathologic complete response, which is used to recalculate the randomization probability of each treatment group for new patients.

regression analysis and thus can more easily describe complex relationships. Designs based on these techniques for determining treatment decision rules have been developed and implemented for chronic diseases such as cancer and have shown the capability of discovering the best treatment for each individual based on a reasonable sample size[142,143]; however, they have not yet been implemented in practice. The machine learning technique is expected to discover new relationships between patient characteristics and response to treatments without any prior knowledge about the true relationship, similar to what the data-driven approach does for identifying biomarkers.

An extension of this idea of developing optimal treatment decision rules to determine treatment for any patient recognizes that, especially in the case of chronic diseases and conditions, "treatment" is often an ongoing process involving a series of decisions made over time. For example, the treatment of cancer may involve selection of a first line of chemotherapy and observation of the patient's response, followed by selection of a second line therapy in the event of no response or of a maintenance or intensification treatment if a positive response is elicited. At each decision point, issues of selection of therapy among available options, choice of dosage and timing of therapy, and so on must be addressed. Identifying the overall strategy for making the entire sequence of decisions to optimize clinical outcome, taking into account the evolving status of the patient at each point, would be a major advance for personalized medicine. It is possible that the treatment that appears "best" with respect to clinical outcome for a single decision point may not be the best choice when viewed in the context of an entire series of decisions. For example, a treatment given early may cause bone marrow toxicity that compromises the dose intensity of future cytotoxic regimens, thus rendering subsequent treatments less effective.

Methods for determining optimal sequential decision rules for personalized medicine using existing databases have been developed[144] but are limited by the quality of the data, as all information relevant to each decision point may not have been recorded. A promising alternative approach is to conduct a prospective clinical trial focused on this goal using the so-called Sequential Multiple Assignment Randomized Trial (SMART) design.[145] SMARTs have been conducted for this purpose in the study of substance abuse and depression, and a similar design suitable for trials involving life-threatening diseases has been developed.[142] In a typical SMART design, participants are initially randomized to treatment options based on their full covariate profiles; at the end of the first treatment segment, patient response to the first treatment and status are reviewed and the second treatment decision is made based on response and status; randomization of treatment may also be employed at this step and later steps; and the steps are repeated until the end of the study. The optimal set of decision rules corresponding to each treatment segment, leading to the best expected outcome for each patient whose treatment is selected according to these rules, can be generated from such designs using artificial intelligence techniques such as reinforcement learning,[122,123] as has been demonstrated for lung cancer.

We contend that this perspective on personalized medicine, focused on development of decision rules to treat optimally the entire population, particularly in the context of a series of treatment decisions, holds considerable promise for the most efficient and effective use of both new and existing treatments.

25.6. CONCLUSION

Personalized medicine has demonstrated considerable promise, although many additional challenges need to be addressed and interpreted in future studies. Even though biomarker and related clinical studies have shown potential application in clinical practice, there is no strong evidence that shows that gene-based biomarkers can completely replace traditional clinical characteristics[146]; and using the biomarkers in clinical trials can cause unbalanced randomization, which can produce biased assessment of treatment.[147] In addition, gene–gene and gene–environment interactions potentially should also be included and modeled using high-dimensional data analysis methods. Taking the broader perspective of identifying optimal decision strategies for treating the entire patient population should be further developed and tested. Addressing all these challenges will require the development of new statistical tools for finding biomarkers, validating results and discovering better decision-making processes for selecting the optimal treatment strategy in an efficient way. This endeavor will not be easy, but the potential gains in human health are enormous.

REFERENCES

1. Adams MD, Kelley JM, Gocayne JD, *et al.* (1991) Complementary DNA sequencing: Expressed sequence tags and human genome project. *Science* **252**: 1651–1656.
2. Leek JT, Scharpf RB, Bravo HC, *et al.* (2010) Tackling the widespread and critical impact of batch effects in high-throughput data. *Nat Rev Genet* **11**: 733–739.
3. Weir BA, Woo MS, Getz G, *et al.* (2007) Characterizing the cancer genome in lung adenocarcinoma. *Nature* **450**: 893–899.
4. Lee SS, Mudaliar A. (2009) Medicine. Racing forward: The genomics and personalized medicine act. *Science* **323**: 342.
5. Haselden JN, Nicholls AW. (2006) Personalized medicine progresses. *Nat Med* **12**: 510–511.
6. Davis JC, Furstenthal L, Desai AA, *et al.* (2009) The microeconomics of personalized medicine: Today's challenge and tomorrow's promise. *Nat Rev Drug Discov* **8**: 279–286.
7. Ng PC, Venter JC, Murray SS, Levy S. (2009) An agenda for personalized medicine. *Nature* **461**: 724–726.
8. Schilsky RL. (2010) Personalized medicine in oncology: The future is now. *Nat Rev Drug Discov* **9**: 363–366.
9. Hayden EC. (2009) Personalized cancer therapy gets closer. *Nature* **458**: 131–132.
10. Harris T. (2010) Gene and drug matrix for personalized cancer therapy. *Nat Rev Drug Discov* **9**: 660.
11. Clayton TA, Lindon JC, Cloarec O, *et al.* (2006) Pharmaco-metabonomic phenotyping and personalized drug treatment. *Nature* **440**: 1073–1077.
12. van 't Veer LJ, Dai H, van de Vijver MJ, *et al.* (2002) Gene expression profiling predicts clinical outcome of breast cancer. *Nature* **415**: 530–536.
13. Schwartz PJ. (2006) The congenital long QT syndromes from genotype to phenotype: Clinical implications. *J Intern Med* **259**: 39–47.
14. Meadows M. (2005) Genomics and personalized medicine. *FDA Consum* **39**: 12–17.
15. Hamburg MA, Collins FS. (2010) The path to personalized medicine. *N Engl J Med* **363**: 301–304.
16. Hayes DF, Thor AD, Dressler LG, *et al.* (2007) HER2 and response to paclitaxel in node-positive breast cancer. *N Engl J Med* **357**: 1496–1506.
17. Rieder MJ, Reiner AP, Gage BF, *et al.* (2005) Effect of VKORC1 haplotypes on transcriptional regulation and warfarin dose. *N Engl J Med* **352**: 2285–2293.

18. Hung SI, Chung WH, Liou LB, *et al.* (2005) HLA-B*5801 allele as a genetic marker for severe cutaneous adverse reactions caused by allopurinol. *Proc Natl Acad Sci USA* **102**: 4131–4139.
19. Fukuoka M, Wu Y-L, Thongprasert S, *et al.* (2011) Biomarker analyses and final overall survival results from a phase III, randomized, open-label, first-line study of gefitinib versus carboplatin/paclitaxel in clinically selected patients with advanced non-small-cell lung cancer in Asia (IPASS). *J Clin Oncol* **29**: 2866–2874.
20. Acharya CR, Hsu DS, Anders CK, *et al.* (2008) Gene expression signatures, clinicopathological features, and individualized therapy in breast cancer. *J Am Med Assoc* **299**: 1574–1587.
21. De Roock W, Jonker DJ, Di Nicolantonio F, *et al.* (2010) Association of KRAS p.G13D mutation with outcome in patients with chemotherapy-refractory metastatic colorectal cancer created with cetuximab. *J Am Med Assoc* **304**: 1812–1820.
22. Gentles AJ, Plevritis SK, Majeti R, Alizadeh AA. (2010) Association of a leukemic stem cell gene expression signature with clinical outcomes in acute myeloid leukemia. *J Am Med Assoc* **304**: 2706–2715.
23. Lynch AI, Boerwinkle E, Davis BR, *et al.* (2008) Pharmacogenetic association of the NPPA T2238C genetic variant with cardiovascular disease outcomes in patients with hypertension. *J Am Med Assoc* **299**: 296–307.
24. Maron BJ, Roberts WC, Arad M, *et al.* (2009) Clinical outcome and phenotypic expression in LAMP2 cardiomyopathy. *J Am Med Assoc* **301**: 1253–1259.
25. Moore J, McKnight AJ, Simmonds MJ, *et al.* (2010) Association of caveolin-1 gene polymorphism with kidney transplant fibrosis and allograft failure. *J Am Med Assoc* **303**: 1282–1287.
26. Mostertz W, Stevenson M, Acharya C, *et al.* (2010) Age- and sex-specific genomic profiles in non-small cell lung cancer. *J Am Med Assoc* **303**: 535–543.
27. Schetter AJ, Leung SY, Sohn JJ, *et al.* (2008) MicroRNA expression profiles associated with prognosis and therapeutic outcome in colon adenocarcinoma. *J Am Med Assoc* **299**: 425–436.
28. Schroth W, Goetz MP, Hamann U, *et al.* (2009) Association between CYP2D6 polymorphisms and outcomes among women with early stage breast cancer treated with tamoxifen. *J Am Med Assoc* **302**: 1429–1436.
29. Shuldiner AR, O'Connell JR, Bliden KP, *et al.* (2009) Association of cytochrome P450 2C19 genotype with the antiplatelet effect and clinical efficacy of clopidogrel therapy. *J Am Med Assoc* **302**: 849–858.

30. Waldman SA, Hyslop T, Schulz S, *et al.* (2009) Association of GUCY2C expression in lymph nodes with time to recurrence and disease-free survival in pN0 colorectal cancer. *J Am Med Assoc* **301**: 745–752.
31. Yang JJ, Cheng C, Yang WJ, *et al.* (2009) Genome-wide interrogation of germline genetic variation associated with treatment response in childhood acute lymphoblastic leukemia. *J Am Med Assoc* **301**: 393–403.
32. Abramson N, Costantino JP, Garber JE, *et al.* (2006) Effect of factor V leiden and prothrombin G20210 → A mutations on thromboembolic risk in the National Surgical Adjuvant Breast and Bowel Project Breast Cancer Prevention trial. *J Natl Cancer Inst* **98**: 904–910.
33. Ansems M, Hontelez S, Looman MWG, *et al.* (2010) DC-SCRIPT: Nuclear receptor modulation and prognostic significance in primary breast cancer. *J Natl Cancer Inst* **102**: 54–68.
34. Asgharzadeh S, Pique-Regi R, Sposto R, *et al.* (2006) Prognostic significance of gene expression profiles of metastatic neuroblastomas lacking MYCN gene amplification. *J Natl Cancer Inst* **98**: 1193–1203.
35. Azzato EM, Tyrer J, Fasching PA, *et al.* (2010) Association between a germline OCA2 polymorphism at chromosome 15q13.1 and estrogen receptor-negative breast cancer survival. *J Natl Cancer Inst* **102**: 650–662.
36. Barry EL, Baron JA, Bhat S, *et al.* (2006) Ornithine decarboxylase polymorphism modification of response to aspirin treatment for colorectal adenoma prevention. *J Natl Cancer Inst* **98**: 1494–1500.
37. Buyse M, Loi S, van 't Veer L, *et al.* (2006) Validation and clinical utility of a 70-gene prognostic signature for women with node-negative breast cancer. *J Natl Cancer Inst* **98**: 1183–1192.
38. Cheang MCU, Chia SK, Voduc D, *et al.* (2009) Ki67 Index, HER2 status, and prognosis of patients with luminal B breast cancer. *J Natl Cancer Inst* **101**: 736–750.
39. Ellis MJ, Tao Y, Luo J, *et al.* (2008) Outcome prediction for estrogen receptor-positive breast cancer based on postneoadjuvant endocrine therapy tumor characteristics. *J Natl Cancer Inst* **100**: 1380–1388.
40. Gordon GJ, Dong LS, Yeap BY, *et al.* (2009) Four-gene expression ratio test for survival in patients undergoing surgery for mesothelioma. *J Natl Cancer Inst* **101**: 678–686.
41. Holm C, Rayala S, Jirström K, *et al.* (2006) Association between Pak1 expression and subcellular localization and tamoxifen resistance in breast cancer patients. *J Natl Cancer Inst* **98**: 671–680.
42. Nielsen M, van Steenbergen LN, Jones N, *et al.* (2010) Survival of MUTYH-associated polyposis patients with colorectal cancer and matched control colorectal cancer patients. *J Natl Cancer Inst* **102**: 1724–1730.

43. O'Malley FP, Chia S, Tu D, *et al.* (2009) Topoisomerase II alpha and responsiveness of breast cancer to adjuvant chemotherapy. *J Natl Cancer Inst* **101**: 644–650.
44. Pine SR, Mechanic LE, Ambs S, *et al.* (2007) Lung cancer survival and functional polymorphisms in MBL2, an innate-immunity gene. *J Natl Cancer Inst* **99**: 1401–1409.
45. Porter PL, Barlow WE, Yeh IT, *et al.* (2006) p27Kip1 and cyclin E expression and breast cancer survival after treatment with adjuvant chemotherapy. *J Natl Cancer Inst* **98**: 1723–1731.
46. Pottier N, Yang W, Assem M, *et al.* (2008) The SWI/SNF chromatin-remodeling complex and glucocorticoid resistance in acute lymphoblastic leukemia. *J Natl Cancer Inst* **100**: 1792–1803.
47. Tryggvadottir L, Vidarsdottir L, Thorgeirsson T, *et al.* (2007) Prostate cancer progression and survival in BRCA2 mutation carriers. *J Natl Cancer Inst* **99**: 929–935.
48. Winnepenninckx V, Lazar V, Michiels S, *et al.* (2006) Gene expression profiling of primary cutaneous melanoma and clinical outcome. *J Natl Cancer Inst* **98**: 472–482.
49. Bang YJ, Van Cutsem E, Feyereislova A, *et al.* (2010) Trastuzumab in combination with chemotherapy versus chemotherapy alone for treatment of HER2-positive advanced gastric or gastro-oesophageal junction cancer (ToGA): A phase 3, open-label, randomised controlled trial. *Lancet* **376**: 687–697.
50. Bleecker ER, Postma DS, Lawrance RM, *et al.* (2007) Effect of ADRB2 polymorphisms on response to longacting β2-agonist therapy: A pharmacogenetic analysis of two randomised studies. *Lancet* **370**: 2118–2125.
51. Collet JP, Hulot JS, Pena A, *et al.* (2009) Cytochrome P450 2C19 polymorphism in young patients treated with clopidogrel after myocardial infarction: A cohort study. *Lancet* **373**: 309–317.
52. Gianni L, Eiermann W, Semiglazov V, *et al.* (2010) Neoadjuvant chemotherapy with trastuzumab followed by adjuvant trastuzumab versus neoadjuvant chemotherapy alone, in patients with HER2-positive locally advanced breast cancer (the NOAH trial): A randomised controlled superiority trial with a parallel HER2-negative cohort. *Lancet* **375**: 377–384.
53. Nanto-Salonen K, Kupila A, Simell S, *et al.* (2008) Nasal insulin to prevent type 1 diabetes in children with HLA genotypes and autoantibodies conferring increased risk of disease: A double-blind, randomised controlled trial. *Lancet* **372**: 1746–1755.
54. Smith I, Procter M, Gelber RD, *et al.* (2007) 2-year follow-up of trastuzumab after adjuvant chemotherapy in HER2-positive breast cancer: A randomised controlled trial. *Lancet* **369**: 29–36.

55. Tutt A, Robson M, Garber JE, *et al.* (2010) Oral poly(ADP-ribose) polymerase inhibitor olaparib in patients with BRCA1 or BRCA2 mutations and advanced breast cancer: A proof-of-concept trial. *Lancet* **376**: 235–244.
56. Wallentin L, James S, Storey RF, *et al.* (2010) Effect of CYP2C19 and ABCB1 single nucleotide polymorphisms on outcomes of treatment with ticagrelor versus clopidogrel for acute coronary syndromes: A genetic substudy of the PLATO trial. *Lancet* **376**: 1320–1328.
57. Wechsler ME, Kunselmon SJ, Chinchilli VM, *et al.* (2009) Effect of β2-adrenergic receptor polymorphism on response to longacting β2 agonist in asthma (LARGE trial): A genotype-stratified, randomised, placebo-controlled, crossover trial. *Lancet* **374**: 1754–1764.
58. Rosell R, Moran T, Queralt C, *et al.* (2009) Screening for epidermal growth factor receptor mutations in lung cancer. *N Engl J Med* **361**: 958–967.
59. Barnetson RA, Tenesa A, Farrington SM, *et al.* (2006) Identification and survival of carriers of mutations in DNA mismatch-repair genes in colon cancer. *N Engl J Med* **354**: 2751–2763.
60. Brock MV, Hooker CM, Ota-Machida E, *et al.* (2008) DNA methylation markers and early recurrence in stage I lung cancer. *N Engl J Med* **358**: 1118–1128.
61. Chen HY, Yu SL, Chen CH, *et al.* (2007) A five-gene signature and clinical outcome in non-small-cell lung cancer. *N Engl J Med* **356**: 11–20.
62. Geyer CE, Forster J, Lindquist D, *et al.* (2006) Lapatinib plus capecitabine for HER2-positive advanced breast cancer. *N Engl J Med* **355**: 2733–2743.
63. Ji J, Shi J, Budhu A, *et al.* (2009) MicroRNA expression, survival, and response to interferon in liver cancer. *N Engl J Med* **361**: 1437–1447.
64. Karapetis CS, Khambata-Ford S, Jonker DJ, *et al.* (2008) K-ras mutations and benefit from cetuximab in advanced colorectal cancer. *N Engl J Med* **359**: 1757–1765.
65. Ley TJ, Ding L, Walter MJ, *et al.* (2010) DNMT3A mutations in acute myeloid leukemia. *N Engl J Med* **363**: 2424–2433.
66. Liu R, Wang XH, Chen GY, *et al.* (2007) The prognostic role of a gene signature from tumorigenic breast-cancer cells. *N Engl J Med* **356**: 217–226.
67. Maemondo M, Inoue A, Kobayashi K, *et al.* (2010) Gefitinib or chemotherapy for non-small-cell lung cancer with mutated EGFR. *N Engl J Med* **362**: 2380–2388.
68. Mallal S, Phillips E, Carosi G, *et al.* (2008) HLA-B*5701 screening for hypersensitivity to abacavir. *N Engl J Med* **358**: 568–579.
69. Marcucci G, Radmacher MD, Maharry K, *et al.* (2008) MicroRNA expression in cytogenetically normal acute myeloid leukemia. *N Engl J Med* **358**: 1919–1928.

70. Mok TS, Wu YL, Thongprasert S, *et al.* (2009) Gefitinib or carboplatin-paclitaxel in pulmonary adenocarcinoma. *N Engl J Med* **361**: 947–957.
71. Mullighan CG, Su XP, Zhang JH, *et al.* (2009) Deletion of IKZF1 and prognosis in acute lymphoblastic leukemia. *N Engl J Med* **360**: 470–480.
72. Pare G, Mehta SR, Yusuf S, *et al.* (2010) Effects of CYP2C19 genotype on outcomes of clopidogrel treatment. *N Engl J Med* **363**: 1704–1714.
73. Poeta ML, Manola J, Goldwasser MA, *et al.* (2007) TP53 mutations and survival in squamous-cell carcinoma of the head and neck. *N Engl J Med* **357**: 2552–2561.
74. Potti A, Mukherjee S, Petersen R, *et al.* (2006) A genomic strategy to refine prognosis in early-stage non-small-cell lung cancer. *N Engl J Med* **355**: 570–580.
75. Pritchard KI, Shepherd LE, O'Malley FP, *et al.* (2006) HER2 and responsiveness of breast cancer to adjuvant chemotherapy. *N Engl J Med* **354**: 2103–2111.
76. Rennert G, Bisland-Naggan S, Barnett-Griness O, *et al.* (2007) Clinical outcomes of breast cancer in carriers of BRCA1 and BRCA2 mutations. *N Engl J Med* **357**: 115–123.
77. Schlenk RF, Dohner K, Krauter J, *et al.* (2008) Mutations and treatment outcome in cytogenetically normal acute myeloid leukemia. *N Engl J Med* **358**: 1909–1918.
78. Schwarz UI, Ritchie MD, Bradford Y, *et al.* (2008) Genetic determinants of response to warfarin during initial anticoagulation. *N Engl J Med* **358**: 999–1008.
79. Simon T, Verstuyft C, Mary-Krause M, *et al.* (2009) Genetic determinants of response to clopidogrel and cardiovascular events. *N Engl J Med* **360**: 363–375.
80. Zethelius B, Berglund L, Sundstrom J, *et al.* (2008) Use of multiple biomarkers to improve the prediction of death from cardiovascular causes. *N Engl J Med* **358**: 2107–2116.
81. Zheng Z, Chen TG, Li XL, *et al.* (2007) DNA synthesis and repair genes RRM1 and ERCC1 in lung cancer. *N Engl J Med* **356**: 800–808.
82. Chibon F, Lagarde P, Salas S, *et al.* (2010) Validated prediction of clinical outcome in sarcomas and multiple types of cancer on the basis of a gene expression signature related to genome complexity. *Nat Med* **16**: 781–788.
83. Farmer P, Bonnefoi H, Anderle P, *et al.* (2009) A stroma-related gene signature predicts resistance to neoadjuvant chemotherapy in breast cancer. *Nat Med* **15**: 68–74.

84. Finak G, Bertos N, Pepin F, *et al.* (2008) Stromal gene expression predicts clinical outcome in breast cancer. *Nat Med* **14**: 518–527.
85. Li Y, Zou LH, Li QY, *et al.* (2010) Amplification of LAPTM4B and YWHAZ contributes to chemotherapy resistance and recurrence of breast cancer. *Nat Med* **16**: 214–218.
86. McKinney EF, Lyons PA, Carr EJ, *et al.* (2010) A CD8(+) T cell transcription signature predicts prognosis in autoimmune disease. *Nat Med* **16**: 586–591.
87. Potti A, Dressman HK, Bild A, *et al.* (2006) Genomic signatures to guide the use of chemotherapeutics. *Nat Med* **12**: 1294–1300.
88. Shedden K, Taylor JMG, Enkemann SA, *et al.* (2008) Gene expression-based survival prediction in lung adenocarcinoma: A multi-site, blinded validation study. *Nat Med* **14**: 822–827.
89. Fellay J, Thompson AJ, Ge DL, *et al.* (2010) ITPA gene variants protect against anaemia in patients treated for chronic hepatitis C. *Nature* **464**: 405–408.
90. Ge DL, Fellay J, Thompson AJ, *et al.* (2009) Genetic variation in IL28B predicts hepatitis C treatment-induced viral clearance. *Nature* **461**: 399–401.
91. Hurtado A, Holmes KA, Geistlinger TR, *et al.* (2008) Regulation of ERBB2 by oestrogen receptor-PAX2 determines response to tamoxifen. *Nature* **456**: 663–666.
92. Sakai W, Swisher EM, Karlan BY, *et al.* (2008) Secondary mutations as a mechanism of cisplatin resistance in BRCA2-mutated cancers. *Nature* **451**: 1116–1120.
93. Schwickart M, Huang XD, Lill JR, *et al.* (2010) Deubiquitinase USP9X stabilizes MCL1 and promotes tumour cell survival. *Nature* **463**: 103–107.
94. Tsai WW, Wang ZX, Yiu TT, *et al.* (2010) TRIM24 links a non-canonical histone signature to breast cancer. *Nature* **468**: 927–932.
95. Tantisira KG, Lasky-Su J, Harada M, *et al.* (2011) Genomewide association between GLCCI1 and response to glucocorticoid therapy in asthma. *New Engl J Med* **365**: 1173–1183.
96. Slamon D, Eiermann W, Robert N, *et al.* (2011) Adjuvant trastuzumab in HER2-positive breast cancer. *New Engl J Med* **365**: 1273–1283.
97. Ramsey BW, Davies J, McElvaney NG, *et al.* (2011) A CFTR potentiator in patients with cystic fibrosis and the G551D mutation. *New Engl J Med* **365**: 1663–1672.
98. O'Shaughnessy J, Osborne C, Pippen JE, *et al.* (2011) Iniparib plus chemotherapy in metastatic triple-negative breast cancer. *New Engl J Med* **364**: 205–214.

99. McCormack M, Alfirevic A, Bourgeois S, *et al.* (2011) HLA-A* 3101 and carbamazepine-induced hypersensitivity reactions in Europeans. *New Engl J Med* **364**: 1134–1143.
100. Chen P, Lin JJ, Lu CS, *et al.* (2011) Carbamazepine-induced toxic effects and HLA-B* 1502 screening in Taiwan. *New Engl J Med* **364**: 1126–1133.
101. Chapman PB, Hauschild A, Robert C, *et al.* (2011) Improved survival with vemurafenib in melanoma with BRAF V600E mutation. *New Engl J Med* **364**: 2507–2516.
102. Bacon BR, Gordon SC, Lawitz E, *et al.* (2011) Boceprevir for previously treated chronic HCV genotype 1 infection. *New Engl J Med* **364**: 1207–1217.
103. Sinicrope FA, Foster NR, Thibodeau SN, *et al.* (2011) DNA mismatch repair status and colon cancer recurrence and survival in clinical trials of 5-fluorouracil based adjuvant therapy. *J Natl Cancer Inst* **103**: 863–875.
104. Iwamoto T, Bianchini G, Booser D, *et al.* (2011) Gene pathways associated with prognosis and chemotherapy sensitivity in molecular subtypes of breast cancer. *J Natl Cancer Inst* **103**: 264–272.
105. Chen DT, Hsu YL, Fulp WJ, *et al.* (2011) Prognostic and predictive value of a malignancy-risk gene signature in early-stage non-small cell lung cancer. *J Natl Cancer Inst* **103**: 1859–1870.
106. Yang D, Khan S, Sun Y, *et al.* (2011) Association of BRCA1 and BRCA2 mutations with survival, chemotherapy sensitivity, and gene mutator phenotype in patients with ovarian cancer. *J Am Med Assoc* **306**: 1557–1565.
107. Mega JL, Hochholzer W, Frelinger III AL, *et al.* (2011) Dosing clopidogrel based on CYP2C19 genotype and the effect on platelet reactivity in patients with stable cardiovascular disease. *J Am Med Assoc* **306**: 2221–2228.
108. Hatzis C, Pusztai L, Valero V, *et al.* (2011) A genomic predictor of response and survival following taxane-anthracycline chemotherapy for invasive breast cancer. *J Am Med Assoc* **305**: 1873.
109. Yaes RJ. (1988) Human genome sequence. *Nature* **331**: 10.
110. Dhanasekaran SM, Barrette TR, Ghosh D, *et al.* (2001) Delineation of prognostic biomarkers in prostate cancer. *Nature* **412**: 822–826.
111. Capdeville R, Buchdunger E, Zimmermann J, Matter A. (2002) Glivec (STI571, imatinib), a rationally developed, targeted anticancer drug. *Nat Rev Drug Discov* **1**: 493–502.
112. George SL, Wang X. (2011) Targeted clinical trials. In: Harrington D, ed. *Designs for clinical trials: Perspectives on current issues* (*Applied bioinformatics and biostatistics in cancer research*). Springer, New York, pp. 157–178.
113. Catchpoole DR, Kennedy P, Skillicorn DB, Simoff S. (2010) The curse of dimensionality: A blessing to personalized medicine. *J Clin Oncol* **28**: 723–724.

114. George SL. (2008) Statistical issues in translational cancer research. *Clin Cancer Res* **14**: 5954–5958.
115. Simon R. (2010) Clinical trials for predictive medicine: New challenges and paradigms. *Clin Trials* 7: 516–524.
116. Yeung KY, Haynor DR, Ruzzo WL. (2001) Validating clustering for gene expression data. *Bioinformatics* **17**: 309–318.
117. van't Veer LJ, Bernards R. (2008) Enabling personalized cancer medicine through analysis of gene-expression patterns. *Nature* **452**: 564–570.
118. Hochberg Y. (1988) A sharper Bonferroni procedure for multiple tests of significance. *Biometrika* **75**: 800–802.
119. Eisen MB, Spellman PT, Brown PO, Botstein D. (1998) Cluster analysis and display of genome-wide expression patterns. *Proc Natl Acad Sci USA* **95**: 14863–14868.
120. Tusher VG, Tibshirani R, Chu G. (2001) Significance analysis of microarrays applied to the ionizing radiation response. *Proc Natl Acad Sci USA* **98**: 5116–5121.
121. Tibshirani R, Hastie T, Narasimhan B, Chu G. (2002) Diagnosis of multiple cancer types by shrunken centroids of gene expression. *Proc Natl Acad Sci USA* **99**: 6567–6572.
122. Yeung KY, Ruzzo WL. (2001) Principal component analysis for clustering gene expression data. *Bioinformatics* **17**: 763–774.
123. Raponi M, Zhang Y, Yu J, *et al.* (2006) Gene expression signatures for predicting prognosis of squamous cell and adenocarcinomas of the lung. *Cancer Res* **66**: 7466–7472.
124. Wang Y, Klijn JG, Zhang Y, *et al.* (2005) Gene-expression profiles to predict distant metastasis of lymph-node-negative primary breast cancer. *Lancet* **365**: 671–679.
125. Haibe-Kains B, Desmedt C, Piette F, *et al.* (2008) Comparison of prognostic gene expression signatures for breast cancer. *BMC Genomics* **9**: 394.
126. van't Veer LJ, Dai HY, van de Vijver MJ, *et al.* (2002) Gene expression profiling predicts clinical outcome of breast cancer. *Nature* **415**: 530–536.
127. Ioannidis JPA, Allison DB, Ball CA, *et al.* (2009) Repeatability of published microarray gene expression analyses. *Nat Genet* **41**: 149–155.
128. Allison DB, Cui X, Page GP, Sabripour M. (2006) Microarray data analysis: From disarray to consolidation and consensus. *Nat Rev Genet* **7**: 55–65.
129. Overington JP, Al-Lazikani B, Hopkins AL. (2006) How many drug targets are there? *Nat Rev Drug Discov* **5**: 993–996.
130. Amado RG, Wolf M, Peeters M, *et al.* (2008) Wild-type KRAS is required for panitumumab efficacy in patients with metastatic colorectal cancer. *J Clin Oncol* **26**: 1626–1634.

131. Vogel CL, Cobleigh MA, Tripathy D, *et al.* (2002) Efficacy and safety of trastuzumab as a single agent in first-line treatment of HER2-overexpressing metastatic breast cancer. *J Clin Oncol* **20**: 719–726.
132. Goldberg P. (2010) JCO retracts key Duke genomics paper: Duke shuts down three phase II trials. *Cancer Lett* **36**: 3.
133. Keith A, Baggerly KRC. (2009) Deriving chemosensitivity from cell lines: Forensic bioinformatics and reproducible research in high-throughput biology. *Ann Appl Stat* **3**: 1309–1334.
134. Dupuy A, Simon RM. (2007) Critical review of published microarray studies for cancer outcome and guidelines on statistical analysis and reporting. *J Natl Cancer Inst* **99**: 147–157.
135. Quackenbush J. (2001) Computational analysis of microarray data. *Nat Rev Genet* **2**: 418–427.
136. Owzar K, Barry WT, Jung SH, *et al.* (2008) Statistical challenges in preprocessing in microarray experiments in cancer. *Clin Cancer Res* **14**: 5959–5966.
137. Zhou X, Liu S, Kim ES, *et al.* (2008) Bayesian adaptive design for targeted therapy development in lung cancer — A step toward personalized medicine. *Clin Trials* **5**: 181–193.
138. Barker AD, Sigman CC, Kelloff GJ, *et al.* (2009) I-SPY 2: An adaptive breast cancer trial design in the setting of neoadjuvant chemotherapy. *Clin Pharmacol Ther* **86**: 97–100.
139. Zhang B, Tsiatis AA, Laber AB, Davidian M. (2012) A robust method for estimating optimal treatment regimes. *Biometrics* **68**: 1010–1018.
140. Zhao Y, Zeng D, Rush AJ, Kosorok MR. (2012) Estimating individualized treatment rules using outcome weighted learning. *J Am Stat Assoc* **107**: 1106–1118.
141. Shipp MA, Ross KN, Tamayo P, *et al.* (2002) Diffuse large B-cell lymphoma outcome prediction by gene-expression profiling and supervised machine learning. *Nat Med* **8**: 68–74.
142. Zhao Y, Kosorok MR, Zeng D. (2009) Reinforcement learning design for cancer clinical trials. *Stat Med* **28**: 3294–3315.
143. Zhao Y, Zeng D, Socinski MA, Kosorok MR. (2011) Reinforcement learning strategies for clinical trials in nonsmall cell lung cancer. *Biometrics* **67**: 1422–1433.
144. Murphy SA. (2003) Optimal dynamic treatment regimes. *J R Stat Soc B* **65**: 331–366.
145. Murphy SA. (2005) An experimental design for the development of adaptive treatment strategies. *Stat Med* **24**: 1455–1481.

146. Boulesteix AL, Sauerbrei W. (2011) Added predictive value of high-throughput molecular data to clinical data and its validation. *Brief Bioinform* 12: 215–229.
147. Elsaleh H, Joseph D, Grieu F, *et al.* (2000) Association of tumour site and sex with survival benefit from adjuvant chemotherapy in colorectal cancer. *Lancet* 355: 1745–1750.

XI. Translational Research Outcomes and Resources

Translational Cancer Research Involving Molecularly Defined Targets: Issues in the Development of Effective Therapeutics

Maurie Markman

26.1. INTRODUCTION

The revolution in our understanding of the fundamental biology of malignant disease is underway and rapidly gaining momentum.[1–5] The profound complexity of the large group of related but unquestionably different human diseases we loosely classify as falling under the general term, *cancer*, is increasingly evident. Further, the cost and time requirements associated with defining specific somatic genetic abnormalities present within individual cancers or demonstrating unique germ line polymorphisms in the particular host have reached the point where such testing is clearly ready to become a component of standard oncologic care (although certainly not within all healthcare systems).[6,7] It is not unrealistic to anticipate that in the very near future it will be possible to routinely obtain such

Cancer Treatment Centers of America, Philadelphia, Pennsylvania, USA
Drexel University College of Medicine, Philadelphia, Pennsylvania, USA
Full address: Maurie Markman, MD, Cancer Treatment Centers of America, Eastern Regional Medical Center, 1331 East Wyoming Avenue, Philadelphia, PA 19124, USA; E-mail: *maurie.markman@ctca-hope.com*

detailed molecular information within 10–15 days from submission of the malignant and normal tissues at a cost of less than US$4,000–5,000.

However, it is also critical to acknowledge here that the ultimate impact of this rapidly expanding knowledge base is currently impossible to define, and the timing of new developments is very difficult to predict. As a result, it is not unreasonable to state that informed and truly objective observers in this arena should not be faulted for expressing more than a little unease with the potential disruption these events may cause in what we consider the "standard" paradigm in clinical oncology.

The following examples of increasingly common scenarios and concerns emphasize the complexity of the issues which must be considered by multiple involved parties (e.g., academics, pharmaceutical/biotech companies, health payers, governmental drug and clinical laboratory regulators) before the genuine promise of molecular medicine can be fully appreciated and implemented to benefit patients with malignant disease.

26.2. THE USE OF ANTI-HER-2 THERAPY IN THE MULTIPLE CANCERS THAT "OVEREXPRESS" THE HER-2 RECEPTOR

The demonstrated clinical experience with anti-HER-2 therapy in several tumor types where there is documented over expression of the HER-2 receptor is an excellent example of the impact of a single molecular abnormality across multiple tumor types. In the US, the Food and Drug Administration (FDA) has specifically "approved" the use of trastuzumab in the treatment of breast and gastric cancer,[8,9] but overexpression of this important molecular target has been observed in other tumor types, including certain B-cell leukemias, lung cancer and gynecologic malignancies.[10–12]

The experience with a clinical trial of trastuzumab in patients with recurrent ovarian cancer whose malignancy was documented to *overexpress* the HER-2 receptor emphasizes the complexity and difficulty associated with moving the concept of treating malignant disease across tumor types based specifically on well-defined molecular abnormalities into routine clinical care.[12]

In this study conducted by the Gynecologic Oncology Group (GOG), a federally funded cooperative cancer group in the US, the cancers of more than 800 patients were required to be screened to find approximately 90 patients (overall approximately an 11 percent rate of overexpression) eligible for entry into the phase II trial.[12] In fact, even finding this modest number of potentially eligible patients both moderately overexpressing ("+2"staining) and highly overexpressing ("+3" staining) ovarian cancers was considered acceptable for treatment. Within this population an objective response rate to trastuzumab of only 7 percent was observed.

Unfortunately, this was a clearly "negative trial" when considering both the objective response rate noted and the logistics required to find the study population (90 percent of potential patients rejected due to the absence of the relevant molecular marker). Further, it is virtually certain there would be very little interest by any pharmaceutical company in conducting a trial examining the efficacy of trastuzumab (or other comparable anti-HER-2 agents) in this clinical setting considering the effort required.

Finally, and of major relevance to the issue of the nature of definitive evidence-based trials in such settings, the observed very low response rate within this population would make it highly unlikely (if not realistically impossible) for a randomized trial to convert this level of activity into an improvement in a population-based endpoint (e.g., median progression free or overall survival). (Note: This statement makes the reasonable assumption that only patients whose tumors possessed this relevant molecular biomarker would have any opportunity to experience clinical benefit from the "targeted" antineoplastic.)

At this point in the discussion, it is critical to again highlight the fact that with the availability of highly cost-effective whole-genome sequencing, such testing will increasingly be appropriate to be routinely performed in the near future. As a result, *the discovery of the rare ovarian cancer that demonstrates HER-2 overexpression will occur as a component of a process that is undertaken to examine for a variety of possible driver mutations within the individual cancer and NOT specifically to search for this specific abnormality.*

It is also relevant to note that while less than 10 percent of patients with ovarian cancer in this trial responded to anti-HER-2 therapy, only a very limited subset of tumors within this group actually possessed a high level of HER-2 overexpression ("+3 staining"). As a result, the level of clinical activity of trastuzumab within even the smaller subgroup (? 1–2 percent) of ovarian cancers that highly over express the HER-2 receptor is unknown, but realistically may be considerably greater that 7 percent. Of course, a study to directly address this critically relevant question is unfortunately, logically, simply not feasible.

26.3. TYROSINE KINASE INHIBITORS OF EGFR IN OVARIAN CANCER

An additional example from the gynecologic cancer experience further highlights the problematic issue of small patient subsets and the inability to conduct evidence-based (phase III randomized) trials required for regulatory approval and third-party payment.

Solid evidence-based data has revealed the clinical relevance of the presence of activating mutations in EGFR in critically defining the non-small cell lung cancer population likely to achieve evidence of a response to tyrosine kinase inhibitors directed at the EFGR receptor.[13]

In a phase II trial of gefitinib, a tyrosine kinase inhibitor of EFGR conducted in a group of patients with recurrent ovarian cancer (not specifically selected for the presence of such a mutation), only 1 of 27 patients achieved an objective response (4 percent response rate).[14] The authors appropriately concluded this was a "negative trial" and further investigation of this agent (and class of agents) in ovarian cancer did not appear to be warranted. [In fact, a subsequently conducted phase III trial exploring another tyrosine kinase inhibitor of EGFR (erlotinib) in an unselected patient (for the presence or absence of an activating mutation in EGFR) employed as a "maintenance strategy" in advanced ovarian cancer also revealed no clinical utility for the strategy.[15]]

However, and of considerable interest, the malignant cell population from the single patient in this phase II trial who responded to gefitinib was documented to contain an activating mutation in EGFR.[14] Again, clearly the low objective response rate observed in this study and the small percentage of patients whose tumors possess such activating mutations in the malignancy would surely prevent any pharmaceutical company sponsor from conducting a randomized phase III trial.

Therefore, in the opinion of this author, it would be inappropriate to conclude that the experience garnered to date with the administration of small-molecule inhibitors of EGFR means this class of drugs is inactive in ovarian cancer. Rather, it would be far more accurate to declare that the percentage of tumors possessing the molecular abnormalities (activating mutations) demonstrated to be required for biological and clinical activity, and the actual number of patients eligible for the conduct of so-called "evidence-based clinical trials," are unquestionably insufficient to draw any definitive conclusions.

26.4. ADDITIONAL EXAMPLES OF MOLECULARLY TARGETED AGENTS WITH POTENTIAL ACTIVITY IN MULTIPLE TUMOR TYPES

Other examples of *molecularly-based* (a specific molecular target present within the cancer being required for biological and clinical activity of the drug) antineoplastic agents recently approved by drug regulatory agencies that have been documented to improve outcome in a particular tumor type but where the "target" appears to be present within other cancer types include: (a) BRAF abnormality in metastatic melanoma[2]; (b) ALK rearrangement in non-small cell lung cancer[16]; and (c) Hedgehog pathway abnormalities in advanced or metastatic basal cell carcinoma.[17]

What does the future hold for potentially treating patients with these other cancers where the individual tumors within the patient possess these specific molecular abnormalities? Will large-scale randomized trials be required despite the fact the percentage of patients with cancers that demonstrate the mutations/rearrangements is insufficient to initiate and complete a randomized trial (or at least within a rational time period)? What will local, regional and national health authorities require before they agree to approve a particular drug for treatment of one of these conditions, and what approach(es) will be employed to determine if payment should be provided (governmental or private insurance) for use of the novel antineoplastic strategies if large randomized trials are not feasible?

26.5. CANCER AS A "CHRONIC ILLNESS"

An additional factor to be considered in the development of novel antineoplastics is the highly provocative new paradigm that characterizes management goals associated with an increasing number of malignancies. While initial treatment of many solid tumors appropriately focuses on a *cure* following the surgical removal of the primary cancer, with or without adjuvant radiation and/or systemic chemotherapy, once metastatic disease is documented (either at presentation or at the time of initial relapse) the opportunity to permanently eliminate the illness is (in most settings) very limited.

However, prolonged survival (often measured in years) may be a realistically achievable goal, even if the ultimate cause of death may be secondary to complications associated with progression of the malignancy. Thus, it is rational to describe management in such settings as being focused on maximizing the duration and quality of life while minimizing disease and treatment-related symptoms. *It is also reasonable to state that this picture is consistent with viewing many cancers as being very serious, but also chronic disease processes.*

The implications of this change in how cancer is approached cannot be overstated. If a cancer in an individual patient is realistically simply unable to be cured, it becomes quite difficult (if not impossible) to justify certain heroic measures that have not been shown to extend survival compared to other less-intensive strategies but are surely likely to result in serious and possibly permanent morbidity (e.g., severe peripheral neuropathy from dose-intensive platinum or taxanes).

Further, in this setting it is important to recognize that the toxicity resulting from a current or past treatment may negatively impact the future ability to safely deliver a potentially beneficial agent (e.g., persistent bone marrow suppression, persistent neuropathy).

In the context of the issues raised in this commentary, the consequences of cancer being objectively viewed as a serious chronic illness have unique implications for clinical trials traditionally focused on overall survival endpoints. For example, in a metastatic disease setting where survival is anticipated to be short, particularly following progression on either the experimental or control arm of a randomized study, it should not be difficult to observe the impact of an effective new treatment on overall survival, assuming that strategy favorably influences the time to subsequent disease progression [progression-free survival (PFS)].

However, if following the completion of treatment on a randomized clinical trial individuals are able to receive one or more strategies that also delay subsequent progression and prolong survival, it may be very difficult to observe a statistically significant difference in overall survival between the patients treated on the *control arm* versus the *experimental arm* of the trial. The magnitude of this effect in settings where rather long survival is anticipated following completion of a specific trial can be substantial.[18]

Thus, as more effective therapy becomes available to manage a particular malignancy, it will realistically become increasingly difficult for the *next agent demonstrating a favorable effect on PFS in that cancer* to be shown to improve overall survival. This is because it is ethically mandated that all patients entered into the trial be given the opportunity (if medically appropriate) to receive known clinically active antineoplastics (assuming the agents had not been delivered prior to study entry).

26.6. "N OF 1" RESEARCH PARADIGM: A STRATEGY TO PERMIT THE OBJECTIVE CLINICAL EVALUATION OF LABORATORY-BASED BIOMARKER RESEARCH

Thus, considering the serious concerns expressed above, it must be asked at this point how in the future it will realistically be possible for investigators to objectively evaluate the clinical utility of a particular molecular marker suggested in pre-clinical studies to be useful in the selection of an effective antineoplastic strategy.

Considering the small sample sizes associated with specific somatic genetic mutations or rearrangements in many tumor types, the time and cost required to initiate, conduct, complete and report on clinical trials, and the substantial number of questions that might be addressed in any given cancer, are there alternative options to examine clinical benefit?

The final section of this chapter briefly discusses a novel clinical trials concept that permits patients with unique molecular profiles (e.g., ovarian cancer patients with tumors over expressing the HER-2 receptor or discovered to contain an activating mutation of EGFR; lung cancer patients with a BRAF mutation, etc.) to serve as single experiments ("N of 1") and for the individual data obtained following treatment based on that specific abnormality to be collected with the experiences of other such individuals to document or refute a favorable effect on the course of the illness.

Consider, for example, the recurrent ovarian cancer patient previously described as having an activating mutation in EGFR who responded to a tyrosine kinase inhibitor of EGFR.[14] What if, through the availability of widespread whole-genome sequencing, it was possible to identify 10 or 20 such patients who might subsequently be treated with a commercially available small molecule EGFR inhibitor. If the particular third-party payer (government or insurance company) agreed to pay for the cost of this therapy under the conditions that the anonymous results (with no possible individual patient identifiers) would be included in a publicly available database, then after this cohort of patients had been treated and followed it would be possible for these individual "N of 1"experiences to be viewed together to determine the utility of this approach.

Further, one could rationally propose various levels of *activity* (biological and clinical) that might be employed to ultimately classify the experience as documenting the agent to be *active* or *inactive* in this specific clinical setting. For example, in the example above, if 7 of 10 or 15 of 20 ovarian cancer patients with an activating EGFR mutation achieved at least a partial response (by RECIST or CA-125 criteria) following treatment with an EGFR inhibitor, one might quite realistically conclude the drug was highly active in this well-defined (by unique individual tumor molecular characteristics) patient population. In addition, based on this reported experience, routine use and third-party payment for such therapy could be strongly and rationally advocated. Conversely, if only 1 of 10 or 3 of 20 patients achieved this level of response, one might reasonably decide that considering the substantial cost and potential toxicity of this class of agents, routine use (outside the confines of a clinical trial) and payment would not be supported.

Of course, many critical details of how such a research program will be organized must be considered, including questions of who will create, organize and maintain the absolutely essential databases required for this purpose; how will reported responses be "validated"; who will "own" the posted clinical data; how will governmental drug regulatory and payer groups view such efforts; how will a "N of 1" strategy impact existing and future academic research (including grants, promotion and tenure); and what effect this effort will have on the pharmaceutical/biotech industry's approach to oncology drug development.

26.7. CONCLUSION

The fundamental goal in presenting this basic outline has been to emphasize that possible solutions to cost-effectively and objectively examining the clinical relevance of novel laboratory-based molecular observations are feasible. However, to realistically accomplish this truly worthy goal to benefit both the quality and quantity of life for cancer patients, major (if not truly revolutionary) changes in the paradigm for the conduct of clinical trials in the oncology arena will unquestionably be required.

REFERENCES

1. Patel JP, Gonen M, Figueroa ME, *et al.* (2012) Prognostic relevance of integrated genetic profiling in acute myeloid leukemia. *N Engl J Med* **366**: 1079–1089.
2. Chapman PB, Hauschild A, Robert C, *et al.* (2011) Improved survival with vemurafenib in melanoma with BRAF V600E mutation. *N Engl J Med* **364**: 2507–2516.
3. Bergethon K, Shaw AT, Ou S-HI, *et al.* (2012) ROS1 rearrangements define a unique molecular class of lung cancer. *J Clin Oncol* **30**: 863–870.
4. Gerlinger M, Rowan AJ, Horswell S, *et al.* (2012) Intratumor heterogeneity and branched evolution revealed by multiregion sequencing. *N Engl J Med* **366**: 883–892.
5. Wheler J, Tsimberidou AM, Hong D, *et al.* (2012) Survival of 1,181 patients in a phase 1 clinic: The MD Anderson Clinical Center for Targeted Therapy experience. *Clin Cancer Res* **18**(10): 2922–2929.
6. Tran B, Dancey JE, Kamel-Reid S, *et al.* (2012) Cancer genomics: Technology, discovery, and translation. *J Clin Oncol* **30**: 647–660.
7. MacConaill LE, Garraway LA. (2010) Clinical implications of the cancer genome. *J Clin Oncol* **28**: 5219–5228.
8. Gianni L, Dafni U, Gelber R, *et al.* (2011) Treatment with trastuzumab for 1 year after adjuvant chemotherapy in patients with HER2-positive early breast cancer: A 4-year follow-up of a randomized controlled trial. *Lancet Oncol* **12**: 236–244.

9. Bang Y-J, Cutsem EV, Feyereislova A, *et al.* (2010) Trastuzumab in combination with chemotherapy versus chemotherapy alone for treatment of HER2-positive advanced gastric or gastro-oesophageal junction cancer (ToGA): A phase 3, open-label, randomized controlled trial. *Lancet* **376**: 687–697.
10. Chevallier P, Robillard N, Charbonnier A, *et al.* (2012) Trastuzumab for treatment of refractory/relapsed HER-2 positive adult B-ALL: Results of a phase 2 GRAALL study. *Blood* **119**(11): 2474–2477.
11. Cappuzzo F, Bemis L, Varella-Garcia M, *et al.* (2006) HER2 mutation and response to trastuzumab therapy in non-small-cell lung cancer. *N Engl J Med* **354**: 2619–2621.
12. Bookman MA, Darcy KM, Clarke-Pearson D, *et al.* (2003) Evaluation of monoclonal humanized anti-HER2 antibody, trastuzumab, in patients with recurrent or refractory ovarian or primary peritoneal carcinoma with overexpression of HER2: A phase II trial of the Gynecologic Oncology Group. *J Clin Oncol* **21**: 283–290.
13. Keedy VL, Temin S, Somerfield MR, *et al.* (2011) American society of clinical oncology provisional clinical opinion: Epidermal Growth Factor Receptor (EGFR) mutation testing for patients with advanced non-small-cell lung cancer considering first-line EGFR tyrosine kinase inhibitor therapy. *J Clin Oncol* **29**: 2121–2127.
14. Schilder RJ, Sil MW, Chen X, *et al.* (2005) Phase II study of gefitinib in patients with relapsed or persistent ovarian or primary peritoneal carcinoma and evaluation of epidermal growth factor receptor mutations and immunohistochemical expression: A gynecologic oncology group study. *Clin Cancer Res* **11**(15): 5539–5548.
15. Vergote IB, Joly F, Katsaros D, *et al.* (2012) Randomized phase III study of erlotinib versus observation in patients with no evidence of disease progression after first-line platin-based chemotherapy for ovarian carcinoma. A GCIG and EORTC-GCG study. *LBA5000, Proceedings of the American Society of Clinical Oncology Annual Meeting*, Chicago, June 1–4.
16. Kwak EL, Bang Y-J, Camidge DR, *et al.* (2010) Anaplastic lymphoma kinase inhibition in non-small-cell lung cancer. *N Engl J Med* **363**: 1693–1703.
17. Sekulic A, Migden MR, Oro AE, *et al.* (2012) Efficacy and safety of vismodegib in advanced basal-cell carcinoma. *N Engl J Med* **366**: 2171–2179.
18. Broglio KR, Berry DA. (2009) Detecting an overall survival benefit that is derived from progression-free survival. *J Natl Cancer Inst* **101**: 1642–1649.

CHAPTER 27

Health Services and Economics in Translational Science

Louise Wideroff

27.1. INTRODUCTION

The term *translational science* is often used synonymously with basic and pre-clinical research to develop new drugs, tests, vaccines, medical devices, and behavioral interventions. However, translational science has also been conceptualized as a continuum that extends beyond the developmental stages to clinical studies of efficacy, and ultimately, post-market research to evaluate and improve effectiveness in community care.[1] Health services research (HSR) is a multidisciplinary field that studies the behavioral, health system, economic and societal factors influencing access to care, as well as the quality and cost of care. The ultimate goal of HSR is to identify the most effective ways to organize, manage, finance and deliver high quality care, reduce medical errors, and improve patient safety.[2]

This chapter will examine the factors influencing integration of new medical technologies, and of health interventions in general, into community practice, and will also describe the vital role of HSR at a time of increased emphasis on evidence-based medicine and expanding access to health care. Current methods to evaluate the effectiveness and

National Institute on Drug Abuse, Bethesda, Maryland, USA
Full address: Louise Wideroff, PhD, MSPH, National Institute on Drug Abuse, 6001 Executive Boulevard, Rm. 4271, MSC 9555, Bethesda, MD 20892-9555, USA; E-mail: *wideroff@nih.gov*; Tel: +1-301-451-8663; Fax: +1-301-594-6043

cost-effectiveness of interventions, monitor their adoption, and improve clinical utility will be discussed. A glossary containing definitions of key HSR terms is provided in Table 1. Topics not addressed in this chapter include consumer needs, delivery or cost factors in the design of new products, and pre-market regulatory approval processes.

Table 1 Glossary of Health Services Research Terms

Term	Definition
Clinical utility	The ability of an intervention to change clinical or public health practice and result in improved health outcomes.
Comparative effectiveness research (CER)	Clinical trials, observational studies, and economic analyses that compare the clinical effectiveness and cost-effectiveness of interventions, in order to improve health care delivery and outcomes.
Cost-effectiveness analysis	A type of economic analysis that compares two or more health interventions on the basis of value, by examining the amount spent to achieve an improvement in survival (i.e., life-years gained) or other health outcome. Each intervention is assigned an incremental cost-effectiveness ratio to compare the cost per life-year gained, which can help guide health system and policy makers decisions to select interventions with the best value.
Cost-utility analysis	A type of cost-effectiveness analysis that adjusts the denominator for quality of life factors (e.g., quality-adjusted life-years gained).
Efficacy	The ability of a new health intervention to produce an acceptable degree of improvement in health in terms of prolonged survival, pain-free interval, etc. Efficacy is assessed in randomized clinical trials and evaluated in the regulatory approval process and/or in decisions regarding use in clinical practice and coverage of costs.
Effectiveness	The ability of an intervention to improve health and health-related quality of life in the context of routine community care.
Evidence synthesis	The evaluation of data from multiple studies, which begins with a systematic review of the literature about a health intervention and also includes a meta-analysis of clinical outcomes data from high-quality randomized clinical trials or other study designs, if such data are available. Economic and psychosocial data may also be included in evidence synthesis, if available.

(*Continued*)

Table 1 (*Continued*)

Term	Definition
Health services research	A multidisciplinary field that studies the behavioral, health system, economic and societal factors influencing access to care, as well as the quality and cost of care, with the goal of improving delivery of services and health-related outcomes.
Health technology assessment	A form of evidence synthesis that uses clinical, economic, psychosocial and other data to help inform clinical guidelines, policy on the coverage of an intervention within a health system, quality of care standards, and additional areas for research.
Incremental cost-effectiveness ratios	See *cost-effectiveness analysis.*
Implementation science	The study of methods to promote the integration of research findings and evidence into health care policy and practice, at the patient, provider and system levels.
Meta-analysis	The simultaneous analysis of outcomes data from multiple studies, to obtain a graphical plot of how closely the findings from different studies match, and a single statistical estimate across all studies that may overcome the individual studies' power limitations.
Patient-reported outcomes	Questionnaire data reported by patients about frequency and severity of pain or other symptoms, functional ability in daily life, psychosocial impact of treatment, economic and time burden, and satisfaction with care. These variables can be incorporated into study questionnaires and evaluated during evidence syntheses, to provide additional information about efficacy and effectiveness that cannot be measured by clinical exams and diagnostic tests.
Practical clinical trials (or pragmatic trials)	Randomized trials of patients under the less controlled conditions of routine care, to test if an intervention is effective in sicker, more diverse patient populations than those recruited for explanatory randomized clinical trials.
Practice guidelines	Systematically developed statements about the most effective way to administer drugs, perform medical procedures or otherwise provide services, usually developed by professional societies and health organizations.
Quality improvement	Structural, organizational, process and other modifications in a health care system to optimize the delivery of care and patient health and safety.

(*Continued*)

Table 1 (*Continued*)

Term	Definition
Quality of care	A conceptual framework for establishing standards and performance measures in health care delivery to achieve care that is effective, efficient, accessible, acceptable, patient-centered, equitable and safe.
Randomized clinical trials (or explanatory trials)	Studies to compare clinical outcomes in groups of patients who are randomly assigned to either receive a new intervention or the standard care. These studies are conducted to test the efficacy of new drugs or other interventions in select patient populations and specific doses that are specifically intended to maximize chances of seeing an effect.
Surveillance research	The systematic collection, analysis and dissemination of descriptive data on health-related outcomes, risk factors and health services cost and utilization, to use in public health and in health care system planning and action.
Systematic review	An extensive methodical search to identify as many studies as possible about an intervention of interest, followed by a review of the studies, selecting those that meet *a-priori* standards of quality and can be used for meta-analysis and evidence synthesis.
Translational science	The continuum of research needed to develop a new health intervention, test it in preclinical and clinical settings, introduce it into health care, and then evaluate and improve its effectiveness.
Willingness-to-pay models	A type of economic analysis that estimates the monetary amount that would be acceptable to pay in order to achieve a given health effect.

27.2. POST-MARKET FACTORS INFLUENCING TRANSLATION

In 1981, Penchansky and Thomas[3] published a paper about healthcare access that provides a framework for understanding many of the post-market challenges to translation of interventions into clinical and public health practice. Access was defined as the "degree of fit" between a person's healthcare needs and what the healthcare system provides, in terms of the availability of services, the organization of services to accommodate patient needs, the affordability of services and medications relative to what patients can pay, the geographic distance to services or other accessibility issues, and the acceptability of these services within the context of consumer preferences and satisfaction. Inadequate access to care remains a major contributor to disparities in disease occurrence and health-related quality of life, whether due to financial, health literacy or language barriers, cultural beliefs, medication or provider shortages, or other factors.[4] The impact of access barriers is particularly acute in low- and middle-income countries, which bear a disproportionate burden of premature global mortality from disease and injury.[5]

Access factors influence the use of many well-established interventions, such as colonoscopy for colorectal cancer screening and highly active antiretroviral treatment for HIV/AIDS, which remain under utilized in some populations despite substantial evidence of effectiveness.[6,7] Access factors also affect the rate of adoption of new interventions. For example, consumer uptake of prophylactic human papillomavirus vaccines, first introduced for pre-teen girls in 2008, has been somewhat limited by parental reluctance to endorse childhood vaccination against a sexually transmitted infection and to return to providers for the full three-dose vaccine series.[8]

In the US, a well-known issue surrounding biomarker diagnostic tests is the reluctance of health systems and third-party payers (e.g., health insurance companies) to cover the costs of testing because of uncertain accuracy in laboratory performance and in predicting clinical outcomes. The very limited pre-market evidence of validity for most tests that become commercially available has been widely attributed to regulatory processes which are less stringent for diagnostic tests than for drugs.[9–14] The practice of genomic medicine incorporates a number of these biomarker tests, such as tumor gene profiling and pre-emptive pharmacogenetic tests to guide therapy, and genome and exome sequencing to diagnose unknown disorders. As testing technologies increase in complexity from single gene tests and multigene expression arrays to whole genome and exome sequencing, issues of validity are compounded by other concerns, including laboratory requirements for specialized equipment and the generation of massive amounts of data that may be difficult to interpret or integrate into decision support tools and electronic medical records.[15,16]

The specific post-market challenges to effective translation vary by intervention and over time. The next section describes HSR methods to assess these challenges at the patient, provider and system levels, and to use the research results to maximize quality of care.

27.3. EVIDENCE GENERATION AND SYNTHESIS

Evidence generation refers to the collection and analysis of new data, or analysis of data from existing sources, to determine the most effective approaches to disease prevention, diagnosis and treatment. The research is conducted to fill an evidence gap for new interventions, or for existing interventions with limited data on effectiveness. The explanatory randomized clinical trial (RCT) has long been the gold standard for evidence generation, particularly for new drugs. The main research question is whether a new drug extends overall survival or symptom-free time with an acceptable level of side effects, compared with existing treatments.[17] To maximize the chances of finding effects, the experimental conditions are strictly controlled: eligibility is restricted to patients with predefined disease severity and limited comorbidities, patients are randomized into blinded treatment groups (new drug versus old drug or placebo), and compliance and adverse effects are closely monitored.

Evidence synthesis is the evaluation of clinical data from multiple studies. The gold standard is the systematic review and meta-analysis of high quality RCTs. The systematic review begins with an extensive methodical search to identify as many RCTs as possible for the intervention of interest, followed by a review of the RCTs to select those that meet *a-priori* standards of quality. A meta-analysis of the data from the selected studies is then performed to graphically plot how closely the findings from different studies match, and to obtain a single statistical estimate of efficacy across all studies that presumably overcomes the power limitations of individual studies.[18]

Evidence synthesis is critical to the development of practice guidelines for healthcare providers and to the establishment of benefit and coverage policies by employers and payers. Where the number of high quality RCTs is insufficient, practice and policy decisions are often based on past experience and consensus opinions, which imply greater levels of uncertainty about the health benefits. Evidence synthesis also helps to identify new areas for research to fill an evidence gap.

Global trends toward evidence-based decision-making and greater focus on value in an era of rising healthcare costs have increased the need for research to clarify the effectiveness and cost-effectiveness of uncertain clinical and public health interventions.[19] Simultaneously, there has been increased recognition of the importance of studying effectiveness in routine community care, where patient demographics, disease severity, prevalence of comorbidities, healthcare access, and delivery factors can significantly influence clinical outcomes.[20] Furthermore, quality of care standards have evolved towards patient-centeredness, placing greater emphasis on improving patient quality of life in addition to expanding survival, and also on accommodating patient preferences and directly engaging patients in medical decision-making.[21] These trends underlie the recent "boom" in comparative effectiveness research (CER),[22] which expands the kinds of health data that are evaluated to guide healthcare practice and policy.

27.3.1. Comparative Effectiveness Research

CER is the conduct and synthesis of research that compares the benefits and harms of different interventions to prevent, diagnose and treat health conditions, and takes into consideration data collected in "real-world" conditions of community care.[22] While RCTs remain the backbone of CER, other research methods have gained increasing attention in the past decade or so, including practical (or pragmatic) clinical trials, observational cohort studies using routinely collected health system data, collection and analysis of patient-centered outcomes within clinical trials and observational studies, and economic decision analysis (Fig. 1).[23–26] Practical clinical trials are randomized trials of patients under conditions of routine care, to test if an intervention is effective in more co-morbid, diverse patient populations than the patients recruited for RCTs.[17] Practice-based physician research networks or large healthcare systems with diverse populations of patients and providers are examples of settings that are amenable to these trials. In addition to studying a wider range of patients, practical clinical trials also tend to study a broader range of outcomes such as those related to quality of life.

Large observational cohort studies that compare non-randomized patients who receive, versus those who do not receive, a particular

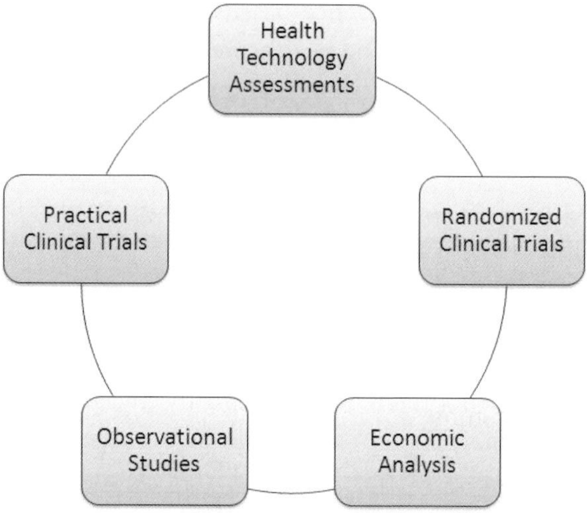

Fig. 1. Comparative effectiveness research.

intervention, are relatively inexpensive and quick to conduct if the researcher uses routinely collected patient information that is stored in electronic databases.[27] Such databases are found in large clinical systems that maintain electronic medical records (EMR) containing patient demographic variables, risk factors such as smoking and family history, screening and diagnostic procedures, treatment, diagnoses, and relapse.[28] Other sources of routinely collected data include large claims databases of organizations managing health services reimbursement, geographically based disease registries used for public health surveillance, and record-linkage databases containing merged data from multiple sources.[29,30]

Patient-centered research expands the breadth of CER to include health-related quality of life variables that are not measurable by clinical examination or diagnostic tests. One major example of this has been the introduction of questionnaires in RCTs or observational studies to assess patient-reported outcomes, such as frequency and severity of pain or other symptoms, functional ability in daily life, psychosocial impact of treatment, financial and time burden, and satisfaction with care.[31,32] The underlying assumption is that some outcomes can only be reported by patients, who can contribute unique and important perspectives to the overall measurement of effectiveness.

Cost-effectiveness analysis is a form of CER that introduces the dimension of value to the concept of effectiveness, where value reflects the health outcomes achieved for a given economic cost.[33,34] As a prominent research tool in health economics and decision analysis, it provides health care systems and policy makers with useful quantitative measures for deciding whether to cover the costs of a health intervention. The main economic question in CER is which interventions can achieve the best health-related outcomes, at an affordable cost that facilitates equitable access to care. The intersection of cost and effectiveness in economic analysis allows for alternative choices to be ranked relative to a standard of care, as either more effective/costs more, more effective/costs less, less effective/costs more, or less effective/costs less.[35] A judgment must be made as to what is an acceptable threshold of cost-effectiveness to justify coverage of the intervention.

The basic cost-effectiveness model estimates the incremental cost-effectiveness ratio, which is the change in costs associated with a particular intervention (compared with standard care), divided by the corresponding change in survival. Costs are expressed in monetary units like dollars or euros, while health effects are typically expressed in life-years gained or some other measure of relevance. Interventions with higher ratios suggest a less efficient choice of care, although cost considerations are not necessarily the main decision factor, as in the case of a more expensive intervention that markedly improves survival. In cost-utility modeling, a form of cost-effectiveness analysis, longevity is not the sole measure of effectiveness, and the model is adjusted for quality of life factors to yield a measure of cost per quality-adjusted life-years.[36] Willingness-to-pay models, another form of economic analysis, estimate the monetary amount that would be acceptable to pay in order to achieve a given health effect. In evidence synthesis, several different types of economic models may be evaluated to provide a broader perspective on the value of an intervention.[37]

Economic decision modeling requires assumptions to be made about costs and health effects, in order for these parameters to be quantified and entered into the simulation software program. The full extent of costs for a cycle of care, and the true range of health effects, may be difficult to quantify, and estimates derived from pre-market RCTs can yield different results than post-market data reflecting costs and clinical outcomes in "real-world" settings.[38] Because of the uncertainty in these parameters, a sensitivity analysis can be performed in which the models are run multiple times using different estimates of cost and effect. Even so, it may be hard to capture cost factors resulting from lost work time, transportation to the point of care, or caretaking expenses,[39] and it is often another challenge to factor in patient-reported outcomes and preferences.[40]

Health technology assessment (HTA) is a type of evidence synthesis that incorporates more kinds of data than just RCT clinical endpoints, including economic analyses if available,[41] data from observational studies, psychosocial impact studies, and so on. Although HTAs usually begin with a systematic review, there is no one standard protocol for the content, which can vary according to the research question, type and amount of data available, and author preferences. HTAs are often conducted by organizations that specialize in this approach, such as the National Institute for Health Research HTA Programme in the UK[42] or the Blue Cross Blue Shield Association Technology Evaluation Center in the US.[43] HTAs are used by healthcare provider organizations to develop evidence-based clinical guidelines, and by healthcare systems and payers to establish coverage and reimbursement policies.

The dissemination of research findings occurs through numerous channels, including medical journals, clinical guidelines, provider workforce education and training, academic and public Internet sites, provider–patient communications, and the popular press. The emerging fields of dissemination and implementation science address how research findings are integrated into health care delivery, policy and health behavior, and how barriers to effective integration can be overcome.

27.4. INTEGRATION OF EVIDENCE INTO PRACTICE

Implementation science is described by the National Institutes of Health as "the study of methods to promote the integration of research findings and evidence into healthcare policy and practice. It seeks to understand the behavior of healthcare professionals and other stakeholders as a key variable in the sustainable uptake, adoption, and implementation of evidence-based interventions."[44] Implementation science also aims to "investigate and address major bottlenecks (e.g., social, behavioral, economic, management) that impede effective implementation, test new approaches to improve health programming, as well as determine a causal relationship between the intervention and its impact."[45] By definition, this covers a broad spectrum of research, such as intervention studies to increase provider adherence to clinical guidelines, practical trials of patient-centered communication tools to increase screening adherence, policy interventions to engage legislators and administrators, and studies examining how health information is relayed in the delivery of care.[46–48] Priorities for implementation research may be identified through surveillance data that reveal clusters of preventable disease or injury, or gaps in health services. Priorities may also be identified through utilization reviews, which evaluate the necessity, appropriateness and efficiency of specific services or facilities. The introduction of new vaccines, diagnostic tests, and other products or procedures also provides opportunities to study the adoption process and design interventions to optimize use. The ultimate goal of implementation research is to identify and test concrete ways to improve the quality of care.

With tremendous global variation in health care systems and populations, there is no one-size-fits-all model of quality healthcare, but the World Health Organization broadly defines it as the effective, efficient, accessible, acceptable, patient-centered, equitable, and safe delivery of services.[49] The results of implementation research can be directly translated into quality improvement (QI) programs, designed to introduce beneficial changes within healthcare systems and communities and to monitor the impact of these changes.[50] The evaluation of QI strategies is itself a form of implementation science. For example, Tricco *et al.*[51] conducted a systematic review and meta-analysis of RCTs testing QI interventions for the management of diabetes. The interventions targeted healthcare systems (provider team management changes, EMR tracking, facilitated relay of laboratory or pharmacy information), clinicians (e.g., audit and feedback, clinical education, reminders, positive or negative financial incentives), and diabetes patients (e.g., education, enabling self-management through equipment or behavioral tools, reminders). Compared with usual care, the QI interventions overall were found to significantly improve some but not all diabetes-related health outcomes, with the effect size largest for patients with poor baseline glycemic control. QI strategies that focused primarily on clinician education were not specifically found to result in significant improvements.

In general, maintaining a knowledgeable and competent provider work force is an essential component of quality, particularly in an era of rapidly expanding medical data and information sources. HSR plays a role in workforce learning through physician surveys to monitor knowledge and skill sets, testing of educational and training interventions, and other approaches. Information technology (IT) tools to support decision-making at the point of care have gained increasing attention in HSR, as a complementary approach to traditional forms of the training and continuing education required for credentialing. For example, "rapid learning"strategies incorporate the use of large relational databases that link individual patient data (i.e., clinical, biomarker, behavioral, demographic) to research evidence, providing decision support to providers in real time.[52] Telemedicine offers the potential to connect consulting specialists to health care workers and/or directly to patients who are located in other geographical areas, which can be a particularly effective strategy in remote and low resource settings.[53,54]

The complementary side to provider learning is patient learning. The field of patient-centered communications studies the exchange of information between patients and providers, as well as the behavioral aspects of their interactions in decision-making.[55,56] A significant amount of health information, however, is disseminated to consumers outside the context of clinical care, though direct-to-consumer advertising, news media, the Internet, and other means. Health communications, therefore, is a very broad field of research that overlaps somewhat with HSR in regards to those communication factors that directly influence healthcare access and effectiveness.

The final section of this chapter describes the critical role of surveillance and monitoring to identify gaps and evaluate the impact of interventions to improve quality.

27.5. POST-MARKET SURVEILLANCE AND MONITORING

Public health surveillance refers to the collection, analysis and dissemination of descriptive data on health-related outcomes that are important for public health, and for healthcare system planning and action.[57] Globally, public health agencies manage a wide range of disease surveillance systems, including sentinel case report networks for tracking epidemics, and geographically based cancer registries for generating incidence, mortality and survival rates. There are also surveillance systems that track behavioral[58] and environmental risk factors[59] and delivery of health services. To manage all these surveillance systems, data are drawn from a variety of data sources, including hospitals, laboratories, surveys and designated provider networks.[60]

From an HSR perspective, the most useful public health surveillance systems are those that track healthcare utilization[61] (e.g., hospital admissions, use of preventive services or treatment, etc.) and costs,[62]and those that electronically link utilization and cost records to individual patient outcomes. The SEER-Medicare system is a notable example of the latter, linking cancer diagnoses from a major US cancer registry surveillance system with a national database of health services reimbursement claims for patients age 65 and older.[63] Health administrative data systems are of varying completeness and validity, and data quality must be evaluated and reported in research findings.[64] Nevertheless, individual and linked databases are a critical resource for monitoring population trends in morbidity and mortality, and for identifying healthcare delivery and access factors that help explain the trends.

The advent of EMR has greatly enhanced the utility of clinical health systems for surveillance of health-related outcomes and service utilization,[65,66] enabling faster access to data and greater clinical detail than in public health surveillance systems (although the latter may be more representative of the general population). There are risks and benefits to the use of clinical EMR databases for various purposes.[67] One area of tremendous potential is the real-time monitoring of adverse events, such as prescription errors, drug–drug interactions, and pharmacogenetic outcomes.[68–70] EMT databases are also very useful for evaluating patterns of care to identify potential barriers. For example, data from the National Comprehensive Cancer Center Network have been used to track race/ethnic differences and other patterns in the use of personalized medicine options for breast cancer diagnosis and treatment.[71–73]

27.6. SUMMARY

HSR plays a vital role in translational science during the clinical and post-market stages. CER compares interventions to identify the most effective and cost-effective choices for care, considering the impact on access to services as well as improvements in health-related quality of life. The full range of CER study designs and resulting data create a body of evidence that can be synthesized in health technology assessments and used to inform clinical practice, coverage policy, and quality improvement programs.

REFERENCES

1. Khoury MJ, Gwinn M, Yoon PW, *et al.* (2007) The continuum of translational research in genomic medicine: How can we accelerate the appropriate integration of human genome discoveries into health care and disease prevention? *Genet Med* **9**: 665–674.
2. National Information Center on Health Services Research and Health Care Technology. *www.nlm.nih.gov/nichsr/ihcm/01whatis/whatis07.html* (Accessed March 4, 2013).
3. Penchansky R, Thomas WJ. (1981) The concept of access. Definition and relationship to consumer satisfaction. *Med Care* **19**: 127–140.
4. Mullins CD, Blatt L, Gbarayor CM, *et al.* (2005) Health disparities: A barrier to high-quality care. *Am J Health Syst Pharm* **62**: 1873–1882.
5. Wang H, Dwyer-Lindgren L, Lofgren KT, *et al.* (2012) Age-specific and sex-specific mortality in 187 countries, 1970–2010: A systematic analysis for the Global Burden of Disease Study 2010. *Lancet* **380** (9859): 2071–2094.
6. Centers for Disease Control and Prevention (CDC). (2012) Cancer screening — United States, 2010. *Morb Mortal Wkly Rep* **61**: 41–45.
7. Agwu AL, Fleishman JA, Korthuis PT, *et al.* (2011) Disparities in antiretroviral treatment: A comparison of behaviorally HIV-infected youth and adults in the HIV Research Network. *J Acquir Immune Defic Syndr* 58: 100–107.
8. Jemal A, Simard EP, Dorell C, *et al.* (2013) Annual report to the nation on the status of cancer, 1975–2009, featuring the burden and trends in human papillomavirus (HPV)-associated cancers and HPV vaccination coverage levels. *J Natl Cancer Inst* **105**: 175–201.
9. McDermott U, Downing JR, Stratton MR. (2011) Genomics and the continuum of cancer care. *N Engl J Med* **365**: 340–350.
10. Lesko LJ, Zineh I, Huang S-M. (2010) What is clinical utility and why should we care *Clin Pharmacol Ther* **88**: 729–733.
11. Quinn B. (2010) Payers and the assessment of clinical utility for companion diagnostics. *Clin Pharmacol Ther* **88**:751–754.

12. Ramsey SD, Veenstra D, Tunis SR, *et al.* (2011) How comparative effectiveness research can help advance "personalized" medicine in cancer treatment. *Health Aff (Millwood)* **12**: 2259–2268.
13. Flockhart DA, Skaar T, Berlin DS, *et al.* (2009) Clinically available pharmacogenomics tests. *Clin Pharmacol Ther* **86**: 109–113.
14. Evans BJ. (2010). Payers and the assessment of clinical utility for companion diagnostics. *Clin Pharmacol Ther* **88**: 751–754.
15. Phimister EG, Feero WG, Guttmacher AE. (2012) Realizing genomic medicine. *N Engl J Med* **366**: 757–759.
16. Manolio TA, Chisholm RL, Ozenberger B, *et al.* (2012) Implementing genomic medicine in the clinic: The future is here. *Genet Med* **5**(4): 258–267.
17. Tunis SR, Stryer DB, Clancy CM. (2003) Practical clinical trials: increasing the value of clinical research for decision making in clinical and health policy. *J Am Med Assoc* **290**: 1624–1632.
18. Egger M, Davey Smith G. (2001) Principles of and procedures for systematic reviews. In: Egger M, Davey Smith G, Altman DG (eds). *Systematic Reviews in Health Care. Meta-analysis in Context.* BMJ Publishing Group, London, pp. 23–42.
19. Institute of Medicine. (2013) *Delivering Affordable Cancer Care in the 21st Century — Workshop Summary.* The National Academies Press, Washington D.C. *www.iom.edu/Reports/2013/Delivering-Affordable-Cancer-Care-in-the-21st-Century.aspx* (Accessed March 4, 2013).
20. Kupersmith J, Sung N, Genel M, *et al.* (2005) Creating a new structure for research on health care effectiveness. *J Invest Med* **53**: 1–6.
21. Torda P, Peikes D, Han E, Genevro J. (2010) *Engaging Patients and Families in the Medical Home.* Publication No. 10-0083-EF. Agency for Health Care Research and Quality, Rockville. *http://pcmh.ahrq.gov/portal/server.pt/community/pcmh_home/1483/PCMH_HTMLConversion_10-0083-EF_v2* (Accessed March 4, 2013).
22. Federal Coordinating Council for Comparative Effectiveness Research. (2009) *Report to the President and the Congress.* U.S. Department of Health and Human Services, Washington D.C. *www.hhs.gov/recovery/programs/cer/cerannualrpt.pdf* (Accessed March 4, 2013).
23. Lyman GH. (2009) Comparative effectiveness research in oncology: The need for clarity, transparency and vision. *Cancer Invest* **27**: 593–597.
24. Lyman GH, Levine M. (2012) Comparative effectiveness research in oncology: An overview. *J Clin Oncol* **30**: 4181–4184.
25. Hahn OM, Schilsky RL. (2012) Randomized controlled trials and comparative effectiveness research. *J Clin Oncol* **30**: 4194–4201.

26. Armstrong K. (2012) Methods in comparative effectiveness research. *J Clin Oncol* **30**: 4208–4214.
27. Langan SM, Benchimol EI, Guttman A, *et al.* (2013) Setting the RECORD straight: Developing a guideline for the REporting of studies Conducted using Observational Routinely collected Data. *Clin Epidemiol* 5: 29–31.
28. Newton KM, Larson EB. (2012) Learning health care systems: Leading through research.The 18th Annual HMOResearchNetwork Conference, April 29–May 2, 2012, Seattle, Washington. *Clin Med Res* **10**: 140–142.
29. Meyerhardt JA, Li L, Sanoff HK, *et al.* (2012) Effectiveness of bevacizumab with first-line combination chemotherapy for Medicare patients with stage IV colorectal cancer. *J Clin Oncol* **30**: 608–615.
30. Källén B, Reis M. (2012) Neonatal complications after maternal concomitant use of SSRI and other central nervous system active drugs during the second or third trimester of pregnancy. *J Clin Psychopharmacol* **32**: 608–614.
31. Food and Drug Administration. (2009) *Guidance for Industry: Patient-Reported Outcome Measures: Use in Medical Product Development to Support Labeling Claims.* U.S. Department of Health and Human Services, Silver Spring. *www.fda.gov/downloads/Drugs/Guidances/UCM193282.pdf* (Accessed March 4, 2013).
32. Lipscomb J, Donaldson MS, Hiatt RA. (2004) Cancer outcomes research: The arenas of application. *J Natl Cancer Inst Monogr* **33**: 1–7.
33. Porter ME. (2010) What is value in health care? *N Engl J Med* **363**: 2477–2481.
34. Thariani R, Veenstra DL, Carlson JJ, *et al.* (2012) Paying for personalized care: Cancer biomarkers and comparative effectiveness. *Mol Oncol* **6**: 260–266.
35. Black W. (1990) A graphical representation of cost-effectiveness. *Med Decis Making* **10**: 212–214.
36. Chapman RH, Berger M, Weinstein MC, *et al.* (2004) When does quality-adjusting life-years matter in cost-effectiveness analysis? *Health Econ* **13**: 429–436.
37. Robertson C, ArcotRagupathy SK, Boachie C, *et al.* (2011) The clinical effectiveness and cost-effectiveness of different surveillance mammography regimens after the treatment for primary breast cancer: Systematic reviews registry database analyses and economic evaluation. *Health Technol Assess* **15**: v–vi, 1–322.
38. Carlson JJ, Ramsey SD. (2012) Proof or principle? On economic modeling to guide genomic testing in metastatic colorectal cancer. *J Natl Cancer Inst* **104**: 1779–1780.
39. Banegas MP, Yabroff KR. (2013) Out of pocket, out of sight? An unmeasured component of the burden of cancer. *J Natl Cancer Inst* **105**: 252–253.

40. Wang G, Kuppermann M, Kim B, *et al.* (2012) Influence of patient preferences on the cost-effectiveness of screening for Lynch syndrome. *J Oncol Pract* **8**(3 Suppl): e24s–30s.
41. McKenna C, Burch J, Suekarran S, *et al.*(2010) A systematic review and economic evaluation of the clinical effectiveness and cost-effectiveness of aldosterone antagonists for postmyocardial infarction heart failure. *Health Technol Assess* **14**: 1–162.
42. National Institute for Health Research HTA Programme. *www.hta.ac.uk* (Accessed March 4, 2013).
43. Blue Cross Blue Shield Association Technology Evaluation Center. *www.bcbs.com/blueresources/tec/tec-assessments.html* (Accessed March 4, 2013).
44. National Institutes of Health. Fogarty International Center. Frequently Asked Questions about Implementation Sciences. *www.fic.nih.gov/News/Events/implementation-science/Pages/faqs.aspx* (Accessed March 4, 2013).
45. National Library of Medicine. National Information Center on Health Services Research and Health Care Technology. *www.nlm.nih.gov/hsrinfo/implementation_science.html* (Accessed March 4, 2013).
46. Quinn GP, Murphy D, Malo T, *et al.* (2012) A national survey about human papillomavirus vaccination: What we didn't ask, but physicians wanted us to know. *J Pediatr Adolesc Gynecol* **25**: 254–258.
47. Main C, Moxham T, Wyatt JC, *et al.* (2010) Computerised decision support systems in order communication for diagnostic, screening or monitoring test ordering: Systematic reviews of the effects and cost-effectiveness of systems. *Health Technol Assess* **14**: 1–227.
48. Acheson LS, Wang C, Zyzanski SJ, *et al.* (2010) Family history and perceptions about risk and prevention for chronic diseases in primary care: A report from the family healthware impact trial. *Genet Med* **12**: 212–218.
49. World Health Oranization. (2006) *Quality of Care. A Process for Making Strategic Choices in Health Systems.* WHO Press, Geneva. *www.who.int/management/quality/assurance/QualityCare_B.Def.pdf* (Accessed March 4, 2013).
50. Varkey P, Reller K, Resar RK. (2007) Basics of quality improvement in health care. *Mayo Clin Proc* **82**: 735–739.
51. Tricco AC, Ivers NM, Grimshaw JM, *et al.* (2012) Effectiveness of quality improvement strategies on the measurement of diabetes: A systematic review and meta-analysis. *Lancet* **379**: 2252–2261.
52. Ginsburg GS, Kuderer NM. (2012) Comparative effectiveness research, genomics enabled personalized medicine, and rapid learning health care: A common bond. *J Clin Oncol* **30**: 4233–4242.
53. Casey M, Hayes PS, Heaney D, *et al.* (2013) Implementing transnational telemedicine solutions: A connected health project in rural and remote areas

of six Northern Periphery countries Series on European collaborative projects. *Eur J Gen Pract* **19**: 52–58.

54. Fortney JC, Pyne JM, Mouden SB, *et al.* (2013) Practice-based versus telemedicine-based collaborative care for depression in rural federally qualified health centers: A pragmatic randomized comparative effectiveness trial. *Am J Psychiatry* **170**(4): 414–425.
55. Epstein RM, Street RL. (2007) *Patient-Centered Communications in Cancer Care: Promoting Healing and Reducing Suffering.* National Cancer Institute, NIH Publication No. 07-6225, Bethesda. *http://outcomes.cancer.gov/areas/pcc/communication/pcc_monograph.pdf* (Accessed March 4, 2013).
56. O'Neill SC, McBride CM, Alford SH, Kaphingst KA. (2010) Preferences for genetic and behavioral health information: The impact of risk factors and disease attributions. *Ann Behav Med* **40**: 127–137.
57. Lee LM, Thacker SB. (2011) Public health surveillance and knowing about health in the context of growing sources of health data. *Am J Prev Med* **41**: 636–640.
58. Cole AM, Jackson JE, Doescher M. (2012). Urban-rural disparities in colorectal cancer screening: Cross-sectional analysis of 1998–2005 data from the Centers for Disease Control's Behavioral Risk Factor Surveillance Study. *Cancer Med* **1**(3): 350–356.
59. Malecki KC, Resnick B, Burke TA. (2008) Effective environmental public health surveillance programs: A framework for identifying and evaluating data resources and indicators. *J Public Health Manag Pract* **14**: 543–551.
60. Hall HI, Correa A, Yoon PW, Braden CR. (2012) Lexicon, definitions and conceptual framework for public health surveillance. *MMWR Surveill Summ* **61**(Suppl): 10–14.
61. Herk-Sukel MP, Lemmens VE, Poll-Franse LV, *et al.* (2012) Records linkage for pharmacoepidemiological studies in cancer patients. *Pharmacoepidemiol Drug Saf* **21**: 94–103.
62. Gipson DS, Messer KL, Tran CL, *et al.* (2013) Inpatient health care utilization in the United States among children, adolescents, and young adults with nephroticsyndrome. *Am J Kidney Dis.* Epub ahead of print.
63. Engels EA, Pfeiffer RM, Ricker W, *et al.* (2011) Use of surveillance, epidemiology, and end results-medicare data to conduct case-control studies of cancer among the US elderly. *Am J Epidemiol* **174**: 860–870.
64. Benchimol EI, Manuel DG, To T, *et al.* (2011) Development and use of reporting guidelines for assessing the quality of validation studies of health administrative data. *J Clin Epidemiol* **64**: 821–829.

65. Nekhlyudov L, Greene SM, Chubak J, *et al.* (2012) Cancer research network: Using integrated health care delivery systems as platforms for cancer survivorship research. *J Cancer Surviv* 7: 55–62.
66. Wagner EH, Greene SM, Hart G, *et al.*(2005) Building a research consortium of large health systems: The Cancer Research Network. *J Natl Cancer Inst Monogr* **35**: 3–11.
67. Walker JM, Carayon P, Leveson N, *et al.* (2008) EHR safety: The way forward to safe and effective systems. *J Am Med Inform Assoc* **15**: 272–277.
68. Moore TJ, Bennett CL. (2012) Underreporting of hemorrhagic and thrombotic complications of pharmaceuticals to the U.S. Food and Drug Administration: Empirical findings for warfarin, clopidogrel, ticlopidine, and thalidomide from the Southern Network on Adverse Reactions (SONAR). *Semin Thromb Hemost* **38**: 905–907.
69. Hennessy S, Flockhart DA. (2012) The need for translational research on drug–drug interactions. *Clin Pharmacol Ther* **91**: 771–773.
70. Avery TR, Kulldorff M, Vilk Y, *et al.* (2013) Near real-time adverse drug reaction surveillance within population-based health networks: Methodology considerations for data accrual. *Pharmacoepidemiol Drug Saf* **22**(5): 488–495.
71. Warner ET, Tamimi RM, Hughes ME, *et al.* (2012) Time to diagnosis and breast cancer stage by race/ethnicity. *Breast Cancer Res Treat* **136**: 813–821.
72. Freedman RA, Hughes ME, Ottesen RA, *et al.* (2012) Use of adjuvant trastuzamab in women with human epidermal growth factor receptor 2 (HER2)-positive breast cancer by race/ethnicity and education within the National Comprehensive Cancer Network. *Cancer* **119**: 839–846.
73. Hassett MJ, Silver SM, Hughes ME, *et al.* (2012) Adoption of gene expression profile testing and association with use of chemotherapy among women with breast cancer. *J Clin Oncol* **30**: 2218–2226.

CHAPTER 28

Translational Brain Tumor Research: The UCSF Experience

Russell O. Pieper[*,†], *Michael D. Prados and Mitchel S. Berger*

28.1. INTRODUCTION

In 2012, more than 20,000 adults and children were diagnosed with primary malignant brain tumors in the US. Patients with less aggressive, low-grade (grade II) gliomas (astrocytomas, oligodendrogliomas and mixed oligo-astrocytomas) have a median survival that ranges from five to more than 10 years, while those with highly aggressive grade IV gliomas (glioblastomamultiforme, GBM) have a five-year survival of only five percent.[1] Despite the best efforts of neurosurgeons and neuro-oncologists, the mortality rates of brain cancer have remained stable over the past 20 years. As such, there are few cancers that are as uniformly fatal and in more need of new therapeutic approaches. The early 1990s marked a shift in the way researchers pursued the development of these new therapies, as well as diagnostic tools for brain cancer. Separate laboratory-based and clinically based approaches shifted to a more integrated, results-driven, team approach that came to be known as "translational science." To be accurate, what is currently known

*Department of Neurological Surgery, The Brain Tumor Research Center, University of California-San Francisco, San Francisco, California, USA,
Neurologic Oncology Program, Helen Diller Family Comprehensive Cancer Center, University of California-San Francisco, San Francisco, CA94158
†Corresponding author: Russell O. Pieper, UCSF Helen Diller Family Cancer Research Building, 1450 S. 3rd St, Rm HD287, Box 0520, San Francisco, CA94158-9001, USA; E-mail: *rpieper@cc.ucsf.edu*; Tel: +1-415-502-7132; Fax: +1-415-514-9792

as "translational science" had been practiced at multiple academic institutions for quite some time prior to the 1990s. As an example, UCSF neurosurgeons in the 1940s collected brain tumor samples for research, and by the 1970s the Department of Neurological Surgery and the Brain Tumor Research Center (BTRC) at UCSF had obtained National Institutes of Health (NIH)-based funding to establish cultures of brain tumors, develop infrastructure, and pursue work directed at improving brain tumor patient survival.

The accelerated pace of translational cancer research in the 1990s was in part motivated by the initiation of a National Cancer Institute (NCI)-based grant mechanism that specifically funded teams of researchers to pursue translational, disease site-specific cancer research (the Specialized Program of Research Excellence or SPORE Program). The awarding of a Brain Tumor SPORE to researchers at UCSF has allowed an established group of basic scientists, neuro-oncologists and neurosurgeons to come together and to use their scientific expertise, clinical trial excellence, and the over 40 years of accumulated resources of the UCSF brain tumor community to perform work focused on making a difference for brain tumor patients. This chapter will describe the experiences of this research group, the problems faced, the solutions found, the problems that still remain, and how the changing landscape of academic science creates both new problems and new opportunities in the effort to provide better outcomes for individuals with brain tumors.

28.2. THE CURRENT STATE OF CARE AND RESEARCH

As noted, brain tumors cover a wide range of subtypes and affect individuals of all ages. Meningioma is the most common type of brain tumor and carries a relatively favorable prognosis. However, patients with most types of gliomas, including anaplastic gliomas and GBM, continue to have universally poor outcomes. Neither the outcomes of patients nor the therapeutic options for the disease have changed significantly in the past 20 years. In 1997 temozolomide, a monofunctional methylating agent, was approved for treatment of anaplastic astrocytoma patients who were refractory to both nitrosourea and procarbazine,[2] and since then, temozolomide in combination with radiation has become the backbone of brain tumor therapy.[3] Recent studies, however, have shown that temozolomide-based therapies have only added approximately two months of median survival for brain cancer patients.[4] The approval of bevacizumab in 2009 provided another therapeutic option for brain tumor patients,[5] but agents such as bevacizumab may prove to be more effective at improving quality of life than extending overall survival.[6] A variety of factors appear to limit the efficacy of therapy, including the relative lack of penetration of new and existing agents into the brain, the lack of complete distribution through the variably perfused tumor, the development of drug resistance, and the lack of definitive targets, the inhibition of which may lead to death of tumor cells.

Despite the fact that relatively little progress has been made therapeutically, our knowledge of brain tumor biology has exploded over the past five years. The underlying molecular drivers of gliomagenesis began to be identified in the 1990s with the discovery of mutations in the p53, Ras, Rb and PTEN-regulated pathways in GBM[7] and chromosomal deletions in oligodendrogliomas that impacted prognosis and chemosensitivity.[8] The importance of these pathways was confirmed in more recent larger studies, including The Cancer Genome Analysis (TCGA) Project, which used cutting-edge expression and sequencing approaches to help define four distinct groups of GBM.[9] In the past two years, the number of events critically involved in brain tumor formation has expanded to include mutations in isocitrate dehydrogenase (IDH), which occur at an early stage in virtually all tumors other than GBM,[10] and mutations in histone H3.3, which occur primarily in pediatric GBM but also in some adult GBM.[11] These findings, as well as the role of stem cells in brain tumor development, have revealed a wealth of new therapeutic targets and new ideas as to how the growth of glioma may be more effectively controlled.

The tremendous growth in information about glioma biology and gliomagenesis has set the stage for a new era of brain tumor therapy. A key challenge now is to determine how the enormous amount of information available about gliomas and their formation can be harnessed into new agents to treat patients, and how these agents can be most effectively tested and tracked to the most appropriate group of brain tumor patients. In essence, how can we best enable the type of translational research that will convert this new knowledge into successful therapies for brain tumor patients?

28.3. FACTORS THAT LIMIT TRANSLATIONAL BRAIN TUMOR RESEARCH

From the academic perspective, there are a variety of factors that limit the ability of the system as it currently exists to reach the desired endpoint of producing improved outcomes for brain cancer patients. None of these problems are new and few are unique to any one institution. Rather, these problems are near universal, have grown over the years with the system, and have now reached a critical stage. Recognizing the problems (discussed below) is the first step in the creation of a system that will better serve translational science.

28.3.1. The Closed Shop

Laboratories focused on cancer research of any kind often resemble small businesses. The principal investigator (PI) of the lab is the CEO, and in this role employs individuals at multiple levels to create, market, and hopefully be compensated for the product. The success of the lab business determines how many different products the lab creates, how many people work in the enterprise, and how many layers of responsibility exist in the lab structure. The product, however, is not a tangible item such as a car or a machine part, but rather knowledge. And the product is not for sale to the public as an item that can be held or directly used, but rather is purchased by larger organizations as part of their mission to improve human health. The most direct example of this, and perhaps the most relevant for the scientific enterprise as it presently exists, is the support of labs by the NIH. Laboratories that are successful by current standards create a research product that is marketed to their peers through scientific journals and meeting presentations, and ultimately paid for by grant support from NIH or any of its branches, such as NCI or the National Institute of Neurological Disorders (NINDS). In this model, the government, and by inference the people, are the consumers of the product, and their purchase of the particular good is the result of competition among scientists to create the most attractive product and the most compelling story around the research.

The pros and cons of this system should be readily apparent. The system clearly rewards innovation and the creation of new ideas and new products. The system also places very few limits on the types of products that can be created and has little to say in the direction the product should take. The system is also somewhat unique in that the consumer has very little say in what the product should be, nor is the consumer necessarily even queried about this. Rather, the participants of the marketplace are free to pursue their own goals with the caveat that the end product needs to be recognized by the consumer (represented by their proxy scientists on study sections) as valuable. A successful sale generates revenue and more product development, while no sale can cause a near immediate readjustment if not outright folding of the lab business. Therefore, the system clearly values innovation, directly rewards success, provides instant feedback, and is free of any directive in terms of what the ultimate product should look like.

While these are all positive attributes, there are many drawbacks of the system as well. Because universities and institutes provide a home for these small businesses and indirectly collect the equivalent of rent, they encourage the businesses to grow and expand as separate entities, and have set up additional reward systems that are based on individual lab achievement. Similarly, individual labs have become very good at making very specific types of products, individual pieces of cars rather than the car as a whole. As a result, the long term goal of human health can often get obscured. The end result of this approach is the selection of successful labs, which in turn build on their success and become nearly entirely self-reliant. Although the products of these labs are shared by the community at large, the products are created with a firm eye on the bottom line and a proprietary attachment to the results generated. Although this system uses entrepreneurial drive and reward to great benefit, what is sacrificed in the pursuit of individual lab accomplishment is the exact behavior that is needed to do successful translational research, namely an effort to integrate knowledge gained in individual labs into the larger setting of human disease.

28.3.2. Lack of Shared Interests and Potentially Shared Solutions

The end result of pure competition is the growth of entities that have only competitive interest in the products that others produce, and even less interest in how cooperation might improve the entire market. In the case of academic science, this takes the form of collections of investigators who may share a similar workspace but have very little knowledge or interest in what neighboring labs and investigators are studying. Most PIs recognize this symptom in their institutions if not in their own labs, and despite the near universal recognition that it is detrimental, seem to have little ability to reverse the process. Again, the university structure contributes to this problem by inadvertently, and in some cases intentionally, forcing investigators to compete for limited resources that ultimately will be awarded to a limited number of competitors. The scientific marketing situation also plays a role in this problem, as the means by which a product or discovery is linked to its creator is codified by a single line in a publication describing in a hierarchical manner who owns the product. Single first authors and single senior authors clearly define ownership of ideas, which in turn limit how these ideas will be used and who can interact. If ownership of the idea as well as the ultimate usage of the idea is linked to a very limited number of people, and if rewards are similarly distributed, what then is the motivation in sharing these ideas at early stages and in working in a collaborative manner to solve problems? In the modern academic setting, the concept of team is not rewarded and could more accurately be said to be suppressed by the reward system established. If individuals gathered to solve problems and generate ideas see their rewards as coming from their individual efforts, they will have little incentive to work together for a common goal.

28.3.3. Clinicians and Basic Scientists often Pursue Separate Goals

What if an institution could assemble the individuals needed to fully address translational brain tumor research problems, and could convince these individuals that common pursuit of a shared goal was desirable and would be rewarded? Wouldn't this be enough to guarantee success? Based on our experience, probably not. Any translational research team, by definition, needs to be composed of clinical investigators closely linked to patient care, basic scientists with a focus on biologic discovery, and, where possible, a limited number of individuals who by training or expertise can bridge these two areas. While a willingness to work together and a reward system that encourages team effort is a good first step, it is important to recognize that clinical and basic scientists do not necessarily see problems the same way, and may not be working toward the same solution. Individuals who work directly with patients are critical to the translational research effort, as they are in a unique position to identify the most important treatment problems and to communicate these to the team. These individuals often have a broader picture of the problems faced and can pinpoint gaps in knowledge. By training, however, these individuals tend to be more focused on solutions for patients, and the knowledge gained by a given study and the better understanding of how an agent works may take a back seat to therapeutic concerns. In contrast, basic scientists, in the absence of direct patient contact, can easily lose focus on the need for the development of effective agents in pursuit of interesting and novel biology. In its purest sense, this dichotomy leaves basic scientists wondering why clinicians don't care about how a drug works and clinicians wondering why basic scientists cannot develop agents that just kill tumor cells. Clearly, both groups and both perspectives are needed in any successful team approach. As a result, it is important to keep in mind that individuals bring different perspectives and different expertise to the team, and that the sharing of these perspectives is exactly what educates the team as a whole and moves the process forward.

28.3.4. Translational Cancer Research Requires Special Tools

Carefully assembled teams of quality individuals ready to do team-based translational science require the tools to do this work. Unfortunately, these tools are not typically present at the outset and take a good deal of effort and expense to generate. In the simplest sense, teams that want to do translational brain tumor research need patient material. Virtually any institution whose mission includes patient care has access to this material, but the number of institutions that have made the financial and administrative commitment to collect and catalog this material over a long period of time is relatively small. While a limited number of institutions, including UCSF, made a commitment to collect this material over 40 years ago, smaller institutions may not have had this luxury. The first critical tool for translational cancer research is therefore a tissue collection, and at the very minimum the commitment to develop a tissue collection that can grow over time with the team. In connection with this is the need for a focused group of individuals who can perform specialized tasks that serve the tissue needs of the group rather than any one individual. As an example, tissue banking requires individuals to collect materials from the operating room, catalog the samples, retrieve the samples when needed, verify the identity of the samples, and distribute material in a rational and fair manner. Similarly, if genome analysis is part of the translational research effort, bioinformatics personnel will be required to turn the mountains of raw data into packages understandable to the larger group. The same also holds true for the biostatisticians needed to help drive the shape of clinical studies that may arise from the team effort. These individuals are both required and difficult to support by traditional funding mechanisms. On the positive side, every translational group faces these same problems, and collecting and supporting these resources may in fact be easier for small groups just starting than large organizations in which the large, immediate need may never be fundable. The special need for translational research tools therefore provides an additional layer of complexity beyond that encountered in forming the translational research team.

28.3.5. Translational Brain Tumor Research Is Expensive and Has a Long Horizon

The course of an individual lab experiment can be measured in days to weeks, while the outcome of individual cancer patient treatment may take months to years to evaluate. It is therefore not surprising that any attempt to move lab-based discoveries to the level of the patient, and to critically evaluate this effort, will be neither inexpensive nor rapid. The movement to begin funding translational cancer research through the SPORE program was in part motivated by the public demand for results. As consumers of our scientific product and as drivers of the system, it is fair for citizens to expect that new knowledge should in turn lead to new and better therapies for cancer, and ultimately to improved patient survival. With this in mind, it is worth remembering that time is of the essence in moving NIH-funded translational brain tumor research to its conclusion, and that the consumers of this work deserve accountability, activity, and our best-faith effort to make a difference, even in the face of the difficulties encountered.

28.4. A FEW SOLUTIONS WITH EXAMPLES

In the face of all the problems encountered by teams interested in doing translational brain tumor research, it is easy to think that the challenges are insurmountable. However, a number of teams of investigators, including those of us at UCSF, have at least gained some experience wrestling with these problems, and have survived long enough to share some ideas and concrete actions that might help others still wondering whether to join the fight.

28.4.1. Open the Shop

As noted, one of the biggest challenges to doing the team-based work needed to make translational advances is moving from an environment in which each lab is its own entity to an environment in which each lab views at least part of its activity as communal. UCSF is no different from most large institutions in having what appears to be an individualistic, "siloed" approach to scientific discovery. And yet a number of changes have occurred that have helped lessen this problem.

First, and perhaps unfortunately, consumer demand for the product of individual labs is flat. The largest consumer of science, the NIH, is facing the end of a period of expanding funding, and depending on the many budget battles yet to come, seems destined to decrease the amount of science it funds. An early effect of this appears to be a new willingness by investigators to consider sources of funding in which they previously had only a modest interest. While R01-based funding will continue to be the most direct and comprehensive way to support a lab, the increased competition for such funding may increase the willingness of successful investigators who are not focused on a specific organ site to participate in translational programs. At UCSF, the Developmental Research Program embedded within the Brain Tumor SPORE provides additional impetus via funds that seed the brain tumor-related efforts of established investigators, while the Career Developmental Program of the SPORE similarly encourages early stage investigators to dedicate at least part of their effort toward translational brain tumor research. These approaches therefore help turn the disadvantage of limited funding into a positive for translational research.

Second, universities currently appear to be placing more value on team-based research than they have previously. While group-based projects such as P01s have always had value, support for translational research from mechanisms such as the SPORE and groups such as Stand Up to Cancer (SUTC) have taken on a special importance to cancer centers, and the presence of such support is now seen to not only add research dollars, but also to add value and visibility to the cancer center enterprise.

Finally, there is increased acceptance of shared work. In an age in which science is expensive and expertise is increasingly fragmented, no one lab can do all the work necessary to prove a concept or answer important translational questions. Consistent with this idea, just 10 years ago it was highly unusual to see scientific articles with shared first authorship, shared senior authorship, or published by a collaborative and separately named group of investigators. A glance at most journals today, however, would show that all three are quite common, and that some journals go as far as to describe (at least in limited detail) what each party contributed to the work. Whether these changes have filtered through to university promotion committees is as of yet uncertain, although the general trend is toward recognizing that a growing number of research projects require a team-based effort. From a translational brain tumor perspective, this approach should be encouraged, and those translational investigators who serve on university evaluation committees should work to educate their colleagues as to the changing face of research and the value of team-based science.

28.4.2. Put People Together, Spend Time Together

An effective translational research team includes individuals with diverse backgrounds and interests, and it is critical to nurture this diversity and encourage interactions that can take advantage of diverse viewpoints. It is worth recognizing from the outset that scientists talk about interacting and collaborating far more than they actually engage in the processes. This undoubtedly goes back to the problem that time is limited for all individuals, and especially clinicians, and that historically investigators willingly engage only in those activities that they see as directly benefitting their own narrow interests. From our perspective, however, there is no substitute for direct face-to-face interaction, especially among individuals with different expertise. Surprisingly, the venue for this interaction and the exact purpose of such meetings may be less important than suspected. While a structured mandatory seminar may generate some interaction, a voluntary non-structured opportunity to sit and talk can open doors that were not thought to exist. At UCSF, the SPORE mechanism offers structured interactions through the SPORE Seminar Series and research updates, as well as less structured interactions that occur in weekly meetings of the SPORE Executive Committee and at monthly breakfast meetings supported by the SPORE. While the former focus on specific research topics, the latter often begin as casual conversations that at a minimum help build a better understanding between team members and often lead to more substantive conversations about the direction of our research and how to accomplish goals within the team concept. Over the years, these less structured meetings have proven to be at least as useful as the structured ones, perhaps because they allowed team members to get to know one another, and based on those friendships, to share data and ideas more freely.

At UCSF we are also very fortunate to have moved into open-structure labs that house nearly all brain tumor researchers on campus. As a result, an enormous wealth of expertise and experience exists in one place, and questions and advice are never more than a few doors away. Similarly, the open lab structure encourages research groups to share space and equipment. In the short time these labs have been occupied, the interaction between groups has increased, as has the number of shared research projects and even shared research personnel, all of which is critical in building team efforts.

In addition to building connections between labs, it is also important to build connections between clinicians and lab based investigators. At UCSF, neuro-oncologists and neurosurgeons, despite their very busy schedules, spend one day a week (Friday in our case) away from clinical responsibilities talking with groups of lab-based scientists. In this manner, clinicians keep abreast of what occurs in the lab, and lab-based investigators get feedback about ideas from clinicians. The benefits of this interaction go both ways, and there are now numerous examples of basic scientists who include clinicians on funded grant proposals, and of clinicians initiating clinically based projects than include lab components. In summary, people who know each other well tend to work together better than people who know each other less well, and from the UCSF experience, it is worth investing effort in building non-scientific as well as scientific relationships.

28.4.3. Core and Tool Investment is a Must

As noted, an adequate collection of patient tumor tissue is essential for translational research. In building this type of resource, a number of issues must be dealt with. First, there is a natural instinct for surgeons to take a proprietary interest in the samples they generate. At UCSF, all samples are deposited into the tissue bank regardless of how they were generated, and all are available for use upon request and approval from a tissue usage committee. There is no ownership of the material and only the Tissue Core and its Usage Committee stand between the user and the sample. Practically, however, it proves useful to involve the surgeon in any study as commitment from the surgeon as well as the neuropathologist provides a wealth of knowledge about the samples, opens doors with regard to what types of samples can be gathered, and in some cases focuses and redefines the work planned.

Second, core investment is expensive. The funding of a core effort is a complicated issue and no one institution handles this matter the same way. There is increased emphasis from the National Cancer Institute to have all cores, including tissue cores, unified across cancer centers. In this scenario, there would be a single tissue core at any given institution, supported entirely by the Comprehensive Cancer Center (CCC). This pure model, however, is more of a goal than a reality, and even at institutions with long-standing CCC support, non-CCC funding is needed. Tissue cores perform billable procedures and can recoup some of their personnel costs from recharge mechanisms. The recharge costs, however, need to be kept low, sometimes artificially low, to encourage usage, and the recharge approach is subjected to a changing funding mix that makes long-term support tenuous at best. Departmental support, if available, continues to be a viable approach for the cores that are needed to do translational research and in the case of new programs is likely to prove essential. Creative approaches to funding, including philanthropy and arrangements with industry, should also be considered, especially in cases in which unique resources are to be generated, such as a collection of rare, specific tumor types. All these issues are also relevant for other cores. At UCSF we are fortunate to have a pre-clinical animal-testing core associated with, and supported in part by, our SPORE and CCC, and this core has proven critical in moving ideas from the bench to the clinic. The funding of this core through a combination of SPORE funds, CCC funds, and outside industrial contracts has also increased the number of personnel available and sped the work the core performs. Finally, no translational research program can be complete without the ability to test agents in patients. Most institutions interested in translational brain tumor research will already have a clinical trials program that is funded by various internal and external sources, although practically this "core" effort, which includes research coordinators, nurses and physicians, may require the largest investment.

28.4.4. Commit to Obtaining Larger Group-based Funding

Although individual translational cancer research projects can be funded at the R01 level, it should be apparent from the types of core facilities and the variety of expertise necessary that the support provided by an R01, or even by multiple R01s, would not adequately fund the work. The UCSF translational brain tumor effort was initiated in the 1970s with support from a P01 award, although this type of award, based on the requirement for a unified theme, is often limiting and lacks the needed flexibility of funding.The initiation of the SPORE program in the early 1990s provided a novel mechanism to specifically fund translational cancer research. The SPORE mechanism provides five years of support for typically four or five research projects at near R01-levels of funding, allowing individual institutions the time and money needed to build translational research teams. The mechanism also encourages flexibility and the possible changing of projects, all of which allows the flow of individuals and projects in and out of the SPORE program. An additional benefit of the SPORE funding mechanism is that projects only need to be united by their goal of translational impact in the cancer of interest, minimizing the risk of recruiting investigators with a relatively narrow area of expertise. As noted, the SPORE mechanism also provides funding for cores that typically cannot be financed by other means. While these qualities make SPORE funding nearly ideal for team-based translational cancer research, a growing number of other sources also exist to fund this type of work. Programs such as SUTC grant awards are typically larger than SPORE awards, although the duration of funding is typically shorter. The SUTC mechanism also requires the inclusion of investigators at multiple institutions, which may increase the diversity and expertise of the team at the risk of less communication between the team members. Smaller funding organizations, such as the Ivy Foundation in the case of brain tumor research, are also moving toward the funding of larger translational projects. Regardless of the mechanism, it is encouraging that funders with diverse interests are all increasingly recognizing the need for, and the value of, team-based translational research.

28.5. TRENDS FOR BETTER AND FOR WORSE

The field of translational research is ever changing, and new challenges as well as new opportunities arrive on a regular basis. A number of changes have already taken place or are currently taking place that will have an impact on our ability to gather investigators to do high-quality translational brain tumor research. A consideration of the impact of these changes at this early stage may help maximize our chances of using these changes to our benefit, and to facilitate the research process.

28.5.1. Open Source Publishing and Reduced Importance of Impact Factor

The Internet has dramatically influenced the way information is stored and shared. A few thousand years ago, the entire knowledge of the world could be found in the few great libraries of the world. As little as 20 years ago, libraries still held most of the information scientists needed to generate new ideas and stay abreast of their field. This is in stark contrast to today, when arguably very few people go to the library as a source of scientific information, instead relying on the Internet and personal computers to access needed data. While it could be argued that the effect of the Internet on the dissemination of information in general has outpaced its effect on the dissemination of scientific information, it already seems quite likely that scientific information will soon be shared much in the same way general information is shared. Where as printed journals, much like newspapers, used to be the gatekeepers of information, it now seems likely that scientific discoveries will find their way to scientists more rapidly in the form of online journals, individual websites, or aggregators of content — services that will deliver a mix of information determined to be of interest to the subscriber. Furthermore, much as one can gather news as a complete story from professional organizations, or in pieces and in real time from blogs, instant messages, and tweets, similarly one may soon be able to follow science in real time. And while peer-review of this information remains the standard today, it is not hard to imagine a scenario in which the reader will be increasingly asked to make up his or her own mind about the validity of the data. One may imagine that this sort of development is far in the future, but already one in six scientific articles is published online in open-access journals.[12] This brave new world opens all sorts of concerns, but may also open the way for better translational team-based research. The primary benefit may be the breakdown of the rigid credit system currently used. Under the present system, credit is assigned primarily to single first and senior authors, and points are tallied in relation to the impact factor of the journal in which the work appeared, itself a poor approximation of how many readers saw and were influenced by the work. By comparison, an open-access, net-based system of publication, whether this takes the form of self-publishing or working through a publishing organization, need not rely on artificial measures of citation but instead can directly and easily measure the number of readers the work attracts. On the whole, these changes will make it much easier for individuals to work together, to share data faster, to try to build a following for their work, to more freely collaborate, and to improve the impact of their work. Given that there are a limited number of programs funded to do team-based translational work, and that this research has a patient-oriented endpoint, it would benefit translational researchers to get ahead of the curve in determining how their work and results can be directly communicated to other scientists and the public, rather than to rely on existing, and perhaps dated, communication methods.

28.5.2. Lab and Office Design

A critical factor in building teams of investigators is putting these individuals in contact with one another. There are multiple schools of thought on how this can be done. With the bias that direct interaction between investigators contributes to optimal efficiency, a few recent trends in lab and office design may facilitate translational team research in the future. At UCSF and at many other institutions, the open lab structure has been featured in most if not all research buildings constructed in the past 10 to 15 years. Labs in these buildings typically feature open spaces with a minimal number of walls separating individual group spaces. Many of these buildings also provide common areas for seating as well as specialized areas in which multiple groups perform specific tasks such as tissue culture or microscopy. This model breaks down the separation between labs and encourages groups to share equipment, share facilities, order supplies jointly, and work more communally. The flexibility this model provides also allows the lab space assigned to any one group to fluctuate as dictated by the work and by funding, minimizing the territorial battles that otherwise may accompany such changes. The increased flexibility also has proven to enhance the usage of the space and to allow more investigators to fit into the same research space. In concrete terms, this may allow multiple lab-based investigators to retain individual desk space but to share the bench space, resulting in an increase in the number of investigators and lab members, and ultimately an increase in the number of ideas that can be pursued. This model suits team-based translational research very well and should be encouraged. Related to this model is the more recent push to move faculty into less structured office space, in some cases into buildings in which individual office space is replaced entirely by communal space, meeting rooms, and cubicles. It may be too early to tell if this trend facilitates or hinders scientific interaction (or how faculty will function without offices), but if the interconnectivity provided by the Internet continues to improve the ability of teams of investigators to communicate and to work together even at great distances, it seems likely that scientists of all stripes will be spending more time with each other.

28.5.3. Cross-Training of Individuals

The American education system tracks individuals into specific areas very early on, and there is increasing recognition that this approach is detrimental to modern science. For example, in college, individuals interested in math are tracked away from biology, while those interested in biology will be tracked away from the type of mathematical and biostatistical classes that could ultimately shape their thought processes and serve their future work.[13] This concern may have seemed somewhat academic 5 to 10 years ago, but with the explosion of genomics, it has become apparent that the modern scientist, and especially the modern translational scientist, needs to have more than a knowledge of biology to make optimal progress. Unfortunately, even at a large institution like UCSF, few individuals have a working knowledge of cancer biology as well as extensive knowledge in bioinformatics or programming. While a few individuals proficient in both can be found, it is striking how inefficiently the worlds of biology and bioinformatics communicate. While it may be too late to retrain senior scientists, it certainly is not too late to require that trainees, regardless of whether they come from clinical or basic science backgrounds, become more broadly proficient in the technologies that will shape how research is done in the future.

Similar problems also exist in creating individuals who can speak both the language of the bench scientist and the clinical scientist. MD/PhD programs have historically been a primary source of such individuals, but the number of people willing to put the time, effort and dollars into completing such programs, as well as the continued pressures on individuals trained in this manner to maintain both lab and clinical existences, has always proved to be a limitation. While support for such programs should continue and be encouraged by the translational research community, it is also worth trying to devise new ways by which clinical scientists can interact with and teach lab-based investigators more about clinical science. In the simplest sense, this may be instruction for all investigators on how to write a clinical trial. At UCSF, we also offer a T32 Training Program in Translational Brain Tumor Research, which includes an overview course that introduces PhD trainees to the clinical faculty, covers the essentials of clinical care of patients with brain tumors, and allows lab-based trainees to begin to think of their work in a clinically relevant manner. These types of efforts should also be encouraged.

28.5.4. Sharing of Data and Materials

In an age in which a dollar value can be placed on nearly anything, it is remarkable that the scientific community has managed to generate large databases full of information about the human genome and of human tumors, and to maintain this information in a free and freely accessible form. Of course, this did not happen by accident and was driven by funds provided by NIH through the TCGA and similar efforts, as well as by the efforts of individual institutions that provided the patient material necessary for these databases. While the way in which this was accomplished is a good lesson for translational researchers about the value of sharing and ownership, the ability of the scientific community to share patient material still needs work. Even within individual institutions, it has been remarkably difficult to develop communal tissue resources, much less to provide systems by which specimens can be shared with other institutions. Some tumor materials require a great deal of effort to collect, and one cannot expect that those who have spent considerable time and effort collecting the samples will or should honor all requests for the material. But just as patients, and subsequently surgeons, turn specimens over to the institution, it is worth considering how individual medical centers can work in a concerted manner to make tissue more freely available to the community at large. There may be no one answer to this problem and commercial interests may ultimately become part of the process as well. The willingness of institutions to provide samples to the TCGA, however, suggests that there may be ways to navigate these somewhat difficult waters.

28.5.5. Ways to Work Faster and Cheaper

Consumers of translational science, namely those individuals who suffer from cancer, want answers quickly. And given the squeeze on federal sources of funding, consumers want the work done for less. The question then arises as to how translational research can be done faster and less expensively. Rather than getting into the minutia of how businesses squeeze cost out of product production, it might be more instructive to focus on where most of the time and money goes in moving a scientific idea into a potential therapeutic gain. Numerous studies have examined this question and to no surprise the vast majority of time and dollars is spent in the final push to move agents and devices into and through clinical trials. With the recognition of this, positive steps are occurring in clinical trial development, and large multi-institution clinical trials are gradually being replaced by smaller trials with sub-selected groups of patients who receive multiple drugs that vary within the trial depending on whether their disease progresses or goes into remission. This approach, although in its infancy, is a step in the right direction, and the knowledge gained will hopefully allow the development of agents that ultimately target small subsets of patients or perhaps even individual patients.

28.5.6. Funding

Finally, it is recognized that no gains in translational research can be made in the absence of financial support. However, the trend for federal funding of research of any kind is at present flat, if not declining. How then can better translational efforts be built in the face of increasing competition for fewer dollars? One possible solution relates to the unique nature of philanthropy in the US. While many cultures take a negative view toward fundraising and philanthropy, a recently completed analysis of charitable giving per capita completed by the Charitable Aid Foundation listed the US in first place, followed closely by Ireland, New Zealand, and other countries historically linked to the British Empire.[14] Although Americans may differ on how they want money to reach scientists, they remain remarkably in favor of donating to a good cause and of supporting cancer research. American corporations seem to be similarly supportive, and any number of companies ranging from arrow manufacturers to the National Football League appear willing to lend their name in service of raising funds for cancer research (and perhaps their own profile). In our focus on our work and our reliance on existing systems of funding, perhaps we have lost sight of the fact that Americans as a whole want scientists to succeed and want to support the cancer research effort. It may be time therefore to consider how translational cancer research can more effectively be presented to the population at large. The SUTC effort that supports a limited number of translational research teams is a good example of how this can be done successfully, although other perhaps more targeted efforts are certainly possible. What appears critical in these efforts is to clearly explain the benefit of the work and to keep the funders involved. Although it may not always be apparent, every translational research team has interesting stories that unfold weekly. Finding new ways to convey our stories and our excitement to the public should therefore be an increasingly important part of what we do.

28.6. CONCLUSIONS

Although what is now called translational cancer research has existed for decades, we have only recently begun to appreciate the incredible promise of this type of work, as well as to begin to face some of the problems in doing this work effectively. Neither academic science nor industry was set up to optimally perform, or to properly reward, translational cancer research, and the systems that have been inherited must change before advances can be made. Funding teams of researchers, keeping these teams together, rewarding their efforts, and allowing them to share their expertise remain critical elements in improving translational research. Similarly, finding ways to do research faster and cheaper must be developed. On the positive side, however, most of the trends in areas related to translational science are positive. There is a growing appreciation of team-based translational science at academic institutions, and systems that limit credit and reward are giving way to mechanisms that reward team effort and allow the freer dissemination of scientific findings. Communal, integrated efforts to solve problems are being emphasized at medical centers, and the American public remains as optimistic and supportive of the research effort as ever. Perhaps most importantly, a new generation of individuals cross-trained in the disciplines necessary to understand the post-genomics world is set to move into research and to provide answers. Therefore, although the way in which translational science is done is changing, these are promising times.

ACKNOWLEDGMENTS

This work was supported in part by National Institutes of Health Grant CA097257 (SPORE).

REFERENCES

1. CBTRUS. (2012) *Statistical Report: Primary Brain Tumors in the United States, 2005–2009.* Central brain Tumors Registry of the United States.

2. Yung WK, Prados MD, Yaya-Tur R, *et al.* (1999) Multicenter phase II trial of temozolomide in patients with anaplastic astrocytoma or anaplastic oligoastrocytoma at firstr elapse. Temodal Brain Tumor Group. *J Clin Oncol* **17**: 2762–2771.
3. Cohen MH, Johnspon JR, Pazdur R. (2005) Food and Drug Administration Drug Approval Summary: Temozolomide plus radiation therapy for the treatment of newly diagnosed glioblastomamultiforme. *Clin Cancer Res* **11**: 6767–6771.
4. Stupp R, Hegi ME, Mason WP, *et al.* (2009) Effects of radiotherapy with concomitant and adjuvant temozolomide versus radiotherapy alone on survival in glioblastoma in a randomised phase III study: 5-year analysis of the EORTC-NCIC trial. *Lancet Oncol* **10**(5): 459–466.
5. National Comprehensive Cancer Network. (2009) *NCCN Practice Guidelines in Oncology: Central Nervous System Cancers.* v.1.2008. *www.nccn.org/professionals/physician_gls/PDF/cns.pdf* (accessed May 21, 2009).
6. Iwamoto FM, Abrey LE, Beal K, *et al.* (2009) Patterns of relapse and prognosis after bevacizumab failure in recurrent glioblastoma. *Neurology* **73**(15): 1200–1206.
7. Furnari FB, Fenton T, Bachoo RM, *et al.* (2007) Malignant astrocyticglioma: Genetics, biology, and paths to treatment. *Genes Dev* **21**: 2683–2710.
8. Cairncross JG, Ueki K, Zlatescu MC, *et al.* (1998) Specific genetic predictors of chemotherapeutic response and survival in patients with anaplastic oligodendrogliomas. *J Natl Cancer Inst* **90**: 1473–1479
9. The Cancer Genome Atlas Research Network (2008) Comprehensive genomic characterization defines human glioblastoma genes and core pathways. *Nature* **455**: 1061–1068.
10. Yan H, Parsons DW, Jin G, *et al.* (2009) IDH1 and IDH2 mutations in gliomas. *New Eng J Med* **360**(8): 765–773.
11. Schwartzentruber J, Korshunov A, Liu XY, *et al.* (2012) Driver mutations in histone H3.3 and chromatin remodelling genes in paediatric glioblastoma. *Nature* **482**: 226–231.
12. Bjork B-C, Laakso M. (2012) Anatomy of open access publishing: A study of longitudinal development and internal structure. *BMC Med* **10**: 124–127.
13. Gitschier J. (2006) Willing to do the math: An interview with David Botstein. *PLoS Genet.* **2**(5): e79.
14. Charities Aid Foundation. (2011) *World Giving Index 2011* (Report). Kent, UK.

Index